Recent Developments in Ruminant Nutri

Recent Developments in Ruminant Nutrition 4

Editors

PC Garnsworthy

J Wiseman

School of Biosciences, University of Nottingham

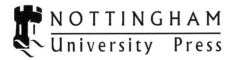
NOTTINGHAM
University Press

Nottingham University Press
Manor Farm, Main Street, Thrumpton
Nottingham, NG11 0AX, United Kingdom

NOTTINGHAM

First published 2002
Reprinted 2007
© The several contributors names in the list of contents 2002

British Library Cataloguing in Publication Data
Recent Developments in Ruminant Nutrition 4:
I. Garnsworthy, Philip C. II. Wiseman, J.

ISBN 10: 1-897676-45-X
ISBN 13: 978-1-897676-45-5

Typeset by Nottingham University Press, Nottingham
Printed and bound by Hobbs the Printers, Hampshire, England

CONTENTS

INTRODUCTION

The chapters of this book have all been previously published in *Recent Advances in Animal Nutrition*, which is the annual proceedings of the University of Nottingham Feed Manufacturers Conference. They are gathered together in this volume to provide a convenient reference book for ruminant specialists. All chapters were written by leading authorities and most have been updated slightly to reflect changes in concepts or to cite material that was unpublished in the original version.

There have been major changes to ruminant production systems in recent years, following increased globalisation of markets for animals and their products. Particularly noticeable, have been the increased genetic merit of dairy cows in many countries and the demand for closer control of product quality. These changes have necessitated major reconsideration of nutrient supply and responses to nutrients in terms of milk composition, health and fertility, all of which are addressed in this book.

The first section of this book covers the supply of forages to dairy cows, particularly the use of maize silage and the problem of maintaining physical structure in the diet. Other chapters discuss raw materials that can be used to supplement forages. The next section considers energy and nutrient requirements and responses. The previous volume in this series covered the period when the Metabolisable Protein system was introduced in the UK. Many of the chapters in the current volume consider the practical application of this system, developments of the system to include amino acid nutrition, and alternative systems used in Europe and the USA. There are also chapters on the manipulation of milk composition to meet the requirements for a healthier product. The next section considers methods of monitoring cow health and the effects of nutrition on health and fertility. The final chapter looks at systems of rearing heifers for optimum lifetime performance.

This book provides a collection of excellent reviews on ruminant nutrition that will be valuable to students, teachers, research workers, advisory staff, farmers and many others.

1

FEEDING DAIRY COWS OF HIGH GENETIC MERIT

L.E. CHASE
Department of Animal Science, Cornell University, Ithaca, NY 14853, USA

Introduction

The genetic base for milk production continues to increase in both the individual cow and total herd milk production. The current world record milk production for an individual cow is in excess of 26, 700 kg. The highest producing herd in the US has a herd average of 14,700 kg/cow/year from 440 milking cows. Average herd milk production for US Holstein herds on Dairy Herd Improvement recording programmes increased from 4,160 to 8,1 78 kg/cow/year from 1950 to 1990. What will herd averages be 10 years from now?

A challenge exists in developing feeding and management programmes for these herds. The herd manager expects and demands nutrition programmes that control the feed cost per unit of milk while supporting high levels of milk production. At the same time, herd health and reproductive performance must be maintained. Milk components must also be considered, based on the formulae used to determine the price of milk. Milk pricing systems in the US are shifting from milk-fat based to either a protein or nonfat solids basis. These shifts in pricing structure will alter ration formulation strategies.

One challenge is to define the appropriate requirements to use in formulating rations for high producing dairy cows. A number of nutrient requirement systems are used throughout the world (AFRC, 1993; NRC, 1989), based on research data where available. The majority of the data used as a base for developing these requirements were obtained using cows producing less than 9,000 kg of milk per lactation. Can these requirements be used when designing rations for high producing herds?

Nutrient utilization

Energy and nutrients consumed by the dairy cow must be partitioned to meet demands for maintenance, growth, reproduction and milk production. These requirements will be met in a priority order by the cow depending upon the quantity of energy and nutrients available. A mature cow will have maintenance as the highest priority followed by milk production and then reproduction. As dry matter intake (DMI) increases, a smaller proportion of the total energy and nutrient intake is used for maintenance. Figure 1.1 shows the proportion of the net energy (NE) and crude protein (CP) available to support milk production levels. The proportions of the protein and energy intake available for milk production are 73 and 49% for a cow producing 15 kg of milk/day. These figures increase to 89 and 74% in a cow producing 45 kg of milk.

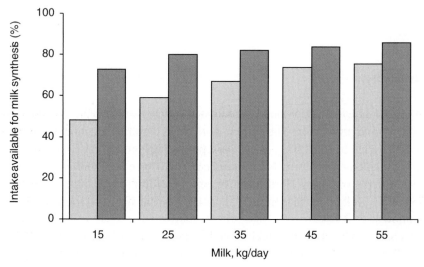

Figure 1.1 Proportion of total net energy (☐) and crude protein (■) intake used for milk production.

Dry matter intake

The single most important variable which influences productivity in dairy cows is DMI (Mertens, 1987; Waldo, 1986). Surveys of high producing herds in England and Wales indicated that attaining high levels of DMI was a key management attribute (Neilson, Whittemore, Lewis, Alliston, Roberts, Hodgson-Jones, Mills, Parkinson and Prescott., 1983; Wood and Wilson, 1983). There have been a number of equations proposed to predict DMI of dairy cows (Roseler, Fox, Chase and Stone, 1993; NRC, 1989). However, none of these have been validated with data from high producing dairy cows. An additional consideration is the rate of increase in DMI in early lactation. A depression of 18% from predicted DMI is indicated for early lactation cows (NRC, 1989) and weekly adjustment factors for DMI have been developed (Kertz, 1991; Roseler *et al.,* 1993). In the first week postcalving, DMI is about 67% of the maximum attained at 8 weeks into lactation. This depressed DMI in early lactation presents a challenge in terms of meeting energy needs while maintaining fibre intake and rumen function.

The energy value of feeds is also altered by DMI. A positive relationship exists between DMI and rate of passage of feed through the cow (Colucci, Chase and Van Soest, 1982; Mertens, 1987). This depression in digestibility with increasing DMI is not uniform for all feeds and feed fractions. Feed composition tables containing discounts for individual feeds are available (Van Soest and Fox, 1992). Computer modelling approaches may be needed to make these adjustments in a more systematic and practical manner (Sniffen, O'Connor, Van Soest, Fox and Russell, 1992). Current nutrient requirement publications do provide for adjustments in feed energy values based on level of intake (AFRC, 1993; NRC, 1989).

Forage quality

Forages provide the base for designing dairy rations. Potential forage intake is at least partially related to neutral-detergent fibre (NDF) content (Kawas, Jorgensen and Danelon, 1991; Waldo, 1986). Kawas *et al.* (1991) indicated that dietary concentrations should be less than 20% acid-detergent fibre (ADF) or 29% NDF for cows between weeks 10 and 26 of lactation. The cows in this study were producing more than 35 kg of 4% fat-corrected milk (FCM). The relationship between forage quality, concentrate supplementation and milk production has been examined with alfalfa forages (Kaiser and Combs, 1989; Kawas *et al.,* 1991; Llamas-Lamas and Combs, 1990 and 1991). Fibre digestion was more rapid in early vegetative hay than in either late bud or full bloom hay (Llamas-Lamas and Combs, 1990). No differences were detected in milk production when rations contained similar dietary fibre contents with three qualities of alfalfa and varying forage to concentrate ratios (Kaiser and Combs, 1989). Similar levels of milk production were reported in mid-lactation dairy cows fed rations with either high quality orchard-grass or alfalfa silages (Weiss and Shockey, 1991). There are differences in the composition and digestion of the NDF fractions of legume and grass forages. Total NDF is higher in legumes than grasses. However, the cell-soluble fraction is lower in grasses. Ruminal and total tract digestibilities for both ADF and NDF were higher in rations containing orchard grass than those containing alfalfa (Holden *et al.,* 1994). A forage source with high digestibility and intake is still the key to development of rations to support high levels of milk production.

Carbohydrate and protein

Energy and nutrient utilization and microbial protein synthesis in the rumen are the keys to designing efficient and profitable dairy rations. A number of review articles have examined the protein and carbohydrate considerations in optimizing rumen fermentation (Clark, Klusmeyer and Cameron, 1992; Chalupa and Sniffen, 1994; Hoover and Stokes, 1991; Nocek, 1994).

The carbohydrate components of feeds can be divided into structural and nonstructural fractions. The structural component includes pectin, cellulose, hemicellulose and lignin. The ADF fraction consists of cellulose plus lignin. The ADF plus hemicellulose comprises NDF. The non-fibrous carbohydrate (NFC) fraction is calculated as follows:

$$NFC = 1000 - (g\ CP/kg + g\ NDF/kg - g\ Ash/kg + g\ EE/kg)$$

where EE = ether extract.

The NFC fraction is also termed nonstructural carbohydrate (NSC) in some publications. The main components of this fraction are sugars, starches, pectin, galactans and beta-glucans. In fermented feeds, volatile fatty acids and lactic acid are in this fraction. The calculated NFC values should be adjusted for the presence of the organic acids (AFRC, 1993). More information is needed on the rates of digestion of the carbohydrate fractions. Depending upon the proportion of sugars and starches, degradation rates would be expected to vary significantly. Currently published digestion rates are based on very limited data (Sniffen *et al.*, 1992). There are also digestion rate differences between feed types. *In vivo* ruminal starch degradation values for wheat, oats and barley are about 84-90% of the total starch. Similar values for com and sorghum grain were 67-76%. Differences also exist due to processing method and particle size. Relative rates of degradation (fastest to slowest) are steam-flaked > high moisture > dry ground > dry rolled > dry whole for com and sorghum grains.

The protein components of feeds are divided into rumen degradable (DIP) and rumen undegradable (UIP) in the new dairy requirement system (NRC, 1989). In some sectors, a soluble protein (SIP) fraction is also used. This is the rapidly available portion of DIP as determined in a borate- phosphate buffer with a 1 hour incubation. This subdivision of protein fractions is similar in concept to the AFRC (1993) system. Amino acid nutrition is an integral component of the protein utilization system. This area has been recently reviewed (Chalupa and Sniffen, 1994; Schwab, 1994). The available knowledge in this area continues to grow. However, there are still significant questions relative to amino acid nutrition of dairy cattle which require additional research. The amount of microbial protein synthesized in the rumen and its contribution to the amino acid supply requires better quantification. Additional information on the amino acid content of the UIP fraction of feeds is also needed. A recent paper determined the amino acid profiles in the original feedstuff and the UIP fraction (Erasmus *et al.*, 1994). The lysine concentration in the UIP fraction was lower than in the original feed for 9 out of 12 feeds. The intestinal digestibility of the UIP fraction ranged from 56% for blood meal to 98% for soya bean meal. This variation in intestinal digestibility of the UIP fraction has been previously reported in other papers. It appears that the amino acid balance of dairy cows can be estimated using computer models (Sniffen *et al.*, 1992; Chalupa and Sniffen, 1994; Chase, 1991).

The relationship between carbohydrates, proteins, rumen fermentation and milk production has been reviewed (Hoover and Stokes, 1991). The concept of matching the rates of ruminally available carbohydrate and protein should enhance rumen fermentation, microbial protein synthesis (MPS) and animal performance. Nocek (1994) suggested that rations for high producing dairy cows should contain 78% total carbohydrate and 53% ruminally available carbohydrate. Hoover and Stokes (1991) examined the relationships of NSC and DIP needed to optimize rumen microbial yield. In their studies, NSC level as a percentage of total carbohydrates was held constant at 56%. Maximum MPS was attained when rations contained 10-13% DIP on a dry matter basis. Additional research work is needed to examine the impact of NSC subfractions on MPS and milk production.

One challenge in implementing the protein systems proposed by both NRC (1989) and AFRC (1993) is defining the proportion of the total protein in the various fractions. Tabular values are available (NRC, 1989; AFRC, 1993; Chalupa and Sniffen, 1994). However, many of these values are based on limited data. The published tabular values also do not provide an index of the variability which exists. The mean protein degradability for soya bean meal analysed in 23 laboratories was 63% with a standard deviation of 11.1 % (Madsen and Hvelplund, 1994). The variation reported in this paper is primarily laboratory variation. Stern, Calsmiglia and Endres (1994a) reported a UIP value of 25% for soya bean meal with a standard deviation of 3 %. This value was for 5 samples of soya bean meal evaluated by the *in situ* method within the same laboratory.

A second area of ongoing research is to describe better the effect of processing methods on ruminal protein degradation. Heat or chemical treatments will decrease the protein degradability of soya bean meal in the rumen (Stern, Varga, Clarke, Firkins, Huber and Palmquist, 1994b). Heat treating of cereal grains has also been reported to significantly decrease ruminal protein degradability (McNiven *et al.,* 1994). Extensive work has also been reported on the effect of various processing times and temperatures on the UIP value of whole soya beans (Faldet, Satter and Broderick, 1992; Satter, Dhiman and Hsu, 1994). These treatment methods should enhance our ability to control the nitrogen use between the rumen and postruminal segments of the digestive tract.

It is also accepted that the rumen degradability of protein sources varies with. outflow rate. The effective rumen degradability of protein sources tends to decrease as rumen outflow rates increase. Protein degradability of soya bean meal was reported to be 86.9, 74.2 and 66% at fractional outflow rates of 0.02, 0.05 and 0.08 per hour (Erasmus *et al.,* 1988). The protein fraction values listed in AFRC (1993) reflect this situation.

The changes in protein fractions of forages which occur during harvest and storage are important factors in formulating rations. Their importance increases as dairy herds utilize a higher proportion of silages in the ration. During both the wilting and fermentation processes, some of the true protein is converted to soluble protein and non-protein nitrogen (NPN). Field observations indicate that soluble protein may comprise 50-80% of the total protein in silages. The degradation rate of both total and chloroplast membrane proteins were higher for silages than the original, fresh forage (Makoni *et al.,* 1994). Nitrogen metabolism was investigated in dairy cows fed direct-cut or wilted grass silages

(Teller *et al.,* 1992). Organic matter intake was higher for cows fed the wilted grass silage. Nitrogen and amino acid flow to the duodenum was also higher for cows fed wilted silage. An 18% increase in milk production was reported when an UIP source was added to alfalfa based rations (Dhiman *et al.,* 1993). This implies a shortage of intestinally available protein and amino acids even though the base ration contained an excess of total protein.

High producing herds

Field observations of feeding programmes in high producing dairy herds can be useful in examining how nutritional concepts are put into practice. This information must be interpreted cautiously since DMI is estimated rather than measured as in a research context.

A survey of 61 high producing herds in the US was conducted in 1991 (Gordan and Fourdraine, 1993). These herds averaged 231 milking cows. Average annual milk production was 11,096 kg with 394.5 kg of fat and 347.1 kg of protein. In this survey, 67.2 % of the producers used a total mixed ration (TMR) feeding system. Maize silage was fed to 67.2% of the milking herds. Legume hay or haylage was fed to about half of the herds while grass forage was fed to 24.5% of the milking herds. There were also a large number of commodity feeds fed in these herds. The most common ones (with percentage of total herds in brackets) were whole cottonseed (72.1 %), distillers grains (37.7%), blood meal (37.7%), meat and bone meal (34.4%) and fish meal (19.7%). Feed additives used were sodium bicarbonate (75.4%), magnesium oxide (67.6%), yeast (50.8%) and niacin (37.7%). Even though this survey provides useful information, it does not permit a detailed analysis of the feeding programme.

Detailed information on feeding programmes was obtained in 13 high producing Holstein herds (Chase, 1993; Howard and Shaver, 1991). The herds averaged 12,995kg of milk per cow with a range of 11,740 to 14,167 kg. Milk fat percent averaged 3.65% with a range of 3.3 to 3.95%. Milk protein percent averaged 3.15% with a range of 2.97 to 3.4%. One approach was to summarize the types of feeds used in these herds as follows:

Table 1.1 contains milk production and ration nutritional parameters for 8 high producing Holstein herds. As a comparison, NRC (1989) requirement guidelines are provided where possible. It must be emphasized that the data for the 8 herds in Table 1.1 are 'field' data rather than research data. For each of these herds, some pieces of information were estimated. However, this information does provide an overview of ration guidelines used in the field. The average daily total protein intake would be about 4.7 kg for the average DMI in Table 1.1. This would be adequate to support about 50 kg of milk production for second lactation dairy cows.

What is the basis for the high levels of milk production attained by these herds? The ration nutrient parameters in Table 1.1 are similar to those used in routinely formulating

Table 1.1 MILK PRODUCTION AND RATION NUTRITIONAL PARAMETERS FOR SELECTED HOLSTEIN HERDS[a]

Item	Herd								Average	NRC (1989)[c]
	1	2	3	4	5	6	7	8		
Milk, kg/cow	14,167	13,590	13,353	13,103	12,818	13,070	12,260	11,740	13,012	-
Milk fat, %	3.7	3.8	3.5	3.7	3.6	3.4	3.7	3.9	3.7	-
Milk protein, %	3.2	3.4	3.2	3.1	3.0	3.0	3.1	3.1	3.1	-
DMI, kg	26.7	24.0	26.3	25.5	24.7	22.9	23.6	22.3	24.5	-
Ration DM, %	42.5	60.0	-	58.0	60.0	56.0	67.0	58.0	57.4	-
CP, %	18.5	18.0	20.0	18.6	19.6	20.0	19.4	19.0	19.1	18
UIP, % of CP	38.0	41.0	34.0	37.3	37.0	37.3	36.2	34.0	36.8	35
SIP, % of CP	29.0	31.0	32.0	-	-	-	-	-	-	-
NE_l, MCal/kg	1.76	1.76	1.76	1.72	1.80	1.76	1.76	1.69	1.75	1.72[b]
Fat, %	6.9	5.0	5.5	5.1	8.8	7.5	7.3	6.7	6.6	3 (min)
ADF, %	19.1	20.0	17.0	19.2	19.9	19.5	20.4	19.1	19.3	19 (min)
NDF, %	31.2	32.0	27.0	29.0	29.2	29.0	28.6	28.7	29.3	25 (min)
NDF-forage, %	22.1	20.0	19.0	22.1	16.1	23.0	21.6	20.6	20.6	-
NFC, %	35.0	38.0	37.0	39.6	34.0	34.8	36.3	35.8	36.3	-

[a] Adapted from Chase, 1993 and Howard and Shaver, 1991
[b] Equivalent to about 7.3 MJ/kg of NE_l
[c] NRC (1989) guidelines for 600 kg cows producing 50 kg of milk with 4% milk fat

rations for high group rations. However, many of these herds are producing between 8,500 and 10,000 kg of milk per cow per year. The primary difference between these herds and those represented in Table 1.1 is DMI. These high producing herds have developed feeding management strategies to maximize intake. These observations are similar to those made in other high producing herds (Neilson *et al.,* 1983; Wood and Wilson, 1983).

Summary

The challenge of developing rations for high levels of milk production will persist in the future. As nutritionists, we should look forward to this opportunity. The key to attaining high levels of efficient and profitable milk production is to maximize DMI, optimize rumen fermentation and provide postruminal energy and protein supplements to meet tissue needs.

The integration of nutritional concepts into a balanced ration can most easily be done utilizing computer ration programs. There are a large number of programs being successfully utilized in the US. These programs are well suited to routine ration formulation. However, they are not designed to handle many of the newer nutritional concepts such as level of intake, rate of passage, digestion rates, and amino acids. Computer models have been developed which do consider the above concepts (Sniffen *et al.,* 1992). These models are in a continuing state of development, validation and field testing. It is anticipated that this type of approach will become more available in the future.

What guidelines do I use in formulating rations for high producing herds? The following guidelines are provided for consideration and discussion. They are based on both NRC (1989) and field experience. Some of these have not been fully defined by research data at this time.

1. Ration fibre levels
    a. ADF = 19-21% of DM
    b. NDF = 26-30% of DM
    c. Forage NDF = 20-22% of DM

2. NFC = 35-40% of DM

3. Fat = 5-7% of DM

4. Ration protein:
    a. Crude protein = 17-19% of DM
    b. Degradable protein = 60-65 % of CP
    c. Undegradable protein = 35-40% of CP
    d. Soluble protein = 30-35% of CP

5. NE_l = 1.7-1.8 Mcal/kg of DM (7.1-7.5 MJ/kg of DM)

The milk produced using the above guidelines depends on DMI. As an example, assume that a ration with 18% CP is fed. Milk production would be 38 kg if DMI was 20 kg. However, if DMI is 25 kg, then milk production would be 49 kg on a protein basis for a mature cow. DMI needs to average 4% or more of bodyweight if high levels of milk production are to be attained. Individual cows will have DMIs in excess of 5% of bodyweight.

The principles outlined above are currently utilized in formulating rations for dairy herds in the US. These guidelines will continue to be modified as additional research information becomes available. A better understanding of nutrient digestion rates and amino acid nutrition are the key areas in which research is needed. Computer based ration formulation models will be needed to integrate and utilize these concepts. What are the limits to milk production in the dairy cow?

References

AFRC (1993) *Energy and Protein Requirements of Ruminants. An advisory manual prepared by the AFRC Technical Committee on Responses to Nutrients.* Walling- ford, CAB International

Albright, J.L. (1992) Management and Behavior of the high producing dairy cow. *Proceedings of the Tri-State Dairy Nutrition Conference* p. 53

Chalupa, W. and Sniffen, CJ. (1994) Carbohydrate, protein and amino acid nutrition of lactating dairy catde. In *Recent Advances in Animal Nutrition* -1994, pp.265-275. Edited by P.C. Garnsworthy and DJ.A. Cole. Nottingham: Nottingham University Press

Chase, L.E. (1991) Identifying optimal UIP sources to supply limiting amino acids. *Proceedings of the Cornell Nutrition Conference* p. 57

Chase, L.E. (1993) Developing nutrition programs for high producing dairy herds. *Journal of Dairy Science,* **76**, 3287

Clark,j.H., Klusmeyer, T.H. and Cameron, M.R. (1992) Microbial protein synthesis and flows of nitrogen fractions to the duodenum of dairy cows. *Journal of Dairy Science,* **75**, 2304

Colucci, P .E., Chase, L.E. and Van Soest, P J. (1982) Level of feed intake and diet digestibility in dairy cattle. *Journal of Dairy Science,* **65**, 1445

Dhiman, T.R., Cadorniga, C and Satter, L.D. (1993) Protein and energy supplementation of high alfafa silage diets during early lactation. *Journal of Dairy Science,* **76**, 1945-1959

Erasmus, LJ., Prinsloo,j. and Meissner, H.H. (1988) The establishment of a protein de grab ability data-base for dairy cattle using the nylon bag technique I: Protein sources. *South African Journal of Animal Science,* **18**, 23-29

Erasmus, LJ., Botha, P.M., Cruywagen, C.W. and Meissner, H.H. (1994) Amino-acid profile and intestinal digestibility in dairy cows of rumen-undegradable protein from various feedstuffs. *Journal of Dairy Science,* **77,** 541-551

Faldet, M.A., Satter, L.D. and Broderick, G.A. (1992) Determining optimal heat treatment of soybeans by measuring available lysine chemically and biologically with rats to maximize protein utilization by ruminants. *Journal of Nutrition,* **122**,151

Gunderson, S. (1992) How six top Wisconsin herds are fed. *Hoard's Dairyman,* **137**, 686

Holden, L.A., Glenn, B.P., Erdmann, R.A. and Potts, W.E. (1994) Effects of alfalfa and orchardgrass on digestion by dairy cows. *Journal of Dairy Science,* **77**, 2580-2594

Hoover, W.H. and Stokes, S.R. (1991) Balancing carbohydrates and proteins for optimum rumen microbial yield. *Journal of Dairy Science,* **74**, 3630

Howard, W.T. and Shaver, R.D. (1991) Rations fed on selected high Wisconsin herds - 1990. *Report by Department of Dairy Science,* Madison: University of Wisconsin

Jordan, E.R. and Fourdraine, R.H. (1993) Characterization of the management practices of the top milk producing herds in the country. *Journal of Dairy Science,* **76**, 3247

Kaiser, R.M. and Combs, D.K. (1989) Utilization of three maturities of alfalfa by dairy cows fed rations that contain similar concentrations of fiber. *Journal of Dairy Science,* **72**, 2301

Kawas ,J.R. Jorgensen, N.A. and Danelon, J.L. (1991) Fibre requirements of dairy cows: optimum fibre level in lucerne-based diets for high producing cows. *Livestock Production Science,* **28**, 107

Kertz, A.F., Reutzel, L.F. and Thomson, G.M. (1991) DMI from parturition to midlactation. *Journal of Dairy Science,* **74**, 2290

Llamas-Lamas, G. and Combs, D.K. (1990) Effect of alfalfa maturity on fiber utilization by high producing dairy cows. *Journal of Dairy Science,* **73**, 1069

Llamas-Lamas, G. and Combs, D.K. (1991) Effect of forage to concentrate ratio and intake level on utilization of early vegetative alfalfa silage by dairy cows. *Journal of Dairy Science,* **74**, 526

Madsen,J. and Hvelplund, T. (1994) Prediction of *in situ* protein degradability in the rumen. Results of an European ringtest. *Livestock Production Science,* **39**, 201

Makoni, N.F., Shelford, J.A. and Fisher, LJ. (1994) Initial rates of degradation of protein fractions from fresh, wilted and ensiled alfalfa. *Journal of Dairy Science,* **77**, 1598-1603

McNiven, M.A., Hamilton, R.M.G., Robinson, P.H. and deLecuw,J.W. (1994) Effect of flame roasting on the nutritional quality of common cereal grains for non-ruminants and ruminants. *Animal Feed Science and Technology,* **47**, 31

Mertens, D.R. (1987) Predicting intake and digestibility using mathematical models of rumen function. *Journal of Animal Science,* **64**, 1548

National Research Council (NRC: 1989) *Nutrient Requirements of Dairy Cattle. 6th Revised Edition.* Washington: National Academy of Science

Neilson, D.R., Whittemore, C.T., Lewis, M., Alliston, J.C., Roberts, DJ., Hodgson-Jones, L.S., Mills,J., Parkinson, H. and Prescott, J.H.D. (1983) Production characteristics of high-yielding dairy cows. *Animal Production,* **36**, 321

Nocek, J.E. (1994) Effective management of rumen carbohydrates in rations for dairy cattle. *Proceedings 55th Minnesota Nutrition Conference,* p.165.

Roseler, D.K., Fox, D.G., Chase, L.E. and Stone, W.C. (1993) Feed intake prediction and diagnosis in dairy cows. *Proceedings of the Cornell Nutrition Conference,* p. 216.

Satter, L.D., T.R. Dhiman and J.T. Hsu. (1994) Use of heat processed soybeans in dairy rations. *Proceedings of the Cornell Nutrition Conference,* p. 19.

Schwab, C.G. (1994) Amino acid requirements of lactating dairy cows. *Proceedings 55th Minnesota Nutrition Conference,* p. 179.

Sniffen, CJ., O'Connor, J.D., Van Soest, P J., Fox, D.G. and Russell, J.B. (1992) A Net Carbohydrate and Protein System for evaluating cattle diets. II. Carbohydrate and protein availability. *Journal of Animal Science,* **70**, 3562

Stern, M.D., Calsmiglia, S. and Endres, M.I. (1994a) Dynamics of ruminal nitrogen metabolism and their impact on intestinal protein supply. *Proceedings of the Cornell Nutrition Conference,* p. 105

Stern, M.D., Varga, G.A., Clark, J.H., Firkins, J.L., Huber, J.T. and Palmquist, D.L. (1994b) Evaluation of chemical and physical properties of feeds that affect protein metabolism in the rumen. *Journal of Dairy Science,* **77**, 2762

Teller, E., Vanbe1le, M., Foulon, M., Collignon, G. and Matatu, B. (1992) Nitrogen metabolism in the rumen and whole digestive tract of lactating dairy cows fed grass silage. *Journal of Dairy Science,* **77**, 1296-1304

Van So est, P J. and Fox, D.G. (1992) Discounts for net energy and protein- Fifth revision. *Proceedings of the Cornell Nutrition Conference,* p. 40

Waldo, D.R. (1986) Effect of forage quality on intake and forage-concentrate interactions. *Journal of Dairy Science,* **69**, 617

Weiss, W.P. and Shockey, W.L. (1991) Value of orchard grass and alfalfa silages fed with varying amounts of concentrates to dairy cows. *Journal of Dairy Science,* **74**, 1933

Wood, P.D.P. and Wilson, P.N. (1983) Some attributes of very high- yielding British Friesian and Holstein dairy cows. *Animal Production,* **37**, 157

This paper was first published in 1995

2

THE IMPORTANCE OF GRASS AVAILABILITY FOR THE HIGH GENETIC MERIT DAIRY COW

D.A. MCGILLOWAY* and C.S. MAYNE
Agricultural Research Institute of Northern Ireland, Hillsborough, Co. Down, BT26 6DR, UK
Current address: DAFRD Crop Testing Station, Backweston Farm, Leixlip, Co. Kildare, Ireland

Introduction

The introduction of milk quotas in 1984 effectively set ceiling limits to milk production and provided for a commodity price well above world market prices. For the individual farmer this has resulted in increased emphasis on efficiency of production per litre, rather than production *per se*. Efficiency of production can be increased either by reducing inputs whilst maintaining output, or by increasing both inputs and outputs such that the value of the additional output exceeds the cost of the extra input. Adoption of these strategies has resulted in a gradual shift in emphasis on many dairy farms towards maximising milk output per cow, at the expense of output per hectare. A logical extension of this policy is to breed the highest yielding cows to the best available bulls. This has been achieved with considerable success in the USA, Canada and Holland, etc., where the chosen system of production relies heavily on complete diet feeding and intensive feedlot management. The question is - do cows that are genetically predisposed to produce more milk under high input systems have a role to play in low input grass-based systems of production?

The idea that grass might have a role to play in feeding cows of high genetic merit is not a prospect that feed manufacturers are likely to welcome with open arms. However, the reality is that if high merit cows are to make a useful contribution to the farming economies of countries which operate low cost systems of milk production based on grass and grass-silage, then they must do so whilst continuing to utilize pasture grazed *in situ* as the greater portion of the diet. Scope exists for modifying existing management systems to accommodate the high merit cow, but in low input systems, there are fewer alternatives for change than in more complex production systems that use a range of inputs, produced either on the farm, or purchased from outside sources. Innovative grassland management strategies, coupled with supplementation of grazed grass with complementary concentrates of high nutrient concentration, offers the best hope for resolving this dilemma in low input systems, provided it can be achieved without large-scale substitution of grass. Given the suitability of climatic conditions in western regions of the United Kingdom (UK) and Ireland for growing high quality grass at minimal cost, and the more favourable cereal and forage maize growing conditions prevailing elsewhere in Europe, such an approach affords the best opportunity to maintain the competitiveness of low input systems. If this objective cannot be realised, then continued selection for increased genetic merit in grass-based milk production systems must be questioned.

It is also worth noting that given the imposition of GATT and other reforms, milk price in Europe will increasingly reflect the market price for the product. Consequently, the long term viability of systems currently dependent upon high milk prices must be called into question.

Can we feed the high merit cow on a predominantly grass-diet and still achieve satisfactory levels of performance? What are the limitations to intake, and how might they be overcome? These are the issues that the authors have sought to address in this review. Also included are definitions of the principal terms of reference, i.e. herbage availability and high genetic merit.

Definitions

HERBAGE AVAILABILITY

For the purposes of this review, herbage availability is defined as the relative ease or difficulty with which herbage can be harvested by the grazing animal (Wade, 1991). This is a qualitative term and is considered to be distinct from herbage allowance which is a quantitative measure of the herbage on offer, but does not take account of the manner in which herbage is presented to the grazing animal. Herbage availability therefore represents a description of the interaction between the sward and the grazing animal. Sward characteristics known to influence the grazing process include canopy height, leaf length and extended tiller height (Wade, 1991), herbage bulk density (Laca, Ungar, Seligman and Demment, 1992), stem and pseudostem position in the canopy (Flores, Laca, Griggs and Demment, 1993), and leaf orientation, stiffness and tensile strength (Laca, Demment, Distel and Griggs, 1993). Nutritional factors such as protein and carbohydrate fractions must also be considered.

HIGH GENETIC MERIT

The term 'high genetic merit' is used to describe a cow, which as the result of selection for yield traits, is genetically predisposed to produce significantly more milk and milk constituents than a cow of lower merit status. The term is relative: what was considered as being high merit in the mid 80s, is by today's standards more accurately described as of intermediate status. In Ireland and the UK, the rate of genetic progress for yield traits has increased considerably since the mid 1980s. For example the rate of genetic progress in sires for fat plus protein yield has trebled in the ten year period between 1980 and 1990 (Figure 2.1) (UK Statistics for Genetic Evaluation, July 1995).

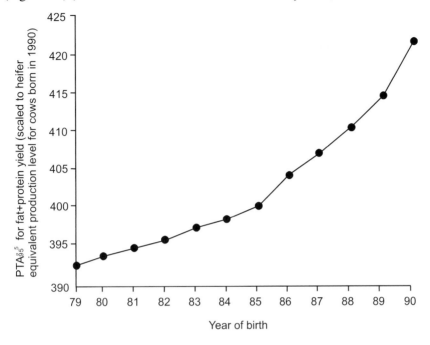

Figure 2.1 Rate of genetic progress in fat+protein yield for sires born over the 12 year period 1979-1990. Source: UK Statistics for Genetic Evaluation (July 1995)

The term Predicted Transmitting Ability (PTA $_{95}$) is a measure of an animals ability to transmit its genes to the next generation, and can relate to production traits, compositional quality, linear type, etc. It is measured relative to a fixed reference point, the genetic base, which is the average PTA of animals born during 1990 and milking in 1995. However, the selection of animals using PTAs for various traits, e.g. fat+protein yield, has now been largely superseded by selection based on indices such as the Profit Index (PIN) and more recently the Index of Total Economic Merit (ITEM). These are overall breeding indices which weight PTAs for various economically important traits, after accounting for the costs of milk production, into an overall financial value. This value therefore indicates the predicted margin over food and quota costs that the animal is expected to pass on to its progeny. A similar index, the Relative Breeding Index (RBI) is used in Ireland, and takes account of the Irish dairy situation to weight PTAs into an overall breeding index. In essence therefore, indices such as PIN, ITEM and RBI enable dairy farmers to select animals that will improve farm profits. Given that many dairy farmers are breeding to a clearly defined goal, selection based on these indices can be expected to further increase the rate of genetic progress. The consequence of this is that although the PIN value of the UK national dairy herd is currently around £17, some breeders have herds with PIN values in excess of £38 (M.Coffey, *pers comm.*). If this trend continues, then by the year 2000 there will be numerous herds with average PIN values greater than £50, and individual animals with PIN values in excess of £100 (A.Cromie, *pers comm.*).

Implications of increased genetic merit for pasture-based production systems

Before considering the importance of herbage availability for the high merit cow, it is worthwhile considering the likely implications of increased genetic merit for pasture based production systems in general.

GENOTYPE X ENVIRONMENT INTERACTIONS

There has been much discussion recently on the possible existence of an interaction between various environmental factors (principally nutrition) and genotype. The existence of such an interaction would have major implications for the dairy industry, since it would mean that an animal performing well in one system of production, e.g. intensive feedlot, might not necessarily be able to hold that production advantage in a low input system. The problem then for producers in opting to select from American and continental bred sires – sires that have been selected and assessed on the basis of daughter performance on complete diets fed indoors, with limited access to grazed grass – is that there is no indication of how well a particular bull will perform in a grass-based system. Considerable time and money could be invested in a selection *cul de sac*.

Evidence of a genotype x environment interaction can be found in the results of a joint New Zealand (NZ) and Canadian study (CANZ) in which the daughters of Canadian and NZ sires were reared and milked in Canada or NZ (Peterson, 1988; Burnside, Graham, Rapitta, McBride and Gibson, 1991; Graham, Burnside, Gibson, Rapitta and McBride, 1991). Overall, progeny of NZ sires produced fractionally less milk and milk solids than the Canadian daughters in both countries, though differences between sire groups were greater when evaluated in Canadian herds, i.e. NZ daughters produced more milk fat in Canada than in NZ, due primarily to the more generous feeding in Canada (heifers weighed 530 kg in Canada compared with 390 kg in NZ) (Table 2.1). Further analysis of the data revealed considerable differences in the ranking of Canadian sires based on the performance of their daughters in NZ, compared to that predicted from evaluation in Canada (Table 2.2). This suggests that sire proofs for milk, fat and protein made under Canadian feeding and management conditions are not good predictors

Table 2.1 PERFORMANCE OF PROGENY OF CANADIAN OR NEW ZEALAND SIRES EVALUATED EITHER IN CANADA OR NEW ZEALAND.

Trait	Location (for evaluation)	Canadian	New Zealand
Milk (kg)	Canada	6097	5469
	New Zealand	3395	3157
Fat (kg)	Canada	231	226
	New Zealand	140	138
Protein (kg)	Canada	206	192
	New Zealand	109	105
Fat + Protein (kg)	Canada	437	418
	New Zealand	249	243

Sire Group spans the Canadian and New Zealand columns.

Source : Peterson (1988); Burnside, Graham, Rapitta, McBride and Gibson (1991).

Table 2.2 CORRELATION BETWEEN SIRE RANKINGS IN CANADIAN/NEW ZEALAND TRIAL WITH THOSE IN COUNTRY OF ORIGIN.

Trait	Canadian sires	New Zealand sires
Milk (kg)	0.22[+]	0.80
Fat (kg)	0.25[+]	0.79
Protein (kg)	0.36[+]	0.80
Fat (g/kg)	0.69	0.75
Protein (g/kg)	0.68	0.54
Expected correlation	0.68	0.65

[+]Values significantly different to expected values

Source : Peterson (1988).

of a bull's relative merit in the NZ environment. According to Peterson (1988), the fact that the Canadian sires ranked differently in the NZ environment implies that the trait limiting production in the two countries is different. Given the almost total dependence on grazed grass in NZ, the results suggest that daughters of some Canadian sires performed significantly better on a pasture-based diet (when compared to daughters of other Canadian sires) than would be predicted from their performance in Canada, i.e. on a diet with a high energy and nutrient concentration. This could reflect differences in grazing behavioural characteristics between daughters of different sires. Choice of appropriate sires is therefore of considerable importance in situations where reliance on grazed grass is high. This subject has been discussed in further detail by Holmes (1995), and Mayne and Gordon (1995).

Further evidence of a genotype x nutrition interaction was presented by Veerkamp, Simm and Oldham (1994), who undertook a regression analysis (based on Langhill data from Scotland) of animal performance against pedigree index (PI), and tested regression coefficients for possible PI x diet (proportion of forage) interactions. Significantly different regression coefficients were observed between PI and milk yield for the low and high forage diets respectively, indicating that differences between merit groupings vary with the forage content of the diet.

Given the existence of genotype x nutrition interactions, it is possible that high genetic merit heifers and cows (bred to perform on diets of high nutrient concentration fed indoors), such as those imported into Hillsborough (N. Ireland) and Moorepark (Ireland), will not be as well suited to a grass-based diet as animals evaluated under grass-based production systems. Consequently, the response of these animals in a grazing situation is likely to underestimate the true potential of high merit cows that have been selected on the basis of intake and foraging characteristics.

Possible genotype x nutrition interactions on fertility and animal health have not been studied, though it is likely that they exist and are of some importance (Holmes, 1995). Cows producing higher volumes of milk are under more physiological stress than lower producing cows (Funk, 1993). Several studies (Shanks, Freeman, Berger and Kelley, 1978, and Bertrand, Berger, Freeman and Kelley, 1985) have shown that health costs tend to increase as production increases. Hansen, Freeman and Berger (1983) and Oltenacu, Frick and Lindhe (1991) have shown a negative genetic correlation between cow reproductive performance and production, suggesting that continual selection for production will result in poorer reproductive performance. In a grazing trial at Moorepark with cows of low to intermediate merit status, grazing to residual sward heights of 40, 60 and 80 mm resulted in an inverse linear relationship between residual sward height and calving to pregnancy interval (Ryan, Snijders, McGilloway and O'Farrell, *unpublished*). It can be expected that high merit cows in the same situation would be seriously disadvantaged. Veerkamp *et al.* (1994) make the point that because tissue reserves in dairy cows are substantial (Butler-Hogg, Wood and Bines, 1985; Gibb, Ivings, Dhanoa and Sutton, 1992), high merit cows might use these reserves to buffer against nutritional adversity in the short term, with interactions only becoming evident in the longer term (i.e. in subsequent lactations).

FOOD INTAKE

Given the high merit dairy cow as previously defined, there is a lack of data with regard to food intake at pasture. Consequently, it is necessary to look to the indoor environment to gain an insight into intake potential and feed conversion efficiency.

It is now generally accepted that improvements in milk production with increasing genetic merit stem from a change in nutrient partitioning within the cow, whereby a greater proportion of nutrient intake is diverted towards milk production at the expense of liveweight gain (Sejrsen and Neimann-Sorensen, 1994; Veerkamp *et al.*, 1994; Patterson, Gordon, Mayne, Porter and Unsworth, 1995). A summary of indoor feeding trials at Langhill (Scotland) and more recently at Hillsborough are presented in Table 2.3. In both studies, animals of intermediate or high merit status produced significantly more milk, and fat plus protein, than low merit animals. However, intake of energy did not differ significantly between the various genetic groupings. In the Hillsborough study, although high merit cows produced almost 22 per cent more fat plus protein per unit food consumed, intakes of dry matter (DM) were only slightly higher than with cows of intermediate genetic merit. In addition the high merit cows lost up to 1 kg liveweight per day over the first 60 days of lactation, despite being on a high level of concentrate input (14 kg concentrate DM/d).

Table 2.3 EFFECTS OF INCREASED GENETIC MERIT ON FEED EFFICIENCY (SILAGE BASED SYSTEMS).

	Langhill studies (182 days)		*Hillsborough studies* (160 days)
Genetic merit (PTA$_{90}$ kg F + P)	4.3 *vs* 18.8		5 vs 45
Comparative treatment	High conc.	Low conc.	High conc.
Animal performance (% change)			
Food intake	+5.0	+4.3	+6.3
Fat + protein yield	+11.5	+12.2	+29.6
Food conversion efficiency (% change)			
Fat + protein yield/unit food intake	+6.2	+7.6	+21.8

Source : Veerkamp, Simm and Oldham (1994); Patterson, Gordon, Mayne, Porter and Unsworth (1995).

Similar responses have been observed in grazing trials carried out in NZ. At pasture, cows of 'high' merit produced more milk (by 20-40%), consumed more herbage (by 5-20%), were more efficient converters of food into milk (by 10-15%) and produced higher milk yields per hectare than low merit cows (Grainger, Holmes and Moore, 1985; Holmes, 1988; Holmes, 1995). It is important to note that the difference in genetic merit of the high and low groups used in these NZ experiments was small compared to that in the Langhill and Hillsborough studies.

Voluntary food intake is a major factor influencing total nutrient intake and hence degree of body tissue mobilization in early lactation (Forbes, 1995). Undoubtedly the physical capacity of the digestive tract and/or the rate of substrate utilization are important aspects of intake regulation, but other factors also exert influence. For example, metabolic control is thought to be mediated via chemo- and osmo- receptors in the rumen, intestines and liver, which are sensitive to volatile fatty acids (VFAs). Higher yielding cows absorb VFAs more quickly than low yielders, principally via a greater demand from the mammary gland, resulting in weaker negative feedback from these receptors and hence increasing food intake (Gill and Beever, 1991; Forbes, 1995). Nevertheless, the available data indicate that although high merit cows have higher intake characteristics than animals of lower merit, the difference is small in comparison with the large differences observed in milk production.

Future selection strategies

Selection for yield traits without due consideration of food intake may well be seen as a major oversight by breeders in the years to come. According to Veerkamp, Emmans, Cromie and Simm, (1995) food intake in dairy cattle (under winter feeding regimes) has a heritability of 0.36, indicating that direct selection will result in considerable genetic improvement for this trait. However, in most situations it is not possible to measure intake directly, so other indirect traits may have to be considered, e.g. chest width, body depth and muzzle size, etc. Higher intakes might well partially offset the greater loss of live weight and condition observed with high merit cows in early lactation.

ENERGY AND NUTRIENT REQUIREMENTS AT PASTURE

Mayne and Gordon (1995) calculated a theoretical energy balance for cows of medium and high merit (assuming yields of 25 and 32.5 kg milk/day respectively in early lactation) at pasture (Table 2.4). Assuming similar live-weight loss, herbage intakes of 15.0 and 18.7 kg DM/cow/d were predicted to meet the energy requirements for medium and high merit cows respectively. Work by McGilloway and Stakelum (*unpublished*) at Moorepark indicates that where cows were grazed exclusively on grass, to residual sward heights of 40, 60 and 80 mm, intake of DM up until mid July averaged 13.8, 14.3 and 15.8 kg/cow/day respectively (as measured using the n-alkane technique). Previous studies in the Netherlands (Meijs and Hoekstra, 1984) indicate that 16.9 kg DM/cow/day is an upper limit to the intake of grass under 'ideal' grazing conditions. Consequently, under good grassland management practices, herbage intake at pasture is normally sufficient to meet the requirements of the medium merit cow.

Table 2.4 THEORETICAL ENERGY BALANCE FOR MEDIUM AND HIGH GENETIC MERIT COWS ON GRAZED PASTURE.

Genetic merit	Medium	High
(Predicted Transmitting Ability (kg Fat + Protein))	*(+5)*	*(+60)*
Live-weight (kg)	550	650
Live-weight loss (kg/day)	0.5	0.5
Milk yield[+] (kg/day)	25.0	32.5
Metabolisable energy requirements (MJ/day)		
Maintenance[++]	55.4	62.5
Total requirement	180	225
Dry matter required (kg/day) assuming ME of 12.0 MJ/kg DM)	15.0	18.7

[+]   Assuming milk composition of 39.4 g/kg butterfat, 31.9 g/kg protein and 44.2 g/kg lactose
[++]   Maintenance energy requirements as estimated by Agricultural and Food Research Council (1993).

Source: Mayne and Gordon (1995).

It is now generally accepted that milk yield drives intake demand. Indirect evidence in support of this hypothesis can be found in the milk production response of cows treated with the hormone bST. In trials in the USA, milk production increased within days of treatment initiation, but DM intake did not respond until after four to six weeks had elapsed (Bauman, Eppard, DeGeeter and Lanza, 1985). The slower increase in intake relative to milk yield post-calving also lends support to this hypothesis. Data from grazing studies at Moorepark suggest that for each kg increase in milk yield (over the range 15-30 kg milk/day) cows will consume an extra 0.4-0.5 kg DM/day (Stakelum, 1993; Stakelum and Dillon, 1995). This relationship is depicted graphically in Figure 2.2. However for cows yielding in excess of 30 kg milk/d the nature of this relationship is unknown, but it is speculated that because of sward and animal behaviour constraints that restrict intake, the slope of the line will tend towards a plateau. The challenge in managing the high merit cow at grass, is to seek to arrest this decline in intake at high levels of animal performance, by manipulating grassland management and supplementation strategies. This implies presenting the grazing animal with herbage in a form that will maximise intake/bite and hence daily DM intake. It is accepted however, that the provision of complementary concentrates with high nutrient concentration will be a necessary component of any grazing strategy developed with high genetic merit dairy cows in early lactation. It is also important to highlight the fact that the current research work being undertaken at Hillsborough and Moorepark is unique within the UK and Ireland, with regard to feeding the high merit cow in a predominantly grass-based system.

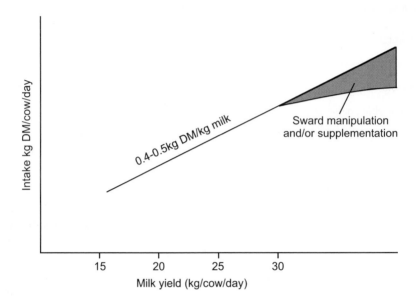

Figure 2.2 Relationship between milk yield (kg/cow/day) and dry matter intake (kg/cow/day)

Constraints to food intake at pasture

Limitations to the intake of herbage by the grazing animal exist at many levels. At the sward/animal interface, herbage availability and quality are the main factors constraining herbage intake. These factors are largely under the control of the farmer, but ultimately, climate and soil fertility factors exert far more powerful influences on the production system than any management strategies imposed by the farmer.

MACRO-FACTORS

Climate and location

Climatic factors largely determine the start and duration of the growing and grazing seasons, how much grass is produced, how this production is distributed across the season, and how it varies between locations and years (Brereton, 1995). Within Europe, the grass growing season can vary from 365 days in lowland coastal areas, to less than 200 days in inland continental and upland areas (Thran and Broekhuizen, 1965). Even within relatively small areas there is considerable variation. For example, Connaughton (1973) and Brereton (1995) examined the geographical variation in the start and length of the growing season in Ireland. In southern coastal areas the date of start of growth is February 1 and the length of the growing season is up to 340 days. This contrasts with inland northern areas where the equivalent values are March 20 and 240 days respectively.

Under optimum conditions, potential production from grass swards in the UK and Ireland is high, varying from 15 tDM/ha in the extreme southwest of Ireland to less than 11 tDM/ha in the northeast (Brereton, 1995). Estimates of total annual production however obscure some important effects of climate on the seasonal distribution of DM. Where the total annual production is concentrated over a short growing season, the system of herbage utilization must place relatively greater emphasis on forage production during the growing season for winter feeding. Similarly where summer drought occurs the bulk of annual production tends to be concentrated in the spring period (Brereton, Danielov and Scott, 1995).

Climate can also have quite dramatic short term effects, both within and between days, e.g. on herbage quality, where temperature and sunlight hours can affect soluble sugar concentrations within the plant. These are known to display diurnal variation, being highest around 17:00 and lowest around 08:00 (Kingsbury, 1965; Wilkinson, Price, Russell and Jones, 1994).

In effect therefore, climatic variation means that the farmer cannot predict precisely how much grass will be produced over the season, or what kind of conditions will prevail for utilization. This is in stark contrast to the situation pertaining to indoor feeding systems where diets of known quality and quantity are fed. At pasture a 'best estimate' based on feed budgeting and a retrospective examination of cow performance is often all that is available.

Herbage varieties

Herbage varieties are considered here because it is through the plant that the production potential of a given sward is realized (Brereton *et al.*, 1995). Any species or variety will be most productive on warm, humid, highly fertile sites, but only one or two varieties will be capable of expressing the full site potential (Brereton *et al.*, 1995). The inherent characteristics of a species or variety, e.g. date of flowering, formal growth habit (erect or prostrate), the tensile strength of the leaves, etc., largely reflect the breeding policy employed in the original selection process. These factors are largely outside the sphere of influence of the farmer, and therefore cannot be manipulated in the same way as for example herbage allowance. However, selection for reduced shear strength, increased persistency, higher DM content, etc., may be desirable management objectives, and in the long term could prove of greater benefit to increasing the intake of DM by the high merit cow, than breeding strategies designed to produce more total DM per annum.

GRASSLAND MANAGEMENT FACTORS

Poor utilization of herbage in the conventional grazing systems of the mid 80s has often been cited as a major factor limiting efficiency of production, and is closely related to the economic performance of dairy herds (Leaver, 1983; Leaver, 1987). In this scenario, herbage utilization can be increased by producing more grass per ha and /or by cows eating a greater proportion of the herbage on offer. However, from the perspective of the high merit cow, to even approach the degree of herbage utilization achieved by low to medium merit cows would result in serious energy balance deficits. If high merit cows are to achieve their potential at grass, they must have virtually unrestricted access to high quality herbage over the lactation. The implication is that utilization per hectare by the high merit cow *per se* will be poor, and therefore a major challenge in grazing management is to develop alternative strategies to utilize residual herbage to a degree commensurate with maintaining sustainable, high quality swards over the grazing season.

Grazing system

Providing grass of high quality over the grazing season can only be achieved by attention to detail in grassland management. We will go one step further and say that to provide quality herbage for the high merit cow, rotational grassland management systems based on fertilizer nitrogen (N) are essential. Rotational grazing has been widely advocated in countries where pasture plays a significant role in livestock production (McMeekan and Walsh, 1963). Furthermore, Evans (1981) observed a more uniform pattern of herbage intake and increased animal performance with rotational grazing relative to continuous grazing, with February-April calving dairy cows grazed at similar stocking rates. Under rotational grazing the area of pasture is divided into paddocks, the animals spending only one or two days in each, eventually coming back to the start after approximately 15-30 days. The alternative approach (continuous grazing) involves animals remaining on the same area of pasture for protracted periods.

Unless at high stocking rates, herbage production from both systems is similar (McMeekan and Walsh, 1963: Grant, Barthram and Torvell, 1981). So what is the advantage of rotational grazing over continuous? Essentially rotational grazing facilitates identification of grass surpluses and deficits far more readily than is the case where cows are continuously grazed. For example, if in a 'normal' year it takes one day to graze out paddocks to between 60 and 70 mm residual sward height (given the normal stocking rate for the farm and optimum usage of N), then reaching this same height in 0.5 days or 1.5 days would indicate that supply is failing to meet demand in the former case, and is surplus to demand in the latter. Rotational grazing permits greater flexibility, extra paddocks can be maintained as 'buffers' allowing cows to be moved onto these paddocks if conditions deteriorate (Illius, Lowman and Hunter, 1986; Brereton, 1987). Similarly, during periods of surplus growth, paddocks can be taken out of the system via big bale silage, and then fed back again towards the end of the grazing season when grass growth rates are in decline. Furthermore, rotational grazing facilitates management practices designed to utilise high residual herbage masses following grazing by high merit cows. Flexibility is the key and it is not present to the same extent in continuous grazing systems. However, the most important characteristic of rotational grazing systems is that they facilitate presentation of herbage to the animal in an 'optimum' form for prehension – see later sections.

Within rotational grazing systems, several options are available for controlling high residual sward masses which will result from under utilization by the high merit cow. Swards could be topped in order to control stem extension and maintain quality, or alternatively a leader-follower system could be implemented to utilize residual herbage. A combination of the two is the most desirable option, since topping alone is wasteful, but if the topped grass was then eaten by either cows of lower genetic merit, heifers or other dry-stock, then utilization will be enhanced, and sward quality ensured for subsequent rotations. The Dutch system of alternating grazing with cutting might also offer scope for maintaining sward quality.

Nitrogen fertilizer

Earlier, it was stated that fertilizer-N was an essential component of the system, implying there is no role for clover. This is not necessarily the case. Clover has many merits (both nutritionally and environmentally), and has been shown to sustain higher levels of animal performance than pure grass swards (Thomson, Beever, Haines, Cammell, Evans, Dhanoa and Austin, 1985). However, it neither fixes enough N, nor does so reliably enough over the grazing season to sustain the intensive system needed to consistently meet the demands of the high merit cow. Also, there is considerable year-to-year variation in the clover content of swards, and unpredictability with sward establishment. Stewart (1985) in a review paper states 'The authors experience in managing a low N grass-clover (cv. Blanca) sward over the last 7 years, involving integrated cuts for silage with rotational grazing by beef cattle, would indicate that it may take many years for a satisfactory stable equilibrium to be reached between the grass and clover components of the sward'.

Fertilizer N is the cornerstone of current systems of rotational grazing, producing between 15 to 25 kg DM/kg N applied (Holmes, 1968; Reid, 1978). However, under farm conditions some studies have measured a response much less than this, typically in the region of 8 kg DM/kg N applied (Ball, Molloy and Ross, 1978; Leaver, 1985). Nevertheless, within the limitations imposed by the environment, fertilizer N is the most important management input 'controlling' herbage yield (Morrison, Jackson and Williams, 1974). Furthermore, when applied strategically throughout the season it can be used to improve 'mid-season' production without reducing annual yield (Morrison, 1977; Morrison, Jackson and Sparrow, 1980) thereby producing a more uniform growth pattern through the grazing season.

Stocking density

Stocking density defines the number of animals contained within a particular paddock at any time. Production per hectare increases with increased stocking density to a maximum, and then declines rapidly. Conversely, as stocking density is increased, production per animal declines. Journet and Demarquilly (1979) estimated that for each increment in stocking density of one cow per hectare, milk production per cow was reduced by 10%, but production per hectare was increased by over 20%.

The effects of stocking density on milk production and animal live weight are exhibited through effects on herbage allowance and therefore intake. At high stocking densities animals are forced to graze deeper in the sward, i.e. to lower residual sward heights, and therefore consume a diet of lower digestibility and nutrient value than those at lower stocking densities. Interanimal space is reduced at high stocking density, thus competition for food is potentially increased (Phillips, 1993). Increased levels of social interaction may also alter grazing patterns and subsequent production levels. Stocking density will also impinge on sward dynamics, since with less time to select, animals cannot be as selective with regard to species and/or morphological characteristics (Struth, Brown, Olson, Araujo and Alijoe, 1987).

Grazing frequency

Under conditions of good grassland management, the dairy cow is allocated fresh grass once or twice daily. In any grazing period, as time progresses, less pasture is available due to a diminishing supply of herbage, and as a result of fouling. For the individual cow, it is to her advantage to consume as much of her daily requirement as possible within a few hours of being given a fresh allowance. Thus cows with an aggressive appetite are likely to have higher intake rates than more passive eaters, or those with a lesser capacity to consume large volumes of herbage, due to constraints such as satiety and rumen fill. In conditions where cows graze in close proximity to each other, aggressive animals will be further advantaged relative to more placid animals. However, whilst 'aggressive' traits may be desirable with regard to intake levels, ingestion of large amounts of feed in infrequent feeding bouts will tend to lower digestive efficiency and nutrient utilization. In a review of the effects of feeding frequency (in indoor feeding systems) on the growth and efficiency of food utilization of ruminants, Gibson (1981) found that increasing the frequency of feeding of cattle improved utilization and liveweight gain by 16%.

FACTORS INFLUENCING HERBAGE INTAKE ON A DAILY BASIS

On a day to day basis, the main factors restricting herbage intake, are herbage availability (see earlier definition) and herbage quality.

Grazing behaviour

Spedding, Large and Kydd, (1966) considered the daily intake of herbage by the grazing cow to be the product of three variables;

a)   the total time spent grazing per day,
b)   the biting rate per minute, and
c)   DM intake per bite.

Total time devoted to grazing varies between 420-700 min/day (Arnold, 1981; Fitzsimons, 1995). Biting rate generally varies in the range 45-65 bites/min (Chacon and Stobbs, 1976; Phillips, 1993; Fitzsimons, 1995), but is influenced by intake per bite, tending to increase when intake per bite is depressed. Other studies have suggested that cows are constrained to a maximum of 4000 bites per day, which effectively restricts the ability of a cow to compensate for large reductions in intake per bite (Hodgson, 1981). Consequently, it is evident that intake per bite (bite size) is the principal determinant of daily intake, and as such is sensitive to changes in sward composition and character. Stobbs (1974) measured bite size using oesophageal-fistulated animals grazing tropical pastures of varying canopy structure, and concluded that sward bulk density and the relationship between stem content and leaf:height ratio was the major factor determining bite size. Maximum biting rates have been recorded at minimum forage availability (Chacon and Stobbs, 1976), but as herbage availability increases, biting rate declines as individual bite size increases (Scarnecchai, Nastis and Malechek, 1985). Chacon and Stobbs (1976) considered the presence (i.e. acceptability) and density (i.e. accessibility) of leaf in the grazed horizon as the major factors determining daily herbage intake.

Fitzsimons (1995) calculated the bite size of British Friesian dairy cows from fistula samples collected over three or four day residency periods. Bite size varied from 0.42 to 0.81 g DM per bite, and tended to decline over time as the herbage on offer was depleted. Earlier work by Stobbs (1974) reported that a range between 0.31 and 0.71 g DM per bite is more typical of the smaller breeds such as the Jersey. Whether bite size variation is a breed characteristic, or a reflection of animal size is not known.

In more recent trials at Hillsborough, intake rates of dairy cows allowed access to swards varying in sward height and bulk density were assessed over short (1 hour) grazing periods. Data presented in Figure 2.3 illustrated the overriding importance of intake/bite in achieving high intake rates. Intake/bite increased linearly with increasing sward height between 80 and 180 mm, varying from 0.39 to 1.19 g DM/bite (Cushnahan, McGilloway, Laidlaw and Mayne, *unpublished*). Irrespective of sward height, intake per bite was greatest on the most dense sward (Figure 2.4).The relationship between sward height, bulk density and intake (kg DM/hr) is illustrated in Figure 2.5. Intake rates in excess of 3 kg DM/hr were achieved either with a dense sward at a sward height of 120 mm, or with an open sward at approximately 155 mm. These data suggest that cows of medium genetic merit have the potential to consume upwards of 3.5 kg DM/hr.

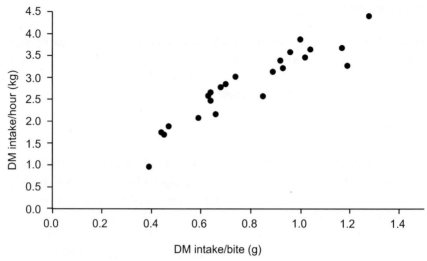

Figure 2.3 Relationship between intake rate (kg DM/hr) and intake/bite (g DM)

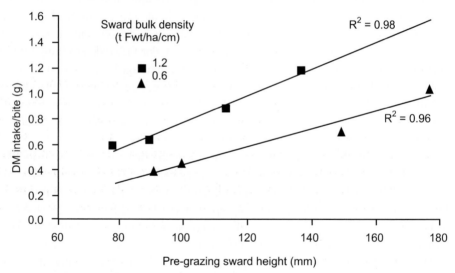

Figure 2.4 Relationship between pre-grazing sward height (mm), DM intake/bite (g) and sward bulk density (t Fwt/ha/cm)

Whilst this represents the upper potential to intake rate, it suggests that cows can consume almost 0.25 of their daily requirement (15 kg DM/cow/day) within one hour when given access to dense swards of readily prehendable green leaf. This highlights the marked superiority of rotational grazing systems relative to continuous grazing systems which are generally managed at lower sward heights. It is also evident from these data that intake per bite is markedly reduced at sward heights of 80 mm relative to 180 mm (irrespective of bulk density) (Figure 2.4). From observations in the field it appears that

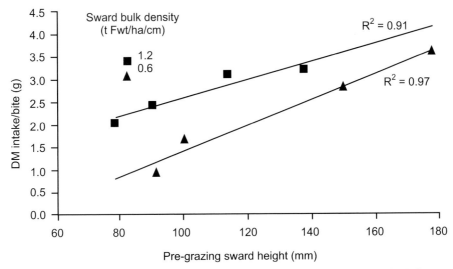

Figure 2.5 Relationship between pre-grazing sward height (mm), DM intake (kg/hr) and sward bulk density (t Fwt/ha/cm)

if the herbage on offer is too tall, then the animal is presented with difficulties in manipulating the bite into the mouth, thus biting rate is reduced.

With large herbivores such as cows, plant structure is a major determinant of selection and therefore acceptability. Cows graze green leaf preferentially and even when herbage allowance is low, the proportion of green leaf in the diet remains high. For example, Fitzsimons (1995) has shown that cows spending either three or four days per residency period, still managed to maintain a leaf fraction in the diet of approximately 0.85 on the final day of residence, although this was accompanied by a small but steady increase in the dead and stem content of the diet. Other data indicate that where the physical accessibility of the leaf is reduced, energy expenditure of the grazing animal is increased (O'Reagain and Mentis, 1989). Leaf accessibility also directly affects bite size and therefore intake rates (Stobbs, 1973).

Whilst individual bites are the smallest unit of feeding behaviour, a more frequently studied unit is the meal or grazing bout (Baile and Della-Fera, 1981), which is defined as the period from when grazing commences until rest. There are generally two grazing bouts between a.m. and p.m. milking, and one grazing bout between p.m. milking and one to two hours after dusk. During the night, and up until a.m. milking there are between one and two grazing bouts.

Large animals will experience greater restrictions in bite depth and bite volume on short swards than small animals, and there is a clear effect of body size on the ability to obtain adequate energy intake from short herbage (Illius and Gordon, 1987). Cows grazing short swards are unable to eat sufficient quantities of DM, even if the area of pasture offered is large. Allden and Whittaker (1970) associated the inability of animals to graze swards of low herbage mass with reduced height, and not with any inherent characteristics of the sward such as lack of leaf material.

Combellas and Hodgson (1979), Hodgson and Jamieson (1981) and Brereton and Carton (1988) have all shown that cattle grazing swards of *L. perenne* in which the leaf material is exhausted, will reduce grazing time or even cease grazing altogether. However Wade (1991) made the point that this is just as likely to be the result of prehension difficulties, as opposed to a lack of herbage mass. However, the hypothesis that rate of intake is determined by sward height is contradicted to some extent by Le Du, Combellas, Hodgson and Baker (1979), who concluded that intake restriction occurs when 50% of the herbage mass has been consumed. This would suggest that the residual sward height in rotational grazing systems should vary in direct proportion to the herbage mass and sward height on offer.

Sward Structure

Sward structure describes the proportion of leaf, stem and dead material in the sward, and the relative vertical distribution of these in the sward profile. Four components can be identified. There is a horizontal separation into an upper potentially grazed horizon and a lower ungrazed horizon, and a vertical separation of the grazed and rejected area of the pasture. Swards are composed of a collection of tillers, which in turn comprise a vertical axis bearing leaves. In the flowering tiller the vertical axis is formed by stem, and in the vegetative tiller by sheath bundles. Leaf, stem and/or pseudostem length determine the potential height of the canopy, whilst leaf angle determines orientation of the photosynthetic material. Swards therefore comprise an upper leaf canopy of highly digestible material, presented over a lower layer of relatively low digestibility. Consequently, forcing cows to graze to low residual sward heights reduces the overall nutritive value of the herbage consumed.

On dense swards, Jamieson (1975 – cited by Hodgson, 1982) found an apparently linear relationship between herbage intake and sward height with grazing cattle. This was considered by Hodgson (1982) to be due to tall swards being more prehendable, but he conceded that the presence of leaf sheath in the grazed horizon may have contributed to, or caused, the decline in herbage intake that was found with declining sward height.

Herbage dry matter content

The DM content of the herbage on offer can have a significant effect on herbage intake rates at pasture. In a pasture diet, the energy and nutrient content will be markedly diluted by the presence of water, which can vary from 850 g/kg in early spring to around 750 g/kg in mid-summer. This water is predominantly intracellular in nature, and thus makes a large contribution to the bulk of the diet. Evidence that voluntary intake of DM is limited by the DM content of fresh forage comes from several studies over a range of

DM contents (Johns, 1954; Duckworth and Shirlaw, 1958; Arnold, 1962; Halley and Dougall, 1962; Lloyd-Davies, 1962; Moral, 1982). For dairy cows the threshold at which forage water content limits voluntary intake is thought to be between 150 and 180 g/kg DM, with an estimated depression of 0.34 kg DM intake/10 g/kg decline in DM below this level (Vérité and Journet, 1970). It is postulated that the mechanism is due to a bulk effect on rumen fill, but this is only poorly understood.

John and Ulyatt (1987) reported results of a series of studies which examined the influence of plant composition and the role of rumen fill with fresh grasses in sheep. They found a positive relationship between voluntary intake of fresh grass DM and forage DM content over a wide range (120-250 g/kg) of DM concentration, but there was no correlation between intake of fresh weight and forage DM concentration (Figure 2.6). Limitations to fresh food intake due to bulk were not attributed to negative feedback from distension of the rumen.

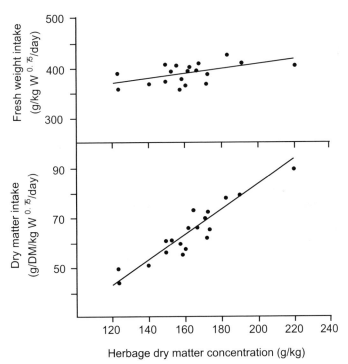

Figure 2.6 Relationship between voluntary consumption (g/kg live wt$^{0.75}$/day) on wet feed and dry matter basis and feed dry matter content (g/kg) for perennial ryegrass.
Source: John and Ulyatt (1987)

A system of feed intake based on the grinding and pelleting of fresh herbage is not feasible with regard to costs, but it may be possible to cut herbage at a sward height of 60 to 70 mm (thereby avoiding the bulk of stem and pseudostem material) and allow to wilt prior to grazing. Selection for herbage varieties with higher DM concentrations might also prove fruitful.

Leaf tensile strength

Leaf tensile strength may also be an important selection criteria influencing herbage intake in the grazing animal. Tough leaves require greater expenditure of energy to harvest (O'Reagain and Mantis, 1989). Furthermore passage of dietary residues out of the rumen requires comminution to a critical particle size (approximately 2 mm). Consequently any plant attribute that aids particle size reduction will have an impact on intake and nutritive value. Grasses are known to vary with respect to leaf strength (Evans, 1964), and it has been demonstrated that low leaf tensile and shear strength results in higher intake rates in sheep (Inoue, Brookes, John, Barry and Hunt, 1993). Both tensile and sheer strength are known to be highly heritable and so offer the possibility of breeding for superior intake characteristics based on these traits (Henry, MacMillan, Roberts and Simpson, 1993). The primary tissue influencing leaf strength is the sclerenchyma bundle (John, Inoue, Brookes, Hunt and Easton, 1989), and therefore reduction of sclerenchyma tissue could reduce leaf tensile/shear strength and so increase feeding value.

Ulyatt and Waghorn (1993) also make the case for breeding for reduced protein solubility, e.g. by including condensed tannins in the plant, which will reduce the degradation of protein in the rumen and thereby improve nutritive value. Selection can also be made for cultivars with a slower rate of nutrient release during chewing (Kudo, Cheng, Hanna, Howarth, Goplen and Costerton, 1985).

Supplementation at pasture

The provision of supplementary feeds to dairy cows at pasture is normally undertaken either to improve animal performance over and above that which can be produced from pasture alone, or to maintain performance during periods of grass deficit. Improvement in milk yields of dairy cows at pasture (either as a result of increasing genetic merit or changes in production system, e.g. summer calving dairy herds) has meant that these considerations are becoming increasingly important.

The major challenges in supplementary feeding at pasture relate to difficulties in estimating dry matter intake and herbage composition on a daily basis. This information is an essential prerequisite in aiding decisions such as level and composition of concentrate feeds, timing of feeding and the role of supplementary forages. Furthermore, the effect of provision of supplementary feeds on herbage intake, i.e. substitution rate, is critical in determining whether production responses to supplementation are economic. However unlike the indoor feeding situation, there is relatively little information on the relationship between milk output and level of supplementary feeding at pasture.

CONCENTRATE SUPPLEMENTS

Level of feeding

Mayne (1991) summarized the effects of concentrate feeding on herbage substitution rates and milk production responses over a range of herbage allowances as shown in Table 2.5. These data indicate marked increases in substitution rate, and reductions in milk production responses with increases in herbage allowance.

Table 2.5 EFFECT OF SUPPLEMENTATION AT DIFFERENT HERBAGE ALLOWANCES ON SUBSTITUTION RATE AND RESPONSE.

Herbage allowance (kg OM+/day)	Substitution rate (kg herbage OM/ kg concentrate OM)	Increase in ME intake (MJ/day/kg concentrate OM)	Predicted milk response (kg/day/kg concentrate OM)
15	0.11	12	1.0
20	0.30	9	0.8
25	0.50	7	0.6
30	0.69	4	0.4

+ Organic matter

Source : Mayne (1991).

The large substitution effects observed at generous herbage allowances can be attributed to effects on grazing behaviour, with reductions in time spent grazing of 15-22 min/kg DM concentrate offered per day (Sarker and Holmes, 1974; Cowan, Byford and Stobbs, 1975). However it is interesting to speculate whether such large reductions in grazing time would be obtained at similar herbage allowances with high genetic merit cows, given the increased nutrient demand, and consequently intake drive, associated with higher levels of milk production.

Holden, Muller and Fales (1994) estimated pasture and total DM intake for high genetic merit cows grazing Orchardgrass, Kentucky-bluegrass and Smooth-broomegrass pastures in the US. Cows in mid-lactation at turnout were supplemented at the rate of 1 kg concentrate DM/5 kg milk, with a maximum of 10 kg and minimum of 4 kg of concentrate DM/day. Over the period 30 April-1 July, mean concentrate, pasture and total DM intakes averaged 7.3, 14.5 and 21.8 kg/day respectively with a mean milk yield of 33 kg milk/cow/day.

In more recent studies at Hillsborough (Ferris, Gordon, Patterson and Mayne *unpublished*) high genetic merit cows (PTA$_{90}$ fat+protein yield = 53.2 kg; sd 9.6) (on average 90 days after calving at turnout) receiving 5.5 kg concentrate fresh-weight/day produced 31.5 kg milk/d during the first 112 days at pasture. In contrast, a group of medium genetic merit cows (PTA_{90} fat+protein yield = 10.9 kg; sd 10.7) receiving a similar level of concentrate, produced 26.8 kg milk/day over the same time period at pasture. These data clearly illustrate the potential to achieve higher levels of performance with high merit cows at pasture, feeding only moderate levels of concentrate supplementation, relative to that attainable with indoor housing and grass-silage based diets at similar concentrate inputs.

Again, attention is drawn to the fact that much of the research on the effect of concentrate supplementation at pasture on animal performance has been undertaken with animals of moderate milk yield potential (generally in the range 15-25 kg milk/day). Consequently, caution must be exercised in extrapolating these results to the pasture-based environment with animals of higher milk production potential.

Concentrate allocation systems

Whilst there is no published information on the effect of concentrate allocation systems to dairy cows at pasture, extrapolation from indoor feeding studies suggests that feed-to-yield systems rather than flat rate feeding systems may be justified with concentrate feeding at pasture. This reflects the fact that in the grazing situation, sward and/or animal behaviour constraints may limit herbage intake with higher producing animals. Results of indoor feeding studies (Broster and Thomas, 1981) indicate that, where forage intake is restricted, cows of higher production potential produced a greater milk yield response to incremental increases in concentrate feeding.

Recent studies in the US (Buckmaster, Muller, Hongerholt and Gardner, 1995) have examined the effect of frequency of feeding of complementary concentrates, offered in addition to grazed pasture, on performance of high yielding (mean 38.4 kg milk/day) dairy cows. Concentrates were offered either at pasture over four meals/day (via a mobile concentrate feeder), or twice daily at milking. Preliminary results indicate that increased frequency of concentrate feeding had no effect on milk yield, although increases in milk fat concentration and milk fat yields were obtained at high concentrate feed levels (mean concentrate intake 12.2 kg/cow/d). However, timing of concentrate feeding may have important implications on herbage substitution rate. For example at relatively low concentrate feed levels it may be beneficial to offer a greater proportion of concentrates after peak grazing periods (i.e. at p.m. rather than a.m. milking).

Concentrate type

A wide range of concentrate supplements are fed to dairy cows at pasture. These vary from supplements that are high in sugar (molasses), to starch (cereal grains) and digestible fibre (beet pulp, citrus pulp, brewers' grains, etc.).

Energy source

The effects of concentrate energy source on substitution rate and animal performance of dairy cows at grass are inconsistent. For example Meijs (1986) observed higher substitution rates and lower animal performance responses with high starch (350 g starch+sugars/kg DM) relative to high fiber (100 g starch+sugars/kg DM) concentrates. However, Van Vuuren, Van der Koelen and Vroons-de Bruin (1993) observed no effect of concentrate energy source on herbage intake, although organic matter digestion in the fore stomach was reduced and duodenal amino acid flow increased with high starch (487 g starch+sugar/kg DM) relative to high fiber (94g starch+sugar/kg DM) concentrates. Van Vuuren *et al.*, (1993) concluded that the efficiency of microbial protein synthesis was increased with high starch concentrates, even when relatively high levels of concentrate (7.1 kg DM/day) were offered in addition to herbage.

The apparent conflict between these studies may be related to changes in the chemical composition of herbage throughout the season. More information is required on the effect of concentrate energy source on rumen fermentation characteristics, herbage substitution rate and animal performance with a range of herbage types.

Protein

Whilst the crude protein content of perennial ryegrass based swards is high (particularly in spring and autumn) less than 30% of the ingested grass protein reaches the duodenum (Beever, Losada, Cammell, Evans and Haines, 1986). A high proportion of the rumen degradable protein in fresh herbage is absorbed from the rumen and excreted as urea in urine, resulting in increased potential for nitrate leaching. Consequently supplementation strategies should be designed to increase utilization of rumen degradable nitrogen by improving the synchronization of energy and protein supply to the rumen microflora. Possible options include feeding supplements with high levels of starch and sugars, or alternatively varying the timing of supplementary feeding during the day.

Recent evidence (Hongerholt, 1995) indicates that, as a result of reduced N flow to the duodenum with herbage-based diets, substantial responses in pasture intake, milk and milk protein yield can be obtained with high genetic merit cows through increases in the undegradable protein content of supplementary concentrates. The potential benefits of protected proteins arise from reduced degradation in the rumen, allowing a greater amount of dietary protein to reach the small intestine and become available to the animal (Kaufmann, 1979).

FORAGE SUPPLEMENTS

With the increase in the levels of animal performance during the grazing season, there is a developing trend towards feeding conserved forage either once or twice daily post milking (buffer feeding), or in more extreme cases feeding forage supplements to animals housed overnight (partial storage feeding) (Phillips and Leaver, 1985).

Adequate grass availability

In situations where grass supply is adequate, offering grass silage as a buffer feed results in large substitution effects (up to 0.89 kg herbage DM/kg grass silage DM), and reductions in both milk and milk protein yield (Mayne, 1991). It is important to note that substitution effects with grass silage supplementation are much greater than that with concentrate supplements (0.69 kg herbage DM/kg supplement DM) in situations where adequate herbage is available. This appears to be related to a greater depression in grazing time/day with grass silage (43 min/d/kg forage DM) than with concentrate supplements (20-23 min/d/kg forage DM).

Maize silage has also been examined as a buffer feed for grazing dairy cows. Bryant and Donnelly (1974) observed a reduction in animal performance with buffer feeding of maize silage when adequate pasture was available. However, Holden, Muller, Lykos and Cassidy (1995), reported that feeding 2.3 kg maize silage DM/day to high yielding (29.0 kg milk/day) dairy cows grazing grass pastures and receiving 8.7 kg concentrate DM/day had no effect on milk production or total DM intake.

The data presented above suggest that in situations where adequate grass is available, shortfalls in nutrient supply from herbage, relative to nutrient requirements for high producing dairy cows, should be rectified by supplementation with complementary concentrates of high nutrient concentration, rather than forage supplements. Given that high quality grazed grass has the potential to support milk yields up to 27.0 kg/day in spring, declining to 20.0 kg/day in late August, the appropriate level of concentrate supplementation for high producing dairy cows can be calculated as shown in Table 2.6. These data relate to a rotational grazing system with a daily herbage allowance of 25.0 kg DM/cow, and assume a typical substitution rate of 0.40 kg herbage DM/kg supplement DM (Mayne, 1991). They also assume an incremental increase in herbage intake of 0.125 kg DM/kg increase in milk yield, well below the 0.4-0.5 kg incremental increase in intake normally observed in animals yielding between 15.0-25.0 kg milk/day (Stakelum, 1993; Stakelum and Dillon, 1995).

Grass shortages

The use of conserved forage as a supplement to grazed grass during periods of grass shortage, or when herbage quality is poor (e.g. swards in late season that have been undergrazed in spring) generally results in increased total DM intake and improved animal performance (Phillips, 1988). In these situations it is important to continue to

Table 2.6 SUGGESTED CONCENTRATE FEED LEVELS FOR HIGH YIELDING DAIRY COWS IN EARLY AND LATE SEASON WITH HIGH HERBAGE ALLOWANCE (25 KG DM/COW/DAY).

	Mid May Target yield (kg milk/day)			Late August Target yield (kg milk/day)	
	25.0	35.0	40.0	25.0	35.0
Potential production from grass (kg milk/day)[+]	27.0	29.4	30.9	20.0	24.5
ME required from supplement (MJ/cow/day)[++]	0.0	28.0	45.5	25.0	52.5
Supplement feed level required (kg DM/cow/day)[+++]	0.0	3.9	6.3	3.5	7.3

[+]   Assumes increase in herbage intake of 0.125 kg DM/kg additional milk.

[++]   Assumes ME required for milk production of 5.0 MJ/kg milk.

[+++]   Assumes substitution rate of 0.4 kg herbage DM/kg supplement DM and ME concentration of herbage and supplement of 12.0 MJ/kg DM.

monitor grass utilization on the grazing area, e.g. through sward height measurement, and either eliminate or restrict access to the buffer feed when sward conditions improve.

Conclusions

Management of high genetic merit dairy cows at pasture presents a major challenge to the dairy industry in the UK and Ireland. The future profitability of milk production and milk processing will be highly dependent upon maintaining low cost, grass-based production systems. Whilst there are considerable opportunities to increase the potential contribution of grazed grass in the diet of high merit cows, full exploitation of this potential will require grazing management systems designed to present herbage to the animal in a form that will maximise intake/bite and daily DM intake. Critical factors influencing herbage intake include herbage DM content (specifically intracellular water), and sward characteristics that determine bite size. Bite size is optimized with tall, dense, leafy swards, and this can best be achieved by rotational grazing systems. Even in these systems, high merit cows will require supplementation with complementary concentrates of high nutrient concentration in order to fully exploit their genetic potential for milk production. Buffer feeding of forages and partial storage feeding systems have a role in overcoming periodic shortages in grass supply, but do not have a major role in increasing animal performance above that attainable from well managed rotationally grazed swards.

References

Agricultural and Food Research Council (1993) *Energy and Protein Requirements of Ruminants*. An advisory manual prepared by the AFRC Technical Committee on Responses to Nutrients. CAB International, Wallingford.

Allden, W.G. and Whittaker, A.M. (1970) The determinants of herbage intake by grazing sheep : the interrelationship of factors influencing herbage intake and availability. *Australian Journal of Agricultural Research* **21** : 755-766.

Arnold, G.W. (1962) Effects of pasture maturity on the diet of sheep. *Australian Journal of Agricultural Research* **13** : 701-706.

Arnold, G.W. (1981) Grazing behaviour. In: *World Animal Science 1. Grazing Animals* pp.79-104. Ed. F.H.W. Morley. Elsevier Scientific Publishing, New York

Baile, C.A. and Della-Fera, M.A. (1981) Nature of hunger and satiety control systems in ruminants. *Journal of Dairy Science* **64** : 1140-1153.

Ball, R., Molloy, L.F. and Ross, D.J. (1978) Influence of fertilizer nitrogen on herbage dry matter and nitrogen yields, and botanical composition of a grazed grass-clover pasture. *New Zealand Journal of Agricultural Research* **21** : 47-55.

Bauman, D.E., Eppard, P.J., DeGeeter, M.J. and Lanza, G.M. (1985) Responses of high producing dairy cows to long-term treatment with pituitary somatotropin and recombinant somatotropin. *Journal of Dairy Science* **68** : 1352-1362.

Beever, D.E., Losada, H.R., Cammell, S.B., Evans, R.T. and Haines, M.J. (1986) Effects of forage species and season on nutrient digestion and supply in grazing cattle. *British Journal of Nutrition* **56** : 209-225.

Bertrand, J.A., Berger, P.J., Freeman, A.E. and Kelley, D.H. (1985) Profitability in daughters of high versus average Holstein sires selected for milk yield of daughters. *Journal of Dairy Science* **68** : 2287-2294.

Brereton, A.J. (1987) Efficient utilization of pasture requires flexible management. In: *Agricultural Pasture Improvement* Ed. L. Miro-Granada Gelabert. Commission of the European Community, Madrid, Spain. pp.147-154.

Brereton, A.J. (1995) Regional and year-to-year variation in production. In: *Irish Grasslands-their Biology and Management* pp.12-22. Eds. D.W. Jeffery, M.B. Jones, and J.H. McAdam. Royal Irish Academy, Dublin.

Brereton, A.J. and Carton, O.T. (1988) Sward height, structure and herbage use. In: *Research Meeting No. 1*, British Grassland Society, Edinburgh

Brereton, A.J., Danielov, S.A. and Scott, D. (1995) Agrometeorology of grasslands for the middle latitudes. *World Meteoroology Organisation Technical Note*, Geneva

Broster, W.H. and Thomas, C. (1981) The influence of level and pattern of concentrate input on milk output. In: *Recent Advances in Animal Nutrition 1981* pp. 49-69. Ed. W. Haresign. Butterworths, London.

Bryant, A.M. and Donnelly, P.E. (1974) Yield and composition of milk from cows fed pasture herbage supplemented with maize and pasture silages. *New Zealand Journal of Agricultural Research* **27** : 491-493.

Buckmaster, D., Muller, L., Hongerholt, D. and Gardner, M. (1995) Mobile computer controlled concentrate feeder for lactating cows. *Summaries of Pasture Research and Extension Activities* Penn State University, University Park PA.

Burnside, E.B., Graham, N., Rapitta, A.E., McBride, B.W. and Gibson, J.P. (1991) The Canadian approach to breeding efficient dairy cows. In: *Proceedings British Cattle Breeders Club Winter Conference, Cambridge* pp.25-28.

Butler-Hogg, B.W., Wood, J.D. and Bines, J.A. (1985) Fat partitioning in British Friesian cows; the influence of physiological state on dissected body composition. *Journal of Agricultural Science*, Cambridge **104** : 519-528.

Chacon, E. And Stobbs, T.H. (1976) Influence of progressive defoliation of a grass sward on the eating behaviour of cattle. *Australian Journal of Agricultural Research* **27** : pp.709-718.

Combellas, J. and Hodgson, J. (1979) Herbage intake and milk production by grazing dairy cows 1. The effect of variation in herbage mass and daily herbage allowance in a short-term trial. *Grass and Forage Science* **34** : 209-214.

Connaughton, M.J. (1973) The grass-growing season in Ireland. *Agrometeorological Memorandum No. 5.* Dublin Meteorological Service.

Cowan, R.T., Byford, I.J.R. and Stobbs, T.H. (1975) Effects of stocking rate and energy supplementation on milk production from tropical grass-legume pasture. *Australian Journal of Experimental and Animal Husbandry* **15** : 740-746.

Duckworth, J.E. and Shirlaw, D.W. (1958) A study of factors affecting feed intake and the eating behaviour of cattle. *Animal Behaviour* **6** : 147-154.

Evans, P.S. (1964) A study of leaf strength in four ryegrass varieties. *New Zealand Journal of Agricultural Research* **7** : 508-513.

Evans, B. (1981) Production from swards grazed by dairy cows. *Grass and Forage Science* **36** : 132-134.

Fitzsimons, E. (1995) Influence of sward structure on the grazing behaviour of dairy cows. *M.Sc. Thesis*, University College Cork, Ireland.

Flores, E.R., Laca, E.A., Griggs, T.C. and Demment, M.W. (1993) Sward height and vertical morphological differentiation determine cattle bite dimensions. *Agronomy Journal* **85** : 527-532.

Forbes, J.M. (1995) Voluntary intake - A limiting factor to production in high-yielding dairy cows? In: *Breeding and Feeding the High Genetic Merit Cow* British Society of Animal Science Occasional Publication No. 19. pp.13-19.

Funk, D.A. (1993) Optimal genetic improvement for the high producing herd. *Journal of Dairy Science* **76** : 3278-3286.

Gibb, M.J., Ivings, W.E., Dhanoa, M.S. and Sutton, J.D. (1992) Changes in body components of autumn calving Holstein-Friesian cows over the first 29 weeks of lactation. *Animal Production* **55** : 339-360.

Gibson, J.P. (1981) The effects of feeding frequency on the growth and efficiency of food utilization of ruminants : An analysis of published results. *Animal Production* **32** : 275-283.

Gill, M. And Beever, D.E. (1991) Modeling as an aid to nutrition research. In: *Isotope and related techniques in animal production and health* pp.171-182. IEAE, Vienna.

Graham, N.J., Burnside, E.B., Gibson, J.P., Rapitta, A.E. and McBride, B.W. (1991) Comparison of daughters of Canadian and New Zealand Holstein sires for first lactation efficiency of production in relation to body size and condition. *Canadian Journal of Animal Science* **71** : 293-300.

Grainger, C., Holmes, C.W. and Moore, Y.F. (1985) Performance of Friesian cows with high and low breeding indexes 2. Energy and nitrogen balance experiments with lactating and pregnant, non lactating cows. *Animal Production* **40** : 389-400.

Grant, S.A., Barthram, G.T. and Torvell, L. (1981) Components of regrowth in grazed and cut *Lolium perenne* swards. *Grass and Forage Science* **36** : 155-168.

Halley, R.J. and Dougall, B.M. (1962) The feed intake and performance of dairy cows fed on cut grass. *Journal of Dairy Research* **29** : 241-248.

Hansen, L.B., Freeman, A.E. and Berger, P.J. (1983) Yield and fertility relationships in dairy cattle. *Journal of Dairy Science* **66** : 293-305.

Henry, D.A., MacMillan, R.H., Roberts, F.M. and Simpson, R.J. (1993) Assessment of the variation in shear strength of leaves of pasture grasses. *Proceedings 17th International Grassland Congress*, Palmerston North, New Zealand. pp.533-555.

Hodgson, J. (1981) Variations in the surface characteristics of the sward and the short-term rate of herbage intake by calves and lambs. *Grass and Forage Science* **36** : pp.49-57.

Hodgson, J. (1982) Influence of sward characteristics on diet selection and herbage intake by the grazing animal. In*: Nutritional Limits to Animal Production from Pasture* pp.153-166, Commonwealth Agricultural Bureaux, St Lucia, Australia.

Hodgson, J. and Jamieson, W.S. (1981) Variations in herbage mass and digestibility, and the grazing behaviour of adult cattle and weaned calves. *Grass and Forage Science* **36** : 39-48.

Holden, L.A., Muller, L.D. and Fales, S.L. (1994) Estimation of intake in high producing Holstein cows grazing grass pasture *Journal of Dairy Science* **77** : 2332-2340.

Holden, L.A., Muller, L.D., Lykos, T. And Cassidy, T.W. (1995) Effect of corn silage supplementation on intake and milk production in cows grazing grass pasture. *Journal of Dairy Science* **78** : 154-160.

Holmes, C.W. (1988) Genetic merit and efficiency of milk production by the dairy cow. In: *Nutrition and Lactation in the Dairy Cow* pp.195-215. Ed. P.C. Garnsworthy, Butterworths, London.

Holmes, C.W. (1995) Genotype x environment interactions in dairy cattle: a New Zealand perspective. In: *Breeding and Feeding the High Genetic Merit Cow* British Society of Animal Science Occasional Publication No. 19. pp.51-58, Edinburgh

Holmes, W. (1968) The use of nitrogen in the management of pasture for cattle. *Herbage Abstracts* **38** : 265-277.

Hongerholt, D.D. (1995) Grain supplementation strategies for dairy cows grazing grass pastures and their effects on milk production and microbial fermentation. *Ph.D. Thesis, Pennsylvania State University.*

Illius, A.W. and Gordon, I.J. (1987) The allometry of food intake in grazing ruminants. *Journal of Animal Ecology* **56** : 989-999.

Illius, A.W., Lowman, B.G.and Hunter, E.A. (1986) The use of buffer grazing to maintain sward quality and increase late season cattle performance. In: *Grazing* pp.119-128. Ed. J. Frame. British Grassland Society Occasional Symposium No. 19, BGS, Hurley.

Inoue, T., Brookes, I.M., John, A., Barry, T.N. and Hunt, W.F. (1993) Effect of physical resistance in perennial ryegrass leaves on feeding value for sheep. *Proceedings 17th International Grassland Congress*, Palmerston North, New Zealand. pp.570-572.

Jamieson, W.S. (1975) Studies on the herbage intake and grazing behaviour of cattle and sheep. *Ph.D. Thesis*, University of Reading.

John, A., Inoue, T., Brookes, I.M., Hunt, W.F. and Easton, H.S. (1989) Effects of selection for shear strength on structure and rumen digestion of perennial ryegrass. *Proceedings of the New Zealand Society of Animal Production* **49** : 225-228.

John, A. and Ulyatt, M.J. (1987) Importance of dry matter content to voluntary intake of fresh grass forages *Proceedings of the New Zealand Society of Animal Production* **47** : 13-16.

Johns, A.T. (1954) Bloat in cattle on red clover. *New Zealand Journal of Science and Technology* **36** : 289-320.

Journet, M. and Demarquilly, C. (1979) Grazing In: *Feeding strategies for the high yielding dairy cow* pp.295-321. Eds. W.H. Broster and H. Swan. Granada Publishing, London.

Kaufmann, W. (1979) In: *Feeding Strategies for the High Yielding Dairy Cow* pp.90-113. Eds. W.H. Broster and H. Swan. Granada Publishing, London

Kingsbury, L.R. (1965) Pasture quality in terms of soluble carbohydrates and volatile fatty acid production. *Proceedings of the New Zealand Society of Animal Production* **25** : 119-136.

Kudo, H., Cheng, K.J., Hanna, M.R., Howarth, R.E., Goplen, B.P. and Costerton, J.W. (1985) Ruminal digestion of alfalfa strains selected for slow and fast initial rates of digestion. *Canadian Journal of Animal Science* **65** : 157-161.

Laca, E.A., Demment, M.W., Distel, R.A. and Griggs, T.C. (1993) A conceptual model to explain variation in ingestive behaviour within a feeding patch.

Proceedings 17th International Grassland Congress, Palmerston North, New Zealand. pp.710-712.

Laca, E.A., Ungar, E.D., Seligman, N.G. and Demment, M.W. (1992) Effects of sward height and bulk density on bite dimensions of cattle grazing homogenous swards. *Grass and Forage Science* **47** : 91-102.

Leaver, J.D. (1983) Feeding for high margins. In: *Recent Advances in Animal Nutrition - 1983* pp.199-207. Ed. W. Haresign. Butterworths, London.

Leaver, J.D. (1985) Milk production from grazed temperate grassland. *Journal of Dairy Science* **52** : 313-344.

Leaver, J.D. (1987) The potential to increase production efficiency from animal-pasture systems. *Proceedings of the New Zealand Society of Animal Production* **47** : 7-12.

Le Du, Y.L.P., Combellas, J., Hodgson, J. and Baker, R.D. (1979) Herbage intake and milk production by grazing dairy cows 2. The effects of level of winter feeding and daily herbage allowance. *Grass and Forage Science* **34** : 249-260.

Lloyd-Davies, H. (1962) Intake studies in sheep involving high fluid intake. *Proceedings of the Australian Society of Animal Production* **4** : 167-171.

Mayne, C.S. (1991) Effects of supplementation on the performance of both growing and lactating cattle at pasture. In: *Management Issues for the Grassland Farmer in the 1990s* pp.55-71. Ed. C.S. Mayne. Occasional Symposium No. 25. British Grassland Society, Hurley.

Mayne, C.S. and Gordon, F.J. (1995) Implications of genotype x nutrition interactions for efficiency of milk production systems. In: *Breeding and Feeding the High Genetic Merit Cow* British Society of Animal Science Occasional Publication No. 19. Edinburgh pp.67-77.

McMeekan, C.P. and Walsh, M.J. (1963) The inter-relationships of grazing method and stocking rate in the efficiency of pasture utilisation by dairy cattle. *Journal of Agricultural Science* **61** : 147-166.

Meijs, J.A.C. (1986) Concentrate supplementation of grazing dairy cows 2. Effect of concentrate composition on herbage intake and milk production. *Grass and Forage Science* **41** : 229-235.

Meijs, J.A.C. and Hoekstra, J.A. (1984) Concentrate supplementation of grazing dairy cows 1. Effect of concentrate intake and herbage allowance on herbage intake. *Grass and Forage Science* **61** : 147-166.

Moral, M.M.C. del (1982) Study of the nutritive value of a mixed pasture: variations in digestibility and intake. *Pastos* **12** : 119-133. (Summarised in *Nutrition Abstracts and Reviews (series B)* **56** (4)).

Morrison, J. (1977) The growth of *Lolium perenne* and response to fertilizer-N in relation to season and management. *Proceedings XIII International Grassland Congress,* Leipzig. pp.943-946.

Morrison, J., Jackson, M.V. and Williams, T.E. (1974) Variation in the response of grass to fertilizer N in relation to environment. *Proceedings of the Fertilizer Society* **142** : 28-38.

Morrison, J., Jackson, M.V. and Sparrow, P.E. (1980) The response of perennial ryegrass to fertilizer nitrogen in relation to climate and soil : report of the joint ADAS/GRI grassland manuring trial GM20 *Technical Report No. 27* Grassland Research Institute, Hurley.

Oltenacu, P.A., Frick, A. and Lindhe, B. (1991) Relationship of fertility to milk yield in Swedish cattle. *Journal of Dairy Science* **74** : 264-268.

O'Reagain, P.J. and Mentis, M.T. (1989) The effect of plant structure on the acceptability of different grass species to cattle. *Journal of the Grassland Society of South Africa* **6** : 163-170.

Patterson, D.C., Gordon, F.J., Mayne, C.S. Porter, M.G. and Unsworth, E.F. (1995) The effects of genetic merit on nutrient utilization in lactating dairy cows. In: *Breeding and Feeding the High Genetic Merit Cow* British Society of Animal Science Occasional Publication No. 19. pp.97-98.

Peterson, R. (1988) Comparison of Canadian and New Zealand sires in New Zealand for production, weight and conformation traits (Unpublished Report). 12pp.

Phillips, C.J.C. (1988) The use of conserved forage as a supplement for grazing dairy cows. *Grass and Forage Science* **43** : 215-230.

Phillips, C.J.C. (1993) *Cattle Behaviour* Farming Press Books, Ipswich.

Phillips, C.J.C. and Leaver, J.D. (1985) Supplementary feeding of forage to grazing dairy cows. 2. Offering grass silage in early and late season. *Grass and Forage Science* **40** : 193-199.

Reid, D. (1978) The effect of frequency of defoliation on the yield response of a perennial ryegrass sward to a wide range of nitrogen application rates. *Journal of Agricultural Science, Cambridge* **90** : 447-457.

Ryan, D.P., Snijders, S., McGilloway, D.A. and O'Farrell, K.J. (1996) Effects of grazing pressure on dry matter intake, ovarian follicular populations, and reproductive performance in lactating cows. *Journal of Animal Science* (submitted).

Sarker, H.B. and Holmes, W. (1974) The influence of supplementary feeding on the herbage intake and grazing behaviour of dry cows. *Journal of the British Grassland Society* **29** : 141-143.

Scarnecchia, D.L., Nastis, A.S. and Malechek, J.C. (1985) Effects of forage availability on grazing behaviour of heifers. *Journal of Range Management* **38** : 177-180.

Sejrsen, K. and Neimann-Sorensen, A. (1994) Sources of genetic variation in efficiency of cattle : biological basis. *Proceedings 45th Meeting of European Association of Animal Production,* Edinburgh pp 140.

Shanks, R.D., Freeman, P.J. Berger, P.J. and Kelley, D.H. (1978) Effects of selection for milk production on reproductive and general health of the dairy cow. *Journal of Dairy Science* **61** : 1765-1772.

Spedding, C.R.W., Large, R.V. and Kydd, D.D. (1966) The evaluation of herbage species by grazing animals. *10th International Grassland Congress*, Helsinki pp.479-483.

Stakelum, G. (1993) Achieving high performance from dairy cows on grazed pastures. *Irish Grassland and Animal Production Association Journal* **27** : 9-18.

Stakelum, G. and Dillon, P. (1995) Supplementary feeding of grazing dairy cows. *Technical Bulletin, Issue No. 2*, R & H Hall , Dublin

Stewart, T.A. (1985) Utilising white clover in grass based animal production systems. In: *Forage Legumes* pp.93-103. Ed. D.J. Thomson. Occasional Symposium No. 16, British Grassland Society, Hurley.

Stobbs, T.H. (1973) The effect of plant structure on the intake of tropical pastures 2. Differences in sward structure, nutritive value and bite size of animals grazing *Setaria anceps* and *Chloris gayana* at various stages of growth. *Australian Journal of Agricultural Research* **24** : 821-829.

Stobbs, T.H. (1974) Rate of biting by Jersey cows as influenced by the yield and maturity of pasture swards. *Tropical Grasslands* **8** : 81-86.

Struth, J.W., Brown, J.R., Olson, P.D., Araujo, M.R. and Alijoe, H.D. (1987) Effects of stocking rate on critical plant animal interactions in a rotationally grazed *Schizachyrium-Paspalum savannah*. In: *Grazing-lands Research at the Plant-animal Interface* pp.115-139. Eds. F.P. Horn, J. Hodgson, J.J. Mott and R.W. Brougham. Winrock International, Morriton, Arkansas, USA

Thomson, D.J., Beever, D.E., Haines, M.J., Cammell, S.B., Evans, R.T., Dhanoa, M.S. and Austin, A.R. (1985) Yield and composition of milk from Friesian cows grazing either perennial ryegrass or white clover in early lactation. *Journal of Dairy Research* **52** : 17-31.

Thran, P.S. and Broekhuizen, S. (1965) *Agro-climatic Atlas of Europe* Pudoc., Wageningen. Elsevier, Amsterdam.

UK Statistics for Genetic Evaluation (1995) Animal Data Centre Ltd, Rickmansworth

Ulyatt, M.J. and Waghorn, G.C. (1993) Limitations to high levels of dairy production from New Zealand pastures. In: *Improving the Quality and Intake of Pasture Based Diets for Lactating Dairy Cows* pp.11-32. Eds. N.J. Edwards and W.J. Parker. Department of Agricultural and Horticultural Systems Management, Occasional Publication No. 1, Massey University, Palmerston North, New Zealand.

Van Vuuren, A.M., Van der Koelen, C.J. and Vroons-de Bruim, J. (1993). Ryegrass versus corn starch or beet pulp fibre diet effects on digestion and intestinal amino acids in dairy cows. *Journal of Dairy Science* **76** : 2692-2700.

Veerkamp, R.F., Emmans, G.C., Cromie, A.R. and Simm, G. (1995) Variance components for residual feed intake in dairy cows. *Livestock Production Science* **41** : 111-120.

Veerkamp, R.F., Simm, G. and Oldham, J.D. (1994) Effects of interaction between genotype and feeding system on milk production, feed intake, efficiency and body tissue mobilization in dairy cows. *Livestock Production Science* **39** : 229-241.

Vérité, R. And Journet, M. (1970) Influence de la teneur en eau et la deshydration de l'herbe sur la valeur alimentaire pour les vaches laitiers. *Annales de Zootechnie* **19** : 255-268.

Wade, M.H. (1991) Factors affecting the availability of vegetative *Lolium perenne* L. to grazing dairy cows with special reference to sward characteristics, stocking rate and grazing method. Thése de Docteur Ingénieur, Université de Rennes.

Wilkinson, J.M., Price, W.R., Russell, S.R. and Jones, P. (1994) Diurnal variation in dry matter and sugar content of ryegrass. *British Grassland Society, 4th Research Conference*, University of Reading. pp.61-62.

This paper was first published in 1996

3

EVALUATION OF PHYSICAL STRUCTURE IN DAIRY CATTLE NUTRITION

D.L. DE BRABANDER, J.L. DE BOEVER, J. M. VANACKER, CH.V. BOUCQUÉ and S.M. BOTTERMAN
Department Animal Nutrition and Husbandry, Agricultural Research Centre - Ghent, Ministry of Small Enterprises, Traders and Agriculture, Scheldeweg 68, B-9090 Melle-Gontrode, Belgium

Introduction

Optimum feeding of dairy cattle requires the maintenance of good rumen function. A disturbed rumen fermentation is the main outcome of a shortage of physical structure. This results in depressed feed intake, reduced digestion, decreased production efficiency, health problems like rumen acidosis and parakeratosis, and lowered fat milk content. Although physical structure is difficult to define, it could be considered as an expression of "the extent to which a feedstuff, through its content and properties of the carbohydrates, contributes to an optimum and stable rumen function". Feed containing physical structure stimulates chewing activity and this in its turn increases saliva secretion. Since saliva buffers the rumen contents, it reduces acidosis and helps to achieve an optimum pH and ratio of volatile fatty acids. Roughage creates a fibrous layer in the rumen, which is important for frequent and strong rumen contractions. It is generally accepted that physical structure deficiency depresses milk fat content. Most likely, this is mainly caused by a lower acetic acid:propionic acid ratio in the rumen.

Due to breeding, improved nutrition and better management, the milk production level of dairy cattle has increased considerably and will no doubt increase still further in the future. Although feed intake capacity increases with increasing milk production potential, the higher feed intake of certain rations is insufficient to meet the increased energy requirements. Consequently, the quality of the diet has to improve. This can be achieved by raising the proportion of concentrates in the ration, and/or by supplementing with energy-rich byproducts, and/or by using better roughages. All these measures reduce the structure value of the ration. Hence, problems with physical structure occur more frequently now than in the past and will increase still further in the future. Therefore the need for an adequate physical structure system has become more and more important.

Different methods have been proposed to optimise dairy cattle diets with regard to rumen activity. Some authors suggested minimum roughage:concentrate ratios e.g. 40:60 (Flatt, Moe, Munson and Cooper, 1969) or 45% long roughage (Sutton, 1984). Due to the great variation in chemical and physical characteristics of roughages, such standards are useless. Other authors suggested crude fibre (CF) content as a standard. The big variation among the proposed CF levels, i.e. 100-160 g/kg (Hoffmann, 1983), 130-140 g/kg (Kesler and Spahr, 1964), 170 g/kg (NRC, 1978), 180 g/kg (Kaufmann, 1976) and 180-220 g/kg in the German technical literature (Guth, 1995), as well as the wide ranges, support the conclusion that CF is not appropriate as a general standard. Moreover, CF is not a nutritional, chemical or physically uniform entity (Van Soest, Robertson and Lewis, 1991). Nevertheless, within a type of roughage with well-defined physical characteristics, CF content could be a suitable criterion. In the USA, a system based on NDF is used (NRC, 1988). However, it was recognised that NDF as such could not be used as a general parameter for physical structure (Weiss, 1993). Therefore, the system was modified by attributing an effectivity coefficient to the NDF of feedstuffs, and the unit became "effective NDF" (Sniffen, O'Connor, Van Soest, Fox and Russell, 1992; Mertens, 1997). Besides eNDF, which is aimed at providing a normal milk fat content, peNDF (physical effective NDF) was also introduced (Armentano and Pereira, 1997; Mertens, 1997). The latter takes the physical properties as well as particle size into account, and is related to chewing activity. However, the standards are vague and a modification was suggested. Because most factors influencing rumen activity are related to chewing activity, the latter became an important research topic (Balch, 1971; Sudweeks, Ely, Mertens and Sisk, 1981; De Boever, 1991; Sauvant, 1992; Dulphy, Rouel, Jailler et Sauvant, 1993; Nørgaard, 1985, 1993).

Conscious of the need for a scientifically-based system for evaluation of physical structure for dairy cattle, a research programme was started some years ago at our Department to determine the physical structure value of feedstuffs in current use on the one hand and to derive physical structure standards for dairy cattle on the other. It is an important step towards an innovative system for evaluation of physical structure for dairy cattle. Obviously, the system may need further adjustments with the evolution of knowledge in this field.

Materials and methods

CHEWING ACTIVITY

Several arguments support a relationship between physical structure and chewing activity. Therefore, eating and ruminating time were measured for a large number of feeds according to a standardised experimental design. Chewing activity was measured continuously during 4 days, according to the method described by De Boever, De Smet, De Brabander and Boucqué (1993). An adaptation period of 10 days between batches of the same forage type was considered sufficient, whereas this period was 17 days for transition to another type of forage. The recordings enabled a clear distinction between eating and ruminating activity. In the following, eating, ruminating and chewing time, expressed per kg dry matter (DM) intake, are indicated as the indices EI, RI and CI, respectively.

In each trial, 8 low-yielding Holstein cows were used. Because of the moderate milk production level, the amount of concentrates could be restricted without risks to metabolism. First lactation cows were avoided, except when they had attained the age of 2nd lactation cows, because of the less efficient chewing behaviour of primiparous cows (Dehareng and Godeau, 1991; Dado and Allen, 1994; Beauchemin and Rode, 1994, 1997).

The roughage under investigation was fed *ad libitum*. To meet requirements for minerals and vitamins, and to assure a good rumen function, the basal ration was supplemented with 3 kg balanced concentrates or, in case of protein shortage, with 2 kg soya bean meal and 200 g of a mineral-vitamin mixture. By-products or other feeds, that could not be fed as single feedstuffs, were combined with maize or grass silage and chewing indices were derived by difference.

Eighty-one chewing trials, carried out according to the standardised experimental design, produced 644 cow observations from 95 different cows.

CRITICAL ROUGHAGE PART

The physical structure requirements were derived from trials (standard trials), in which the roughage (R) part of the diet of Holstein cows was decreased weekly until symptoms of physical structure deficiency appeared (decreased milk fat content, decreased milk yield, off feed). The roughage part just before problems occur, is called "the critical roughage part (R_{crit})". Thus, a lower R_{crit} corresponds with a higher structure value. These data in combination with the chewing indices were also used to derive structure values.

During the first two weeks of the standard trials, the roughage part of the diet was always ± 600 g/kg on DM basis. Then, the proportion was changed weekly to a lower roughage part: 500, 450 or 400 g/kg and further in steps of 50 g/kg. After the problematic ratio, most cows received the ration with 600 g R/kg again for one week. Cows were fed approximately *ad libitum*, though without appreciable refusals.

Milk yield was measured at each milking and the last 4 milkings of each week were sampled for determination of milk fat and protein content. A decrease in milk fat content was the main indicator to terminate the experiment. The concentrate (C) was always the same, except in trials concerning the nature of the concentrate. The main ingredients were sugar beet pulp (300 g/kg), wheat (180 g/kg), soya bean meal (140 g/kg), malt sprouts (100 g/kg), maize gluten feed (100 g/kg) and sugar beet molasses (70 g/kg). The ingredients were ground through a sieve of 6 mm, whereas the concentrates were pelleted (6 mm). Concentrates were supplied twice daily, except in trials where the effect of more frequent feeding was studied.

Because the R:C-ratios were changed in steps of 50 g/kg, the R_{crit} could not be determined precisely. Statistically, it is likely that the exact mean R_{crit} of a ration is 20 g/kg lower than the observed value. Therefore, all values of R_{crit} were diminished by 20 g/kg. The values of R_{crit} were also corrected for the effects of milk yield, milk fat content and age, so that they are valid for a standard cow producing 25 kg milk with 44 g fat/kg in the 1st, 2nd or 3rd lactation.

The R_{crit} was determined for 56 rations, resulting in 510 cow observations. The average milk yield, when the diets contained 600 g roughage/kg was 25.1 kg. The mean fat and protein concentrations amounted to 43.8 and 33.0 g/kg, respectively. Total DM intake averaged 18.1 kg/d.

General results

CHEWING ACTIVITY

The average eating, ruminating and chewing time for all observations was 287, 487 and 774 min/day with a SD of 64, 85 and 104 min/day. Ruminating generally lasts longer than eating, and usually takes between 7 and 9 hours per day (Welch, 1982; Sniffen, Hooper, Welch, Randy and Thomas, 1986; Beauchemin, Farr, Rode and Schaalje, 1994; Dado and Allen, 1994). The observed EI, RI and CI of the basal rations (C not included) averaged (SD) 25.2 (11.6), 41.4 (12.2) and 66.6 (21.7) min/kg DM. When animal species or live-weight classes are compared, chewing time is usually expressed in minutes per gram DM per kg $LW^{0.75}$. On average for the 644 observations, the chewing time was 8.4 min/kg DM/kg $LW^{0.75}$.

The main parameters representing the eating and ruminating behaviour for rations with preserved grassland products, fresh grass and maize silage as the sole roughage are presented in Table 3.1.

The chewing indices are corrected to a live weight of 600 kg based on metabolic weight. The EI, RI and CI averaged 26.2, 47.4 and 73.6 min/kg DM for 30 preserved grassland products, 33.5, 37.3 and 70.8 min/kg DM for 13 samples of fresh grass and 19.9, 39.3 and 59.3 min/kg DM for 23 maize silages. Variation was usually at least as high between cows as between samples of the same kind of roughage. Mean number of meals per day was 9.2, 8.6 and 8.5, respectively, with an average duration of 34.8, 43.5 and 34.6 minutes. Feeding is followed by a long eating time. For preserved grassland products and maize silage the first meal after the 2 feeding times represented 51% and 53% of the total eating time. The mean number of ruminating periods was 14.8, 14.1 and 15.0 per day, and lasted on average 36.6, 28.7 and 35.6 minutes, respectively. Other experiments confirm the higher frequency of ruminating compared with eating (Nørgaard, 1989; Dado and Allen, 1994). The longer eating time after feeding is generally found, whereas ruminating is more regularly spread over the day (Rémond and Journet, 1972; Dado and Allen, 1994).

Table 3.1 EATING AND RUMINATING BEHAVIOUR FOR RATIONS BASED ON GRASSLAND PRODUCTS AND MAIZE SILAGE

Roughage	Preserved grassland products	Fresh grass	Maize silage
Number of samples	30	13	23
NDF content (g/kg DM)	471	432	386
CF content (g/kg DM)	261	230	202
Roughage intake (kg DM/day)	11.8	11.0	14.1
Chewing time[1] (min/day)			
Eating	301	356	273
Ruminating	526	391	522
Chewing	827	746	795
Chewing indices[1] (min/kg DM)			
EI mean	26.2	33.5	19.9
SD_f - SD_c	4.9 – 4.5	4.4 – 6.6	2.2 – 3.1
RI mean	47.4	37.3	39.3
SD_f - SD_c	6.4 – 6.0	3.9 – 4.5	4.2 – 5.1
CI	73.6	70.8	59.3
SD_f - SD_c	10.1 – 8.6	7.7 – 9.5	5.9 - 6.7
Meals			
Number/day	9.2	8.6	8.5
SD_f - SD_c	1.8 – 1.9	1.1 – 1.5	1.5 – 1.9
Duration/meal (min)	34.8	43.5	34.6
SD_f - SD_c	7.5 – 7.5	4.6 – 7.7	7.1 – 8.1
Duration 2 main meals (min)	154	-	146
Ruminating periods			
Number/day	14.8	14.1	15.0
SD_f - SD_c	0.8 – 1.9	1.6 – 1.8	0.8 – 1.8
Duration/period (min)	36.6	28.7	35.6
SD_f - SD_c	2.8 – 7.0	2.8 – 5.5	3.1 – 5.0

[1] Chewing time and chewing indices refer to the roughage

SD_f: standard deviation of forages

SD_c: standard deviation of cow data within each trial

CRITICAL ROUGHAGE PART

With an increasing proportion of concentrates, milk yield increased until the R:C-ratio just before the R_{crit}. When physical structure appeared to be deficient, daily milk yield decreased by an average of 0.4 kg in one week. At that moment, the decrease in milk fat content averaged 5.8 g/kg. In the subsequent (recovery) week with 600 g roughage/

kg, fat content rose by 5.6 g/kg, whereas milk yield was 2.6 kg lower due to the depressed feed intake. Consequently, it can be assumed that the rumen function of most cows is normalised within one week.

For the 510 cow observations, average R_{crit} amounted to 299 g/kg, with a SD of 115 g/kg. The wide variation illustrates that a "fixed roughage proportion" in the ration cannot be a useful standard in a structure evaluation system. The R_{crit} seems to depend to a great extent on the cow as well as on the type of ration. The values for R_{crit} of the rations with a grassland product or maize silage as the sole roughage are presented in Table 3.2. The R_{crit} was appreciably higher for maize silage than for grassland products. The difference is greater than would be expected based on the difference in chewing indices.

Table 3.2 CHARACTERISTICS AND R_{CRIT} OF GRASSLAND PRODUCTS AND MAIZE SILAGE

| *Roughage* | *Grassland products* | | *Maize silage* | |
Number of samples	*17*		*14*	
	Mean	*$SD_f^{(1)}$*	*Mean*	*$SD_f^{(1)}$*
Characteristics				
NDF (g/kg DM)	495	56	397	31
CF (g/kg DM)	259	24	208	14
Chewing index (min/kg DM)	74.9	8.8	59.3	7.1
R_{crit} (g/kg)	205	39	348	56
$SD_c^{(1)}$	52	21	65	18

[1] SD_f : standard deviation for samples of forages
  SD_c: mean of standard deviations for cow data within each trial

Variation between samples of forages was relatively higher for R_{crit} than for chewing indices. The standard deviation of the individual cow data within each trial amounted to 52 and 65 g/kg for grassland products and maize silage, respectively. This relatively large individual variation necessitates a large safety margin in the structure evaluation system.

Animal-linked factors

CHEWING ACTIVITY

To make the results (n=644) of the different trials useful for studying the effect of animal characteristics, all chewing indices, as well as potential influences (live weight, milk yield, roughage intake), were expressed as a percentage of the mean for each trial. Relationships were studied by means of regression analysis.

The EI, RI and CI, were negatively correlated (P<0.001) with live weight(LW). This is in agreement with the results of Bae, Welch and Gilman (1983). To eliminate the effect of LW, all chewing indices were corrected to a LW of 600 kg, based on metabolic LW, (x $LW^{0.75}/600^{0.75}$). However, CI appeared to be overcorrected since a positive relationship was found between the corrected CI and LW. A log-transformation of both variables led to the choice of 0.3 as exponent rather than 0.75. The corrected index CI x $LW^{0.3}/600^{0.3}$ was independent of LW. The other animal-linked factors were studied for chewing indices corrected for $LW^{0.3}$.

In the present experimental circumstances, where young primiparous cows were not involved in the trials, age had no effect on chewing activity.

The results demonstrate a weak but significant negative relationship between milk yield and chewing index. When milk yield was expressed as the absolute difference (x) from the mean milk yield in each trial, the following regression equation was obtained:

$$y = 100.0 - 0.32 * x \text{, where y is the CI (in \%)} \hspace{2cm} \text{(Eq. 3.1)}$$

Since feed intake capacity is related to LW, the correction of CI for LW probably implies some correction for differences in feed intake capacity. Nevertheless, a highly significant negative effect of feed intake on the corrected ($LW^{0.3}$) chewing indices was obtained. EI, RI and CI were depressed by 0.5, 0.4 and 0.5% per one per cent higher feed intake. Consequently, total chewing time per day increased 0.5% for each increase of feed intake by one per cent. The negative relationship between chewing indices and feed intake is confirmed by Coulon, Doreau, Rémond and Journet (1987), Deswysen, Ellis and Pond (1987), Deswysen and Ellis (1990) and Dado and Allen (1994).

From the results of cows (n=76), which were involved in several chewing experiments, it appeared that 0.31, 0.50 and 0.46 of the total variance in EI, RI and CI was due to differences between cows.

CRITICAL ROUGHAGE PART

To study the animal linked factors, R_{crit} and the independent variables were also expressed as a percentage of the mean of each trial. First the independent variables were considered within each of five age groups (1st, 2nd, 3rd, 4th and 5th+ lactation) with respectively 188, 126, 97, 53 and 46 cow observations.

For each age group, relative milk yield was positively correlated with the relative R_{crit}, whereas milk fat content was negatively correlated with R_{crit} in four of the five age groups. The effect of LW was not consistent and feed intake capacity seemed to have no effect.

Subsequently, the effects of milk yield, fat content, live weight and age were studied using a regression model with categorical (dummy) variables which enables detection of the fixed effects of variables (age). From this analysis it was concluded that live weight has no effect on physical structure requirements. Regression equations with milk yield and/or milk fat content were highly significant (P<0.001). This was the case irrespective of whether these variables were expressed as a percentage of, or as absolute differences from the average of each trial. As milk yield and fat content are negatively correlated, their regression coefficients were lower when both were considered in a multiple regression than when each was separately included in a single regression. When both parameters were taken into account, the R_{crit} was 1.2% higher per kg higher milk yield, and 0.7% lower per g/kg higher milk fat content. Considered separately, these effects were 1.5 and 1.1%, respectively.

After correcting for the effect of milk yield and milk fat content, the relative R_{crit} in the first 6 lactations were 103, 105, 99, 94, 83 and 79%. Differences were not significant between cows in the first three lactations, nor between the cows in the 5th and 6th lactations, whereas these two groups differed significantly from each other. Therefore, the first three lactations were considered as a reference group, cows in the 5th lactation and older as another group and the 4th lactation cows as a separate group. Compared with the reference group, R_{crit} in the 4th and 5th+ lactation was 9 and 20% lower, respectively. Considering the 5th lactation cows separately, the difference was 19%.

Three-hundred and forty-six R_{crit} values, from 67 cows, were used to study the effect of individual cows on physical structure requirements. 0.21 of the total variance in R_{crit} could be explained by differences between cows. This highly significant effect was lower than for chewing activity.

Feed-linked factors

GRASSLAND PRODUCTS

Growth stage

Three trials were carried out with prewilted grass silage, originating from grass that was cut at two different growth stages. Mean NDF content was 437 and 515 g/kg DM respectively, for the young and older growth stage. Consequently, EI, RI and CI (corrected to a LW of 600kg based on metabolic weight) were significantly higher for the latter. These indices averaged 23.0, 44.0 and 67.0 min/kg DM for the young growth stage vs. 26.9, 52.7 and 79.6 min/kg DM for the more advanced growth stage.

The relationships between chewing index and characteristics depending on growth stage, such as CF, NDF, ADF, OM digestibility and roughage intake, were studied using the results of 13 prewilted grass silages that were chopped to a nominal length of 24 mm. All these parameters were significantly (P < 0.05) related to the chewing index; CF content was the best predictor.

Regression analysis to estimate R_{crit} from parameters reflecting the growth stage, was carried out using the results of 12 rations, of which 10 used prewilted and 2 used direct-cut grass silage as the sole roughage. Here too, CF content was the best predictor, whereas the relationship between R_{crit} and CI was not significant (P = 0.16). The main regression equations to estimate CI and R_{crit} are given in Table 3.3. Figure 3.1 represents the relationship between CF content and R_{crit}.

Table 3.3 REGRESSION EQUATIONS TO ESTIMATE CHEWING INDEX AND CRITICAL ROUGHAGE PART OF GRASS SILAGE

Regression equation	P	R²	RSD
CI (min/kg DM) n = 13			
- 15.1 + 0.326 * CF [1]	0.000	0.86	3.6
- 18.7 + 0.188 * NDF [1]	0.001	0.64	5.7
9.7 + 0.197 * ADF [1]	0.014	0.44	7.1
230.1 - 2.13 * Dig.OM [2]	0.000	0.77	4.5
135.8 - 5.422 * Rint. [3]	0.001	0.68	5.4
R_{crit} (g/kg) n = 12			
406 - 0.79 * CF	0.03	0.40	20
342 - 0.29 * NDF	0.05	0.34	21
- 475 + 3.24 * Dig.OM	0.07	0.29	21
301 - 1.40 * CI	0.16	0.19	23

[1] CF, NDF, ADF in g/kg DM
[2] Dig.OM = *in vitro* organic matter digestibility in % (Tilley and Terry, 1963)
[3] Rint. = roughage intake in kg dry matter/day

The present results, as well as data from the literature (Castle, Gill and Watson, 1981; Dulphy and Michalet-Doreau, 1983; Nørgaard, 1985; Kaiser and Combs, 1989; Beauchemin, 1991; Kamatali, 1991; Sauvant, 1992; Dulphy *et al.*, 1993) clearly demonstrate an increased CI when grass is cut at a later growth stage.

Particle length

The effect of chopping grass at harvest versus long silage on chewing activity was investigated in five trials. In four trials the grass was either chopped at a nominal length of 24 mm or harvested with a self-loading wagon equipped with 16 knives, whereas in one trial, three lengths were compared, i.e. 3.5 mm, 24 mm and long material.

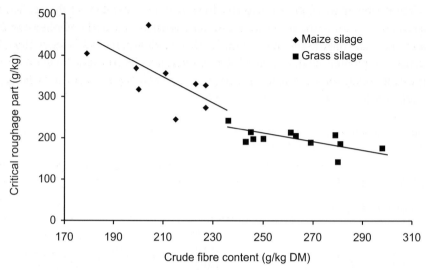

Figure 3.1 Relationship between crude fibre content and critical roughage part

The effect of particle length on chewing index is ambiguous. In three of the five trials CI significantly (P < 0.05) increased with increasing particle length, but in most trials fibre content tended to be higher in the longer silage. When chewing indices were corrected to equal CF contents, the differences became negligible, except for one trial. Corrected to the CF content of the long silages, EI, RI and CI averaged, for the five trials, 23.9 and 24.7, 47.3 and 49.6, and 71.1 and 74.3 min/kg DM, respectively for the 24 mm and the long silage. Compared with the large difference in measured particle length between treatments, the effect on CI was very small. Chewing time, expressed per kg NDF, increased by an average of only 0.1 min per mm increase in particle length.

In two trials the R_{crit} was compared for rations with either chopped or long prewilted grass silage from the same origin as the sole roughage. The nominal chopping length was 24 mm, whereas a self-loading wagon with 16 knives was used for the long material. Although CI was lower for the chopped silage in both trials, the R_{crit} was by no means higher for that silage. A third long silage was used in this research, whereas all other silages were chopped. The R_{crit} of all three long silages was situated around the regression line which represents the relationship between CF content and R_{crit}. This again indicates no effect of particle length of grass silage on structure value. One has to keep in mind that for grass silage, particle length is several centimetres.

Fine chopping (< 20 mm), which is rarely used in practice for grass silage , mostly resulted in a depressed EI and CI (Voskuil and Metz, 1973; Piatkowski, Nagel und Bergner, 1977; Castle, Retter and Watson, 1979; Deswysen, 1980; Dulphy, Michalet-Doreau and Demarquilly, 1984). However, it appears that beyond a certain limit, increasing particle length does not further stimulate chewing activity. According to the review of Beauchemin *et al.* (1994), that upper limit should be situated between 6.4 and 10 mm.

Clark and Armentano (1997) tend to conclude from their literature study that the critical particle length with regard to chewing activity, rumen pH and acetic acid:propionic acid ratio is situated between 4 and 8 mm. Lammers, Heinrichs and Buckmaster (1996) suggest a length of $\pm$ 2 cm as critical. Therefore it may be concluded that the structure value of normal grass silages in practice (> 20 mm) is independent of particle length.

Preservation method

In five trials, chewing indices of direct-cut and prewilted grass silages were compared. As expected, DM intake of the prewilted grass silages exceeded intake of the direct-cut silages by an average of 1.1 kg. The direct-cut silages were mainly characterised by a higher EI. On average for the five comparisons of direct-cut and prewilted grass silage, EI amounted to 31.1 and 23.6, RI to 49.0 and 46.2 and CI to 80.1 and 69.8 min/kg DM, respectively. The higher EI for direct-cut silage is supported by other researchers (Teller, Vanbelle, Kamatali and Wavreille, 1989; Teller, Vanbelle, Kamatali, Collignon, Page and Matatu, 1990). This is probably due to the higher volume of feed that has to be eaten, as well as to reduced palatability, which is a result of the stronger silage fermentation.

Two trials were carried out to compare direct-cut with prewilted grass silage; with regard to the R_{crit}, EI and CI were considerably higher for the direct-cut silages. The R_{crit} values for the diets with direct-cut silage and prewilted silage amounted to 214 and 191 g/kg in the first trial, and to 215 and 198 g/kg in the second one. Contrary to the EI and CI, R_{crit} does not demonstrate a higher structure value for direct-cut grass silage. Meyer, Bartley, Morrill and Stewart (1964) showed that during eating of fresh grass, saliva secretion per kg DM intake decreases with decreasing DM content; the same may be true for silage. Moreover, direct-cut silage has a lower pH and a higher acid content. Therefore direct-cut silage has a higher base buffer capacity than prewilted silage (Playne and McDonald, 1966). The reduced saliva secretion and the higher base buffer capacity could probably compensate for the higher CI.

Chewing activity was compared between grass hay and prewilted silage in two trials. CF content was higher for the hay, whereas the difference in NDF content seems to depend on DM content of silage. It appears that drying the grass to a high DM content or hay making considerably increases NDF content. EI was significantly higher for hay, whereas RI did not differ. After correction to the same CF content, CI was on average approximately 1.06 times higher for hay. Brouk and Belyea (1993) obtained both a higher RI and EI for alfalfa hay than for prewilted silage. Moreover, Meyer *et al.* (1964) observed a 1.2 times higher saliva secretion per kg DM during eating of alfalfa hay compared with alfalfa silage with 200 g/kg DM. In the first trial R_{crit} was considerably lower (157 vs. 186 g/kg) for the ration including hay instead of prewilted silage, whereas no difference was noted in the second trial. Obviously, a higher structure value can be attributed to hay than to silage.

Fresh grass

Thirteen samples of fresh grass, containing on average 432 g NDF and 230 g CF per kg DM, had a mean EI, RI and CI of 33.5, 37.3 and 70.8 min/kg DM. Eight and five chewing trials with respectively spring and autumn grass, each originating from two different years, were carried out. Although fibre content did not differ, chewing indices were markedly lower for the spring grass, i.e. EI: 31.1 vs. 37.4 , RI: 36.0 vs. 39.3, and CI: 67.1 vs. 76.7 min/kg DM. The differences could perhaps be explained by the higher digestibility, the lower milling resistance and the higher intake level of the spring grass.

R_{crit} was determined in two concurrent trials with spring grass and in one trial with autumn grass. Spring grass was supplemented with either Concentrate 1 or Concentrate 3 (Table 3.6), whereas autumn grass was supplemented only with Concentrate 1. The R_{crit} values were 310, 380 and 212 g/kg, respectively. The higher R_{crit} of the spring grass diets, although they contained more fibre, clearly indicate a lower structure value of spring grass. The difference between the two first trials illustrates the effect of concentrate composition (Table 3.7).

MAIZE SILAGE

Stage of maturity

The effect of the stage of maturity of whole crop maize on chewing activities was studied in three trials. Three stages were compared in the first trial, and two in each of the other two. As fibre content decreased with advancing stage of maturity, CI significantly decreased. On average for the three trials, maize silage harvested in the milk dough and the hard dough dent stage had a DM content of 271 and 353 g/kg and a NDF content of 395 and 372 g/kg DM, respectively. The mean chewing indices were 61.6 and 57.4 min/kg DM, respectively.

Regression analysis with 17 maize silages, chopped at a length of 8 mm, confirms the dependence of chewing activity on stage of maturity. The main relationships between CI and parameters reflecting stage of maturity are presented in Table 3.4. CI was best related to roughage intake level. Among the chemical parameters, CF seems to be the best predictor.

Relationships between R_{crit} and other parameters, were investigated using nine maize silages (Table 3.4, Figure 3.1). Here NDF seems to be a somewhat better predictor than CF, whereas CI was not significantly related to R_{crit}.

Chopping length

Five chewing trials were carried out to study the effect of chopping length of maize silage. Four trials were carried out to compare a nominal length of 4 and 8 mm; in one of

Table 3.4 REGRESSION EQUATIONS TO ESTIMATE CHEWING INDEX AND CRITICAL ROUGHAGE PART FOR MAIZE SILAGE

Regression equation		P	R^2	RSD
CI (min/kg DM)	n = 17			
4.7 + 0.272 * CF [1]		0.001	0.50	4.5
- 10.5 + 0.182 * NDF [1]		0.014	0.34	5.1
18.6 + 0.176 * ADF [1]		0.013	0.35	5.1
219.9 - 2.16 * Dig.OM [2]		0.001	0.57	4.3
127.4 - 4.789 * Rint. [3]		0.000	0.70	3.5
R_{crit} (g/kg)	n = 9			
844 - 2.38 * CF		0.11	0.32	58
783 - 1.09 * NDF		0.07	0.39	55
607 - 4.37 * CI		0.19	0.23	62

[1] CF, NDF, ADF in g/kg DM
[2] Dig.OM = in vitro organic matter digestibility in % (Tilley and Terry, 1963)
[3] Rint. = roughage intake in kg dry matter/day

these trials a 16 mm treatment was also used. In a fifth trial, 6.5 mm was compared with 8 mm. Chopping length had no effect on EI, except for the 16 mm treatment. In three of the four trials, chopping at 8 mm significantly increased RI compared with 4 mm. Mean CI for the 4 and 8 mm comparisons were 54.2 and 58.2 min/kg DM, respectively. Expressed per mm increase in particle length, chewing time per kg NDF was approximately 8 minutes longer, compared with only 0.1 minutes for prewilted grass silage. Chopping at 16 mm length also significantly increased CI compared with 8 mm. The comparison of 6.5 with 8 mm resulted in chewing indices of 63.9 and 66.7 min/ kg DM, which were not significantly different. The observed effect of the chopping length of maize on chewing activity agrees with other experiments (Rohr, Honig and Daenicke, 1983; Kuehn, Linn and Jung, 1997).

The maize silages of the trial with the 6.5 and 8 mm treatments were also used to compare R_{crit} values. The latter were 397 and 368 g/kg, respectively, indicating a higher structure value for the more coarsely chopped maize silage. Demarquilly (1994) also concluded that fine chopping of maize can reduce milk fat content. In contrast to grass silage, chopping length of maize affects its structure value, probably because particle size is smaller.

SUPPLEMENTS

The physical structure of fodder beets, raw potatoes, ensiled pressed sugar beet pulp and ensiled brewers grains was evaluated by determining the chewing indices and the critical roughage part in the ration. Two samples of brewers grains were tested – conventional brewers grains (A) and pressed brewers grains (B). The latter had a higher DM content (280 vs. 236 g/kg) and originated from ground malt, resulting in a smaller particle size. In the chewing trials, beet pulp was used as a supplement to either grass silage or maize silage A, and beets were supplemented to the same grass silage and maize silage B, each time in two ratios of 20:80 and 35:65 on DM basis. Potatoes and brewers grains A and B were used as supplements to maize silage C, C and D respectively in a fixed amount of 5 to 6 kg DM. In addition, cows received a restricted amount of concentrates. The chewing indices of the test feeds were derived by difference.

The critical roughage part was determined for rations including plus concentrates either the control roughage alone or the roughage and one of the supplements. Supplements were given in constant amounts of 4.9, 4.2, 4.0, 4.3 and 4.6 kg DM respectively for beet pulp, fodder beets, potatoes and brewers grains A and B.

Chewing indices derived for the experimental feeds are presented in Table 3.5. Data obtained by difference are mostly characterised by a great variation. The CIs of beet pulp and beets were hardly affected by the nature of the roughage or by the inclusion ratio, and amounted on average to 32.3 and 34.3 min/kg DM. The CI of potatoes, brewers grains A and B were 23.7, 56.6 and 40.7 min/kg DM, respectively.

Table 3.5 CHEWING INDICES (MIN/KG DM) OF THE SUPPLEMENTS – R_{CRIT} (G/KG)

Diet[1]	Chewing trials			Critical roughage part		
	R:S[2]	CI (SD)		Diet	R_{crit} (SD)	
GS+PBP	80:20	35.0	(18.9)	GS	206	(44)
	65:35	33.3	(9.3)	GS+PBP	102	(40)
				GS+FB	115	(43)
MS A+PBP	80:20	30.1	(12.1)			
	65:35	30.6	(8.4)	MS A	369	(63)
				MS A+PBP	229	(75)
GS+FB	80:20	32.4	(15.9)	MS A+FB	276	(96)
	65:35	40.0	(11.9)			
MS B+FB	80:20	29.8	(40.2)			
	65:35	35.0	(22.4)	MS C	473	(45)
				MS C+PO	385	(77)
MS C+PO	64:36	23.7	(7.5)	MS C+BG A	380	(38)
MS C+BG A	65:35	56.6	(17.5)			
				MS D	405	(78)
MS D+BG B	64:36	40.7	(14.6)	MS D+BG B	321	(85)

[1] GS = grass silage, MS = maize silage, PBP = ensiled pressed beet pulp, FB = fodder beet, PO = potatoes, BG = ensiled brewers grains,
[2] R:S = roughage:supplement

The critical grass silage part was 206 g/kg and decreased to 102 and 115 g/kg when fed in combination with beet pulp and beets, respectively. Also the critical maize silage part was markedly lower when these two supplements were added. In agreement with the chewing activity, the R_{crit} values also decreased by adding potatoes or brewers grains to the diet. Although the R_{crit} indicates a similar structure value for potatoes and brewers grains A, chewing indices were very different. In agreement with the findings of Vérité and Journet (1973), Rohr, Daenicke, Honig and Lebzien (1986), Dulphy *et al.* (1993) and Swain and Armentano (1994), these results clearly demonstrate that the supplements investigated here contain physical structure.

STRUCTURE CORRECTORS

Straw

Because straw is often used as a structure corrector in dairy rations, three chewing experiments were carried out, two with wheat and one with barley straw. The NDF and CF contents were 813 and 469 g per kg DM on average. Mean eating, ruminating and chewing indices were 72.5, 85.8 and 158.3 min/kg DM. Barley straw had higher NDF and CF contents as well as a higher CI. In one standard trial with wheat straw, a R_{crit} of 155 g/kg was obtained.

Dehydrated chopped alfalfa

The alfalfa used was chopped to a mean particle length of 11.8 mm and was pressed in big bales. NDF and CF contents were 524 and 367 g/kg DM. EI, RI and CI were 21.6, 29.4 and 51.0 min/kg DM, whereas a R_{crit} of 249 g/kg was found.

CONCENTRATES

Acidotic effect

Concentrates could, on the one hand, contribute to rumen buffering by the chewing activity they induce and by their intrinsic buffering capacity. On the other hand, rapid degradation of the carbohydrates can cause rumen acidosis. The structure value of concentrates will mainly depend on these two characteristics.

In a chewing trial with maize silage and dried sugar beet pulp, an EI, RI and CI of 7.7, 14.0 and 21.6 min/kg DM were derived for beet pulp. This illustrates how concentrate ingredients could even be ruminated. According to Mertens (1997), chewing index is mainly related to NDF content, particle size and physical form. CI of pelleted concentrates could be estimated by CI = 150 * 0.01 * 0.3 * NDF(%/DM) (Mertens, 1997). This equation assumes a chewing time of 150 minutes per kg NDF and a physical effectivity of 0.3 for pelleted concentrates.

The acidotic effect of three concentrates and nine ingredients was studied by *in sacco* and *in vitro* incubations (De Smet, De Boever, De Brabander, Vanacker and Boucqué, 1995). DM degradation was determined *in sacco* and pH decrease *in vitro*. Even though pH decrease is also influenced by the intrinsic buffering capacity, a close relationship between both parameters could still be expected. The ingredients were used to formulate three concentrates with different composition and rates of carbohydrate degradation (Table 3.6).

Table 3.6 COMPOSITION OF THE CONCENTRATES

Concentrate	1	2	3
Starch + sugar content	Low	High	High
DM Degradation rate	Low	Low	High
Main ingredients (g/kg)			
Beet pulp	357	-	-
Soya bean hulls	120	-	-
Maize	-	230	-
Sorghum	-	230	-
Barley	-	-	200
Wheat	-	-	170
Manioc	-	-	140
Soya bean meal	205	185	207
Maize gluten feed	140	207	120
Chemical composition (g/kg DM)			
Crude protein	194	203	192
NDF	291	137	143
Crude fibre	143	41	54
Starch	56	377	342
Sugars	100	68	78
DM degraded 3h (g/kg)	490	480	670

Two lactating Holstein cows, fitted with rumen cannulae, were used to determine the *in sacco* DM degradation of the feedstuffs. Sets of bags were incubated in the rumen for 0, 3, 6, 12, 24 and 48 hours. The *in vitro* pH decrease was determined using a rumen fluid / buffer solution (50/50 v/v). The buffer solution was prepared according to the method described by Tilley and Terry (1963).The rumen fluid was taken from the two previously mentioned fistulated cows. Figures 3.2 and 3.3 show the DM degradation and pH decrease, respectively. Based on the degradation after 3h incubation, ingredients

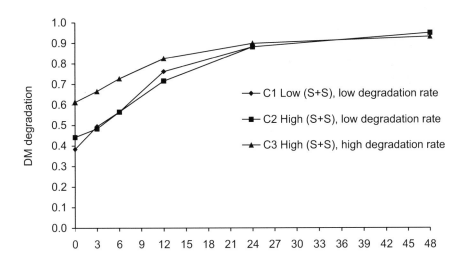

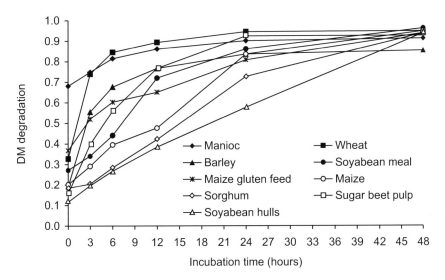

Figure 3.2 *In sacco* dry matter degradation of concentrates and ingredients

could be placed in order of decreasing DM degradation: manioc, wheat, barley, maize gluten feed, beet pulp, soya bean meal, maize, sorghum, soya bean hulls. After 5h *in vitro* incubation, ingredients were placed in order of declining pH decrease: manioc, wheat, beet pulp, maize gluten feed, barley, maize, soya bean meal, sorghum, soya bean hulls. The best correlation was obtained between DM degradation after 3 or 6h and *in vitro* pH decrease after 5h incubation. Between 3h degradation and 5h pH decrease (Figure 3.4) a correlation coefficient of 0.91 was found.

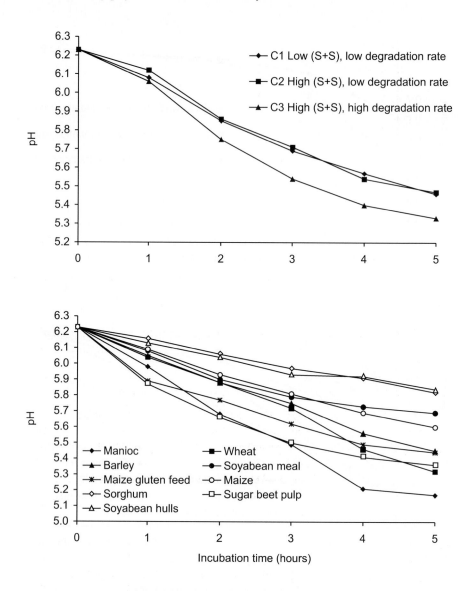

Figure 3.3 pH of *in vitro* incubated concentrates and ingredients

Critical roughage part – type of concentrate

The effect of the composition (starch + sugar: S+S) and the degradation rate of the compound feed on R_{crit} was investigated in five experiments with three different concentrates (Table 3.6). The R_{crit} values are shown in Table 3.7.

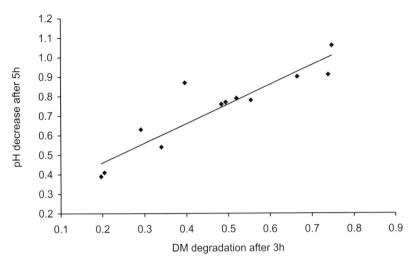

Figure 3.4 Relationship between *in sacco* DM degradation and *in vitro* pH decrease of concentrates and ingredients

Table 3.7 EFFECT OF CONCENTRATE COMPOSITION ON R_{CRIT}

Concentrate	1	2	3	
Starch + sugar content	Low	High	High	SD
Degradation rate	Low	Low	High	
Trial 1 - Maize silage	262 g DM/kg, 468 g NDF/kg DM, CI: 72.8 min/kg DM			
R_{crit} (g/kg)	305[a]	331[ab]	391[b]	68
Trial 2 - Pre-wilted grass silage	317 g DM/kg, 479 g NDF/kg DM, CI: 61.0 min/kg DM			
R_{crit} (g/kg)	204[a]	262[ab]	329[b]	64
Trial 3 - Maize silage 2 concentrate meals	334 g DM/kg, 406 g NDF/kg DM, CI: 59.0 min/kg DM			
R_{crit} (g/kg)	299		375*	58
Trial 4 - Maize silage 6 concentrate meals	see Trial 3			
R_{crit} (g/kg)	240		344*	92
Trial 5 - Fresh grass	198 g DM/kg, 460 g NDF/kg DM, CI: 70.8 min/kg DM			
R_{crit} (g/kg)	310		380[ns]	79

[a,b]: means on a same line with the same superscript letter are not significantly different (P>0.05)
* : significantly different (P≤0.05)
[ns] : not significantly different (P>0.05)

The trials were carried out with an average of eight cows per treatment. Concentrates were given twice daily, except in Trial 4. The R_{crit} was consistently lower when concentrates with a low (S+S)-content were used. However, due to high individual variation, differences were not always significant. The mean difference between the two extreme concentrates was 92 g/kg, corresponding to 29% of the average R_{crit}. Taking into account the fact that increasing the proportion of concentrates in a diet increases the ingestibility of the total diet, markedly more concentrate can be incorporated in the diet when the concentrate has a low (S+S)-content. In the present trials 3.9 kg more concentrate was given in the critical phase when C1 was given instead of C3. These results, as well as results from similar trials with fewer cows not discussed here, indicate that *in sacco* DM degradation after 3h and *in vitro* pH decrease after 5h incubation are closely related to the acidotic effect of concentrates.

Critical roughage part – Number of concentrate meals

It is well-documented that more frequent feeding of concentrates results in a more stable pH and fatty acid concentration in the rumen and consequently reduces the risk of critical values (Satter and Baumgardt, 1962; Bath and Rook, 1963; Kaufmann, 1976; Malestein, van 't Klooster, Counotte and Prins, 1981; Sutton, Hart, Broster, Elliott and Schuller, 1986; Robinson, 1989). The effect of 6 versus 2 concentrate meals per day on R_{crit} was investigated in three trials. Two trials are mentioned in Table 3.7 (Trials 3 and 4). A third trial was linked to Trial 2 in Table 3.7, where concentrate 3 was given in 2 and 6 meals per day, resulting in R_{crit} values of 329 and 299 g/kg, respectively. On average for the 3 trials the R_{crit} was 40 g/kg lower when the concentrates were given in 6 meals, corresponding to a higher concentrate intake of 1.8 kg in the critical phase.

Formation of a structure evaluation system

WHICH STANDARD?

The following parameters, related to physical structure, were investigated as potential standards in the structure system:
1.   chewing time, ruminating time + half the eating time
2.   NDF, effective NDF, crude fibre
3.   derived unit

For a standard to be perfect, its value in the critical phase of the present trials has to be the same independent of the ration type. This critical value, including a safety margin to allow for individual variation, could be considered as the minimum structure requirement. However, some variation in critical values is acceptable, as the R_{crit} values could not be determined precisely. The values of the parameters concerned in the critical phase were calculated for the 510 observations. The chewing indices of the concentrates were estimated according to the formula proposed by Mertens (1997), i.e. CI = 150 * 0.01 * peNDF with NDF expressed as % of DM and assuming a pe-factor of 0.3 for pellets. Besides CI, RI + 0.5 * EI was also considered, because there are reasons for reducing the weighting of eating index. A summary of the results is given in Table 3.8. The average critical chewing time for all the rations concerned was 26.5 min/kg DM with a standard deviation of 4.0 min.

Table 3.8 VALUE OF SOME PARAMETERS IN THE R_{CRIT} PHASE

		$n^{(1)}$	$CT^{(2)}$	RT+0.5ET	NDF	eNDF	CF
			(min/kg DM)			*(g/kg DM)*	
All rations	Mean	56	26.5	21.7	302	161	136
	SD		4.0	3.2	32	13	18
Grassland products[3]	Mean	21	24.1	19.6	295	160	130
	SD		2.7	1.9	218	13	17
Maize silage[4]	Mean	21	27.4	22.7	300	160	137
	SD		2.7	2.3	30	12	18
Individual trials							
Grass silage			22.3	18.4	301	154	130
Grass silage + PBP[5]			22.0	18.2	329	148	137
Grass silage + FB			22.4	18.0	249	129	107
Maize silage A			25.5	21.1	304	168	134
Maize silage A + PBP			25.8	21.4	325	159	145
Maize silage A + FB			26.7	21.6	261	153	116
Maize silage C			31.8	25.9	304	172	147
Maize silage C + PO			30.7	24.2	261	157	127
Maize silage C + BG A			37.4	30.8	354	169	155
Maize silage C + MCH A			34.6	28.2	295	171	141
Maize silage D			27.2	22.8	325	173	144
Maize silage D + BG B			30.7	25.2	372	168	144
Maize silage D + grass silage			25.9	21.5	33.7	176	140
Maize silage D + grass silage + MCH B			34.0	28.1	307	184	139
Straw			35.1	26.9	340	194	153

[1] n : number of rations
[2] : CT, RT, ET: chewing, ruminating, eating time
[3] : results of rations with a grassland product as the sole roughage
[4] : results of rations with maize silage as the sole roughage
[5] : PBP = pressed beet pulp, FB = fodder beet, PO = potatoes, BG = brewers grains, MCH = maize cobs + husks

For rations with a grassland product or maize silage, the critical chewing time was 24.1 and 27.4 min/kg DM, respectively. This parameter also varied considerably between rations with brewers grains, potatoes or maize cobs + husks. For the ration with straw, the critical chewing time was 35.1 min/kg DM. When only half the eating time was taken into account, similar results were found. The generally high SD, the difference between grassland products and maize silage and the difference between other types of diets, lead to the conclusion that chewing time is not an ideal standard for physical structure. This is supported by some data from the literature and other considerations. Beauchemin, Farr and Rode (1991) found structure deficiency when a ration with a CI of 36.8 min/kg DM was fed, whereas this was not the case with similar rations with a lower CI. The structure-deficient diets contained more barley. The rapidly degradable barley could have depressed microbial digestion in the rumen, which is probably compensated by a higher chewing activity. Grummer, Jacob and Woodford (1987), De Boever (1991) and Dulphy (1995) also obtained a higher CI as a result of compensation due to a high proportion of concentrates in the ration. We also found that certain animal-linked factors, such as live weight and feed intake level, influence chewing indices, but not R_{crit}. Moreover we could not demonstrate an individual relationship between chewing activity and physical structure requirements. In addition, the chewing index can only be considered as a measure of rumen buffering through saliva but does not take the acidotic effect and the intrinsic buffering capacity of the feed into account.

The R_{crit} of grass and maize silage was more closely related to NDF content than to CI (Tables 3.3 and 3.4). The critical NDF content amounted on average to 302 g/kg DM with a SD of 32 g, which is relatively low compared with the SD for critical CI. This is not surprising as the standard compound feed already contained 254 g NDF per kg DM. Therefore, this parameter is not sensitive enough to detect changes in the roughage:concentrate ratio. Moreover the minimum requirement should mainly depend on the NDF content of the concentrate. In the trials with three concentrates (Table 3.7), critical NDF contents amounted to an average of 311, 237 and 256 min/kg DM, respectively.

Both the chewing trials and the standard trials attribute a similar structure value to pressed beet pulp as to fodder beets. However, since beet pulp contains markedly more NDF, critical NDF content was also a lot higher for the rations with beet pulp. A similar observation was made for the rations containing brewers grains. On the other hand, the structure value of beets and potatoes based on NDF content would be considerably underestimated. The high variation in critical NDF content between different rations, as well as the dependence of it on the NDF content of the concentrate lead to the conclusion that NDF is also not a suitable parameter for physical structure. Data from the literature support this conclusion. This is not surprising because NDF content does not take particle size and physical form of feedstuffs into account, nor the acidotic effect of ingredients. The different chewing times per kg NDF also make NDF doubtful as a suitable structure index (Kaiser and Combs, 1989; Beauchemin and Buchanan-Smith, 1990; Beauchemin, 1991; Beauchemin *et al.*, 1991; Beauchemin and Iwaasa, 1993; Okine, Khorasani and Kennelly, 1994). Due to other influences on structure value, NDF has recently been replaced by effective NDF. This necessitates the attribution of an effectivity coefficient to the NDF of feedstuffs (Sniffen *et al.*, 1992; Armentano and Pereira, 1997; Mertens, 1997). For a lot of feedstuffs these coefficients are missing or are estimated through extrapolation. Table 8 again demonstrates great differences in critical eNDF content between certain types of rations. Although an effectivity coefficient of 1.0 was attributed to fodder beet and potatoes, the critical eNDF contents of the ration with those feeds were clearly lower than the mean value. Furthermore, the two experimental compound feeds with a high starch + sugar content clearly affect R_{crit} in a different way, despite similar eNDF content (49 and 47 g/kg DM). Hence there are few reasons to use eNDF as a standard in a structure evaluation system.

From the critical crude fibre contents, it can also be concluded that CF is not suitable as a general standard for physical structure. This explains why in the past, strongly diverging standards, ranging from 100 to 220 g CF/kg DM were proposed.

Considering the above, a structure evaluation system with a derived unit was chosen. Primarily, this system is based on the obtained R_{crit} results, but chewing indices, NDF and eNDF contents are also taken into account for several feedstuffs.

PRINCIPLE FOR DERIVING THE STRUCTURE VALUES (SV)

With a derived unit, it does not matter what the unit is. The feeding values simply have to correspond to the requirements. For practical reasons, the minimum structure requirements of a standard cow is assumed equal to 1. A standard cow is presumed to be a cow in 1st, 2nd or 3rd lactation, producing 25 kg milk daily with a fat content of 44 g/kg and receiving concentrates in two meals a day.

It was postulated that in the critical phase of the experiments the minimum requirement was met precisely. Then, roughage, concentrates and eventually supplements provided just enough structure.

Principle: $(R_{crit}/1000 * SV_R) + (C_{crit}/1000 * SV_C) = 1$ R_{crit} in g/kg

When a supplement was also fed, a third term was added i.e. $S_{crit} * SV_S$, with S_{crit} being the proportion of the supplement in the critical phase and SV_S the structure value of the supplement. The critical R-, C- and S-proportions were determined individually in the experiments. If for the rations with only a roughage and a concentrate, the SV of the concentrate is known, the SV of the roughage can be derived from the equation. For that purpose, the concentrate poorest in structure, the one with the high (S+S) content and rapidly degradable, Concentrate 3 (Table 3.6), was attributed a SV of 0.05 per kg DM. Once the SV of the roughage was known, the SVs of the other two experimental concentrates, which were given in combination with the same roughage (Table 3.7), could be deduced. Following this procedure, the SV of Concentrate 1 was derived five times and the SV of Concentrate 2 twice. If a higher or lower SV was attributed to Concentrate 3, only a small effect on SV of the concentrates and roughages was noticed.

Consequently, the SV of 0.05 for concentrate 3 was maintained. From the SV of the 3 concentrates, the SV of the ingredients were estimated. This was based on the buffering effect of the concentrates and ingredients on the one hand and on their acidotic effect on the other hand. The rumen buffering from saliva secretion during mastication was estimated from NDF content according to the system proposed by Mertens (1997). The acidotic effect was mainly based on the determined *in vitro* pH decrease after 5h incubation. Once the SVs of the ingredients had been estimated, the SV of the standard concentrate, which was used in most trials, could be calculated. Finally, the SVs of the roughages and supplements were derived by means of the equation mentioned above.

SAFETY MARGIN

Because of the great individual variation in structure requirements, and the variation in structure value among samples of the same forage type, a large safety margin has to be built in to minimise the risks for cows fed at the limit (according to the system). However, a larger safety margin lowers the tolerable concentrate proportion in the ration, which could jeopardise the energy supply of high yielding cows. As a compromise, a risk of 5% was chosen. In principle, this implies that, when the system is applied strictly, 5% of the cows fed at the limit would show physical structure deficiency. Based on individual variation and variation among samples of forages, the safety margin could be based on a standard deviation of 25% of the R_{crit}. At a risk of 5%, the R_{crit} have to be increased by $1.65 * 25\% = 41\%$. Statistically, 5% of the R_{crit} exceed the value given by the average $+ 1.65*SD$. This safety margin would increase the physical structure requirements by 0.3. Because a requirement for a standard cow equal to 1 was preferred, the SVs were divided by 1.3.

STRUCTURE VALUES

Roughages and supplements

The derived structure values, shown in Table 3.9, are the so-called "safe" structure values. The SV of grassland products and maize silage are mainly based on the R_{crit} values, although the chewing indices were taken into account to adjust the intercept and regression coefficients somewhat, when desirable. CF and NDF contents seem to be the best predictors of SV. The SV of maize silage can also be estimated with the same precision from starch content. Chewing index was a poor predictor of SV. From the R_{crit} values, no difference appeared between direct-cut and prewilted grass silage, nor between normal chopped and longer grass silage. The same regression equations can be used for hay as for silage. If the CF formula is used, the SV obtained has to be increased by 0.06. This correction is not necessary when the SV of hay is calculated from NDF, because

Table 3.9 STRUCTURE VALUES (PER KG DM) OF CURRENTLY USED FEEDSTUFFS

1. Grassland products
   Grass silage

$SV = +0.15 + 0.0060 * NDF^{(1)}$	$(R^2 = 0.26; RSD = 0.40)$
$SV = -0.20 + 0.0125 * CF$	$(R^2 = 0.40; RSD = 0.35)$

   Direct cut grass silage = pre-wilted grass silage
   Chopped silage = longer silage
   Hay
   NDF equation for grass silage without correction
   CF equation for grass silage * 1.06

2. Maize silage   chopping length 6 mm

$SV = -0.57 + 0.0060 * NDF$	$(R^2 = 0.33; RSD = 0.25)$
$SV = -0.10 + 0.0090 * CF$	$(R^2 = 0.26; RSD = 0.26)$

   Correction for deviating chopping length: +(-) 2% / +(-) 1 mm length

3. Straw
   $SV = 4.30$

4. Supplements

	SV
Ensiled pressed beet pulp	1.05
Fodder beet	1.05
Ensiled brewers grains	1.00
Ensiled pressed brewers grains	0.85
Raw potatoes	0.70

5. Concentrates and ingredients
   Ground ingredients incorporated in pelleted concentrates

   $$SV = 0.175 + 0.00082 * NDF + 0.00047 * USt.^{(2)} - 0.00100 * (SU + a*DSt.)$$
   $$(R^2 = 0.97; RSD = 0.04)$$
   $$SV = 0.321 + 0.00098 * CF + 0.00025 * USt. - 0.00112 * (SU + a * DSt.)$$
   $$(R^2 = 0.91; RSD = 0.07)$$

   $a = 0.90 - 1.3 *$ starch resistance

   [1]Contents in g/kg DM
   [2]USt. = undegradable starch, DSt. = degradable starch, SU = sugars

NDF content increases during the hay making process. At present, the number of trials with fresh grass is too small to propose structure values. Six trials were carried out with fresh grass containing 205, 239, 249, 244, 231 and 257 g CF per kg DM. The derived SVs were 2.57 1.85, 1.96, 2.94, 2.41 and 3.45 respectively. The CF regression equation for grass silage estimates a SV of 2.36, 2.79, 2.88, 2.85, 2.69 and 3.01 per kg DM, respectively. Why the SVs of Trials 2 and 3, both originating from the same spring grass 1994, were markedly overestimates is unclear.

The regression equations to estimate the SV of maize silage are valid for a theoretical chopping length of 6 mm. A correction of 2% per mm deviation in chopping length is proposed.

From the R_{crit} values of 3 trials with wheat straw, and taking into account chewing index and eNDF contents, a SV of 4.30 per kg DM was derived. Although the barley straw used in the trials had a higher NDF content, a higher milling resistance and a higher chewing index than wheat straw, it is not justified to make a distinction between barley and wheat straw, since only one sample of barley straw was used. Fodder beets and ensiled pressed sugar beet pulp were studied extensively. Although NDF contents differed markedly, both chewing indices and R_{crit} values demonstrate similar SVs for the two supplements. Two recent trials with pressed beet pulp confirm the SV of 1.05. For pressed brewers grains, with its smaller particle size than conventional brewers grains, a SV of 0.85 could be derived, compared with 1.00 for conventional brewers grains. The R_{crit} as well as chewing index of rations containing raw potatoes demonstrated a SV of approximately 0.70 per kg DM.

Concentrates and ingredients

According to the principle already described, the SV of the concentrates used and their ingredients were derived. Subsequently, a method was sought to estimate the SV of these feedstuffs on the basis of known or currently determined parameters. The latter were chosen for logical reasons. They imply characteristics which are related to the rumen buffering capacity on the one hand and to the rumen acidotic effect on the other hand. NDF or CF content, as well as undegradable starch content, were considered as rumen stabilising factors, whereas sugars and degradable starch were considered as acidifying factors in the rumen. As sugar content was low and less variable, sugar and degradable starch content were considered as one term. Since the acidifying effect of degradable starch is lower compared with sugars, the first was only partially taken into account. This fraction "a" can be considered as the sugar equivalent of the degradable starch in terms of affecting rumen acidosis. It is logical to assume that this acidifying effect "a" is not a fixed value but depends on the degradation rate, which is related to the solubility of the degradable starch. From solubility results published by Tamminga, van Vuuren, van der Koelen, Ketelaar and van der Togt (1990), Nocek and Tamminga (1991) and Sauvant, Chapoutot and Archimède (1994), we derived the solubility of the degradable starch fraction. For manioc, wheat, barley, maize gluten feed, sorghum and maize, mean solubilities were 0.75, 0.73, 0.62, 0.65, 0.42 and 0.40, respectively. These solubility coefficients could be considered as the sugar equivalent (a) of the degradable starch. However, this parameter is not reported in current feed tables. Expecting an inverse relationship between the solubility of degradable starch and starch resistance to rumen degradation, a relationship between both parameters was sought. Based on the data from Tamminga *et al.* (1990), Nocek and Tamminga (1991), Sauvant *et al.* (1994)

and the Dutch feed tables (Centraal Veevoederbureau, 1998), as well as on a database of 56 concentrates from this Institute, the following relationship, valid for pelleted concentrates, could be derived: a = 0.90 – 1.3 * starch resistance. Regression analysis using the calculated SV of 13 ingredients and concentrates from the present experiments, resulted in the equations shown in Table 3.9. The formulae are valid for ground ingredients (6 mm) which are incorporated into pelleted concentrates. Recent experiments demonstrated that grinding, as well as pelleting, depresses SV. Based on one trial, a SV of 7.0 was attributed to sodium bicarbonate.

Example: maize grain NDF: 139 g, St.: 676 g, SU: 12 g, starch resistance: 0.42
    USt. = 676 g * 0.42 = 284 g, DSt. = 676 g * 0.58 = 392 g
    a = 0.90 – 1.3 * 0.42 = 0.35
    SV = 0.175 + 0.00082 * 139 + 0.00047 * 284 – 0.00100 * (12 + 0.35 * 392)
        = 0.27 /kg DM

The relationship between estimated and the derived SV of the ingredients and concentrates is presented in Figure 3.5.

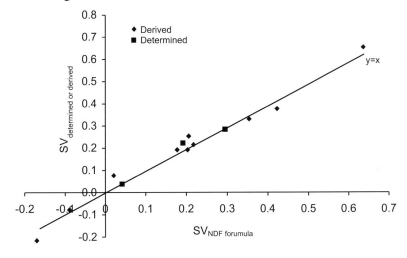

Figure 3.5 Relationship between estimated (NDF formula) and determined or derived structure value of concentrates and ingredients

STRUCTURE REQUIREMENTS

In the system it is assumed that the structure value of the diet has to be at least 1 per kg DM for a standard cow (25 kg milk, 44 g/kg fat, 1st, 2nd, 3rd lactation), when concentrates are provided in two meals (Table 3.10). For other situations, the following corrections have to be applied. Under circumstances similar to the present experiments, a correction to the R_{crit} of 1%, modified the structure requirements by 0.8%.

Table 3.10 STRUCTURE REQUIREMENTS

$$SV_{ration} \geq 1 \text{ per kg DM}$$

Cow 25 kg milk; 44 g/kg fat; 1st, 2nd, 3rd lactation; two concentrate meals

Corrections for
1) - Milk yield and fat content
   +(-) 0.01 / kg milk higher (lower) than 25 kg
   +(-) 0.005 / g fat lower (higher) than 44 g/kg
   - Only milk yield
   +(-) 0.012 / kg milk higher (lower) than 25 kg

2) Age
   4th lactation: -0.07
   $\geq 5^{th}$ lactation: -0.15

3) Frequent concentrate feeding (at least 6 meals): -0.10

Milk yield and fat content

Cows with a higher daily milk yield and/or a lower fat content need a ration with a higher structure value. The effect of both parameters on R_{crit} resulted in an increase (decrease) of the SV requirement by 0.01 per kg higher (lower) milk yield, and by 0.005 per g/kg lower (higher) fat content. If a correction is made for milk yield alone, the requirement has to be increased (decreased) by 0.012 per kg higher (lower) milk yield.

Age (number of lactations)

From the experimental data it could be concluded that the R_{crit} for cows in their 4th or 5th lactation is 9 or 19% lower respectively than for cows in the 1st, 2nd or 3rd lactation. This corresponds with a decrease in structure requirement of 0.07 and 0.15.

Frequent concentrate feeding

Three trials were carried out to study the effect of frequent feeding of concentrates on structure requirements. Six concentrate meals per day resulted in structure requirements of 0.91, 0.92 and 0.88 compared with 1 when the concentrates were given in 2 meals. Hence, the structure requirements with at least 6 meals are assumed to be 0.10 lower.

APPLICATION OF THE SYSTEM

The structure evaluation system allows calculation of the minimum roughage portion in the ration necessary to maintain normal rumen function.

Example: a cow in the 4th lactation producing 35 kg milk with 38 g fat/kg receives concentrates with a SV of 0.20/kg DM in two meals, and roughage consisting of 30% pre-wilted grass silage and 70% maize silage (6 mm chopping length) containing respectively 460 and 380 g NDF per kg DM.

Structure requirement: $1 - 0.07 + (35 - 25) * 0.01 - (38 - 44) * 0.05 = 1.06$
$SV_{pre\text{-}wilted\ grass\ silage}$ $: +0.15 + 0.0060 * 460 = 2.91$
$SV_{maize\ silage}$ $: -0.57 + 0.0060 * 380 = 1.71$
$SV_{roughage}$ $: (2.91 * 0.30) + (1.71 * 0.70) = 2.07$
$(R_{crit}/1000 * SV_R) + (C_{crit}/1000 * SV_C) = 1.06$
$R_{crit}/1000 = x$ $C_{crit}/1000 = 1\text{-}x$
$x * 2.07 + (1\text{-}x) * 0.20 = 1.06$
$x * (2.07 - 0.20) = 1.06 - 0.20$
$x = 0.86/1.87 = 0.46$

The roughage proportion in the diet has to be at least 0.46.

If the concentrates are fed in at least 6 meals per day:

Structure requirements: $1.06 - 0.10 = 0.96$
$x * 2.07 + (1 - x) * 0.20 = 0.96$
$x * (2.07 - 0.20) = 0.96 - 0.20$
$x = 0.76/1.87 = 0.41$

When concentrates are spread, a roughage proportion of 0.41 is sufficient.

Acknowledgements

The authors wish to thank A. Opstal and all the personnel of the Department for their excellent technical assistance. The Institute for the Encouragement of Scientific Research in Industry and Agriculture is gratefully acknowledged for funding this research.

References

Armentano, L. and Pereira, M. (1997) Measuring the effectiveness of fiber by animal response trials. *Journal of Dairy Science*, **80**, 1416-1425.

Bae, D.H., Welch, J.G. and Gilman, B.E. (1983) Mastication and rumination in relation to body size of cattle. *Journal of Dairy Science*, **66**, 2137-2141.

Balch, C.C. (1971) Proposal to use time spent chewing as an index to the extent to which diets for ruminants possess the physical property of fibrousness characteristic of roughages. *British Journal of Nutrition*, **26**, 383-392.

Bath, I.H. and Rook, J.A.F. (1963) The evaluation of cattle foods and diets in terms of the ruminal concentration of volatile fatty acids. *Journal of Agricultural Science*, **61**, 341-348.

Beauchemin, K.A. (1991) Effects of dietary neutral detergent fiber concentration and alfalfa hay quality on chewing, rumen function, and milk production of dairy cows. *Journal of Dairy Science*, **74**, 3140-3151.

Beauchemin, K.A. and Buchanan-Smith, J.G. (1990) Effects of fiber source and method of feeding on chewing activities, digestive function, and productivity of dairy cows. *Journal of Dairy Science,* **73**, 749-762.

Beauchemin, K.A., Farr, B.I. and Rode, L.M. (1991) Enhancement of the effective fiber content of barley-based concentrates fed to dairy cows. *Journal of Dairy Science*, **74**, 3128-3139.

Beauchemin, K.A., Farr, B.I., Rode, L.M. and Schaalje, G.B. (1994) Effects of alfalfa silage chop length and supplementary long hay on chewing and milk production of dairy cows. *Journal of Dairy Science*, **77**, 1326-1339.

Beauchemin, K.A. and Iwaasa, A.D. (1993) Eating and ruminating activities of cattle fed alfalfa or orchard-grass harvested at two stages of maturity. *Canadian Journal of Animal Science*, **73**, 79-88.

Beauchemin, K.A. and Rode, L.M. (1994) Compressed baled alfalfa hay for primiparous and multiparous dairy cows. *Journal of Dairy Science*, **77**, 1003-1012.

Beauchemin, K.A. and Rode, L.M. (1997) Minimum versus optimum concentrations of fiber in dairy cow diets based on barley silage and concentrates of barley or corn. *Journal of Dairy Science*, **80**, 1629-1639.

Brouk, M. and Belyea, R. (1993) Chewing activity and digestive responses of cows fed alfalfa forages. *Journal of Dairy Science*, **76**, 175-182.

Castle, M.E., Gill, M.S. and Watson, J.N. (1981) Silage and milk production: a comparison between grass silages of different chop lengths and digestibilities. *Grass and Forage Science*, **36**, 31-37.

Castle, M.E., Retter, W.C. and Watson, J.N. (1979) Silage and milk production: comparisons between grass silage of three different chop lengths. *Grass and Forage Science*, **34**, 293-301.

Centraal Veevoederbureau - Nederland (1998) *Veevoedertabel 1998 - Chemische samenstelling, verteerbaarheid en voederwaarde van voedermiddelen.* Editor Centraal Veevoederbureau, 8203 AD Lelystad, The Netherlands.

Clark, P.W. and Armentano, L.E. (1997) Influence of particle size on the effectiveness of beet pulp fiber. *Journal of Dairy Science*, **80**, 898-904.

Coulon, J.B., Doreau, M., Rémond, B. andJournet, M. (1987) Evolution des activités alimentaires des vaches laitières en début de lactation et liaison avec les quantités d'aliments ingérées. *Reproduction, Nutrition et Développement*, **27**, 67-75.

Dado, R.G. and Allen, M.S. (1994) Variation in and relationship among feeding, chewing, and drinking variables for lactating dairy cows. *Journal of Dairy Science*, **77**, 132-144.

De Boever, J. (1991) Roughage evaluation of maize and grass silage based on chewing activity measurements with cows. Ph. D. Diss., Univ. Ghent, Belgium, 171 pp.

De Boever, J.L., De Smet, A., De Brabander, D.L. and Boucqué, Ch.V. (1993) Evaluation of physical structure. 1. Grass silage. *Journal of Dairy Science*, **76**, 140-153.

Dehareng, D. and Godeau, J.M. (1991) The durations of masticating activities and the feed energetic utilisation of Friesian lactating cows on maize silage-based rations. *Journal of Animal Physiology and Animal Nutrition*, **65**, 194-205.

Demarquilly, C. (1994) Facteurs de variation de la valeur nutritive du maïs ensilage. *INRA Productions Animales*, **7**, 177-189.

De Smet, A.M., De Boever, J.L., De Brabander, D.L., Vanacker, J.M. and Boucqué, Ch.V. (1995) Investigation of dry matter degradation and acidotic effect of some feedstuffs by means of in sacco and in vitro incubations. *Animal Feed Science and Technology*, **51**, 297-315.

Deswysen, A. (1980) Influence de la longueur des brins et de la concentration en acides organiques des silages sur l'ingestion chez les ovins et bovins. Ph. D. Dissertation, Univ. Louvain-la-Neuve, Belgique, 254 pp.

Deswysen, A.G. and Ellis, W.C. (1990) Fragmentation and ruminal escape of particles as related to variations in voluntary intake, chewing behavior and extent of digestion of potentially digestible NDF in heifers. *Journal of Animal Science*, **68**, 3861-3879.

Deswysen, A.G., Ellis, W.C. and Pond, K.R. (1987) Interrelationships among voluntary intake, eating and ruminating behavior and ruminal motility of heifers fed corn silage. *Journal of Animal Science*, **64**, 835-841.

Dulphy, J.P. (1995) L'indice de fibrosité des aliments des ruminants. Intérêt et utilisation. Personal communication.

Dulphy, J.P. and Michalet-Doreau, B. (1983) Comportement alimentaire et mérycique d'ovins et de bovins recevant des fourrages verts. *Annales de Zootechnie*, **32**, 465-474.

Dulphy, J.P., Michalet-Doreau, B. and Demarquilly, C. (1984) Etude comparée des quantités ingérées et du comportement alimentaire et mérycique d'ovins et de bovins recevant des ensilages d'herbe réalisés selon différentes techniques. *Annales de Zootechnie*, **33**, 291-320.

Dulphy, J.P., Rouel, J., Jailler, M. and Sauvant, D. (1993) Données complémentaires sur les durées de mastication chez des vaches laitières recevant des rations riches en fourrage: influence de la nature du fourrage et du niveau d'apport d'aliment concentré. *INRA Productions Animales*, **6**, 297-302.

Grummer, R.R., Jacob, A.L. and Woodford, J.A. (1987) Factors associated with variation in milk fat depression resulting from high grain diets fed to dairy cows. *Journal of Dairy Science*, **70**, 613-619.

Flatt, W.P., Moe, P.W., Munson, A.W. and Cooper, T. (1969) Energy utilization by dairy Holstein cows. In Energy metabolism of farm animals. Publication n° 12 Symposium European Association of Animal Production - sept. 1969, Warsaw, 235-251. Edited by K.L. Blaxter, J. Kielanowski and G. Thorbek.

Guth, N. (1995) Unterschiedliche Häckselgutstruktur von Halmfutter: Einfluß auf Futteraufnahme, Leistung und Kauverhalten von Rindern, Silagequalität und Häckselleistungsbedarf sowie bildanalytische Vermessung der Futterstruktur. Dissertation, Editor Rosa Fischer - Löw Verlag, Gieben, 305 pp.

Hoffmann, M. (1983) Tierfütterung. *VEB Deutscher Landwirtschaftsverlag*, DDR-Berlin.

Kaiser, R.M. and Combs, D.K. (1989) Utilization of three maturities of alfalfa by dairy cows fed rations that contain similar concentrations of fiber. *Journal of Dairy Science*, **72**, 2301-2307.

Kamatali, P. (1991) L'ingestion volontaire d'ensilages d'herbe, l'efficience digestive et le comportement alimentaire et mérycique chez les bovins. Doctoral thesis, Louvain-la-Neuve, Belgium, 297 pp.

Kaufmann, W. (1976) Influence of the composition of the ration and the feeding frequency on pH-regulation in the rumen and the feed intake in ruminants. *Livestock Production Science*, **3**, 103-114.

Kesler, E.M. and Spahr, S.L. (1964) Physiological effects of high level concentrate feeding. *Journal of Dairy Science*, **47**, 1122-1128.

Kuehn, C.S., Linn, J.G. and Jung, H.G. (1997) Effect of corn silage chop length on intake, milk production, and milk composition of lactating dairy cows. *Journal of Dairy Science*, **80**, (Suppl. 1), 219 (Abstr.).

Lammers, B., Heinrichs, J. and Buckmaster, D. (1996) Method helps in determination of forage, TMR particle size requirements for cattle. *Feedstuffs*, September 30, 14-16.

Malestein, A., van't Klooster, A.Th., Counotte, G.H.M. and Prins, R.A. (1981) Concentrate feeding and ruminal fermentation. 1. Influence of the frequency of feeding concentrates on rumen acid composition, feed intake and milk production. *Netherlands Journal of Agricultural Science*, **29**, 239-248.

Mertens, D.R. (1997) Creating a system for meeting the fiber requirements of dairy cows. *Journal of Dairy Science*, **80**, 1463-1481.

Meyer, R.M., Bartley, E.E., Morrill, J.L. and Stewart, W.E. (1964) Salivation in cattle. I. Feed and animal factors affecting salivation and its relation to bloat. *Journal of Dairy Science*, **47**, 1339-1345.

Nocek, J.E. and Tamminga, S. (1991) Site of digestion of starch in the gastrointestinal tract of dairy cows and its effect on milk yield and composition. *Journal of Dairy Science*, **74**, 3598-3629.

Nørgaard, P. (1985) Physical structure of feeds for dairy cows. (A new system for evaluation of the physical structure in feedstuffs and rations for dairy cows). *CEC-workshop. New developments and future perspectives in research on rumen function*, 25-27 June, Ørum Sønderlyng, Denmark.

Nørgaard, P. (1989) The influence of physical form of ration on chewing activity and rumen motility in lactating cows. *Acta Agriculturae Scandinavica*, **39**, 187-202.

Nørgaard, P. (1993) The effect of carbohydrate composition and physical form of feed on chewing activity and rumen motility in dairy cows. *44ᵗʰ Annual Meeting of the European Association for Animal Production*, Aarhus, Denmark 16-19 August, CN 2.2.

NRC (1978) *Nutrient requirements of dairy cattle*. Fifth Revised Edition. National Academy of Sciences, Washington, 76 pp.

NRC (1988) *Nutrient requirements of dairy cattle*. Sixth Revised Edition. National Academy Press, Washington, 158 pp.

Okine, E.K., Khorasani, G.R. and Kennelly, J.J. (1994) Effects of cereal grain silages versus alfalfa silage on chewing activity and reticular motility in early lactation cows. *Journal of Dairy Science*, **77**, 1315-1325.

Piatkowski, B., Nagel, S. and Bergner, E. (1977) Das Wiederkauverhalten von Kühen bei unterschiedlicher Trockensubstanzaufnahme und verschiedener physikalischer Form von Grasheu. *Archiv für Tierernährung*, **27**, 563-569.

Playne, M.J. and McDonald, P. (1966) The buffering constituents of herbage and of silage. *Journal of the Science of Food and Agriculture*, **17**, 264-268.

Rémond, B. and Journet, M. (1972) Alimentation des vaches laitières avec des rations à forte proportion d'aliments concentrés. *Annales de Zootechnie*, **21**, 191-205.

Robinson, P.H. (1989) Dynamic aspects of feeding management for dairy cows. *Journal of Dairy Science*, **72**, 1197-1209.

Rohr, K., Honig, H. and Daenicke, R. (1983) Zur Bedeutung des Zerkleinerungs-grades von Silomaïs. 2. Mitteilung: Einflub des Zerkleinerungsgrades auf Wieder-kauaktivität, Pansenfermentation und Verdaulichkeit der Rohnährstoffe. *Das Wirtschaftseigene Futter*, **29**, 73-86.

Rohr, K., Daenicke, R., Honig, H. and Lebzien, P. (1986) Zum Einsatz von Prebschnitzelsilage in der Milchviehfütterung. *Landbauforschung Völkenrode*, **36**, 50-55.

Satter, L.D. and Baumgardt, B.R. (1962) Changes in digestive physiology of the bovine associated with various feeding frequences. *Journal of Animal Science*, **21**, 897-900.

Sauvant, D. (1992) Compléments sur la fibrosité des rations des ruminants. *Journées CAAA-AFTAA*, Tours, 26-27/02/1992.

Sauvant, D., Chapoutot, P. and Archimède, H. (1994) La digestion des amidons par les ruminants et ses conséquences. *INRA Productions Animales*, **7**, 115-124.

Sniffen, C.J., Hooper, A.P., Welch, J.G., Randy, H.A. and Thomas, E.V. (1986) Effect of hay particle size on chewing behavior and rumen mat consistency in steers. *Journal of Dairy Science*, **69**, 135 (Suppl. 1).

Sniffen, C.J., O'Connor, J.D., Van Soest, P.J., Fox, D.G. and Russell, J.B. 1992. A net carbohydrate and protein system for evaluating cattle diets: II. Carbohydrate and protein availability. *Journal of Animal Science*, **70**, 3562-3577.

Sudweeks, E.M., Ely, L.O., Mertens, D.R. and Sisk, L.R. (1981) Assessing minimum amounts and form of roughages in ruminant diets: roughage value index system.

Journal of Animal Science, **53**, 1406-1411.

Sutton, J.D. (1984) Feeding and milk fat production. In Milk compositional quality and its importance in future markets. Occasional publication No.9 of the *British Society of Animal Production* - 1984, pp. 43-52. Edited by M.E. Castle and R.G. Gunn.

Sutton, J.D., Hart, I.C., Broster, W.H., Elliott, R.J. and Schuller, E. (1986) Feeding frequency for lactating cows: effects on rumen fermentation and blood metabolites and hormones. *British Journal of Nutrition*, **56**, 181-192.

Swain, S.M. and Armentano, L.E. (1994) Quantitative evaluation of fiber from nonforage sources used to replace alfalfa silage. *Journal of Dairy Science*, **77**, 2318-2331.

Tamminga, S., van Vuuren, A.M., van der Koelen, C.J., Ketelaar, R.S. and van der Togt, P.L. (1990) Ruminal behaviour of structural carbohydrates, non-structural carbohydrates and crude protein from concentrate ingredients in dairy cows. *Netherlands Journal of Agricultural Science*, **38**, 513-526.

Tilley, J.M.A. and Terry, R.A. (1963) A two-stage technique for the in vitro digestion of forage crops. *Journal of the British Grassland Society*, **18**, 104-111.

Teller, E., Vanbelle, M., Kamatali, P., Collignon, G., Page, B. and Matatu, B. (1990) Effects of chewing behavior and ruminal digestion processes on voluntary intake of grass silages by lactating dairy cows. *Journal of Animal Science*, **68**, 3897-3904.

Teller, E., Vanbelle, M., Kamatali, P. and Wavreille, J. (1989) Intake of direct cut or wilted grass silage as related to chewing behavior, ruminal characteristics and site and extent of digestion by heifers. *Journal of Animal Science*, **67**, 2802-2809.

Van Soest, P.J., Robertson, J.B. and Lewis, B.A. (1991) Methods for dietary fiber, neutral detergent fiber, and nonstarch polysaccharides in relation to animal nutrition. *Journal of Dairy Science*, **74**, 3583-3597.

Vérité, R. and Journet, M. (1973) Utilisation de quantités élevées de betteraves par les vaches laitières: étude de l'ingestion, de la digestion et des effets sur la production. *Annales de Zootechnie*, **22**, 219-235.

Voskuil, G.C.J. and Metz, J.H.M. (1973) The effect of chopped hay on feed intake, rate of eating and rumination of dairy cows. *Netherlands Journal of Agricultural Science*, **21**, 256-262.

Weiss, W.P. (1993) Fiber requirements of dairy cattle: emphasis NDF. *54th Minnesota Nutrition Conference & National Renderers Technical Symposium*, September 20-22, Bloomington, Minnesota.

Welch, J.G. (1982) Rumination, particle size and passage from the rumen. *Journal of Animal Science*, **54**, 885-894.

This paper was first published in 1999

4

PARTICLE SIZE IN DAIRY RATIONS

D.R. BUCKMASTER
Department of Agricultural and Biological Engineering, The Pennsylvania State University, University Park, PA 16802, USA

Introduction

As production per animal continues to increase, the role of proper particle size in dairy rations seems to become more important. Smaller particles are desired because of their much larger surface area which leads to more rapid digestion and a consequential increased rate of passage. Too many small particles, however, leads to poor pH control in the rumen and besides digestion disorders, can become a serious health problem. While requirements for protein, energy, vitamins and minerals can be identified as functions of animal characteristics and performance, the particle size issue is confounded by the interaction between particle size and chemical fibre. Furthermore, even an effective fibre "requirement" which accounts for the interaction between physical and chemical traits may be elusive because the requirement, in part, depends upon the diet. While the particle size distribution of the primary energy sources in a dairy ration are also important, this chapter focuses on that of the primary forage sources.

The objectives in this chapter are to:

- Discuss the measurement and reporting of particle size in forages and total mixed rations (TMR),
- Review some recommendations on particle size,
- Examine the effects of feed mixing on forage particle size, and
- Identify some areas for short-term future research.

Measurement of particle size in forage and TMR

There have been many methods proposed to measure the particle sizes of feedstuffs. A special conference on the subject was held in 1984 with proceedings generated (Kennedy,

1984). Methods fall into either dry or wet sieving techniques, with most variation among methods being the types of sieves used and the mechanics of separation. When the interest is in particle size distribution of particles which are approximately spherical, stacked two dimensional (mesh) sieves with sequentially smaller openings are adequate (Figure 4.1). When particles of elongated or odd shapes are to be evaluated, other means should be employed since these particles can move through openings much smaller than their largest, or even mean, dimension.

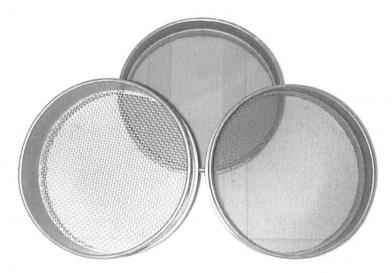

Figure 4.1 Mesh sieves useful for determining particle size distribution when particles are approximately spherical

Gale and O'Dougherty (1982) developed and evaluated an apparatus for assessing particle size distribution of forages which combined mechanical and aerodynamic separation. The unit included sorting gates to separate samples into 8 groups from <4.5 mm to >90 mm. By example, they suggested particle size data be reported on a mass basis. Since the data generally fit the logarithmic normal distribution, the use of cumulative plots on log-normal axes seemed most appropriate for displaying or representing results from a whole sample.

Finner *et al.* (1977) developed a forage particle size separator based solely on mechanical separation through three dimensional sieves (with significant thickness). Their research with square hole sieves, round hole sieves, and wire mesh sieves led to the current ASAE Standard S424 (ASAE, 1998). The ASAE standard method uses 5 sieves and a bottom pan (Figure 4.2). The top 4 sieves have square holes punched in aluminum plate with thickness and percent open area related to the sieve opening size. The thickness and closed area of the upper sieves inhibit long slender particles from falling through these sieves. The fifth sieve is a wire mesh screen that separates finer particles. The entire sieve set is shaken in a horizontal plane for 2 minutes to sort particles in a 9 to 10 litre sample. Sieve openings range from 1.17 to 19.0 mm in nominal dimensions.

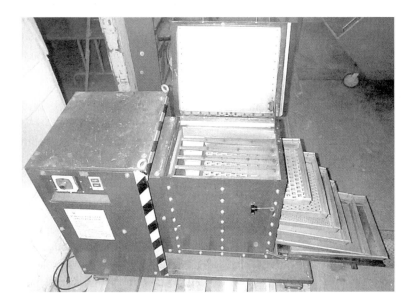

Figure 4.2 ASAE Standard separator with 5 sieves and a bottom pan used for forage and TMR particle size analysis (opened for a view of the sieves; ASAE, 1998)

The current ASAE Standard suggests that forage particle size data be reported using logarithmic normal data analysis and that geometric mean size be calculated. Pitt (1987) suggests that the Weibull distribution is more applicable; Lammers *et al.* (1996a) also found the Weibull distribution to be better when dealing with forage and TMR samples. As will be discussed below, the importance of having a distribution in particle sizes in the ration necessitates that particle size data be reported more completely than just the mean particle size. One could formulate a ration with a mean particle size (e.g. 5 mm) with either a narrow or wide distribution (low or high standard deviation) around that mean size. Depending on the ration ingredients and the target animal performance, there may be more variation in animal performance due to the difference in standard deviation of particle size than the difference in mean particle size.

Murphy and Zhu (1997) compared 9 different methods for evaluating particle size distribution of feedstuffs. Based on median particle size estimates (central tendency), they concluded that 6 of those 9 had relatively consistent estimates of particle size distribution. One of these methods was developed by Finner *et al.* (1977) and adopted as an ASAE Standard (ASAE, 1998). Murphy and Zhu (1997) also noted that measures of dispersion are important to describe particle size. However, more uniform expression of dispersion requires wider agreement on which distribution to use. Until (and even after) there is agreement on the preferred distribution (probably logarithmic normal or

Weibull), it would be wise to report the complete particle size analysis in cumulative probability plots or suitable tables to maximize the utility of published research.

Kammel *et al.* (1995) used the ASAE Standard (ASAE, 1998) separator in research and extension teaching programmes related to TMR delivery and particle size distribution. These efforts have been very successful in getting producers and advisors to quantify this important feed attribute. However, the shortage of laboratories with appropriate analytical capability has limited the extent of impact. In order to facilitate rapid and frequent particle size measurement, Lammers *et al.* (1996a) developed a simplified, on-farm or in-lab method for evaluating particle size distribution of forages and TMRs.

This simplified method (Lammers *et al.*, 1996a) is based on the ASAE Standard S424(1998) and has been proven to generate similar results. This method was not foreseen as a research method, but has rapidly become a method of choice in North America. The device contains 2 sieves and a bottom pan (Figure 4.3). A 1.5 litre sample can be evaluated within minutes, with very repeatable results. We have advocated the use of the Weibull distribution (if any), but many choose to report simply the proportion of the samples in each of the three fractions. Once the simplified separator became commercially available, nutritionists, veterinarians, educators and producers rapidly put it to use. Applications of this device and method have been widespread and include assessment of physical forage treatments (Harrison *et al.*, 1997), assessment of mixer performance (Rippel *et al.*, 1998), assessment of bunk behavior and feed sorting (Hutjens, personal communications), and as a management tool at both harvest and feeding time (Stokes, 1997). Instructions and recommendations for use of the device can be found on the internet (Heinrichs, 1996).

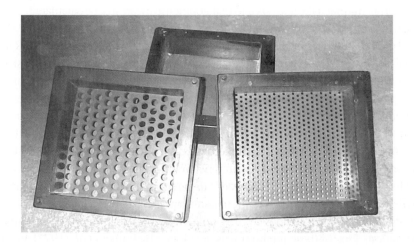

Figure 4.3 Simplified (Penn State) separator for forage and TMR particle size analysis (Lammers *et al.* 1996a).

Heinrichs *et al.* (1999) reported particle size distributions for thousands of samples evaluated at a commercial laboratory (Table 4.1). While these distributions cannot be used to directly determine particle size requirements, they do suggest what is typical on many Northeastern U.S. farms. These data show that there is a tremendous amount of variation in particle size distribution in forages and TMRs. This variation points to the need for standard methods of evaluation and accompanying recommendations.

Table 4.1 MEAN PROPORTION IN THREE PARTICLE SIZE FRACTIONS FOR A VARIETY OF SAMPLES (HEINRICHS *et al.*, 1999)

	Grass silage	*Mixed, mostly grass silage*	*Mixed grass and legume silage*	*Mixed, mostly legume silage*	*Legume silage*	*Small grain silage*	*Maize silage*	*Total mixed rations*
Number of samples	582	280	882	1606	2815	529	5395	831
Proportion > 19 mm								
mean	0.181	0.184	0.174	0.164	0.160	0.146	0.080	0.071
std.	0.135	0.134	0.129	0.123	0.116	0.094	0.064	0.054
Proportion 8 to 19 mm								
mean	0.413	0.384	0.375	0.372	0.405	0.484	0.508	0.352
std.	0.132	0.120	0.116	0.108	0.110	0.139	0.123	0.106
Proportion < 8 mm								
mean	0.406	0.432	0.452	0.465	0.435	0.370	0.411	0.577
std.	0.161	0.150	0.156	0.149	0.138	0.163	0.141	0.122

Kammel *et al.* (1995) tried to correlate mean particle length and the amount of "long" material (proportion > 38 mm) in forage samples; they found the correlation to be poor. Although mean particle length is related to the theoretical length of cut setting of a forage harvester, they are not identical (Savoie *et al.*, 1989); feed rate, moisture content, knife condition, and crop variety are a few factors affecting the difference. Because of these issues and the many alternatives on farms for crop processing, mixer types, etc., it will become increasingly important to characterize the particle size distribution quantitatively. The biological interaction between chemical fibre and particle size necessitates particle size analysis. Laboratory and standard research methods, complemented by an on-farm analysis tool should make particle size analysis as common, as repeatable, and as cost effective as other nutritive evaluations of feedstuffs (via wet chemistry or near infrared spectroscopy). Commercial analysis laboratories are now regularly reporting particle size as a feed attribute (Lammers *et al.*, 1996b).

Dairy ration particle size recommendations

Any particle size recommendations made regarding forage sources or TMRs must be made in the context of fibre "requirements" and fibre sources. Actually, requirements should be formulated using terms such as effective fibre, which encompass the particle size distribution. Current NRC (1989) recommendations are that rations should contain a minimum of 250 to 280 g/kg neutral detergent fibre (NDF) and that 0.75 of this should come from forage sources. This should be refined because effectiveness of fibre and identification of fibre requirement requires attention to particle size, since particle size and chemical fibre are partially interchangable (Allen, 1995; Weiss, 1993).

The literature is rich with published studies regarding effects of particle size on animal health and performance. Lammers *et al.* (1996b) and Weiss (1993) summarized this information nicely. In summary, small particles are desired for:

- Increased surface area for more rapid digestion
- Decreased retention time in the rumen
- Increased rumen turnover rate
- Potentially increased dry matter intake (due to the turnover rate)

Sufficient supply of long particles (or chemical fibre) must be in the ration to:

- Increase chewing activity
- Maintain rumen pH
- Optimize rumen environment for digestion
- Increase acetate to propionate ratio
- Increase milk fat concentration
- Avoid displaced abomasums
- Decrease incidence of parakeratosis, laminitis, and acidosis.
- Potentially increase dry matter intake (due to better rumen and animal health)

Clearly, particle size should be incorporated into fibre requirements because forage amount and particle size interact with non-forage fibre sources to affect the rate of ruminal digestion and the rate of passage (Grant, 1997). Forage particle size must be sufficient to stimulate rumination, avoid a reduction in ruminal pH, and entrap small particles (Grant, 1997); but, this is dependent upon the chemical fibre attributes of the ration (i.e., ration NDF). Physical effectiveness of fibre varies dramatically for different feeds, primarily due to differences in particle size distribution (Allen, 1995).

Prior to common measurement of particle size on farms and consistent measurement of particle size in research studies, Shaver (1990) developed some recommendations for forage particle size. These were stated with regard to theoretical length of cut (a forage harvester setting), which is not the same value as mean particle length. He suggested a theoretical length of cut of 9 mm, which supposedly yields 15 to 20% of particles longer than 38 mm. The data of Savoie *et al.* (1989) shows, however, this is not always true for wilted grass or alfalfa silage; they found that theoretical length of cut needed to be approximately 13 mm to achieve this distribution (15 to 20% > 38 mm). Additionally, the particle size reduction that can occur after chopping (due to roll processing and other mechanical handling) requires that recommendations focus on actual particle size distribution delivered to the animal rather than individual machine settings.

Kammel *et al.* (1995) seemed to be the first to identify particle size recommendations based on measurements of the actual particle size distribution. The application of the ASAE Standard (ASAE, 1998) separator and the use of the Penn State simplified separator (Lammers *et al.*, 1996a) by others in research and educational programs fueled the debate and development of suitable recommendations. Particle size recommendations are still in a state of development and resolution.

Sudweeks *et al.* (1981) proposed an index system whereby the roughage value of a feedstuff could be estimated from mean particle size (as determined with mesh sieves such as those depicted in Figure 4.1), NDF concentration, and dry matter intake. A roughage value index requirement for the ration was proposed. For ration formulation, it would be preferable to avoid feed characteristics, such as the roughage value index, which are functions of the animal response or diet traits such as dry matter intake.

Mertens (1997) proposed a system for determining effectiveness of fibre, but identified eight areas of research needed to bring the system into full utility; the first area dealt with particle size measurement and relating particle size to chewing activity. Mertens (1997) did some simple analysis which distinguished between particles larger and smaller than 1.18 mm, but this does not adequately address forage particle size since 80 to 90% of forage particles are typically in the range of 5-30 mm. De Boever *et al.* (1993) found that material retained above a 2.38 mm screen was a main determinant of chewing index, and therefore fibre effectiveness.

De Boever *et al.* (1993) found that total chewing index (total time spent chewing per unit of forage dry matter) increased as theoretical length of chopping increased from 4 to 16 mm, but ruminating index (RI, time spent ruminating per unit of forage dry matter) was not increased with lengths of cut over 8 mm. While nutritionally there may be no advantage to increasing particle size above a certain point (Allen, 1995), there could be advantages from energy, feed harvest, feed storage, or feed delivery perspectives. Long hay or coarsely chopped silage allows lower NDF levels in the ration (Allen, 1995). Because high energy forages are generally lower in NDF, use of physical length to increase fibre effectiveness can help to achieve high energy concetration in rations for high producing cows. Allen (1995) gave specific recommendations for altering ration NDF concentration as particle size varied. Starting with a baseline NDF level of the ration being 300 g/kg, Allen (1995, as interpreted by Varga *et al.*, 1998) suggests:

- No adjustment if 5 to 10% of the ration is longer than 19 mm.
- Decrease ration NDF content if more than 15% of ration mass is longer than 19 mm.
- Increase ration NDF content up to 40g/kg with very finely chopped silage.

Further indicating the interactions related to particle size and fibre requirements, Allen (1995) and Weiss (1993) give similar adjustments to ration NDF for the use of by-product feeds, changes in grain feeding frequency, ruminal starch digestibility, use of buffers, digestibility of fibre, and fat addition. With some substitutive effect of particle size for chemical fibre, it is clear that there are also interactions between particle size "requirements" and these other feeding factors.

Heinrichs and Lammers (1997) have put particle size recommendations together to complement an on-farm method for particle size measurement (Lammers *et al*, 1996a). While these recommendations differ from those initially suggested by Allen (1995), most of the disagreement appeared to be in interpretation of particle size distribution rather than disagreement in the recommendation itself. Heinrichs and Lammers (1997) suggest:

- 6 to 10% of the whole TMR should be longer than 19 mm.
- If 3 to 6% is longer than 19 mm, the ration may still work successfully if there is sufficient focus on total NDF and forage NDF.
- No more than 60% of the ration particles be smaller than 8 mm to ensure a distribution in size of particles.

Heinrichs and Lammers (1997) also gave broad targets for forage particle size distribution, but cautioned against focusing on individual ration ingredients. The real application of forage particle size measurement is to determine the combination of forages needed to achieve proper particle sizes in the total ration. The focus must remain on the particle size distribution that the cow actually consumes (Allen, 1995; Heinrichs and Lammers, 1997).

Linear and nonlinear programming have been used extensively in ration formulation. Requirements and sources of nutrients, such as energy, degradable or undegradable protein and minerals lend themselves nicely to these optimizing mathematical techniques. Even if nutritionists agreed on effective fibre "requirements", the interaction between (chemical) NDF and (physical) particle size makes optimal ration formulation difficult. One method of incorporating the interaction is to compute a fibre characteristic as "adjusted" by particle size, such as proposed by Mertens (1997); he proposed physically effective NDF or peNDF. A similar, but not identical alternative is to capture the interaction with a calculated index. The advantage of the index is the explicit nature of the adjustment of effectiveness.

The index concept is not new. After introduction of the roughage value index concept (Sudweeks *et al.*, 1981), Santini *et al.* (1983) proposed an alternative roughage index that was adjusted for particle length as well as intake. They used the ASAE Standard (1998) method of measuring particle size and calculated an adjusted forage intake by multiplying forage intake by forage mean particle size. These methods did not fully account for NDF and particle size interactions nor did they account for the dispersion characteristics of particle size distribution (small or large variation). They were, however, early attempts to link actual particle size measurements to the effectiveness of fibre.

Buckmaster *et al.* (1997) proposed an effective fibre index for individual feeds that explicitly links particle size distribution to NDF. The index, which simply weights NDF concentration by particle size, is defined as:

$$EFI = \frac{E_{>19mm} - NDF_{>19mm} - X_{>19mm} + E_{8-19mm} - NDF_{8-19mm} - X_{8-19mm} + E_{<8mm} - NDF_{<8mm} - X_{<8mm}}{X_{>19mm} + X_{8-19mm} + X_{<8mm}}$$

(Eq. 4.1)

where:

EFI = effective fibre index
E = relative effectiveness of particles in each size range
NDF = neutral detergent fibre concentration of each size range, fraction of DM
X = fraction of total mass in each size range

The relative effectiveness coefficients (E) reflect the effectiveness of each particle length range to stimulate rumination and contribute to a rumen mat. More research is needed to establish these coefficients, but a review of the literature suggests coefficients of $E_{>19mm} = 2$, $E_{8-19mm} = 1$, and $E_{<8mm} = 0.2$. These coefficients imply that the top sieve material is twice as effective for stimulating rumination and contributing to a rumen mat than lower sieve material, and that the particles < 8 mm have one fifth the effectiveness for contributing to a rumen mat and stimulating rumination as lower sieve material (Van Soest, 1982; Welch, 1982). This is in contrast to the peNDF method proposed by Mertens (1997) which equally weights particle mass > 1.18 mm, but neglects the rest. Buckmaster *et al.* (1997) showed that the EFI results in a range of values approximately equal to the mean (Table 4.2); such variation will aid in discriminating between feed sources. This simple index does not capture the differences in effectiveness of particles from different sources. Weiss (1993) suggested that grasses may provide more effective fibre per unit of NDF than legumes; if this is true, and if the effect is due to reasons other than particle size, the effectiveness coefficients (E) in the equation above may need some adjustment based on the feed type.

Research such as that done by De Boever *et al.* (1993a, 1993b) could be very valuable in refining effective fibre requirements. For grass silage, growth stage (hence chemical fibre) had far more effect than particle size on ruminating index (RI) (De Boever *et al.*, 1993a). However, the median particle sizes were 11 to 70 mm; if finely chopped silage had been tested, particle size may have become more important. For corn silage, they were able to predict a RI reasonably well based solely on particle size distribution information and *in vitro* digestibility (De Boever *et al.*, 1993b). They have recently used a similar approach to characterize physical structure of alternative feeds (De Brabander *et al.*, 1999).

Table 4.2 ILLUSTRATION OF EFFECTIVE FIBRE INDEX VALUES FOR CORN, MIXED MOSTLY GRASS, AND MIXED MOSTLY LEGUME SILAGES (BUCKMASTER *et al.*, 1997)

	Maize silage	*Mixed mostly grass silage*	*Mixed mostly legume silage*
Number of samples	26	22	43
Whole samples			
Minimum NDF[a]	298	374	323
Mean NDF	415	535	461
Maximum NDF	542	652	577
Means for separated fractions			
NDF of particles > 19 mm	640	590	529
NDF of particles 8 to 19 mm	408	536	473
NDF of particles < 8 mm	394	529	446
Effective fibre index (EFI[b])			
Minimum EFI	15.4	21.8	22.5
Mean EFI	31.4	35.0	35.9
Maximum EFI	49.6	54.2	54.0

[a] NDF = neutral detergent fibre concentration, g/kg DM
[b] EFI = effective fibre index as defined in the text ($E_{>19mm} = 2$, $E_{8-19mm} = 1$, $E_{<8mm} = 0.2$)

As methods for dairy ration formulation and feeding become more refined, it is clear that effective fibre will become increasingly important. Index methods which link physical measures (particle size distribution) and chemical measures (most likely NDF) into one index inherently contain more information; they more accurately reflect the effects on animal function than the expression of mean particle length or fibre concentration alone. It would be straightforward to implement the EFI concept or the RI concept into a linear constraint for ration balancing. For example, a constraint for the balanced ration to satisfy could be:

$$\sum_{i-1}^{\# feeds} A_i - EFI_i \geq EFI^{required}$$

OR

$$\sum_{i-1}^{\# feeds} A_i - RI_i \geq RI^{required}$$

(Eq. 4.2)

where:

A = amount of feed i

Rapidly digested starch sources, such as barley grain, increase the need for effective fibre (Beauchemin and Rode, 1997); this phenomenon could be accommodated by a negative EFI_i value in the formulation matrix (left hand side) for such an ingredient in the ration.

Mixing of total mixed rations

Blending (mixing) of a TMR requires motion; this motion causes reduction in particle size (Kammel *et al.*, 1995). For this reason, particle size and TMR uniformity must be jointly considered (Stokes and Berthard, 1999). The goal of TMR preparation is uniformity, but this is often achieved at the expense of unwanted reduction in particle size (Stokes, 1997).

The type and duration of mixing affect particle size distribution. In a survey of commercial farmers, Kammel *et al.* (1995) reported that mixing time varied from 2 to 60 minutes, with a typical mixing time of 16 minutes. Most mixer manufacturers recommend 4 to 8 minutes, so any particle size reduction that occurs after 8 minutes is unnecessary. Among the TMR samples evaluated in educational programmes, Kammel *et al.* (1995) identified 65% as having too few large particles. Lammers *et al.* (1996b) found a very large variation in amount of long particles in TMRs delivered on farms; they suggested that animals receiving rations at both the low and the high end of the variation are probably performing below their potential. It is likely that improvements in mixer management could help alleviate health and performance problems through better control of particle size distribution in the ration.

For both vertical and horizontal mixers, Rippel *et al.* (1998) noted an average of 9% reduction in "long" particles (>19 mm) when the mixers were operated 15 minutes longer than normal. However, in one case with a silage-based ration, the 15 minutes of excessive mixing time reduced the proportion of long (>19 mm) particles by 28%. In a case with a hay-based ration, the 15 minutes of excessive mixing caused a 39% reduction in long (>19 mm) particles. In these two cases, the mass of fine particles (<8 mm) increased by 20 and 25%, respectively. Figure 4.4 illustrates the particle size reduction reported by Heinrichs *et al.* (1999) for a four-auger horizontal mixer. It is worth noting from this controlled experiment that mixing reduced the size of particles regardless of their initial length (i.e., both long and medium particles became smaller).

Mixer type can have a large effect on particle size reduction, but Stokes and Berthard (1995) illustrated that, if properly managed, both vertical and horizontal mixers can be used to achieve good rations with regard to particle size. Kammel *et al.* (1995) also demonstrated that several types of mixers can be used effectively. Even so, Heinrichs *et al.* (1999) suggested that different mixing mechanisms can have a large effect on particle size reduction (Table 4.3). These data were not collected from a controlled

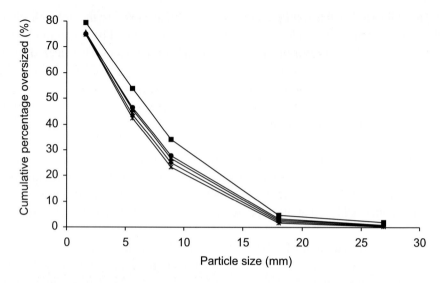

Figure 4.4 Effect of mixing time on particle size distribution of a TMR prepared with a 4-auger mixer (Heinrichs *et al.*, 1999) (■ = 0 min; ● = 4 min; ▲ = 8 min; ♦ = 16 min; ✳ = 32 min)

study, but were collected from farms with mixing performed as it is usually done on the farm. No attempt was made to improve fill order or mixing time prior to sampling. Overall, for the rations that did not include long hay, an average of 19% of the particle mass that was longer than 19 mm when entering the mixer was smaller than 19 mm after mixing. The data for the batches with hay may be misleading because the particle size of the hay could not be determined; therefore, when the overall average reduction is reported as 5%, that means there was 5% less "long" (>19 mm) particle mass after mixing and addition of hay than there was before mixing without the hay considered. In nearly every case, the mixer did more to decrease the amount of long particle mass than the addition of hay did to increase it.

Because the data in Table 4.3 were not generated from controlled experiments with similar feeds, filling sequences, and mixing times, care should be taken in interpreting the numbers. Generally, however, it appears that as farmers operate the machines (not necessarily as the manufacturers intended), mixers that rely on tumbling action of the feed for mixing retain more long particle mass than auger mixers that have much more binding, squeezing, and crushing action. This shows that regardless of mixer type, some particle size reduction occurs. Kammel *et al.* (1995) showed a similar (26%) decrease in long particle mass with a tumble mixer operated for 10 minutes.

It is the material flow within a mixer that accomplishes the blending. For some mixers, material flow is significantly hindered when the mixer is too full or nearly empty. For example, tumble and reel type mixers typically require 30 to 40% "empty" space for the feed to move. If the mixer is improperly sized, mixing time must be increased to accomplish adequate uniformity; this excessive mixing time causes excessive reduction in particle size. Similarly, some auger type mixers will not effectively mix a small batch.

Table 4.3 EFFECT OF MIXER TYPE ON REDUCTION IN LONG PARTICLE MASS
(HEINRICHS *et al.*, 1999)

Mixer type	With hay		Without hay		Overall	
	Number of Batches	*Reduction in particles > 18 mm (%)*	*Number of batches*	*Reduction in particles > 18 mm (%)*	*Number of batches*	*Reduction in particles > 18 mm (%)*
Auger	2	28	4	37	6	34
Chain and slat	2	2	7	2	9	2
Reel	4	7	2	35	6	16
Tumble	1	19	3	22	4	3
Overall	9	5	16	19	25	13

Mixer selection, therefore, can have an effect on particle size and mixers should be selected for both the maximum and minimum batche sizes (Buckmaster, 1998; Stokes and Berthard, 1999)

Besides mixing time and mixer type, mixer management can affect particle size distribution. Operation of the mixer during filling and an improper fill order can reduce particle size significantly. Rippel *et al.* (1998) compared different fill sequences with a three-ingredient ration and found one sequence to cause a 22% reduction in long (>19 mm) particle mass compared to the others. Closer examination of the data presented also suggests that one of the sequences reduced variation in the mix (lowest coefficient of variation among samples) by about 50% while achieving the highest retention of long particle mass.

Modelling particle size reduction

To begin development of a model of particle size reduction during mixing, three forage sources were "blended" in a mixer alone. The mixer was a Rotomix model 354 reel type mixer with a total capacity (level full) of 11.3 cubic metres. The forage sources were grass silage, alfalfa silage, and corn (maize) silage. In nine separate batches (three of each forage source), each forage was "mixed" for a total of 30 minutes. The mixer was not operated until all forage was placed into the mixer. The mixer power-take-off input shaft was operated at 440 rpm. The mixer was filled to approximately 75% of rated volumetric capacity (1200 kg grass silage, 1240 kg alfalfa silage, or 2440 kg corn silage).

Forage was sampled as it entered the mixer. The maize silage was taken from a bunker silo and was not processed with a roll processor. The grass and alfalfa silages were taken from top unloaded tower silos. Samples were taken from the discharge chute of the mixer after 5, 10, 15, 22, and 30 minutes of mixing. Care was taken to avoid sampling forage which may have been "stuck" near the discharge chute and not blended. Particle size distributions of the forage samples were evaluated in duplicate using ASAE Standard S424 (ASAE, 1998). Table 4.4 contains descriptions of the forages before mixing.

Table 4.4 INITIAL FORAGE CHARACTERISTICS FOR THE FORAGE-ONLY MIXING EXPERIMENT

	Grass silage	Alfalfa silage	Maize silage
Dry matter content (g/kg)	*320*	*410*	*330*
Particle size distribution (mass basis)[*]			
> 26.9 mm	0.152	0.112	0.038
18.0 to 26.9 mm	0.097	0.106	0.089
8.98 to 18.0 mm	0.482	0.372	0.631
5.61 to 8.98 mm	0.168	0.193	0.144
1.65 to 5.61 mm	0.084	0.155	0.077
< 1.65 mm	0.017	0.062	0.021

[*] Measured as per ASAE Standard S424 (ASAE, 1998)

Figures 4.5, 4.6, and 4.7 show the particle size distributions of the individual forages after being tumbled in the reel mixer for varying lengths of time. The plot for the grass silage (Figure 4.5) shows that reduction in particle size continued

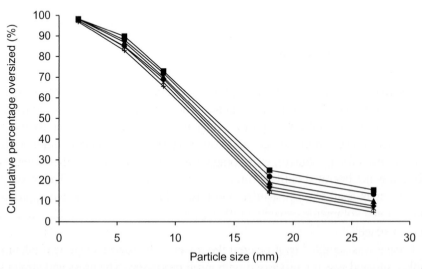

Figure 4.5 Effect of mixing time on particle size distribution of grass silage blended in a reel mixer (■ = 0 min; ● = 5 min; ▲ = 10 min; ◆ = 15 min; ＊ = 22 min; + = 30 min)

for up to 30 minutes of mixing. The curves illustrate that all particles were reduced in size. For example, from 0 to 30 minutes, the mass percentage larger than 26.9 mm (initially large particles) decreased from 15 to 4.5%. Additionally, from 0 to 30 minutes, the mass percentage of particles larger than 5.61 mm decreased from 90 to 83%. The rate of particle size reduction appears approximately steady, neither increasing nor decreasing over time. The rate of elimination of large particles (>19 mm) was 2 to 3% per minute over the 30 minute test period. Comparatively, the reduction in particle size for alfalfa silage occurred primarily during the first five minutes of mixing. Particle size reduction between 5 and 30 minutes was small (Figure 4.6). The rate of large (>19 mm) particle mass began at 9% per minute for alfalfa, then dropped to 2% per minute.

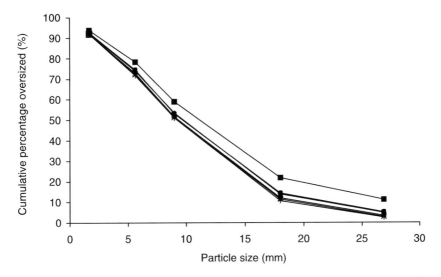

Figure 4.6 Effect of mixing time on particle size distribution of alfalfa silage blended in a reel mixer (■ = 0 min; ● = 5 min; ▲ = 10 min; ♦ = 15 min; ✳ = 22 min; + = 30 min)

The maize silage was relatively finely chopped to begin with (Table 4.4). As a result, the tumble action mixing of the reel mixer did little to further reduce the particle size of the corn silage (Figure 4.7). The retention of approximately 5% large (>25 mm) particle mass was almost exclusively due to cob chunks which would probably only be broken down by grinding or chopping action. Particles like these should not be considered when evaluating effective fibre of corn silage because they would probably be rejected by animals during feeding.

Based on these limited data, a few guidelines can be be regarding mixer management for retention of large particle size — at least with this type of mixer. It would be important to minimize the mixing time with grass in the mixer; it would be best to stop blending after 5-10 minutes because, at this point, TMR uniformity should be acceptable. If liquid ingredients or a small amount of a concentrate ingredient necessitated a longer duration of mixing (>10 minutes), addition of the grass silage after some premixing may

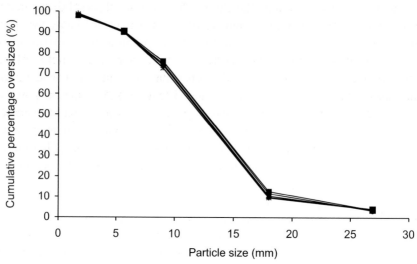

Figure 4.7 Effect of mixing time on particle size distribution of corn silage blended in a reel mixer (■ = 0 min; ● = 5 min; ▲ = 10 min; ♦ = 15 min; ✳ = 22 min; + = 30 min)

help to retain the long particles. Extended mixing of alfalfa will probably do little to reduce particle size; most of the "damage" was done during the first few minutes of mixing.

Efforts are currently underway to use this type of information to model particle size reduction during mixing and other processes between the field and feeding cows. The modelling approach is to consider "pools" of foarge particle size according to the ASAE Standard (ASAE, 1998) sieve size openings. A reduction of particle size can be quantified as a movement from one pool into a pool one size smaller. Rates of movement from one pool to the next, in the case of mixing, are likely to be expressed as a function of mixer type, crop type, crop moisture, and cumulative mixing time. If models can be developed to account for particle size reduction, we will be able to predict actual ration particle size distributions from feedstuff characteristics.

Short-term research focus

Over the next few years, the thrust relative to forage particle size in dairy rations should be on determining requirements and identifying the means to meet the requirements. Complete reporting of particle size distribution of ingredients and rations fed will be necessary if the utility of published studies is to be maximized. There is a wide range in the sizes of forage particles. For research purposes, distribution of particle size in feed and forage should be recorded from <1 to 30 or 40 mm. Recommendations and field application may involve a narrower range. Because mixing and other processes can cause significant reduction in particle size, it is important to know what cows are actually offered and eat.

Sufficient effective fibre assures sufficient rumination to control rumen pH, maintain rumen health, and avoid metabolic disorders; therefore, models that integrate NDF concentration, particle size, and rumination will be needed to establish requirements for effective fibre. The use of an index that links particle size distribution and chemical fibre attributes (most likely NDF) should be helpful in this process. Like most attempts to model or quantify biological phenomena, we will start with simple approximations and assumptions, then add appropriate detail as more insight is gained.

Once effective fibre (particle size and NDF) requirements for the whole ration are identified, it will be possible to work backwards from the whole ration to requirements for particle size of individual forage sources by considering the dilution of effective fibre by concentrate ingredients. The final step in reverse engineering particle size targets of feedstuffs will be to work backwards from the forage as fed to forage as harvested (feed trough back to field), and to account, via modelling or other means, for particle size reductions due to processes such as ensiling, transport, and mixing.

References

Allen, M. 1995. Fiber requirements: Finding an optimum can be confusing. *Feedstuffs.* May 8, 1995: 13-16.

ASAE. 1998. S424: Method of determining and expressing particle size of chopped forage materials by screening. In: *ASAE Standards.* American Society of Agricultural Engineers. St. Joseph, MI.

Beauchemin, K.A., and L.M. Rode. 1997. Minimum versus optimal concentrations of fiber in dairy cow diets based on barley silage and concentrates of barley and corn. *Journal of Dairy Science.* **80(8)**:1629-1639.

Buckmaster, D.R. 1998. TMR Mixer Management. In: *Dairy Feeding Systems: Management, Components, and Nutrients.* Northeast Region Agricultural Engineering Service, Ithaca, NY. pp. 109-119.

Buckmaster, D.R., A.J.Heinrichs, R.A. Ward, and B.P. Lammers. 1997. Characterizing effective fiber with particle size and fiber concentration interactions. *Proceedings of the 18th International Grassland Congress.* 17:53-54. ID: 886.

De Boever, J.L., D.D. De Brabander, A.M. De Smet, J.M. Vanacker, and C.V. Boucque. 1993. Evaluation of physical structure. 2. Maize silage. *Journal of Dairy Science.* **76(6)**:1624-1634.

De Brabander, D.L., J.L. De Boever, A.M. De Smet, J.M. Vanacker, and C.V. Boucque. 1999. Evaluation of the physical structure of fodder beets, potatoes, pressed beet pulp, brewers grains, and corn cob silage. *Journal of Dairy Science.* **82(1)**:110-121.

Finner, M.F., J.E. Hardzinski, and L.L. Pagel. 1977. Measuring particle length of chopped forages. In: *Grain and Forage Harvesting, Proc. of the First Int'l Grain and Forage Conference.* ASAE. St. Joseph, MI. pp. 265-269,273.

Gale, G.E. and M.J. O'Dougherty. 1982. An apparatus for the assessment of the length of distribution of chopped forage. *Journal of Agricultural Engineering Research.* **27(1)**:35-43.

Grant, R.J. 1997. Interactions among forages and nonforage fiber sources. *Journal of Dairy Science.* **80(7)**:1438-1446.

Harrison, J.H., L. Johnson, C. Hunt, J.Siciliano-Jones, and K.J. Shinners. 1997. Use of kernel-processed silage in diary rations. In: *Silage: Field to Feedbunk.* Northeast Region Agricultural Engineering Service, Ithaca, NY. pp. 95-110.

Heinrichs, A.J. 1996. Evaluating particle size of forages and TMRs using the Penn State particle size separator. Extension mimeo DAS 96-20. Located at: www-das.cas.psu.edu/dcn/catforg/particle/index.html

Heinrichs, A.J., D.R. Buckmaster, and B.P. Lammers. 1999. Processing, mixing, and particle size reduction of forages for dairy cattle. *Journal of Animal Science.* **77(1)**:180-186

Heinrichs, A.J. and B.P. Lammers. 1997. Particle size recommendations for dairy cattle. In: *Silage: Field to Feedbunk.* Northeast Region Agricultural Engineering Service, Ithaca, NY. pp. 268-277.

Kammel, D.W., R.T. Schuler, and R.D. Shaver. 1995. Influence of mixer design on particle size. In: *Proc. of the 2nd National Alternative Feeds Symposium.* Univ. Of Missouri. pp. 271-297.

Kennedy, P.M., editor. 1984. *Techniques in particle size analysis of feed and digesta in ruminants.* Occasional Publ. No. 1. Canadian Society of Animal Science.

Lammers, B.P., D.R. Buckmaster, and A.J. Heinrichs. 1996a. A simple method for the analysis of particle sizes of forage and total mixed rations. *Journal of Dairy Science.* **79(5)**:922-928.

Lammers, B., J. Heinrichs, and D. Buckmaster. 1996b. Method helps in determination of forage, TMR particle size requirements for dairy cattle. In: *Feedstuffs.* **68(41)**:14-20.

Mertens, D.R. 1997. Creating a system for meeting the fiber requirements of dairy cows. *Journal of Dairy Science.* **80(7)**:1463-1481.

Murphy, M.R. and J.S. Zhu. 1997. A comparison of methods to analyze particle size as applied to alfalfa haylage, corn silage, and concentrate mix. *Journal of Dairy Science* **80(11)**:2932-2938.

NRC. 1989. Nutrient requirements of dairy cattle, 6th revised edition. National Research Council. National Academy Press. Washington, DC.

Pitt, R.E. 1987. Theory of particle size distributions for chopped forages. *Transactions of the ASAE.* 30(5):1246-1253.

Rippel, C.M., E.R. Jordan, and S.R. Stokes. 1998. Evaluation of particle size distribution and ration uniformity in total mixed rations fed in Northcentral Texas. *Professional Animal Scientist* **14**:44-50.

Santini, F.J., A.R. Hardie, N.A. Jorgensen, and M.F. Finner. 1983. Proposed use of an adjusted intake based on forage particle length for calculation of roughage indexes. *Journal of Dairy Science* **66(4)**:811-820.

Savoie, P., D. Tremblay, R. Theriault, J.M. Wauthy, and C. Vigneault. 1989. Forage chopping energy versus length of cut. *Transactions of the ASAE.* **32(2)**:437-442.

Shaver, R.D. 1990. Forage particle length in dairy rations. In: *Dairy Feeding Systems.* Northeast Region Agricultural Engineering Service, Ithaca, NY. pp. 58-64.

Stokes. S.R. 1997. Particle Size and Ration Uniformity: Is it Important to the Cow? Western Canadian Dairy Seminar, Red Deer, Alberta, Canada.

Stokes, S.R. and G. Bethard. 1999. Selecting and Managing TMR Mixers for Dairy Operations. Minnesota Nutrition Conference, Minneapolis, MN.

Sudweeks, E.M., L.O. Ely, D.R. Mertens, and L.R. Sisk. 1981. Assessing minimum amounts and form of roughages in ruminant diets: roughage value index system. *Journal of Animal Science.* **53(5)**:1406-1411.

VanSoest, P.J. 1982. *Nutritional ecology of the ruminant.* O. & B. Books, Inc. Corvallis, OR.

Varga, G.A., H.M.Dann, and V.A. Ishler. 1998. The use of fiber concentrations for ration formulation. *Journal of Dairy Science.* **81(11)**:3063-3074.

Weiss, W.P. 1993. Dietary fiber requirements of dairy cattle explored. *Feedstuffs.* Nov. 8, 1993. pp 14-17.

Welch, J.G. 1982. Rumination, particle size, and passage from the rumen. *Journal of Animal Science.* **54(4)**:885-894.

This paper was first published in 2000

5

PREDICTION OF THE INTAKE OF GRASS SILAGE BY CATTLE

R.W.J. STEEN[1,2], F.J. GORDON[1,2], C.S. MAYNE[1,2], R.E. POOTS[3], D.J. KILPATRICK[2], E.F. UNSWORTH[2], R.J. BARNES[4], M.G. PORTER[1] AND C.J. PIPPARD[1]

[1] *Agricultural Research Institute of Northern Ireland, Hillsborough, Co. Down, UK*
[2] *Department of Agriculture for Northern Ireland, Newforge Lane, Belfast, UK*
[3] *Greenmount College of Agriculture and Horticulture, Antrim, UK*
[4] *Perstrop Analytical Ltd, Highfield House, Roxborough Way, Maidenhead, UK*

Introduction

Efficient production of high quality milk and beef is highly dependent on dairy cows and beef cattle receiving the correct intake of nutrients. However grass silage, which forms the basis of winter rations for the vast majority of dairy and beef cattle in the United Kingdom and other countries in North Western Europe, varies greatly in terms of chemical and biological composition due to the impact of factors such as sward type, fertilisation, climate and ensiling technique on the fermentation process in the silo and nutritive value. This in turn results in major variation in silage intake, which affects both the quantity and quality of milk and beef produced. The improvement in the genetic potential of dairy and beef cattle has increased the economic benefits of achieving optimal inputs of nutrients. There is also currently considerable concern about the impact of animal production on the environment, especially with regard to reducing losses of nitrogen and phosphate from animals, which adds further impetus to the need for accurate prediction of food and nutrient intakes. An effective method for predicting silage intake from its chemical and biological compositions is essential if animals are to be allocated the correct amounts of concentrates to provide the optimum inputs of nutrients.

Control of food intake in cattle

The commonly accepted theories of the control of food intake by cattle date back at least 50 years ago when Lehmann (1941) proposed that the food intake of ruminants was limited by the amount of indigestible material that they were able to consume. Since then much research has contributed to the understanding of the factors controlling the food intake of cattle and the roles of both physiological and physical restriction of intake (e.g. Conrad, Pratt and Hibbs, 1964; Conrad, 1966; Dinius and Baumgardt, 1970). This led to the concept that the drive for cattle to consume food is related to their requirements for energy as determined by their genetic capacity for growth or milk production (e.g. Jones, 1972; Conrad *et at.,* 1964) and that restriction or control of intake of forage-based diets is determined largely by the rate of degradation of food in the rumen, which in turn limits the rate at which the animal can ingest additional food (Balch and Campling, 1962; Conrad, 1966). In addition to the rate of degradation in the rumen, food intake is also influenced by the extent to which an animal can moderate both its tolerance for different degrees of rumen fill and the rate of passage of digesta through the alimentary tract (Ketelaars and Tolkemp, 1992). The tolerance for rumen fill generally increases with increasing demand for nutrients while the rate of passage is generally increased by factors such as lactation and cold stress.

Despite the importance of the rate of degradation in the rumen, control of food intake by cattle is highly complex involving a wide range of factors in both the animal (such as milk yield, stage of lactation, pregnancy, previous plane of nutrition, body condition, age, breed and sex) and the feed (such as degradability, digestibility, rate of passage, physical form and chemical composition), and the totality of negative and positive effects and their interactions determine the overall level of food intake achieved by the animal (Ketelaars and Tolkamp, 1992). Furthermore patterns of food intake during pregnancy (especially late pregnancy) and lactation do not match requirements and there is evidence that this discrepancy is not caused purely by physical constraints, suggesting a more complex physiological regulation of food intake which may be related to the efficiency of utilization of metabolisable energy and changes in basal metabolism (Ketelaars and Tolkamp, 1992). From a recent review of the literature on factors affecting food intake and a re-assessment of data from earlier studies, Ketelaars and Tolkamp (1992) question the validity of the concept that cattle have a feeding drive which aims at maximising food intake to the extent that they can as far as possible achieve their genetic capacity for milk or meat production. The fact that cattle often exhibit compensatory growth and eat more, following a period of restricted growth, and that animals treated with a number of hormones have a higher level of performance and eat more, suggests that 'normal fed' or untreated animals do not achieve maximum intake or performance, and therefore, that if physical fill is a major factor controlling intake, its controlling effect can be considerably altered by the over-riding effect of the endocrine system of the animal. It is also not clear from the literature whether food intake increases in response to increased rate of passage or *vice-versa* (Journet and Remond, 1976). Intake has been shown to increase with increasing nitrogen content in the diet even when nitrogen content far exceeds that which might be expected to limit microbial fermentation in the rumen, and it has recently been suggested that feed characteristics which are commonly associated with the rumen filling effect of a feed also profoundly affect the metabolism of the animal which in turn may influence the hormonal control of food intake (Ketelaars and Tolkamp, 1992).

Gill, Rook and Thiago (1988) reviewed the results of their studies to examine the extent of rumen fill after individual meals in cattle offered grass and legume hays and grass silage once daily either *ad libitum* or in restricted quantities. The extent of rumen fill at the end of individual meals varied greatly between forages and between individual meals over the 24 hour period. From their results these authors concluded that both physical distension of the rumen and one or more end products of fermentation have important roles in the control of forage intake and that the relative importance of the different factors varies considerably between forages and over the 24 hour feeding period. Factors such as offering leguminous rather than grass hay reduced the extent of rumen fill at the end of an individual meal but this appeared to have little influence on overall intake, while offering silage rather than hay had a similar effect on meal size, but with the slower rate of disappearance of silage from the rumen, would appear to have had greater long-term effects on intake.

Control of silage intake

The intake of grass silage is generally lower than that of comparable hay or fresh forage (e.g. Demarquilly, 1973; Cushnahan and Gordon, 1995) although similar intakes of silage and comparable fresh forage have been recorded (Flynn, 1978; Cushnahan and Mayne, 1994). Silage intake has also been particularly variable and prediction of its intake highly problematic (Rook and Gill, 1990a). The lower intake of silage than that of fresh or dried forage has often been attributed to the end products of fermentation in silage. A number of authors have used simple or multiple regression analyses to examine the relationships between individual parameters or groups of parameters and voluntary intake of silage (e.g. Wilkins, Hutchinson, Wilson and Harris, 1971; Wilkins, Fenlon, Cook and Wilson, 1978; Flynn, 1979; Jones, Larsen and Lanning, 1980; Lewis, 1981; Gill *et al.,* 1988; Rook and Gill, 1990; Rook, Dhanoa and Gill, 1990a). Wilkins *et al.* (1971, 1978) analysed data for 70 and 142 silages respectively which were given to growing sheep over a wide range of experiments, while Jones *et al.* (1980) analysed data for 11 silages given to non-pregnant, non-lactating ewes. Flynn (1979) analysed the data from 37 beef production experiments carried out in Ireland and Rook and Gill (1990) and Rook *et al.* (1990a) used data from a wide range of experiments undertaken at three research centres in the UK in which silages were offered to growing beef cattle. Lewis (1981) reviewed the literature on dairy cow feeding experiments up to 1979, and analysed the data from 78 experiments while Gill *et al.* (1988) analysed data from dairy cow feeding experiments collected over seven years at Hurley and which involved 206 lactations.

Factors affecting silage intake

EFFECT OF SILAGE DRY MATTER CONTENT

There have been significant and positive relationships between silage dry matter content and intake in studies which have involved a wide range of silage dry matter contents (Wilkins *et al.,* 1971; Flynn, 1979; Lewis, 1981; Gill *et al.,* 1988; Rook and Gill, 1990). The R^2 values for linear or quadratic relationships between dry matter content and intake ranged from 0.12 (Gill *et at,* 1988) to 0.44 (Rook and Gill, 1990). Rook and Gill (1990) reported a significant curvilinear relationship between dry matter content and intake which suggested that there was little increase in intake when dry matter content increased above 250 g/kg.

EFFECT OF TOTAL NITROGEN CONTENT

Wilkins *et al.* (1971) and Gill *et al.* (1988) obtained significant positive relationships between silage nitrogen content and intake, R^2 values for linear regressions being 0.33 and 0.13 respectively, while Wilkins *et al.* (1978),Flynn (1979), Jones *et al.* (1980) and Lewis (1981) were unable to detect a significant effect of total nitrogen content on silage intake. However, Rook and Gill (1990) found that the relationships between nitrogen content and silage intake were small in linear regression analyses but that nitrogen content had strong positive relationships with intake in all of their models when collinearity between nitrogen content and other parameters was removed.

AMMONIA-N CONTENT

Wilkins *et al.* (1971, 1978), Flynn (1979), Lewis (1981), Gill *et al.* (1988) and Rook and Gill (1990) all found significant negative relationships between ammonia-N as a proportion of total nitrogen in silage and silage intake. Wilkins *et al.* (1971, 1978) reported that ammonia-N as a proportion of total-N accounted for 38 and 42% of the variation in the intake of non-formaldehyde-treated silages given to sheep, while Rook and Gill (1990) reported R^2 values of 0.16 to 0.44 for relationships between ammonia-N as a proportion of total N and intake by cattle in different data sets. The latter authors also found that the relationship between ammonia content and intake was curvilinear, with the effect on intake increasing as ammonia-N content increased. However, there is no evidence in the literature that ammonia content *per se* affects silage intake, and consequently the negative relationships between ammonia content and intake may be due to strong relationships between ammonia content and the causal agents. This is supported by the fact that the relationship between intake and ammonia content was not as strong when ammonia content was expressed as g/kg dry matter rather than on a g/kg total nitrogen basis. Furthermore, when Rook *et al.* (1990a) carried out further analyses of the data, coefficients for ammonia-N became very small in all models when collinearity between ammonia content and other parameters was removed, indicating that there was little effect of ammonia content *per se* on intake. They also found a strong correlation between ammonia and volatile fatty acid contents, and the fact that the relationship between ammonia content and intake was removed when collinearity with volatile fatty acid content was removed led them to suggest that volatile fatty acid content was the casual agent.

PH AND TOTAL ACIDITY

Wilkins *et al.* (1971, 1978), Flynn (1979), Jones *et al.* (1980) and Lewis (1981) obtained no significant effect of pH on silage intake, while Gill *et at.,* (1988) and Rook and Gill (1990) obtained significant quadratic effects of pH, the general pattern being a positive relationship at low pH followed by a negative relationship as pH increased, with an inflexion at 4.15. However Rook and Gill (1990) state that this result should be treated with caution as there was confounding between the pH of the silages and level of concentrate supplementation. Any relevance of pH in the control of silage intake is also likely to vary according to the relative content of different acids and the buffering capacity of the silage. McLeod, Wilkins and Raymond (1970) examined the effects of adding sodium bicarbonate to silage and found that a reduction in acidity was accompanied by increased voluntary intake by sheep. However in recent studies involving a wide range of low dry matter silages (< 220 g dry matter/kg) with pH values in the range 3.5 to 4.0, offering sodium bicarbonate did not affect the intake of any of the silages when they were offered to cattle (Steen and Gordon, unpublished results; P. O'Keily, personal communication). Wilkins *et al.* (1971,1978) did not find any significant relationship between total acid content and intake by sheep while Rook and Gill (1990) obtained a significant negative relationship in only one out of three sets of data ($R^2 = 0.13$).

LACTIC ACID

The effects of lactic acid content of silage on intake have been variable. Wilkins *et al.* (1971, 1978) did not obtain a significant relationship between lactic acid content and silage intake by sheep while Jones *et al.* (1980) and Gill *et al.* (1988) found significant negative correlations with the intakes of sheep and dairy cows ($R^2 = 0.07$) respectively. Rook and Gill (1990) obtained a significant positive relationship ($R^2 = 0.07$) in one of three sets of data. Furthermore when Rook and Gill (1990) further analysed their data and removed collinearity, the coefficients for lactic acid became very small, indicating that lactic acid content had little direct effect on intake.

VOLATILE FATTY ACIDS

In a number of studies there have been negative relationships between the contents of individual or total volatile fatty acids in silage and voluntary intake. Wilkins *et al.* (1971)

found that acetic acid content was negatively correlated with intake ($R^2 = 0.25$) while Gill *et al.* (1988) obtained negative relationships between acetic and butyric acid contents and intake by dairy cows (R^2 values 0.15 and 0.03 respectively) and Rook and Gill (1990) obtained negative relationships between acetic, butyric and total volatile fatty acid content and intake (R^2 values 0.20, 0.31 and 0.24 respectively). When collinearity was removed from the data of Rook and Gill (1990), butyric acid content was still strongly correlated with intake, which would suggest that it had an important depressing effect on intake independent of other components within the silages.

There is some evidence that infusion into the rumen or addition to the diet of either acetic (Ulyalt, 1965; Simkins, Suttie and Baumgardt, 1965; Buchanan-Smith, 1990) or butyric acid (Simkins *et al.,* 1965) can depress intake. However when combinations of two volatile acids or one acid plus another nutrient have been added, effects on intake have been inconsistent. For example, when butyric or lactic acids were added to the diet with acetic acid, the depressive effect of acetic added alone was eliminated or even reversed (Buchanan-Smith, 1990). Similarly, when propionic acid was infused into the rumen with acetic, the depression in intake due to acetic alone was eliminated (Bhattacharya and Warner, 1968). The effects of the concentrations of volatile acids in the diet on intake and the interactions between them and other dietary components are complex and the mechanisms involved are likely to include osmotic as well as chemoreceptors (Buchanan-Smith and Phillip, 1986).

AMINES AND OTHER NITROGENOUS COMPOUNDS

Few studies have examined the relationships between the contents of amines or other nitrogenous compounds such as gamma amino butyric acid in silages and their intake. Neumark, Bondi and Volcani (1964) found a negative correlation between tryptamine content of silage and intake, but it is not clear if this was due to the amine content *per se* or an association of higher amine content with other factors. In more recent studies the addition of high levels of putrescine, cadaverine or gamma amino butyric acid to the diet, or infused into the rumen did not significantly affect silage intake by cattle (Dawson and Mayne, 1994a, b). Similarly, Buchanan-Smith (1990) found that the addition of a mixture of putrescine, cadaverine and gamma amino butyric acid to the diet of sham-fed sheep did not depress intake. In fact, intermediate levels of addition tended to increase intake while the highest level of addition had little effect on intake, giving a quadratic response.

DIGESTIBILITY AND FIBRE CONTENT

Studies which have examined the relationship between the digestibility and intake of silage by cattle have generally shown significant positive relationships between digestibility and intake (e.g. Flynn, 1979; Lewis, 1981; Gill *et al.,* 1988; Rook and Gill, 1990). However in studies with sheep there has generally been no significant effect of digestibility on silage intake (e.g. Wilkins *et al.,* 1971, 1978; Jones *et al.,* 1980). This may indicate that compared to digestibility, other components such as products of fermentation and chop length are more important determinants of intake in sheep than in cattle.

Osbourn, Terry, Outen and Cammell (1974) found that intake was more closely related to neutral-detergent fibre (NDF) content than to digestible organic matter content of a range of forages. Mertens (1985) has suggested that NDF content should be a better parameter for predicting forage intake than either acid detergent fibre (ADF) or digestible organic matter content, as it is more closely related to cell wall content of the plant, rate of fibre digestion and hence to digesta volume. He subsequently suggested (Mertens, 1987) that data such as lignin concentration and particle size would also be needed to refine predictions in situations in which physical fill was limiting intake. Mertens' hypothesis is supported by the results of Jones *et al.* (1980) who found that the intakes of high dry matter silages were much more closely related to cell wall content and rate of dry matter disappearance in acid pepsin (correlation coefficients, -0.50 and 0.54 respectively) than to ADF content or dry matter digestibility (correlation coefficients -0.10 and 0.03 respectively).

EFFECTS OF CHOP LENGTH

Studies which have examined relationships between the composition of silages and intake have generally not included consideration of the effects of chop length on intake, possibly because there has been little objective data available on the chop length of the silages involved in the experiments. However there have been many experiments in which silages have been made with different types of equipment to produce silages with different nominal chop lengths and the effects of these on intake and animal performance have been recorded.

The results of an extensive series of studies at Hillsborough involving beef cattle, dairy cows and sheep have been reviewed by Steen (1984), Gordon (1986) and Chestnutt and Kilpatrick (1989) respectively. Grass was harvested with a flail forage harvester producing material with a mean chop length of approximately 85 mm and with a precision-chop harvester producing material with a mean chop length of 25 mm. Shorter chopping increased silage intake by 2%, 4% and 32% with dairy cows, beef cattle (400 to 550 kg live weight) and pregnant/lactating ewes respectively. In these studies the silages offered to the dairy cows, beef cattle and sheep were not harvested simultaneously from the same swards although they were harvested with the same equipment. However in one study, the results of which have been reported by Gordon (1982) and Apolant (1982), silages which had been harvested simultaneously from the same sward were offered to dairy cows and finishing lambs (35 kg live weight). In this case offering finely chopped, precision chopped silage rather than material which had been harvested with a double-chop machine or with a precision-chop machine with some of the blades removed to produce a longer particle length, did not affect the intake of dairy cows but increased the silage intake of lambs by 43 and 59% compared to the double chopped and long precision chopped silages respectively.

Prediction of silage intake

Wilkins *et al.* (1971, 1978), Flynn (1979), Jones *et al.* (1980), Lewis (1981), Rook and Gill (1990) and Rook *et al.* (1990a) have all produced multifactor relationships to predict the silage dry matter intake of sheep or cattle. However each of these models has been based on historical data from a range of experiments and consequently the effects of factors within the silages on intake have been confounded with other factors such as the breed, age, weight, physiological state, previous nutritional history and body condition of the animals, the prevailing environmental conditions at the time of each experiment, feeding management and in some cases also with the effects of level and type of concentrate supplementation and milk yield and stage of lactation of the animals. These confounding effects have reduced the accuracy of the predictive relationships. The value of the relationships produced in a number of the studies has also been limited by a lack of comprehensive data on the chemical compositions of the silages, a limitation which was recognised by Lewis (1981) and Rook, Dhanoa and Gill (1990b). In most cases there has also been no attempt made to validate the models in terms of their ability to predict silage intake.

More recently, work undertaken by Offer, Dewhurst and Thomas (1994), which involved the determination of the intakes of 57 silages by sheep, resulted in stronger relationships between the chemical and biological compositions of the silages and intake. Silage intake by lambs was best predicted by an eight-term principle components regression involving the live weight of the animals and digestible organic matter, crude protein, soluble protein, lactic acid and total volatile acid contents of the silages, and total volatile acids as a proportion of total acids and soluble protein as a proportion of crude protein in the silages. This relationship had an R^2 value of 0.81. However when 16 of the silages were fed to dairy cows the model for lambs poorly predicted silage intake by the cows ($R^2 = 0.31$). When additional parameters were taken into consideration the R^2 value for prediction of intakes by cows from intakes by lambs was improved to 0.79. Offer *et al.* (1994) did not present data on the validation of this model and no information was given on the chop length of the silages or on whether or not the data set involved silages of more than one chop length. This is particularly important in view of the very different effects of chop length on the intakes of silages by sheep and cattle as discussed earlier. There is also further evidence that data relating to the intake of silages by sheep is unlikely to be applicable to cattle (Cushnahan, Gordon, Ferris, Chestnutt and Mayne, 1994).

Direct prediction of intake of forages using near infrared reflectance spectroscopy

Near infrared reflectance spectroscopy (NIRS) has been used successfully for several years to predict, not only the chemical composition of feedstuffs, but also biological parameters such as organic matter digestibility (Norris, Barnes, Moore and Stenk, 1976; Barber, Givens, Kridis, Offer and Murray, 1990). Although there would appear to be no information in the literature on the direct prediction of silage intake using NIRS, it has been used to predict the intake of dried forages (Coelho, Hembry; Barton and Saxton, 1988). Coelho *et al.* (1988) reported an R^2 value of calibration of 0.84 for a multiple-linear regression relationship between second derivative NIRS data and the intake of hays by steers. The R^2 values for relationships between NIRS data and crude protein, NDF and ADF contents and dry matter digestibility of the hays used in the same experiment were 0.97, 0.98, 0.96 and 0.69 respectively. The lower R^2 values for the *in vivo* determinations reflect the greater variability in animal responses to the forages (Coelho *et al.,* 1988). The use of NIRS to directly predict intake also has the advantage that the problems of major collinearity between factors should be minimised by the use of partial least squares analysis or differencing between wavelengths.

Research programme at Hillsborough on the prediction of silage intake

In view of the limitations of previous models based on historical data or data obtained with sheep to predict silage intake by dairy cows and beef cattle, a research programme was initiated at Hillsborough in 1992 with the aim of improving the prediction of silage intake by cattle. The intakes of 136 silages from Northern Ireland farms were determined using 192 individually-fed beef cattle with a mean live weight of 415 kg. The silages were selected on the basis of their pH and dry matter, ammonia and metabolisable energy (predicted by NIRS) contents with the aim of obtaining a wide range of chemical compositions. Approximately seven tonnes of each silage was brought to the Institute by covered lorry. Each lot of silage was mixed in a mixer wagon to achieve uniformity and was then stored in polythene-lined, sealed and evacuated boxes as described by Pippard, Porter, Steen, Gordon, Mayne, Agnew, Unsworth and Kilpatrick (1996) until feeding one to four weeks later. There was no deterioration of the silages during storage and their chemical composition remained constant (Pippard *et al.,* 1996). They were offered to the cattle in two linked change- over design experiments, with each silage being offered as the sole feed to ten animals for a period of two weeks. Eight silages were offered in each of 17 periods and in addition a further 16 animals were offered a standard hay in each period to enable variation in intake due to periods to be removed. Detailed chemical and biological compositions of the silages were determined including *in vivo* digestibility and the use of NIRS and electrometric titration. The ranges in the chemical compositions and intakes of the 136 silages are summarised in Table 5.1. These confirm that the silages had a wide range of chemical compositions.

Table 5.1 RANGES OF CHEMICAL COMPOSITONS AND INTAKES OF SILAGES

Parameter	Range	SD
Dry matter (g/kg)	155 to 413	43.2
Crude protein (g/kg DM)	77 to 212	24.5
Ammonia-N (g/kg total N)	45 to 385	63.5
pH	3.5 to 5.5	0.40
Metabolisable energy (MJ/kg (predicted by NIRS)	8.8 to 12.3	0.8
Silage dry matter intake		
(kg/day)	4.3 to 10.9	1.13
(g/kg $W^{0.75}$)	45 to 113	12.0

Thirteen of the 136 silages were also offered unsupplemented to dairy cows to provide a basis by which the intake system developed from the data produced with beef cattle could be translated for use with dairy cows. In addition sixteen of the silages were offered to dairy cows and growing beef cattle with a range of concentrates. Each silage was supplemented with high-starch and high-fibre concentrates, each with three protein contents and at three levels of supplementation, to examine the interactions between silage type and concentrate type/level of supplementation in terms of their effects on silage intake.

Data from the main study involving the 136 silages offered without supplementation have been used to develop relationships between individual parameters or groups of parameters and intake using simple and multiple-regression analyses. Samples of each of the silages which had been dried at 85°C for 20 hours and allowed to equilibrate under normal laboratory conditions were also presented to a Perstrop Analytical Near Infrared Spectrometer. The spectrum for each sample was recorded over the full range of 400 to 2500 nm at 2 nm intervals. In addition the samples were scanned immediately following re-drying. Modified partial least squares regression analyses was used to investigate the relationship between the spectra for each sample and silage intake. Standard normal variate and detrend mathematical transforms were used to minimise any effects of particle size, temperature or residual moisture. Calibration models were developed separately for the equilibrated and re-dried sample sets and also for the combined sample set.

The relationships between individual parameters and intake have been produced to provide an overview of the extent to which individual parameters were correlated with intake. The R^2 values for these relationships are presented in Table 5.2. However it should be noted that, while these results provide an overall picture of the main groups of

Table 5.2 R^2 VALUES FOR RELATIONSHIPS BETWEEN INDIVIDUAL PARAMETERS AND INTAKE

Parameter (g/kg dry matler unless otherwise stated)	R^2 Linear	Quadratic
Dry matter	0.21	0.22
Crude protein	0.19	0.32
Acid insoluble N	0.08	0.19
Soluble-N (total N minus acid insoluble N)	0.19	0.28
Amino acid-N	0.15	0.16
True protein	0.03	0.09
Ammonia-N (g/kg total N)	0.10	0.09
Soluble-N minus ammonia-N	0.34	0.35
Total N minus ammonia-N	0.33	0.35
Lactic acid	0.01	0.09
Acetic acid	0.05	0.08
Propionic acid	0.07	0.08
Butyric acid	0.04	0.03
Total volatile fatty acids	0.07	0.07
Lactic acid as a proportion of total acids	0.08	0.08
Ethanol	0	0.06
Propanol	0.08	0.08
pH	0	0.08
Buffering capacity (m equiv/kg DM)	0.02	0.02
Total free acids	0.02	0.03
Ether extract	0.12	0.15
Residual sugars	0.08	0.22
Neutral detergent fibre	0.38	0.38
Acid detergent fibre	0.36	0.35
Acid detergent lignin	0.34	0.49
Ash	0	0.08
Digestible organic matter content (predicted by NIRS)	0.19	0.19
Organic matter digestibility (*in vivo*)	0.30	0.29
Dry matter degradability	0.28	0.29
Electrometric titration	0.53	

parameters which are closely related to intake and those which are poorly correlated with intake, excessive emphasises should not be placed on the significance of individual values due to the likelihood of the existence of collinearity between individual parameters.

DRY MATTER CONTENT

The increase in dry matter intake as dry matter content increased is in agreement with the results of previous studies (Wilkins *et al.,* 1971; Flynn, 1979; Lewis, 1981; Gill *et al.,* 1988; Rook and Gill, 1990). However there was no indication of major curvilinearity in the response, in contrast to the findings of Rook and Gill (1990) who found that there was little further increase in intake when dry matter content increased above 250 g/kg.

NITROGEN COMPONENTS

The relationship between crude protein content and intake was much stronger than that found in most previous studies, but was in agreement with the results of Wilkins *et al.* (1971). The pronounced curvilinear nature of the relationship would indicate that there was a strong positive relationship with intake at low nitrogen contents, little increase in intake at nitrogen contents above 140 g/kg dry matter, and a slight decrease above 160 g/kg. The response in intake to increasing protein content is likely to have been at least partly due to low nitrogen supply from the low protein silages reducing digestibility of the fibre components of the diet and hence rate of disappearance and intake due to rumen fill effects. This is in line with the strong relationships between intake and soluble-N, soluble-N minus ammonia-N and amino acid nitrogen contents. Alternatively, an inadequate absorption of nitrogen from the small intestine and supply of nitrogen to the animal's tissues may create an effective energy surplus and reduce intake (Egan, 1965). This is a possible contributing factor to the positive relationship between insoluble-N content and intake. The relationship between ammonia content and intake was weaker than those reported previously (Wilkins *et al.,* 1971, 1978; Rook and Gill, 1990). Furthermore the fact that the R^2 value for the relationship between ammonia-N content, expressed on a g/kg total N basis and intake was 0.10, while the R^2 value was only 0.01 when ammonia content was expressed on a g/kg dry matter basis, would indicate that the former relationship was not due to ammonia content *per se,* but rather to an association between ammonia content and some other parameter(s) within the silages which was the causal agent.

DIGESTIBILITY, DEGRADABILITY AND FIBRE FRACTIONS

The positive relationship between *in vivo* organic matter digestibility and intake is in agreement with the results of previous studies involving cattle (Flynn, 1979; Lewis, 1981; Gill *et al.,* 1988; Rook and Gill, 1990). However the relationship was much stronger than those reported previously. For example, Gill *et al.* (1988) and Rook and Gill (1990) reported R^2 values of 0.03 to 0.12 for relationships between digestibility and intake compared to the value of 0.30 in the Hillsborough studies. The relationship between digestibility and intake indicates that intake increased by 1.5% of the mean intake of all 136 silages for each 10 g/kg increase in digestibility. This is close to the response in intake of 1.7 % per 10 g/kg increase in digestibility reported by Steen (1988) from a review of the results of eight experiments which examined the effects of predetermined differences in digestibility (by cutting grass at different stages of growth), on the intake and performance of beef cattle offered the silages as the sole diet. The fact that very similar relationships between digestibility and intake have been obtained for experimentally produced silages and silages from farms is particularly reassuring, and provides strong evidence for the validity of this relationship.

Osbourn *et al.* (1974) found that intake was more highly correlated with NDF content than with digestible organic matter content, while Mertens (1985) suggested that NDF content would be a better predictor of intake than either ADF or digestible organic matter content, as NDF is more closely related to the cell wall content of the plant and hence to rate of digestion and digesta volume. However in the Hillsborough study relationships between intake and ADF and NDF were similar ($R^2 = 0.36$ and 0.38) while the quadratic relationship for acid detergent lignin (ADL) was strongest ($R^2 = 0.49$). Intake was also strongly related to *in vivo* dry matter degradability, R^2 values being 0.28 and 0.26 for assumed rumen outflow rates of 0.05 and 0.08 per hour respectively. Data on degradabilities of NDF and ADF and hemicellulose in this study are not yet available but should be of particular interest in terms of contributing to the understanding of the parameters which controlled intake in this study.

LACTIC AND VOLATILE FATTY ACID CONTENTS

The contents of lactic, acetic, propionic and butyric acids and total volatile fatty acids were very weakly related to intake ($R^2 = 0.01$ to 0.09). This was despite the fact that there were wide ranges in the contents of these acids in the silages, these being 0 to 144 (S.D. 34.7); 4 to 63 (S.D. 12.7); 0 to 13 (S.D. 3.1) and 0 to 32 (S.D. 7.0) g/kg dry matter respectively. As discussed previously, the mechanisms through which an increase in the concentrations of lactic or volatile fatty acids in the diet may affect intake are complex and poorly understood. However, unless there was strong collinearity between these and other factors within the silages, the results of the studies at Hillsborough would indicate that the concentrations of lactic and volatile fatty acids in silage or their relative proportions, are of little importance in determining intake.

PH AND TOTAL ACIDITY

The pH, total free acid content and buffering capacity of the silages were also very weakly related to intake (R^2 0 to 0.08). The quadratic relationship between pH and intake, followed a similar trend to that produced by Rook and Gill (1990), in that there was a slight positive relationship at low pH followed by a negative relationship at high pH and maximum intake at pH 4.3. However the relationship was much weaker than that reported by Rook and Gill (1990).

OTHER PARAMETERS

Relationships between ethanol and propanol contents and intake were weak($R^2 = 0.06$ and 0.08 respectively). The relationship with residual sugar content was strongly curvilinear ($R^2 = 0.22$), with a strong positive relationship at low sugar contents and a decreasing response in intake at higher sugar contents. However it is not clear to what extent relationships with parameters such as oil and sugar content are direct effects and to what extent they are due to collinearity with other factors.

The best relationship between electrometric titration and intake had an R^2 value of 0.53. This would appear to have been largely attributable to strong relationships between the contents of total soluble-N, amino acid-N and reducing sugars on a fresh basis (estimated by electrometric titration) and intake. The R^2 values for the relationships between these three parameters and intake were 0.35, 0.32 and 0.30 respectively. These were partly attributable to the relationship between silage dry matter content and intake, as the relationships for the contents of soluble-N, amino acid-N and reducing sugars expressed on a dry matter basis had R^2 values of only 0.17, 0.16 and 0.04 respectively.

MULTIPLE REGRESSION RELATIONSHIPS

Multiple regression analyses have been used to produce relationships between intake and a range of chemical parameters in the silages. For this purpose the 136 silages were divided into two groups, one of 91 and the other of 45 silages. Relationships were produced using the 91 silages and the other 45 silages were used for validation of the relationships. The best of these relationships had an R^2 value of calibration of 0.69 and an R^2 of prediction of 0.63. However this relationship involved parameters such as ether extract and ADL which would not normally be determined in routine silage analyses. A relationship involving only dry matter, nitrogen and ammonia contents and pH had an R^2 of calibration of 0.63 and an R^2 of prediction of 0.56. When ADF content and electrometric titration were added to these four parameters, the best relationship had an R^2 of calibration of 0.65 and an R^2 of prediction of 0.61.

DIRECT PREDICTION OF INTAKE BY NIRS

The best overall relationship was between NIR spectra and intake. When calibration models were developed separately for the equilibrated and re-dried sample sets and for the combined sample set, R^2 values were 0.85, 0.85 and 0.86 respectively and the standard error of calibration was 4.3 g/kg $W^{0.75}$ for all three relationships. Two approaches to validation of the relationships were undertaken. Firstly cross validation of the model for the re-dried samples was also undertaken. For this purpose the spectra for one of the 136 silages was removed from the set and a model produced using the spectra for the remaining 135 silages. The intake of the remaining silage was then predicted using the model based on the other 135 samples. This procedure was repeated for each of the 136 silages. The R^2 of prediction was 0.73 and the standard error of cross validation was 6.1 g/kg $W^{0.75}$. In the second approach to validation the spectra for the equilibrated and re-dried samples were divided at random into two batches, one of 94 and one of 42. A calibration model was produced using the larger set of spectra and this was then used to predict the intakes of the other 42 silages. This procedure gave an R^2 of prediction of 0.71 and a standard error of prediction of 5.5 g/kg$W^{0.75}$ Although this standard error, at 7.7% of the mean intake of the 136 silages, is numerically large in comparison with the standard errors obtained when the chemical composition or organic matter digestibility of silages have been predicted by NIRS, it is not large relative to the accuracy with which silage intake can be determined *in vivo*. For example, the typical standard error for the determination of organic matter digestibility is 0.007 while Barber *et al.* (1990) and Baker, Givens and Deaville (1994) reported standard errors of prediction of 0.026 and 0.0235 respectively for the prediction of organic matter digestibility by NIRS. Thus the standard error of prediction of organic matter digestibility by NIRS is 3-4 times the typical standard error of determination. By comparison if the typical standard error for the determination of silage dry matter intake is taken as 2.8 g/kg $W^{0.75}$ (i.e. 4% of the mean intake), then the standard error of prediction of intake by NIRS was less than twice the standard error of determination.

APPLICATION OF THE PREDICTION OF SIIAGE INTAKE BY NIRS

Prediction of silage intake by cattle has now been commissioned on a commercial basis in Northern Ireland, and routine laboratory analyses of silage samples now includes a prediction of the intake potential of each silage. Intake is predicted on a g dry matter/kg metabolic live weight basis. This value is then used directly to calculate the potential intake by beef cattle of various live weights. In the case of dairy cows, a conversion relationship has been produced, based on the intakes of the 13 silages which were offered unsupplemented to both beef cattle and dairy cows, which enables the intake value to be converted into an actual predicted daily intake for dairy cows. Feeding models are currently being produced for both beef cattle and dairy cows which will use the predicted silage intakes to calculate total metabolisable energy intakes and predict performance for different inputs of concentrates, or alternatively, predict the inputs of concentrates required to sustain given levels of performance.

INTERACTION BETWEEN CONCENTRATE AND SILAGE TYPE

As outlined previously 16 of the silages used in the main study were also offered to dairy cows and beef cattle with a wide range of levels and types of concentrate supplementation. Statistical analyses of the data for these 16 silages which were supplemented with different levels and types of concentrates have shown linear relationships between concentrate intake level and silage intake. Overall there was a tendency for substitution rate to be higher at the higher inputs of concentrates but this curvilinear effect was not significant. The mean substitution rate decreased with increasing crude protein content in the concentrates, the mean overall substitution rates being 0.46, 0.43 and 0.36 for the concentrates containing 120, 190 and 260 g crude protein/kg respectively. There was no overall difference in the mean substitution rates for the high-starch and high-fibre concentrates. However there were important interactions between silage type and concentrate type in terms of substitution rate. For example, silages A and B had very different patterns of fermentation but similar intakes when offered without supplementation as shown in Table 5.3. Yet silage A had a much lower intake (higher substitution rate) when supplemented with the high- starch concentrate than when supplemented with the high-fibre concentrate, while for silage B the two concentrate types had the opposite effect on silage intake. Prediction of these interactions is vitally important and research in this area is currently being pursued further at Hillsborough. In addition research is also aimed at elucidating the mechanisms involved in producing these interactions, with a view to providing a scientific basis on which different types of silages can be supplemented with the most appropriate type of concentrates.

Table 5.3 INTERACTION BETWEEN SILAGE TYPE AND CONCENTRATE TYPE

	Silage	
	A	B
Silage intake without supplement (kg DM/day)	11.2	11.4
Substitution rate		
High-starch concentrate	0.48	0.39
High-fibre concentrate	0.28	0.55

Conclusions

Silage intake was strongly related to the contents of a number of nitrogen and fibre components, digestibility, dry matter degradability and residual water soluble carbohydrate content ($R^2 = 0.19$ to 0.49).

Intake was either unrelated to, or only weakly related to, pH, buffering capacity, total acidity and the concentrations of lactic acid and volatile fatty acids ($R^2 < 0.09$).

The use of NIRS is a very simple and low-cost method of providing the most accurate prediction of silage intake.

Current research is elucidating the interactions between silage type and concentrate type, in terms of substitution rate, and this must be central to any approach to designing diets, particularly for dairy cows receiving moderately high levels of concentrates.

Acknowledgements

The authors wish to express their thanks to the Northern Ireland Grain Trade Association, the Milk Marketing Board for Northern Ireland and Strathroy Milk Marketing Ltd for financial support for the programme of research at Hillsborough on the prediction of silage intake.

References

Apolant, S.M. (1982) *A study on the value of grass silage-based diets for sheep with particular reference to the breeding ewe.* PhD Thesis, The Queen's University of Belfast

Baker, C.W., Givens, D.I. and Deaville, E.R. (1994) Prediction of organic matter digestibility *in vivo* of grass silage by near infrared reflectance spectroscopy: effect of calibration method, residual moisture and particle size. *Animal Feed Science and Technology,* **50**, 17-26

Balch, C.C. and Campling, R.C. (1962) Regulation of food intake by ruminants. *Nutrition Abstracts and Reviews,* **32**, 669-686

Barber, G.D., Givens, D.I., Kridis, M.S., Offer, N.W. and Murray, I. (1990) Prediction of the organic matter digestibility of grass silage. *Animal Feed Science and Technology,* **28**, 115-128

Bhattacharya, A.N. and Warner, R.G. (1968) Effect of propionate and citrate on depressed feed intake after intraruminal infusions of acetate in dairy cattle. *Journal of Dairy Science,* **51**, 1091-1094

Buchanan-Smith, J.G. (1990) An investigation into palatability as a factor responsible for reduced intake of silage by sheep. *Animal Production,* **50**, 253-260

Buchanan-Smith, J. G. and Phillip, L.E. (1986) Food intake in sheep following intraruminal infusion of extracts from lucerne silage with particular reference to organic acids and products of protein degradation. *Journal of Agricultural Science, Cambridge,* **106**,611-617

Chestnutt, D.M.B. and Kilpatrick, DJ. (1989) Effect of silage type and concentrate supplementation on the intake and performance of breeding ewes. *62nd Annual Report, Agricultural Research Institute of Northern Ireland,* pp. 21-30

Coelho, M., Hembry, F.G., Barton, F.E. and Saxton, A.M. (1988) A comparison of microbial, enzymatic, chemical and near-infrared reflectance spectroscopy methods in forage evaluation. *Animal Feed Science and Technology,* **20**,219-231

Conrad, H.R. (1966) Symposium on factors influencing the voluntary intake of herbage by ruminants: physiological and physical factors limiting feed intake. *Journal of Animal Science,* **25**, 227-235

Conrad, H.R., Pratt, A.D. and Hibbs, J.W. (1964) Regulation of feed intake in dairy cows. I. Change in importance of physical and physiological factors with increasing digestibility. *Journal. of Dairy Science,* **47**, 54-62

Cushnahan, A. and Gordon, F J. (1995) The effects of grass preservation on intake, digestibility and rumen degradation characteristics. *Animal Science* (In press)

Cushnahan, A., Gordon, FJ., Ferris, C.P.W., Chestnutt, D.M.B. and Mayne, C.S. (1994) The use of sheep as a model to predict the relative intakes of silages by dairy cattle. *Animal Production,* **59**, 415-420

Cushnahan, A. and Mayne, C.S. (1994) Effects of ensilage and silage fermentation pattern on the intake and performance of lactating dairy cows. *Animal Production,* **58**, 427 (Abstract)

Dawson, L.E.R. and Mayne, C.S. (1994a) The effects of either dietary addition or intraruminal infusion of amines or juice extracted from grass silage on the voluntary intake of steers offered grass silage. *Animal Production,* **58**, 427 (Abstract)

Dawson, L.E.R. and Mayne, C.S. (1994b) The effect of infusion of amines and gamma amino butyric acid on the intake by steers of grass silage differing in lactic acid content. *Proceedings of the 4th Research Meeting, British Grassland Society,* pp. 69-70

Demarquilly, C. (1973) Chemical composition, fermentation characteristics, digestibility and voluntary intake of forage silages: changes com- pared to the initial green forage. *Annates de Zootechnie,* **22**, 199-218

Dinius, D.A. and Baumgardt, B.R. (1970) Regulation of food intake in ruminants. 6. Influence of caloric density of pelleted rations. *Journal of Dairy Science,* **53**, 311-316

Egan, A.R. (1965) Nutritional status and intake regulation in sheep. III. The relationship between improvement in nitrogen status and increase in voluntary intake of low-protein roughages by sheep. *Australian Journal of Agricultural Research,* **16**, 463-472

Flynn, A. V .(1978) The effect of ensiling on the beef production potential of grass. *Proceedings of the 5th Silage Conference, Ayr,* pp. 48-49

Flynn, A. V. (1979) The effect of silage dry-matter digestibility *in vitro* on live-weight gain and carcass gain by beef cattle fed silage *ad libitum. Animal Production,* **28**, 423 (Abstract)

Gill, M., Rook, AJ. and Thiago, L.R.S. (1988) Factors affecting the voluntary intake of roughages by the dairy cow. *In Nutrition and Lactation in the dairy cow,* pp. 262-279. Edited by P.C. Garnsworthy. London: Butterworths

Gordon, F J. (1982) The effects of degree of chopping grass for silage and method of concentrate allocation on the performance of dairy cows. *Grass and Forage Science,* **37**, 59-65

Gordon, F J. (1986) The influence of system of harvesting grass for silage on milk production. *Jubilee Report, Agricultural Research Institute of Northern Ireland,* pp. 13-22

Jones, G.M. (1972) Chemical factors and their relation to feed intake regulation in ruminants: a review. *Canadian Journal of Animal Science,* **52**, 207-239

Jones, G.M., Larsen, R.E. and Lanning, N.M. (1980) Prediction of silage digestibility and intake by chemical analyses or *in vitro* fermentation techniques. *Journal of Dairy Science,* **63**, 579-586

Journet, M. and Remond, B. (1976) Physiological factors affecting the voluntary intake of feed by cows: a review. *Livestock Production Science,* **3**, 129-146

Ketelaars,JJ .M.H. and Tolkemp, BJ. (1992) Toward a new theory of feed intake regulation in ruminants. 1. Causes of differences in voluntary feed intake: critique of current views. *Livestock Production Science,* **30**, 269-296

Lehmann, F. (1941) Die Lehre vom Ballast. *Jeitschrifl fur T zerernahrung und FuttermittelAunde,5,* 155-173

Lewis, M. (1981) Equations for predicting silage intake by beef and dairy cattle. *Proceedings of the Sixth Silage Conference, Edinburgh,* pp. 35-36

McLeod, D.S., Wilkins, RJ. and Raymond, W.F. (1970) The voluntary intake by sheep and cattle of silages differing in free-acid content. *Journal of Agricultural Science, Cambridge,* **75**, 311-319

Mertens, D .R. (1985) Effect of fibre on feed quality for dairy cows. *Proceedings of the 46th Minnesota Nutrition Conference,* pp. 209-224

Mertens, D.R. (1987) Predicting intake and digestibility using mathematical models of ruminal function. *Journal of Animal Science,* **64**, 1548-1558

Neumark, H., Bondi, A. and Volcani, R. (1964) Amines, aldehydes and keto-acids in silages and their effect on food intake in ruminants. *Journal of the Science of Food and Agriculture,* **15,** 487-492

Norris, K.H., Barnes, R.F., Moore,].E. and Stenk,].S. (1976) Predicting forage quality by infrared reflectance spectroscopy. *Journal of Animal Science,* **43,** 889-897

Offer, N.W., Dewhurst, RJ. and Thomas, C. (1994) The use of electro- metric titration to improve the routine prediction of silage intake by lambs and dairy cows. *Animal Production,* **58,** 427 (Abstract)

Osbourn, D.F., Terry, R.A., Outen, G.E. and Gammell, S.B. (1974) The significance of a determination of cell walls as the rational basis for the nutritive evaluation of forages. *Proceedings of the 12th International Grassland Congress, Moscow,* Vol III, pp. 374-380

Pippard, CJ., Porter, M.G., Steen, R.W.J., Gordon, FJ., Mayne, C.S., Agnew, R.E., Unsworth, E.F. and Kilpatrick, DJ. (1996) A method for obtaining and storing uniform silage for feeding experiments. *Animal Feed Science and Technology,* **57,** 87-95

Rook, AJ. and Gill, M. (1990) Prediction of the voluntary intake of grass silages by beef cattle. 1. Linear regression analyses. *Animal Production,* **50,** 425-438

Rook, AJ., Dhanoa, M.S. and Gill, M. (1990a) Prediction of the voluntary intake of grass silages by beef cattle. 2. Principal component and ridge regression analyses. *Animal Production,* **50,** 439-454

Rook, AJ., Dhanoa, M.S. and Gill, M. (1 990b) Prediction of the voluntary intake of grass silages by beef cattle. 3. Precision of alternative prediction models. *Animal Production,* **50,** 455-466

Simkins, K.L., Suttie, J.W. and Baumgardt, B.R. (1965) Regulation of food intake in ruminants. 4. Effects of acetate, propionate, butyrate and glucose on voluntary food intake in dairy cattle. *Journal of Dairy Science,* **48,** 1635-1642

Steen, R.WJ. (1984) The effects of wilting and mechanical treatment of grass prior to ensiling on the performance of beef cattle and beef output per hectare. *57th Annual Report, Agricultural Research Institute of Northern Ireland,* pp. 21-32

Steen, R.W J. (1988) Factors affecting the utilization of grass silage for beef production. In. Efficient Beef Production from Grass. (Ed.]. Frame). *Occasional Publication No. 22, British Grassland Society,* pp. 129-139

Ulyatt, MJ. (1965) The effects of intraruminal infusions of volatile fatty acids on food intake of sheep. *New Zealand Journal of Agricultural Science,* **8,** 397-408

Wilkins, RJ., Fenlon, J.S., Cook,j.E. and Wilson, R.F. (1978) A further analysis of relationships between silage composition and voluntary intake by sheep. *Proceedings of the 5th Silage Conference, Ayr,* pp. 34-35

Wilkins, RJ., Hutchinson, KJ., Wilson, R.F. and Harris, C.E. (1971) The voluntary intake of silage by sheep. 1. Interrelationships between silage composition and intake. *Journal of Agricultural Science, Cambridge,* **77,** 531-537

This paper was first published in 1995

6

COMPLEMENTARY FORAGES FOR MILK PRODUCTION

R.H. PHIPPS
University of Reading Centre for Dairy Research, Arborfield Hall Farm, Church Lane, Arborfield, Reading RG2 9HX, UK

Introduction

Following the introduction of quotas on milk production in the UK, many farmers reduced the amount of concentrates given to dairy cows and attempted to place greater reliance on high quality, home-produced forage. To achieve this objective they required well-fermented silage with high intake characteristics and a high energy content. These criteria were not easily achieved on a regular basis with grass. The availability of new early-maturing maize hybrids, a growing awareness of environmental issues associated with intensive grassland use and the less aggressive approach of allied commercial organizations also encouraged dairy farmers to consider the potential for integrating complementary forages into diet based on grass silage.

At present, however, the seven million hectares of effective grassland in the UK still provide the most important single source of grazed and conserved forage for ruminant livestock production. This is in marked contrast to mainland Europe where crops such as maize, fodder beet and whole crop cereals have played a major role for the last 25 years in dairy cow rations. In France, Germany and Holland, for example, four million ha of maize are now grown annually for silage, while in Denmark fodder beet and silage made from whole-crop cereals are an integral part of many milk production systems.

In 1492, Christopher Columbus described maize in his log as "a sort of grain like millet, which is very well tasted when boiled, roasted or made into porridge". Early European settlers in North America were equally fulsome in their praise and considered that "it is the best fodder that grows" (Weatherwax, 1954). The benefits associated with feeding roots to dairy cows were described in 1913 by Haecker. He stated that "Roots are excellent feed for dairy cows and are especially desirable as they are palatable, easy to digest, and stimulate the flow of milk. They are especially effective with cows that freshened in the spring and whose flow of milk has been depressed during the summer, because of annoyance by flies and mosquitoes and unfavourable pasture conditions. Less grain is required while roots are being fed."

It is only recently, however, that complementary forages, such as maize or fodder beet, have been taken at all seriously in the UK. This paper will consider the potential role of complementary forages for milk production in the cooler climate of northern Europe. While particular attention will be given to forage maize, since the area grown in the UK has increased from 35,000 ha in 1990 to 77,000 ha in 1993, the role of fodder beet, brewers grains and whole crop wheat will also be reviewed.

Production constraints

FODDER BEET

Although many trials have shown that the inclusion of fodder beet in dairy cow rations will increase feed intake and milk production, and enhance both milk fat and protein concentration (Roberts and Martindale, 1990; Phipps, Sutton, Jones, Allen and Fisher, 1993), the area grown in the Netherlands has decreased from 58,000 ha in 1958 to 2,000 ha in 1988, and only a small area is currently grown in the UK (Kleinhout, 1990). The dairy industry has clearly failed to capitalise on a valuable forage resource. The failure to do so is attributed to the high input requirements both in terms of crop production and in the handling, cleaning and feeding of fodder beet throughout the winter. Kleinhout (1990) has suggested the use of whole-crop fodder beet silage as a means to overcome the management and labour disadvantages currently associated with fodder beet.

WHOLE-CROP WHEAT

Interest in whole-crop wheat as a complementary forage crop was greatly enhanced by the drought years of 1989/1990, when many farmers failed to make sufficient grass silage. Under these conditions whole-crop wheat was either ensiled or preserved through the application of urea. While there are no technical constraints in the production of either form of forage, the application of large quantities of urea is environmentally unattractive. To justify the use of urea it must be established that it is efficiently utilised by the ruminant and not excreted as a pollutant. While large differences have been established between the yield and quality of winter wheat varieties when assessed as a complementary forage (Weller, Cooper and Phipps, 1993), it is doubtful whether varieties will be bred especially for whole-crop conservation as this is unlikely to become a major forage resource in the UK.

MAIZE

The successful utilisation of forage maize depends on the production of maize silage with a high dry matter (DM) content. This is essential as silage intake is positively related to silage DM content (Table 6.1). This relationship was first noted in the USA by Bechdel (1926) and has subsequently been confirmed in many parts of Europe, including a recent study conducted by Phipps, *et al* (2000) which examined not only the effect of crop maturity on feed intake and milk of maize silage for lactating dairy cows, but also the effect of crop maturity on energy and nitrogen utilization (Cammell *et al.,* 2000) and ruminal and post-ruminal digestion (Sutton *et al.,* 2000). Thus, in the relatively cool climatic conditions of Northern Europe, the major constraint to the successful production and subsequent efficient utilisation of maize silage is the availability of suitable plant material. Hybrids must have a maturity rating that will produce crops at harvest with 300 to 350 g DM /kg. Failure to do so must bring into question the strategy of using maize silage as a complementary forage, as the objective of producing cheap, high energy, home-produced forage with high intake characteristics is unlikely to be achieved. Table 6.2 shows that since 1973 the maturity of available hybrids recommended for use in the UK has increased dramatically (National Institute of Agricultural Botany, 1973, 1982, 1993).

Table 6.1 EFFECT OF SILAGE DM CONTENT ON SILAGE DM INTAKE IN LACTATING DAIRY COWS

	Silage DM content (g/kg)			
	200	*250*	*300*	*350*
Silage DM intake (kg/day)	10.5	11.5	13.0	15.0

(Demarquilly, 1988)

Table 6.2 CHANGE IN DM CONTENT (g/kg DM) OF MAIZE VARIETIES GROWN IN THE UK

	Dry matter content (g/kg DM)		
Variety	*1973*	*1982*	*1993*
Pursan			425
Energy			325
LG11		291	
Dorina		264	
Asgrow 88	259		
Inra 321	193		

(National Institute of Agricultural Botany, 1973, 1982, 1993)

This development is the major reason why the area grown in the UK has more than trebled in the last five years. Growers must, however, be aware that the recommended list is a five-year average. Thus the results presented in the 1993 recommended list of hybrids for the UK represents perhaps an unduly optimistic picture as it includes three hot, dry summers. After the more typical English summer of 1993, farmers will no doubt pay increased attention to crop maturity and, in the more marginal areas, may even consider the wisdom of growing forage maize at all. Those who persist should be aware not only of the importance of varietal differences in crop maturity, but also the significant effect that site selection can exert on crop maturity, and the need to avoid adverse growing conditions such as exposed chalk outcrops and cold, wet clays (Carr and Hough, 1979). For the continued expansion northwards of the forage maize crop the production of even earlier maturing hybrids will be required.

Phipps (1992) predicted that the area of maize grown in the UK would increase in 1993 from 50,000 to 65,000 ha, a rise of 30% (Figure 6.1). He also calculated that an annual increase thereafter of 10% would result in 160,000 ha of silage maize in the UK by the turn of the century. The prediction for 1993 was low, as 77,000 ha were grown (Alderton, 1993). It is suggested that although there are serious climatic constraints to the production of forage maize, the area suitable for production is sufficiently large for maize silage to make a major contribution to ruminant livestock production systems. Its importance as a forage resource is only likely to increase.

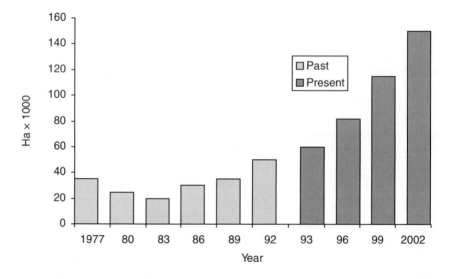

Figure 6.1 The past, present and predicted area of maize grown for silage in the UK

These developments, however, may be overtaken by global warming as climatologists (Parry, Carter and Jones, 1990) have estimated that with an increase in ambient temperature of 2°C, which is predicted by the year 2020, the whole of lowland Britain will be suitable for silage maize and the southern half of England for grain maize (Figure

6.2). We await developments with interest, particularly in the light of earlier comments made by Gerard (1597) who reported that maize "commeth to ripeness when the summer falleth out to be faire and hot."

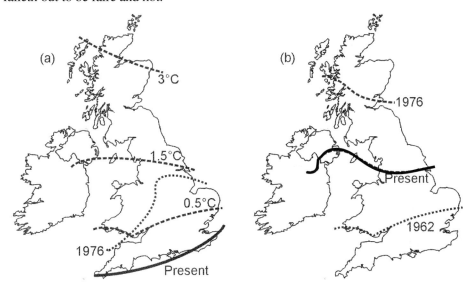

Figure 6.2 The present (solid line) and hypothetical limits (broken line) and individual years (dotted line) for successful ripening in lowland conditions of (a) grain maize and (b) silage maize for arbitrary adjustment in mean temperature.

Chemical composition and nutritive value

VARIATION BETWEEN COMPLEMENTARY FORAGE CROPS

There are major differences between the chemical composition and nutritive value of complementary forages and grass silage. These differences are illustrated in Table 6.3 (Phipps *et al.*, 1993, Phipps, 1993). Grass silage and fermented whole- crop wheat contain only traces of either starch or water soluble carbohydrates so the main source of energy is derived from their fibre component. In marked contrast, starch is the most important energy source in both urea treated whole- crop wheat and maize silage, where it may form over 250 g/kg DM. While starch is the primary energy source for these two complementary forage crops, the nutritional properties of wheat and maize starch vary markedly. De Visser (1993) reported that the effective rumen-resistant starch was 410 g/kg total starch for maize compared with 80 g/kg for wheat. With fodder beet, the main energy component is water soluble carbohydrates, which represents over 600 g/kg DM, while in brewers grains the highly digestible fibre is the primary energy source.

Table 6.3 CHEMICAL COMPOSITION AND NUTRITIVE VALUE OF GRASS SILAGE (GS), MAIZE SILAGE (MS), FERMENTED (FWC) AND UREA-TREATED (UWC) WHOLE-CROP WHEAT, FODDER BEET (FB) AND BREWERS GRAINS (BG)

| | *Forages* | | | | | |
	GS	*FWC*	*UWC*	*BG*	*FB*	*MS*
DM content (g/kg)	266	323	495	277	155	383
DM composition (g/kg)						
Crude protein	141	119	163	245	103	87
Starch	Trace	Trace	280	Trace	Trace	261
Water soluble carbohydrates	Trace	Trace	Trace	Trace	620	Trace
Neutral detergent fibre	525	528	490	468	192	429
Total ash	92				70/157	42
Metabolisable energy						
(MJ/kg DM)	11.0	9.9	10.7	11.5	11.9/10.9	10.9

(Phipps, 1993; Phipps et al., 1993)

Table 6.3 also shows marked variation in the protein content of complementary forages and grass silage. The protein content of fodder beet and maize silage is similar but lower than grass silage. Although of similar protein content, there is evidence that with fodder beet protein is readily degraded in the rumen (Roberts and Martindale, 1990), while with maize it is relatively undegradable (Phipps, Weller and Smith, 1981). Due to the application of urea and its subsequent hydrolysis to ammonia, the protein (total N x 6.25) content of urea-treated whole-crop wheat is higher than that of the fermented product, but similar to that of grass silage. However, the ammonia nitrogen content of urea-treated whole-crop wheat is over three times that of grass silage.

VARIATION WITHIN MAIZE SILAGE

As forage maize matures a number of significant changes occur in its chemical composition and nutritive value. The extent of these changes and how they are influenced by climate is illustrated in Figure 6.3 (Wilkinson and Osbourn, 1975). With advancing crop maturity, the proportion of ear, and therefore the concentration of starch in the total DM increases, as water soluble carbohydrates are translocated from the stover and deposited as starch in the ear component. Thus, as the crop matures, the main energy source changes from sugar to starch. While *in vitro* studies conducted by De Visser (1993) indicated that a proportion of by pass starch increased with advancing crop maturity and that variation exists between hybrids (Table 6.4) recent *in vivo* studies

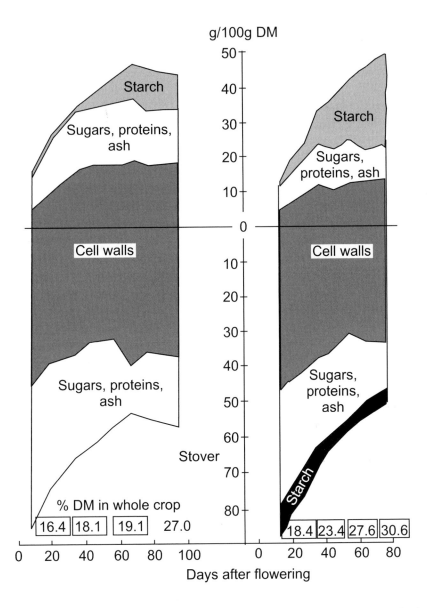

Figure 6.3 Effect of advancing crop maturity and climate on chemical composition of forage maize in two contrasting years.

carried out by Sutton *et al* (2000) suggests otherwise. Their study concluded that while increasing crop maturity resulted in a large increase in the contribution of starch to DM digested in the rumen there were only small differences in rumen fermentation. Although post ruminal starch digestion doubled this was due to the increased starch concentration of the silage rather than major changes in digestion and the amount is small compared with the likely result from feeding maize grain. The movement of nutrients from stover to ear reduces the concentration of cell walls (neutral detergent fibre) in the ear component, but results in an increased concentration of cell walls and thus reduced energy value in the stover. Advancing crop maturity also results in reduced fermentation in the silo that effects a progressive decrease in acid content and a reduction in the proportion of the total nitrogen degraded to non-protein nitrogen (Wilkinson, 1979). The methionine and lysine content of maize silage nitrogen also decreases with increasing crop maturity (Phipps and Oldham, 1979). Although there is conflicting evidence in the literature, Rulquin and Verite (1993) concluded that methionine and lysine were the first limiting amino acids in maize based diets and that correction of this limitation increased milk yield and the true protein content of milk without affecting the concentration of milk fat.

Table 6.4 THE RELATIONSHIP BETWEEN CROP MATURITY, STARCH CONTENT AND PROPORTION OF STARCH RESISTANT TO RUMEN BREAKDOWN

Maize variety	DM matter (g/kg)	Starch (g/kg DM)	Proportion of resistant starch (g/kg DM)
Anjou	198	154	60
	237	270	170
	315	340	390
Scana	228	156	70
	275	233	170
	331	292	250

(De Visser, 1993)

It should be noted that conventional plant selection and breeding techniques have produced strains of maize where the protein content of the grain is over 250 g/kg DM (Dudley and Lambert, 1969) and where the essential amino acid content has been significantly improved by the incorporation of the *Opaque-2* mutant gene (Mertz, Bates and Nelson, 1964). It is interesting to speculate when the genetic engineers will be able to incorporate these genes into commercial plant material, as success in this area will have a profound effect on both animal and human nutrition on a global scale.

The nutritional characteristics of the energy and protein sources provided by complementary forages differ widely and vary markedly compared with those of grass silage. Thus their inclusion as part of the forage component should be capable of providing a more synchronised supply of energy and protein needed to meet the nutritional requirements of the dairy cows, than if only one forage source was available.

Benefits from the use of complementary forage crops

For ruminant livestock producers to consider growing an alternative forage crop there must be some clear positive benefit that will improve the financial viability of the farming enterprise. The possible advantages may include, lower forage production costs, increased forage intake as a result of improved forage quality, reduced concentrate input and improved product quality that will increase output value.

FORAGE PRODUCTION COSTS

Pain and Phipps (1975) established that, when compared with grass silage, the lower inorganic fertiliser requirement for maize silage resulted in lower support- energy inputs, reduced forage costs and a decreased energy input:output ratio. More recent calculations (Straghan and Perry, 1993) have confirmed that maize silage and fodder beet are cheaper sources of energy when compared with grass silage. Mogg (1992) calculated that the Common Agricultural Policy payment for maize silage will further reduce production costs to the point where it is cheaper in 1994 than grazed grass (Table 6.5). It is interesting to speculate how long this ridiculous situation will be allowed to exist. There is no doubt that this policy has contributed to the increased area grown in 1993.

Table 6.5 PRODUCTION COSTS OF A RANGE OF FORAGE CROPS AND THE EFFECT OF THE COMMON AGRICULTURAL POLICY PAYMENT FOR FORAGE MAIZE

Forage	*1992*	*1993*	*1994*
Grass-grazed	2.57	2.57	2.57
Grass-silage	5.80	5.80	5.80
Fodder beet	3.82	3.82	3.82
Whole crop wheat (4% urea)	4.57	3.62	2.70
Maize silage	3.70	2.70	1.66

(Mogg, 1992 unpublished data)

FORAGE INTAKE AND MILK PRODUCTION

Numerous trials have established that the use of fodder beet to replace part of either the forage or the concentrate component of the diet will increase feed intake (Castle, Drysdale, Waite and Watson, 1963; Brabander, Aerts, Boucque and Buysse, 1976; Sabri and Roberts, 1988; Kleinhout, 1990). When reviewing the results of these trials, Roberts and Martindale (1990) concluded that the increased intake was usually reflected in increased milk production.

Trials at both Wye College and at the Centre for Dairy Research at Reading have shown that the inclusion of either urea-treated or fermented whole-crop wheat in grass silage based diets increased forage intake (Leaver and Hill, 1992; Phipps, Weller and Siviter 1992a; Phipps, Sutton, Jones and Fisher, 1993), but that this was rarely reflected in increased milk production. In the case of urea-treated whole-crop wheat, Hill and Leaver (1991) speculated that a considerable proportion of the energy derived from the increased intake was used for the excretion of surplus non-protein nitrogen and was therefore unavailable for milk production. Recent work by Hill and Leaver (1993) has now shown that as the inclusion rate of urea-treated whole-crop wheat in a grass silage based diet increased there was a significant increase in blood urea levels. They also reported that the organic matter and neutral and acid detergent fibre digestibility values all declined as the proportion of urea-treated whole-crop wheat in the diet increased. With fermented whole-crop wheat the lack of response in milk yield is attributed to its relatively low energy value (Adamson and Reeve, 1992). Thus its use to replace part of a high energy, well fermented grass silage is unlikely to increase total energy intake or animal performance. In Denmark, Kristensen (1992) has also reported that the use of fermented whole-crop barley did not increase milk yield when compared with grass silage.

The high intake potential of maize silage has long been recognized in mainland Europe (Demarquilly, 1988). In the UK, short-term studies established that forage intake was increased by approximately 2 kg DM/day when maize silage was used to replace 400 g/kg grass silage DM (Weller and Phipps 1985, 1986). Similar results were recorded in Japan (Izumi, Kurosaura, Ohura, Ishida and Onoe, 1982) and subsequent long-term studies at Reading confirmed these early results (Phipps, Weller, Elliot and Sutton, 1988; Phipps, Weller, Fisher and Poole, 1991; Phipps, Weller and Rook, 1992b).

Phipps *et al.* (1988) showed that as a consequence of increased forage intake concentrate input could be reduced from 9 to 6 kg/day without affecting milk production, provided 600 g/kg grass silage DM was replaced by maize silage (Table 6.6). The use of maize silage in early lactation will result in an improved energy balance of the cow, and it is interesting to speculate whether this enhanced energy status will result in improved reproductive efficiency. While very large numbers of cows would be required to confirm this hypothesis, some farmers have already arrived at this conclusion (Gerring, 1993).

Table 6.6 POTENTIAL FOR REDUCING CONCENTRATE INPUT BY INCOPORATING MAIZE SILAGE IN RATIONS BASED ON GRASS SILAGE

Concentrate (kg/day)	Silage	DM intake	Milk yield
9	Grass	17.7	27.5
6	Grass/maize	17.8	27.2
6	Grass	15.0	24.3

(Phipps *et al.*, 1988)

In order to obtain further information on the effect of mixed forage diets the Milk Marketing Board of England and Wales commissioned a three year study at the Centre for Dairy Research. The results from a preliminary analysis of year 2 are presented in Table 6.7. It shows that when either maize silage (MS), fodder beet (FB) or brewers grains (BG) replaced 330 g/kg DM of well fermented, first cut, high energy, grass silage (GS), forage DM intake was significantly increased by over 2 kg/day and milk yield by at least 3 kg/day (Table 6.7).

Table 6.7 EFFECT OF INCORPORATING 330 g/kg DM OF EITHER MAIZE SILAGE (MS), FODDER BEET (FB) OR BREWERS' GRAINS (BG) OR 750 g/kg DM OF MAIZE SILAGE (MSH) IN A BASAL RATION OF GRASS SILAGE (GS) ON FORAGE INTAKE AND MILK PRODUCTION

	GS	*GS/MS*	*GS/FB*	*GS/BG*	*GS/MSH*
Forage DM intake (kg/day)	10.3	12.2	12.4	12.2	12.8
Milk yield (kg/day)	20.9	24.0	24.0	27.0	27.8
Milk fat (g/kg)	41.5	40.4	42.0	37.8	39.0
Milk protein (g/kg)	30.3	31.4	32.6	31.6	32.1
Value of milk (£/cow per day)	4.18	4.54	4.74	4.96	5.06

(Phipps, 1993 unpublished data)

MILK QUALITY

The use of alternative forage crops can improve milk quality. Roberts (1987) showed that the inclusion of fodder beet as part of a ration based on grass silage increased the concentration of both milk fat and protein by 3.6 and 2.3 g/kg, respectively. Recent studies at Reading (Phipps *et al.,* 1993; Phipps, 1993) have confirmed that the use of a forage mixture based on grass silage and fodder beet will increase both milk fat and protein concentration, when compared with a basal ration of grass silage (Table 6.7). The increased milk fat concentration was attributed to an increased lipogenic to non-lipogenic ratio of volatile fatty acids in the rumen while the increased milk protein concentration associated with fodder beet is often linked to an increased intake of dietary energy.

Although on farm reports state that the inclusion of urea-treated whole-crop wheat resulted in a substantial improvement milk quality (Goddard, 1992; Rea, 1992), trials conducted by Leaver and Hill (1992) and Phipps *et al.(1993)* found only a small and inconsistent effect on milk quality. This discrepancy may be due to the fact that on farms other dietary and management changes may have been implemented at the same time as the introduction of the urea-treated whole-crop silage.

Studies at Reading which compared a range of complementary forage crops, have shown that in contrast to fodder beet, the use of brewers grains to replace 330 g/kg grass silage DM resulted in an increased milk protein but reduced milk fat concentration. The increased milk protein concentration was attributed to an improved intake of dietary protein while the decreased milk fat concentration was attributed to the high level of unsaturated fat in brewers grains, which would reduce fibre digestion (Lewis and Lowman, 1989).

Preliminary short term trials carried out at Shinfield in the mid 1980s (Weller and Phipps 1985, 1986), demonstrated the positive effect of maize silage on milk protein concentration. Subsequent longer term studies (Phipps *et at.,* 1991, 1993) confirmed these results and showed that the increase in milk protein concentration was positively related to its inclusion rate. These studies have also shown an inverse relationship between the inclusion rate of maize silage and milk fat concentration (Table 6.7). Such changes in milk quality, effected by the use of maize silage, illustrate how forage mixtures can be used to manipulate the milk fat:protein ratio. The ability to manipulate this ratio will become increasing important as the price differential between milk fat and protein continues to move in favour of milk protein.

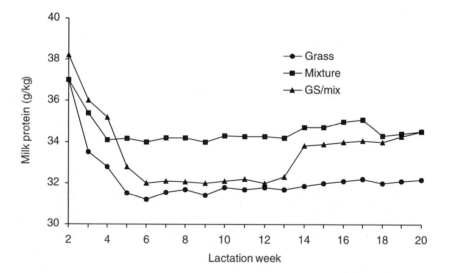

Figure 6.4 Effect of including maize silage (750 g/kg grass silage DM) in early and mid lactation on milk protein content when compared with using grass silage as the sole forage

A limited number of studies have examined the relationship between stage of lactation and the inclusion of complementary forages on milk yield and quality. Working with heifers, Phipps *et al.* (1991) reported that while the inclusion of maize silage in both early or mid-lactation, produced only a small increase in milk yield, it caused a significant increase in milk protein concentration (Figure 6.4) and a concomitant increase in milk protein yield. In a recent review, DeVisser (1993) considered that the partitioning of aminogenic precursors was related to stage of lactation. He referred to work (Valk, van

Vuuren and Langelaar, 1992) which showed that the inclusion of maize silage in early lactation increased milk yield but did not affect milk protein concentration, while its inclusion in late lactation (Meys, 1985) did not affect milk yield but elevated milk protein concentration (Table 6.8). These results show that the inclusion of maize silage in early, mid or late lactation all increased the yield of milk protein, although the increase was derived by different biological routes.

Table 6.8 INFLUENCE OF STAGE OF LACTATION AND INCLUSION OF MAIZE SILAGE ON MILK YIELD AND QUALITY

	Late lactation		*Early lactation*	
	Grass	*Grass/maize*	*Grass*	*Grass/maize*
DM intake (kg/day)	12.9	14.4	18.6	18.7
Milk yield (kg/day)	22.0	22.8	26.9	29.7
Milk protein (g/kg)	32.9	34.2	31.4	31.1
Milk protein (g/day)	683	779	845	923

(De Visser, 1992)

BUFFER FEEDING

By offering premium prices for summer milk production the Milk Marketing Board has encouraged farmers to move away from traditional autumn-calving. Summer milk production requires a consistent supply of good quality forage, which is difficult to obtain from pasture alone. While the use of grass silage as a buffer feed has been studied, the use of complementary forages has received little attention.

Maize silage with its high energy content should be considered as a buffer feed, although the aerobic instability of high DM crops is seen by some as a serious drawback. As a result, few farmers have adopted this feeding strategy and the majority wait for the current season's crop to be harvested before incorporating it into dairy cow rations. This position would change if maize crops could be treated to ensure aerobic stability. Whilst early work established that the application of additives containing the ammonium and/or propionate ion would provide aerobic stability (Leaver, 1975; Phipps and Fulford, 1977) recent studies have concentrated on the efficacy of inoculant additives. Work at Shinfield has shown that the Live System Inoculant can improve aerobic stability of high DM maize silage. This will allow farmers to carry maize silage over and to use it as a buffer feed in the following summer. Indeed this has already started, as the following headline in the Farmers Weekly indicates "Summer calvers go a bundle on maize silage" (Gaisford, 1993). The use of maize silage as a supplement to early spring pasture has also been proposed by Steg (1988). He reported that it reduced urinary nitrogen excretion from 361 to 198 g/cow per day and increased the efficiency of nitrogen utilisation from 17 to 24% and was therefore likely to reduce subsequent pollution.

Hargreaves and Leaver (1993) have reported one of the few studies in which whole crop cereal silage was used as a buffer feed. They reported that in spite of high intake characteristics, the use of whole-crop barley as a buffer feed, between July and October for grazing dairy cows, did little to enhance milk production. This was attributed to the fact that whole-crop barley was only a moderate quality forage, with a low metabolisable energy content and high starch degradability.

ECONOMICS OF MILK PRODUCTION

Using data collected at Shinfield, Doyle and Phipps (1987) carried out a computer simulation study to evaluate the practical and economic consequences of integrating maize and grass silage production on dairy farms in southern England.

They concluded that the economics of the dairy enterprise was positively related to the proportion of the conservation area that was used for maize silage production.

A recent study at Reading (Phipps, 1993) confirmed the results of the computer model. When compared with grass silage, the inclusion of maize silage at 330 and 750 g/kg grass silage DM increased the value of milk produced/cow per day from 4.18 to 4.54 and 5.06, respectively (Table 6.8). The same study also established that the inclusion of either fodder beet or brewers grains at 330 g/kg grass-silage DM improved the value of milk produced per cow per day from 4.18 to 4.74 and 4.96, respectively. These values were calculated by using the basic milk price of 3.293 and 2.223 per percentage unit for milk protein and fat, respectively. The improvement attributed to maize silage has also been demonstrated on commercial farms.

Conclusion

Recent studies carried out at the Centre for Dairy Research have clearly demonstrated the huge potential for UK milk producers of a wide range of complementary forages and forage substitutes. The improvement in forage intake and the resultant increased yield of milk and milk constituents and the enhanced value of milk produced, strongly indicate that dairy farmers should, where possible, replace a significant proportion of the grass silage ration with an appropriate complementary forage resource.

References

Adamson, A.H. and Reeve, A. (1992) Nutritional evaluation of whole-crop wheat. In *Whole-Crop Cereals*. Second Edition, pp. 117-123. Edited by B. A. Stark and J. M. Wilkinson. Marlow: Chalcombe Publications

Alderton, K. (1993) Personal communication

Bechdel, S.I. (1926) Quality of silage for milk production as affected by stage of maturity of corn. *Pennsylvania Agricultural Experimental Station, Bulletin 207*

Brabander, D.L., Aerts, J. V., Boucque, Ch. V. and Buysse, F.X. .(1976) The specific effect of fodder beet on the feed intake of dairy cows. *Revue de l'Agriculture,* **29,** 593-606

Cammell, S.B., Sutton, J.D., Beever, D.E., Humphries, D.J. and Phipps,R.H. (2000) The effect of crop maturity on the nutritional value of maize silage for lactating dairy cows. Part 1. Energy and nitrogen utilisation. *Animal Science,* **71,** 381-390

Carr, M.K. V. and Hough, M.N. (1979) The influence of climate on maize production in North Western Europe. In *Forage Maize,* pp. 15-55. Edited by E.S. Bunting, B.F. Pain, R.H.Phipps, J.M. Wilkinson, and R.E. Gunn. London: Agricultural and Food Research Council

Castle, M.E., Drysdale, A.D., Waite, R. and Watson, J.N. (1963) The effect of replacement of concentrates by roots on intake and production of dairy cows. *Journal of Dairy Research,* **30,** 199-207

De Visser, H. (1993) Characterization of carbohydrates in concentrates for dairy cows. In *Recent advances in Animal Nutrition -1993*, pp. 19-38. Edited by P .C. Garnsworthy and D.J.A. Cole. Nottingham: Nottingham University Press

Demarquilly, C. (1988) Factors that influence the nutritive value of silage maize. In *Quality of silage maize, digestibility and zoo technical performance.* Seminar held in Gembloux, Belgium

Doyle, C.J. and Phipps, R.H. (1987). The practical and economic consequences of integrating maize with grass production on dairy farms in southern England: a computer simulation. *Grass and Forage Science,* **42,** 411-428

Dudley, J. W. and Lambert, R.J. (1969) Genetic variability after 65 generations of selection in Illinois high oil, low oil, high protein and low protein strain of *Zea mays L. Crop Science,* **9,** 179

Gaisford, M. (1993) Livestock. *Farmers Weekly,* 30 July, p 43

Gerard, J. (1597) *The herball or Generall Historie of Plantes.* London: J. Norton. Gerring, J. (1993) The experience of a farmer with a high reliance on maize silage. In *The place of grass in land use systems.* Malvern: British Grassland Society, Winter Meeting

Goddard, R.L. (1992) Whole-crop cereals: a newcomer's experience. In *Whole- Crop Cereals,* Second Edition, pp. 117-123. Edited by B. A. Stark and J. M. Wilkinson. Marlow: Chalcombe Publications

Haecker, J. (1913) *Feeding dairy cows.* Minnesota: Department of Agriculture Experimental Station, University of Minnesota

Hargreaves, A. and Leaver, J.D. (1993) Whole crop barley as a supplementary feed for dairy cows grazing at two sward heights. *Animal Production,* **56,** 442

Hill, J. and Leaver, J.D. (1991) Replacement of whole crop wheat by grass silage in the diet of dairy cows. *Animal Production,* **52,** 606

Hill, J. and Leaver, J.D. (1993) The intake, digestibility and rate of passage of whole crop wheat and grass silage by growing heifers. *Animal Production,* **56**, 443

Izumi, Y., Kurosaura, H., Ohura, N., Ishida, Sand Onoe, S. (1982) Effect of feeding various levels of grass silage and corn silage to lactating dairy cows. *Japanese Journal Zootechnical Science,* **53**, 686-691

Kleinhout, A. (1990) The use of fodder beet as a whole crop: experience in Denmark. In *Meat and Milk from Forage Crops,* pp. 157-172. Edited by G. E. Pollott. British Grassland Society, Occasional Symposium No. 24

Kristensen, V.F. (1992) The production and feeding of whole crop cereals and legumes in Denmark. In *Whole-Crop Cereals,* Second Edition, pp. 21-37. Edited by B. A. Stark and J. M. Wilkinson. Marlow: Chalcombe Publications

Leaver, J. D. (1975) The use of propionic acid as an additive for maize silage. *Journal of the British Grassland Society,* **30**, 17-21

Leaver, J.D. and Hill, J. (1992) Feeding cattle on whole-crop cereals. In *Whole- Crop Cereals,* Second Edition, pp. 59-72. Edited by B. A. Stark and J. M. Wilkinson. Marlow: Chalcombe Publications

Lewis, M. and Lowman, B.G. (1989) Ensiled distillers or brewers grains as the sole diet for beef cattle. *Animal Production,* **48**, 656

Mertz, E. T., Bates, L.S. and Nelson, O.E. (1964) Mutant gene that changes protein composition and increases lysine content of maize endosperm. *Science,* **145**, 279-280

Meys, J.A.C. (1985) Comparison of starchy and fibrous concentrates for grazing dairy cows. *British Grassland Society, Occasional Symposium No.* 19, pp. 129-137

Mogg, J. (1992) Personal Communication National Institute of Agricultural Botany (1973) *Recommended List of Forage Maize Varieties*

National Institute of Agricultural Botany (1982) *Recommended List of Forage Maize Varieties*

National Institute of Agricultural Botany (1993) *Recommended List of Forage Maize Varieties* .

Pain, B.F. and Phipps, R.H. (1975) Energy for maize. *New Scientist,* **16**,394-396

Parry, M.L., Carter, T.R. and Jones, J.H. (1990) The greenhouse effect and the future of UK agriculture. *Ninth Winegarten Memorial Lecture,* presented at Agriculture House, Knightsbridge, London

Phipps, R.H. (1992). Past, present and future of forage maize. Taunton: Maize Growers Association Open Meeting Phipps, R.H. (1993) Unpublished data Phipps, R.H. and Fulford, R.J. (1977) The effect of a non-protein nitrogen additive on the fermentation characteristics of forage maize. *Journal of the British Grassland Society,* **32**, 129-133

Phipps, R.H. and Oldham, J.D. (1979) The amino acid composition of maize silage produced in the UK. *Animal Feed Science and Technology,* **4**, 163-168

Phipps, R.H., Sutton, J.D., Jones, B.A., Allen, D. and Fisher, W. (1993) The effect of mixed forage diets on food intake and milk production of dairy cows. *Animal Production,* **56**, 424

Phipps, R.H., Weller, R.F., Elliot, R.J. and Sutton, (1988). The effect of level and type of concentrate and type of conserved forage on dry matter intake and milk production of lactating dairy cows. *Journal of Agricultural Science,* Cambridge, **111**, 179-186

Phipps, R.H., Weller, R.F., Fisher, W. and Poole, T. (1991) Effect on forage intake and milk production of including maize silage in early or mid-lactation in dairy cow rations based on grass silage. *Animal Production,* **53**, 604

Phipps, R.H., Weller, R.F. and Rook, A.J. (1992b) Forage mixtures for dairy cows: the effect on dry matter intake and milk production of incorporating different proportions of maize silage into diets based on grass silage of differing energy value. *Journal of Agricultural Science,* Cambridge, **118**, 379-382

Phipps, R.H., Weller, R.F. and Siviter, J. W. (1992a) Whole-crop cereals for dairy cows. In *Whole-Crop Cereals,* Second Edition, pp. 51-57. Edited by B. A. Stark and J. M. Wilkinson. Marlow: Chalcombe Publications

Phipps, R.H., Weller, R.F. and Smith, T. (1981) Protein studies with maize silage. *Journal of Agricultural Science,* Cambridge, **96**, 283-290

Phipps, R.H., Sutton, J.D., Beever, D.E. and Jones, A.K. (2000) The influence of crop maturity on the nutritional value of maize silage for lactating dairy cows. Part 3. Food intake and milk production, *Animal Science,* **71,** 401-409

Rea, F. (1992) Recent developments at Kites Nest Farm. In *Whole-Crop Cereals,* Second Edition, pp. 107-115. Edited by B. A. Stark and J. M. Wilkinson. Marlow: Chalcombe Publications

Roberts, D.J. (1987) The effect of feeding fodder beet to dairy cows offered silage ad libitum. *Grass and Forage Science,* **42**, 391-396

Roberts, D.J. and Martindale, J.F. (1990) Fodder Beet: A review of research findings in relation to animal production. In *Meat and Milk from Forage Crops,* pp. 137-156. Edited by G.E. Pollot. British Grassland Society Occasional Symposium No. 24

Rulquin, H. and Verite, R. (1993) Amino acid nutrition of dairy cows: productive effects and animal requirements. In *Recent Advances in Animal Nutrition - 1993,* pp. 55-77. Edited by P.C. Garnsworthy and D.J.A. Cole. Nottingham: Nottingham University Press

Sabri, M.S. and Roberts, D.J. (1988) The effect of feeding fodder beet with two levels of concentrate allocation to dairy cattle. *Grass and Forage Science,* **43**, 427-432

Staghan, Q. and Perry, A. (1993) *Forage Maize.* Wrexham: Genus Management Report No. 77

Steg, A. (1988) Observations on forage maize evaluation in the Netherlands. In *Quality of silage maize digestibility and zoo technical performance.* Seminar held in Gembloux, Belgium, Nov 1988.

Sutton, J.D., Cammell, S.B., Phipps, R.H., Beever, D.E., Humphries, D.J. (2000) The effect of crop maturity on the nutritional value of maize silage for lactating dairy cows. Part 2. Ruminal and post-ruminal digestion. *Animal Science,* **71,** 391-400

Valk, H., van Vuuren, A.M. and Langelaar, S.J. (1992) Bijvoeren verhoogt voederopname en melkproduktie en verlaagt de stikstofuitscheiding in de urine. Wageningen: Mededelingen IVVO-DLO No.8.

Weatherwax, P. (1954) *Indian Corn in Old America.* New York: MacMillan & Co.

Weller, R.F. and Phipps, R.H. (1985) Milk production from grass and maize silages. *Animal Production,* **40**, 560-561

Weller, R.F. and Phipps, R.H. (1986). The effect of silage preference on the .performance of dairy cows. *Animal Production,* **42**, 435

Weller, R.F., Cooper, A. and Phipps, R.H. (1993). The selection of winter wheat varieties for whole-crop cereal. *Animal Production,* **56**, 453

Wilkinson, J.M. (1979) The ensiling of forage maize: effects on composition and nutritive value. In *Forage Maize,* .pp. 201-237. Edited by E.S. Bunting, B.F. Pain, R.H. Phipps, J.M. Wilkinson, and R.E. Gunn. London: Agricultural and .Food Research Council

Wilkinson, J.M. and Osbourn, D.F. (1975) Objectives in breeding forage maize for improved nutritive value. In *Proceedings of the 8th International Congress of the Maize and Sorghum Section of Eucarpia,* pp. 601-639, Versailles

This paper was first published in 1994

7

SUPPLEMENTATION OF MAIZE SILAGE AND WHOLECROP CEREALS

J.D. Leaver
Wye College, University of London, Ashford, Kent TN25 5AH, UK

Introduction

The proportion of forages fed to dairy cows in the UK as maize silage or wholecrop cereals is increasing annually at a substantial rate. This increase is mainly at the expense of grass silage, and several reasons appear to explain this change in nutritional management. In the case of forage maize, plant breeders have been successful in producing early maturing varieties which have a high probability of achieving 300g DM/kg at harvest. As a result, maize can now be successfully grown in a much wider area of the country. Wholecrop cereals are often higher yielding than maize or grass, especially autumn-sown varieties, and can be grown over a wide geographical area. They also have the flexibility of being harvested either as wholecrop or combine harvested for grain. Nevertheless, the two major reasons for the expansion of these forage crops are probably their lower cost of production, and their higher feeding value than grass silage (Phipps, 1994).

These developments in maize silage and wholecrop cereal use have coincided with a rapid rise in the genetic merit of the UK dairy herd, resulting from an increased use of proven bull semen from North American origins. This represents a further factor encouraging farmers to switch from grass silage to forages with high nutritive value and feed intake characteristics.

Supplementation of forage maize and wholecrop cereals with concentrates can have a number of objectives. Firstly, the nutritional deficiencies of the forages must be overcome. It is well established that their protein and mineral/vitamin contents are low compared with grass silages, and these deficiencies must be addressed in supplementation strategies. Secondly, supplementation aims to increase total energy and protein supply to the lactating animal in order to increase milk production. The extent of the milk production response primarily depends on the substitution rate of concentrates for forage. However, the energy source, protein source and protein content of the supplement is also likely to be influential.

139

In general, maize silage and wholecrop cereals are not fed as the sole forage to dairy cattle. They are normally offered in conjunction with grass silage. This can make the quantification of responses to supplementary feeding more complex. There are many challenges therefore for farmers, extension workers and researchers in developing successful nutritional management of high genetic merit cows. Understanding the interrelationships between supplements and forages containing maize silage and wholecrop cereals will be a crucial component of success.

Feeding value of maize silage and wholecrop cereals

NUTRITIVE VALUE

Forage maize and wholecrop cereals have different nutritional characteristics from grass silage, mainly due to the different botanical components of the crops. Grass silage consists predominantly of leaf and stem, whereas grain is an important component of both maize silage and wholecrop cereal forage. Ensiled maize normally has over 500g/kg DM of cob in the total plant if harvested at 300 g DM/kg or more (Table 7.1). Wholecrop wheat has a lower proportion of ear in the total plant, the proportion varying with stage of growth at harvest. The level is in the range 200 to 350 g/kg DM when cut at the ensiling stage (350 to 450 g DM/kg), and 350 to 500 g/kg DM when harvested for urea treatment (450 to 550 g DM/kg). Wholecrop barley is normally harvested for ensiling at 350 to 450 g DM/kg, and the proportion of ear at that time is 350 to 450 g/kg DM (Hargreaves, 1993).

In addition to these differences between maize and wholecrop cereals in the proportion of grain in the total DM, there is also a difference in the digestibility of the vegetative components (Table 7.1). The neutral detergent cellulase digestibility (NCD) of leaf and stem tissue is higher for forage maize than for wholecrop cereals harvested at over 400 g DM/kg. This is probably due to the grain in maize reaching maturity before much of the leaf and stem has senesced, unlike small grain cereals where the leaf and stem tissue is brown at the time of harvesting. Plant breeders of maize are now producing early maturing varieties which attain the 300 g DM/kg target for harvesting when the leaves are still green. The combination of a higher grain proportion and a higher digestibility of leaves and stem of maize leads to a significantly higher digestibility and ME value of the crop than wholecrop wheat and barley (Table 7.2).

These alternative forages to grass silage are characterised by low crude protein (CP), mineral and vitamin contents. The starch content is dependent on the stage of growth of the crop at harvest. In maize, wheat and barley, this can range from nil for crops harvested at the vegetative stage of growth, to over 250 g/kg DM for mature crops of wheat and barley, and 350 g/kg DM for maize. These crops have a low buffering capacity, and consequently when ensiled reach a low pH with a stable fermentation

Table 7.1 COMPONENTS OF MAIZE AND WHOLECROP CEREALS

Forage	Storage system	Crop DM (g DM/kg)	Proportion (g/kg DM)			NCD (g/kg DM)	
			Cob/ ear	Leaf+ sheath	Stem	Leaf+ sheath	Stem
Maize[1]	ensiled	317	545	256	222	610	536
Wholecrop wheat[2]	ensiled	372	260	322	418	602	530
Wholecrop wheat[2]	urea	555	440	220	340	522	411

[1] Mean of four varieties (Leaver, 1994 unpublished)
[2] Variety Haven (Leaver and Hill, 1992 unpublished).

Table 7.2 CHEMICAL COMPOSITION OF MAIZE SILAGE, WHOLECROP WHEAT AND WHOLECROP BARLEY, EACH HARVESTED AT TWO STAGES OF MATURITY

	Maize[1]		Wholecrop wheat[2]		Wholecrop barley[3]	
	low DM	high DM	silage	4% urea	low DM	high DM
Toluene DM (g/kg)	260	356	372	555	362	464
CP (g/kg DM)	86	79	91	152	80	73
NDF (g/kg DM)	401	367	428	459	512	516
ADF (g/kg DM)	271	223	264	309	300	279
Starch (g/kg DM)	93	239	23	258	223	258
NCD (g/kg DM)	689	698	603	619	583	592
ME (MJ/kg DM)*	10.7	10.8	9.8	10.0	9.6	9.5
pH	3.7	3.8	4.0	6.8	4.2	4.5
Ammonia N (g/kg N)	52	51	108	226	126	113

*ME = 0.157 x DOMD. DOMD = 0.65 NCD + 235 (Givens *et al.* 1995)
[1] Leaver (1993 unpublished). [2] Leaver and Hill (1995). [3] Hargreaves (1993)

without the need for acid or acid-stimulating silage additives, providing adequate water soluble carbohydrate is present. This applies to crops up to about 450 g DM/kg, above which water soluble carbohydrate is likely to be limiting for an appropriate fermentation to take place. The low buffering capacity also means that following opening, the silages are very susceptible to aerobic deterioration as the pH can increase rapidly when exposed to air.

The reduced fermentation which occurs with advancing maturity may lead to a reduction in the proportion of nitrogen (N) which is degraded to non-protein nitrogen (Wilkinson, 1978). For all these crops the effective degradability of nitrogen (N) is high at 0.75 to 0.85 (Alderman and Cottrill, 1993).

The ammonia N content is high in urea treated wholecrop wheat (Table 7.2). Leaver and Hill (1992) suggested that the high ammonia intake where urea-treated wholecrop wheat was the sole forage, might be the cause of an apparent inefficiency of energy utilisation of the crop. High blood urea levels (over 60 mg/100 ml blood) were found, and energy balances indicated that the estimated ME intakes were substantially higher than the ME accounted for in animal output. For this reason, maximum inclusion rates in diets of 5 kg DM/day are normally recommended where wholecrop wheat is treated with 40 g urea/kg DM. Recent research by Sutton, Abdalla, Phipps, Cammell and Humphries (1995) did not find this energy inefficiency when urea-treated wholecrop wheat was the sole forage for dairy cows. Givens, Moss and Adamson (1993) have indicated however that the ME of urea-treated wholecrop wheat is equal to 0.0143 DOMD compared with 0.0157 for grass silages, which is an indication of inefficient conversion of DE to ME.

An environmental implication with urea-treated wholecrop is that an application rate of 40 g urea/kg wholecrop DM, represents an N input equivalent to approximately 250 kg N/ha in addition to a typical N fertilizer input to the crop of 150 to 200 kg N/ha. A lower rate of application of 20 g urea/kg wholecrop DM has been investigated (Leaver and Hill, 1995), and found to give an equivalent level of dairy cow performance to a 40 g urea/kg wholecrop DM application rate. It is important that this lower rate of urea is spread evenly throughout the forage.

ROLE OF STARCH

Unlike grass silages, maize silage and wholecrop cereals contain substantial proportions of starch, which is a valuable energy source for the dairy cow. However, the species of crop and the stage of growth at harvest not only influence the quantity of starch, but also substantially affect the rate and extent of starch degradation in the rumen (De Visser, 1993). This has potential consequences for DM intake, FME supply, microbial growth, milk fat and milk protein production (Kung, Tung and Carmean, 1992).

De Visser (1993) reported that for maize silage an increase in DM from 213 to 323 g DM/kg, increased the proportion of starch, resistant to rumen degradation, from 70 to 320 g/kg, and there were differences between maize varieties in this attribute. The same author reviewed research which showed that maize starch had a comparatively low rate of degradation in the rumen and as a consequence 420 g/kg starch by-passed the rumen, compared with 80 g/kg for wheat starch and 70 g/kg for barley starch. Thus there are likely to be differences between maize silage, and wholecrop cereals in FME supply, and potentially in microbial protein production and milk protein content and yield.

The whole tract digestibility of starch is normally greater for maize silage than for wholecrop cereals (Table 7.3). The complete digestion of starch shown for ensiled wholecrop wheat in Table 7.3 has little nutritional significance as the amount of starch in the crop is small. If the crop is very mature the digestibility can be substantially reduced. Sutton *et al.* (1995) with urea-treated wholecrop wheat of 760 g DM/kg reported a starch digestibility of only 755 g/kg. Farmers are naturally concerned about the sight of cereal grain in cow faeces. The present evidence suggests that providing maize silage is harvested below 350 g DM/kg, or a corn cracker is used on the forage harvester if above 350 g DM/kg then high starch digestibility will be attained. For wholecrop wheat a starch digestibility of over 850 g/kg is likely, providing the DM at harvest does not exceed 550 g DM/kg. Wholecrop barley should be ensiled at a stage of maturity not exceeding 450 g DM/kg due to the hardness of the grain. Urea treatment at a higher DM is not appropriate due to the high probability of intact grain passing undigested through the alimentary tract.

Table 7.3 DIGESTIBILITY IN HOLSTEIN FRIESIAN HEIFERS OF STARCH AND FIBRE IN MAIZE SILAGE WHOLECROP WHEAT AND WHOLECROP BARLEY, EACH HARVESTED AT TWO STAGES OF MATURITY

| | *Maize*[1] | | *Wholecrop wheat*[2] | | *Wholecrop barley*[3] | |
	low DM	*high DM*	*silage*	*4% urea*	*low DM*	*high DM*
Forage DM (g/kg)	255	353	372	549	323	452
Starch intake (kg DM/day)	0.84	2.41	0.13	1.70	1.54	2.01
Starch digestibility (g/kg)	979	947	1000	888	880	860
NDF intake (kg DM/day)	3.61	3.71	2.48	3.03	3.53	4.02
NDF digestibility (g/kg)	685	669	637	643	605	551

[1] Leaver (1993 unpublished). [2] Leaver and Hill (1995). [3] Hargreaves (1993)

ROLE OF NDF

The proportion of NDF (cell wall) in these alternative forages is not dissimilar to grass silage of moderate to high digestibility. However, as the crops mature (Table 7.2) the NDF content does not rise substantially as for grass, and may even decline due to the diluting effect of the cob/ear development. The digestibility of the NDF (Table 7.3) normally declines with advancing stage of maturity of the crop, and tends to be higher for maize than for wheat and barley due to the leaves and stem being less mature at harvest.

Information on NDF rumen degradability is of importance because it is influential on FME supply and microbial protein production in the same way as for starch (De Visser, 1993; Overton, Cameron, Elliot, Clark and Nelson, 1995). In addition NDF is an important factor in the control of intake as discussed below.

FORAGE INTAKE

The performance of dairy cattle is strongly influenced by those characteristics of the feed which influence intake. The main reason why maize silage and to some extent wholecrop cereals are advantageous nutritionally compared with grass silage is their high intake characteristics, as is clearly shown in Table 7.4. In mixed forage diets containing 330 to 400 g/kg of maize silage or wholecrop wheat in the total forage, DM intake was increased in all cases compared with grass silage alone. The increases ranged from 3 to 23%, and at higher levels of inclusion of these forages, the advantages in total forage intake can be even greater (Phipps, 1994).

Table 7.4 EFFECTS OF FORAGE TYPE ON FEED INTAKE IN DAIRY COWS

(kg DM/day)	Grass silage		Maize silage		Ensiled wholecrop wheat		Urea treated wholecrop wheat	
1. Concentrates	6.9				6.9		6.9	
Forage	9.4	(100)			11.1	(118)	11.6	(123)
2. Concentrates	6.2				6.2		6.2	
Forage	11.7	(100)			12.1	(103)	12.5	(107)
3. Concentrates	6.0		6.0		6.0		6.0	
Forage	9.3	(100)	10.6	(114)	10.6	(114)	10.2	(110)

1. Leaver and Hill (1995) - mixed forages 40:60 ratio with grass silage.
2. Leaver and Hill (1995) - mixed forages 33:67 ratio with grass silage.
3. Phipps *et al.* (1995) - mixed forages 33:67 ratio with grass silage

There are a number of factors relating to the characteristics of the forage which influence voluntary intake. The higher intakes of maize silage and wholecrop cereals compared with grass silage probably relate both to their botanical characteristics and to their fermentation characteristics in the rumen. Hill and Leaver (1993) reported estimated rumen outflow rates of 0.049 and 0.059/h for grass silage and urea-treated wholecrop wheat respectively. It seems likely therefore that due to the grain content, and possibly due to the higher DM content, these forages have a lower retention time in the rumen, thus allowing a higher forage intake. The lower buffering capacity of these forages when ensiled also means that following consumption, their pH will rise more quickly to the neutral pH of the rumen compared with grass silage. Nevertheless, there are likely to be differences between maize silage and wheat or barley silages in their subsequent effects on rumen pH following fermentation. Maize grain is less degradable in the rumen than small grain cereals and is less likely to depress rumen pH (De Visser, 1993; Kung *et al.*, 1992). The negative effect of starch fermentation in the rumen on intake may therefore be less for maize than for wheat or barley silages. Urea-treated wholecrop cereals are alkaline and therefore have no negative implications for rumen pH, and this may be a useful attribute in rations containing a high proportion of cereals.

MIXED FORAGES AND MILK PRODUCTION

The mixing of maize silage and wholecrop cereals with grass silage has been reviewed by Phipps (1994). He concluded that the 'improvement in forage intake and the resultant increased yield of milk and milk constituents' should enable farmers to 'replace a significant proportion of the grass silage ration with an appropriate complementary forage resource'.

Recent research (Table 7.5) tends to confirm these conclusions. The higher intakes achieved when maize silage or wholecrop wheat were mixed with grass silage (Table 7.4), were in general translated into higher levels of milk yield, although no consistent benefits in milk composition were found. The extent of these responses depends to a large extent on the relative nutritive values of the grass silages and alternative forages used.

Table 7.5 EFFECTS OF FORAGE TYPE ON MILK PRODUCTION IN DAIRY COWS

	Grass silage	*Maize silage*	*Maize silage (H)*	*Ensiled wholecrop wheat*	*Untreated wholecrop wheat*
1. Milk yield (kg/day)	28.0			28.7	29.6
Fat (g/kg)	40.4			40.5	39.8
Protein (g/kg)	31.3			31.3	31.2
2. Milk yield (kg/day)	30.0			29.1	29.9
Fat (g/kg)	41.9			41.0	41.4
Protein (g/kg)	32.5			31.9	32.5
3. Milk yield (kg/day)	23.0	26.4	27.6	24.2	24.0
Fat (g/kg)	41.7	41.8	40.6	41.7	42.1
Protein (g/kg)	29.9	31.2	31.9	30.8	30.8

1 Leaver and Hill (1995) - mixed forages 40:60 ratio with grass silage.

2 Leaver and Hill (1995) - mixed forages 33:67 ratio with grass silage.

3 Phipps *et al.* (1995) - mixed forages 33:67 ratio with grass silage or 75:25 ratio with grass silage (Maize silage (H))

The costs of production of maize and wholecrop cereals have been found to be lower than for grass silage (Leaver, 1991; Phipps, 1994), particularly when in-silo losses are also taken into account. This factor, combined with the higher feeding value of these forages compared with grass silage, makes them increasingly attractive for use by dairy farmers as a partial replacement for grass silage. However, a knowledge of responses to supplements is an integral part of nutritional management, and for these forages much less is known than for grass silage diets.

Supplementation of maize silage and wholecrop cereals

PROTEIN LEVEL AND SOURCE IN SUPPLEMENT

The protein content of maize silage and wholecrop cereals is low (Table 7.2). It is well established that the amount and type of protein supplement influences the supply of amino acids to the small intestine both directly and indirectly, as undegradable and rumen degradable protein respectively (Alderman and Cottrill, 1993). Also there are positive responses in DM intake to increased concentrations of dietary crude protein, due to beneficial effects on DM digestibility (Oldham, 1984) and improved amino acid supply (Egan, 1965). The Metabolisable Protein System (AFRC, 1992) has attempted to quantify animal protein requirements and protein supply from the diet as metabolisable protein.

Oldham (1984) summarised the responses in total DM intake to protein supplementation as 0.42 kg DM/day for maize silage and 0.19 kg DM/day for grass silage based diets per 10 g/kg DM increase in dietary CP. Newbold (1994) concluded for high yielding dairy cows, that as the ERDP:FME ratio was about 6 g/MJ for maize silage and 14 g/MJ for grass silage (compared with the optimum of 11 g/MJ), intake responses to protein were due to both MP and ERDP supply in the case of maize silage, but in the case of grass silage were due to ERDP supply alone.

The benefits from enhancing the ERDP supply were shown by supplementing maize silage offered as 100% of the forage with 175 g urea/day when the supplement consisted of 6 kg sugarbeet, pulp and 2 kg soyabean meal per day (Leaver, 1991 unpublished). This increased the total diet CP from 133 to 155 g/kg DM. The urea supplementation led to an increase in milk fat content from 431 to 452 g/kg, in milk protein content from 315 to 322 g/kg, and in fat plus protein yield from 1.94 to 2.07 kg/day. These effects were probably a result mainly of the increase in forage DM intake from 13.8 to 14.6 kg DM/day.

In total mixed rations (TMR) with 400 g/kg of the DM as maize silage, increasing the total diet CP content using soyabean meal from 110 to 170 g CP/kg DM led to a substantial increase in total DM intake, in milk yield and in milk composition (Table 7.6). The authors (Kung and Huber, 1983) concluded that combinations of NPN and rumen undegradable protein might be the best way to support protein needs at lowest cost (when supplementing low protein forages). More recently (Broderick, Craig and Ricker,

Table 7.6 INFLUENCE OF DIETARY CRUDE PROTEIN CONTENT ON INTAKE AND MILK PRODUCTION IN MAIZE SILAGE BASED DIETS (KUNG AND HUBER, 1983)

Diet CP (g/kg DM)	*110*	*140*	*170*
Total DM intake (kg/day)	16.5	19.4	21.4
Milk yield (kg/day)	31.6	33.7	34.7
Fat (g/kg)	29.0	30.2	30.8
Protein (g/kg)	28.0	29.1	29.8

Maize silage 400 g/kgDM, alfalfa hay 100 g/kgDM

1993) with TMR diets of 163 g CP/kg in the total DM, a supplement of soyabean meal plus meat and bone meal was superior to urea (offered at 18 g/kg DM) as the protein supplement especially with a low DM alfalfa silage offered as the companion forage for maize silage (Table 7.7). Nevertheless, the level of urea in this study might have been too high, and this should not preclude urea making a small contribution to rumen degradable protein supply.

Table 7.7 SUPPLEMENTATION OF MAIZE SILAGE/ALFALFA SILAGE USING DIFFERENT PROTEIN SOURCES, AND WITH DIFFERENT DM CONTENTS OF ALFALFA (BRODERICK *et al.*, 1993).

	Low DM		*High DM*	
Alfalfa silage		*soya bean meal +*		*soya bean meal +*
Protein supplement	*urea*	*meat bone meal*	*urea*	*meat bone meal*
Total DM intake (kg/day)	24.2	26.2	26.0	26.1
Milk yield	35.4	38.5	35.9	36.9
Fat (g/kg)	37.0	34.8	34.7	35.4
Protein (g/kg)	30.9	30.1	30.4	30.2

The supplementation of urea-treated wholecrop wheat offered as the sole forage with protein has led to some responses in milk production, but not in feed intake (Table 7.8). In Experiment 1, supplementation with soyabean meal increased milk protein yield by 6% when the basal diet was 172 g CP/kg DM. In Experiment 2 with a basal diet of 224 g CP/kgDM there was no significant response. However, fishmeal significantly increased milk yield and milk protein yield in spite of the high CP content of the basal diet. The non-protein nitrogen content of the forages was high in both experiments (273 and 289 g ammonia/kg total N respectively) which might indicate the responses were due to the additional UDP. Nevertheless the estimated MP requirements were more than satisfied by the basal diets.

Table 7.8 SUPPLEMENTATION OF UREA-TREATED WHOLECROP WHEAT WITH PROTEIN (HILL AND LEAVER, 1999)

	Experiment 1		*Experiment 2*		
CP of concentrate (g/kgDM)	180	240	165	330	330
Source of supplement	-	soya bean meal	-	soya bean meal	fish meal
Concentrate (kg DM/day)	5.2	5.2	3.5	3.5	3.5
WC wheat (kg DM/day)	14.9	15.0	18.8	19.0	18.2
Milk yield (kg/day)	21.3	22.0	17.3	17.2	19.0
Fat (g/kg)	39.2	39.5	46.1	42.7	42.8
Protein (g/kg)	31.7	32.4	36.8	37.3	36.6
CP content of total diet (g/kg DM)	172	192	224	250	251

A similar conclusion was drawn with growing cattle offered urea-treated wholecrop wheat *ad libitum* (Castejon and Leaver, 1994). Supplementation with fishmeal depressed forage intake, and this was associated with a reduced digestibility of OM and starch (Table 7.9). This indicates that the additional rumen degradable protein supplied by the fishmeal might have been detrimental to rumen conditions in a situation where there was already a massive surplus of ammonia. However, NDF digestibility was increased by both protein supplements which might indicate some enhanced cellulytic activity.

Table 7.9 EFFECT OF ENERGY/PROTEIN SUPPLEMENTS* ON THE INTAKE AND DIGESTIBILITY OF UREA-TREATED WHOLECROP WHEAT (CASTEJON AND LEAVER, 1994)

	Wholecrop wheat	*Wholecrop wheat + SBP*	*Wholecrop wheat + SBP + FM*
Supplement intake (kgDM/day)	0	1.6	1.6
WC wheat intake (kg DM/day)	8.6	8.7	8.2
Digestibility of WC wheat			
DOMD (g/kg)	645	639	626
NDF (g/kg)	634	685	675
Starch (g/kg)	848	829	815

*Mean of two experiments with growing heifers
SBP = molassed sugarbeet pulp. FM = fish meal.

These examples illustrate the complexity of predicting the outcome of supplementation with different levels and sources of protein. One clear conclusion however is that the CP in the total DM should be 160 to 190 g/kgDM, depending on stage of lactation, and that non-protein nitrogen can be used partially, where high proportions of maize and wholecrop silages are in the diet. The observed responses to additional protein up to these levels can be due to a combination of effects; on total DM intake, on MP supply, on body fat mobilisation and on oxidation of MP to enhance energy supply (Newbold, 1994).

AMOUNT OF CONCENTRATE SUPPLEMENTATION

The ME supplied by an increment of concentrate supplement has a number of influences. It may affect milk yield, milk composition, liveweight change and forage intake. An energy balance will reveal for example where the ME from 1 kg concentrate DM is partitioned. Leaver (1988) showed that on average about one third of the ME from an increment of concentrates was partitioned to milk, one third to liveweight and one third substituted for forage intake. Variations in this partition occur due to stage of lactation, quality of forage, and the basal level of concentrates.

Examples of these responses to increments of concentrates are shown in Tables 7.10 and 7.11 for maize silage and urea-treated wholecrop wheat. The substitution rates in Table 7.10 (Phipps *et al.*, 1988) are low, due to a) the poor quality of the grass silage (ME 9.9 MJ/kgDM); and b) the low basal level of concentrates (2.7 kgDM/day). This resulted in high milk yield responses of 1.23 kg milk/kg concentrate DM for grass silage, and 1.08 kg/kg for grass/maize silage mixed. The substitution rate in Table 7.11 for urea-treated wholecrop wheat averaged 0.6 and resulted in an average milk yield response of only 0.5 kg/kg concentrate DM. In both studies the beneficial effects on milk protein content and liveweight change, of incremental increases in concentrates can be clearly seen.

Table 7.10 LEVEL OF CONCENTRATES (186 G CP/KG DM) FED WITH GRASS SILAGE OR A MIXTURE OF GRASS AND MAIZE SILAGES (PHIPPS *et al.*, 1988)

Forage	Grass silage		Grass/maize* silage	
Concentrate level (kg DM/day)	2.7	5.3	2.7	5.3
Forage (kg DM/day)	8.0	7.7	10.0	9.6
Substitution rate		0.12		0.15
Milk yield (kg/day)	16.7	19.9	20.9	23.7
Fat (g/kg)	37.4	38.1	38.2	36.6
Protein (g/kg)	27.9	29.6	29.5	30.2
LW change (kg/day)	-0.40	-0.07	+0.01	+0.12

*ratio 1:2 (DM basis)

Table 7.11 LEVEL OF CONCENTRATES (176 G CP/KG DM) FED WITH UREA-TREATED WHOLECROP WHEAT (HILL AND LEAVER, 1999)

	Concentrate level (kg DM/day)		
	5.2	*7.0*	*8.7*
WC wheat intake (kg DM/day)	14.9	13.8	12.8
Substitution rate		0.61 0.59	
Milk yield (kg/day)	21.3	22.4	23.1
Fat (g/kg)	39.2	40.2	39.8
Protein (g/kg)	31.7	32.6	33.3
LW change (kg/day)	+0.24	+0.17	-0.01

The evidence available indicates that the substitution rates of concentrates for forage are little different for maize silage and wholecrop cereals than for grass silage. Therefore substitution rates will in general fall between 0.33 and 0.67, and milk yield responses are likely to be between 0.7 and 1.2 kg/kg concentrate DM. A review of experiments with grass silage as the basal diet (Thomas, 1980), reported a mean short-term response of 0.79 kg milk/kg concentrate DM.

In evaluating the economic returns to increments of concentrate, caution must be taken in estimating cost/benefits which only compare extra milk value against extra concentrate cost. Firstly, the liveweight change resulting from supplementation has a value either directly as beef or indirectly as condition score for the next lactation, and secondly the substitution of concentrates for forage has an economic return in the cost of forage saved. Finally, where milk quota limitations occur, the financial implications of the extra milk production relative to quota costs must also be included in the cost/benefit analysis.

ENERGY SOURCE IN SUPPLEMENT

The source of energy in the supplement can significantly influence conditions in the rumen especially at high levels of supplementation. At low levels of supplementation eg 5 kg/day of supplement or less, energy source will have little effect on forage intake, milk yield or composition due to its small proportion in the total diet. At higher levels, supplementary energy consisting of starch and sugars will change the balance of microorganisms in the rumen away from cellulytic towards amylolytic activity (Porter, Balch, Coates, Fuller, Latham and Sharpe, 1972; Hoover, 1986). This will reduce the rate and extent of fibre digestion (Terry, Tilley and Outen, 1969) with consequential effects on forage intake (Thomas, 1987).

There has been a large number of experiments to examine starch versus fibre-based concentrates with grass silage and hay diets (e.g. Mayne and Gordon, 1984; Sloan, Rawlinson and Armstrong, 1988; Sutton, Morant, Bines, Napper and Givens, 1993; Aston, Thomas, Daley and Sutton, 1994). Starch supplements have invariably led to a reduction in milk fat content, and to an increase in milk protein content and/or yield. The reduced milk fat content is caused by a higher proportion of propionic acid being produced in the rumen at the expense of acetic acid which is a precursor of milk fat, and is a result of the greater amylolytic activity of the rumen microbes (Thomas and Chamberlain, 1984; De Visser, 1993). The positive responses of milk protein to starch compared with fibre-based concentrates are partly associated with the beneficial effects on microbial protein synthesis (as FME supply), and partly to the supply of additional propionic acid which reduces the necessity for the use of amino acids as glucose precursors, particularly during negative energy balance (De Visser, 1993).

Very few comparisons have been made of starch versus fibre-based concentrates with maize silage or wholecrop cereal forages. Kristensen (1992) compared rolled barley and dried sugarbeet pulp as supplements for ensiled wholecrop barley, offered as the sole forage (Table 7.12). Wholecrop barley intake increased when rolled barley was replaced by sugarbeet pulp, milk fat content increased and milk protein content declined. These results are similar to those reported for grass silages. However, immature wholecrop barley has some similarities to grass silage so this was possibly to be expected.

Table 7.12 ENERGY SOURCE OF SUPPLEMENT FED WITH ENSILED WHOLECROP (WC) BARLEY (KRISTENSEN, 1992)

	RB	*RB/SBP*	*SBP*
Concentrate (kg DM/day)	8.2	8.2	8.2
WC barley (kg DM/day)	9.0	10.6	10.0
Milk yield (kg/day)	28.1	27.6	27.3
Fat (g/kg)	40.0	41.6	41.9
Protein (g/kg)	31.7	31.6	30.0

RB = rolled barley   SBP = molassed sugarbeet pulp

Maize silage and more mature wholecrop cereals have a higher grain content than ensiled wholecrop wheat or barley, and some differences in response to starch versus fibre supplement might be expected. The results for urea- treated wholecrop wheat shown in Table 7.13 indicated no significant differences in milk yield or composition between a high fibre and high starch plus sugar concentrate. Therefore, the source of energy in the supplement may not be influential at a moderate level of alternative forage inclusion (400 g/kg of forage DM) and at a moderate concentrate input (8 kg/day).

Table 7.13 ENERGY SOURCE OF SUPPLEMENT FED WITH UREA-TREATED
WHOLECROP WHEAT AND GRASS SILAGE (LEAVER AND MARSDEN, 1991
UNPUBLISHED)

Supplement*	High fibre	High starch + sugar
Concentrate (kg DM/day)	6.9	6.9
Forage (kg DM/day)+	11.6	12.0
Milk yield (kg/day)	29.6	29.9
Fat (g/kg)	39.8	40.1
Protein (g/kg)	31.2	31.6

* High fibre: 277 g starch + sugar/kgDM and 142 g crude fibre/kg DM
 High starch + sugar: 376 g starch + sugar/kg DM and 76 g crude fibre/kg DM
+ 60:40 ratio of grass silage : urea-treated wholecrop wheat

There is a developing interest in different types of starch as supplements for forages. It
is well established that maize starch has a low rumen degradability compared with
wheat or barley starch (De Visser, 1993), and therefore there are implications for fibre
digestion, forage intake and microbial protein production. In a recent study (Overton *et
al.*, 1995) rolled barley replaced shelled corn (maize grain) as the energy supplement
(Table 7.14). This replacement led to a reduction in total DM intake, a reduction in milk
yield, and an increase in milk fat and protein contents. However the yields of milk fat
and protein declined. A higher proportion of starch was digested in the rumen with
barley than with corn supplements, and this was associated with a decrease in acetic
and an increase in propionic acid production. The higher DM intake of the shelled corn
diets was the explanation for the higher milk yields and for the dilution effect on milk
solids content.

Table 7.14 SHELLED MAIZE AND STEAM ROLLED BARLEY AS SUPPLEMENTS FOR
MAIZE/ALFALFA SILAGE (OVERTON *et al.*, 1995)

	Ratio corn : barley		
	100 : 0	*50 : 50*	*0 : 100*
Total intake (kg DM/day)	22.8	21.3	19.6
% starch intake digested in rumen	42	61	74
% starch intake digested post ruminally	49	33	22
% NDF intake digested in rumen	40	43	35
% NDF intake digested post ruminally	11	3	12
Milk yield (kg/day)	26.9	26.6	22.6
Fat (g/kg)	35.8	35.0	39.1
Protein (g/kg)	33.6	34.4	36.9

TMR with CP 162 g/kgDM, NDF 346 g/kgDM, starch 329 g/kg DM, and forage 400g/kg of
total DM.

The processing of grain (physical and chemical) can also be influential on milk production through its effect on diet digestibility, rate and site of grain digestion and on food intake (Campling, 1991). Processing which leads to an increase in access of rumen microorganisms to the starch, will increase both the rate and extent of digestion in the rumen, particularly for maize grain which is most resistant to microbial attack. Nonetheless the quantification of the effects of processing are not clear due to interactions with the forage and other components of the diet (Owens, Zinn and Kim, 1986; Theurer, 1986). For dairy cattle some processing of cereal grains is recommended except perhaps for oats which can be fed whole (Orskov, 1987; Campling, 1991).

There is no information available on the use of dietary fats specifically as supplements for maize silage or wholecrop cereals. Thomas and Martin (1988) reviewed the role of supplemental fats, and concluded that with 'fat deficient' diets, supplementation leads to increases in milk yield and milk composition, especially in milk fat content. At the other extreme (over 100 g fat/kg total DM) interference of fat in rumen fermentation leads to reduced feed intake and depressed milk yield and composition. For diets between these extremes a range of effects of fat supplementation have been recorded depending on fat source and level, and the type of basal diet (Storry and Brumby, 1980; Palmquist, 1984). Whilst the response in milk fat content to moderate levels of fat supplementation is variable, responses in milk yield are generally positive and in milk protein, negative, even with 'protected fat' products (Thomas and Martin, 1988).

Optimising supplementation

The term "optimising" presents a challenge to whoever is carrying out the task, as it poses the question, optimising for what or whom? Decisions concerning the supplementary feeding of dairy cows offered maize silage or wholecrop cereals could be aimed at optimising rumen conditions for microbial growth, optimising nutrient supply to the cow for reproduction and health, optimising to meet milk quota targets, optimising for profit for the farmer and many more. These objectives would not all require the same type and level of supplement input. Therefore quantification of these relationships is a priority in order to provide the necessary information for nutritional decision making at rumen, cow and farm level.

SUPPLEMENTATION OF THE RUMEN

The development of the MP system (AFRC, 1992) focused attention on the rumen and microbial protein production, and the system has been integrated with the ME system into a practical manual for farmers and advisors (Alderman and Cottrill, 1993). Arising from this, and similar developments in other countries, ruminant nutritionists have become increasingly interested in synchrony between energy and N supply for the rumen microorganisms (Herrera-Saldana, Gomez-Alarcon, Torabi and Huber, 1990; Sinclair, Garnsworthy, Newbold and Buttery, 1993). Newbold (1994) has defined rumen synchrony as 'ensuring the optimal ratio between N and energy supply throughout 24 hours of the day.' He highlighted the problems of confounding differences in rate of degradation with extent of degradation in the rumen, which has occurred in a number of experiments examining synchrony.

The concept of rumen synchrony is potentially useful as an objective for nutritional management. However, with the present state of knowledge, providing advice on optimisation of synchrony is difficult. Although a body of information is being built up on rates and extent of degradation of separate feeds, the outcome of their interactions in the rumen for animals of different production (and therefore intake) levels and with different diurnal feeding patterns is extremely difficult to predict. Nevertheless this is a fruitful area for research.

SUPPLEMENTATION OF THE COW

The objectives of supplementary feeding the cow are to influence milk yield and composition, although the effects on reproduction and health, if known, must also be taken into account.

The effects of amount of concentrates, protein source and level, and energy source have been discussed earlier. Decision making at farm level is normally through ration-formulation procedures which attempt to match nutrient supply to nutrient requirements for individuals or groups of cows. The ME and MP systems have been developed for this purpose, and are more useful in attempting to match diet to cow requirements than to predict responses to changes in diet (Newbold, 1994). This particularly applies to protein where a change in input may affect DM intake as well as the supply of MP.

Systems of feeding are increasingly based on group rather than individual cow concentrate allocation especially through TMR feeding or flat-rate feeding in the milking parlour. TMR feeding should have advantages in rumen synchrony and this might explain why the system has in some instances increased feed intake and milk composition (Phipps, Bines, Fulford and Weller, 1984; Nocek, Steele and Braund, 1986). Nevertheless comparisons of mixed diets with forages and concentrates fed separately have in general not produced clear effects on milk production but where large quantities of concentrates are fed, TMR or out-of-parlour feeding systems become a necessity. Infrequent feeding of large amounts of concentrates gives asynchrony in the rumen by reducing rumen pH, which in turn reduces feed intake and this may reduce milk production especially milk fat content and fat yield (Gibson, 1984).

The effects of supplementation on reproduction and health are complex and not well understood. In early lactation, concentrate supplementation may alleviate the mobilisation of body tissues and this may be beneficial to reproductive efficiency (Garnsworthy and Haresign, 1989). Evidence from the USA indicates that high dietary protein levels (190 to 210 g CP/kg DM) can lead to reduced conception rates, an increased incidence of cystic ovaries, endometritis and dystocia (Carroll, Barton, Anderson and Smith, 1988). The reduced conception rates could be due to an enhanced body tissue mobilisation or to high levels of blood urea. Ferguson and Chalupa (1989) have indicated that the effects are mainly accounted for by rumen degradable protein intake. If this is confirmed, the high levels of ammonia in urea-treated wholecrop cereals, if fed as a large proportion of the diet, could be detrimental to fertility. Also, the level and degradability of the protein supplement offered in early lactation could be influential on fertility.

The prevalence of lameness in herds can be affected by the source and level of supplementation (Leaver, 1990), although this has not been shown with maize silage or wholecrop cereal diets. High protein diets in early lactation (196 g CP/kg DM) have been shown to increase the prevalence of lameness compared with lower protein diets (160 g CP/kg DM). This appeared to be due to faster and softer hoof growth, and which led to adverse effects on locomotion and clinical lameness (Manson and Leaver, 1988). High starch compared with high fibre concentrates also increase the prevalence of lameness due to an increase in the incidence of solar ulcers resulting from laminitis and poor quality horn growth (Kelly and Leaver, 1990). Avoidance of extreme diets in CP content, and starch content may therefore be beneficial to both reproduction and lameness.

Targets for diet formulation change with time, partly due to new knowledge arising and partly to fashion. The present trend is towards USA targets for total diet specification, such as those shown in Table 7.15. There is a need to test the validity of such targets in animal response experiments and to determine cost/benefits of alternative approaches. For example the ration shown in Table 7.16 has a diet specification very different from those in Table 7.15, yet for a farmer with ample quantities of forage available, this may be a perfectly satisfactory nutritional solution.

Table 7.15 RATION SPECIFICATIONS FOR LACTATING DAIRY COWS (POND *et al.*, 1995)

	Stage of lactation		
	Early	*Mid*	*Late*
DM intake (kg/100 kg LW)	>4.0	3.5-4.0	3.0-3.5
(g/kg DM)			
CP	170-180	160-170	140-160
SIP	300-350	350-400	350-400
UIP	350-400	350-400	350-400
NDF	260-300	320-340	340-360
ADF	180-200	210-230	220-240
NSC	350-400	350-400	350-400
Fat (maximum)	60-80	40-60	40-50

SIP = soluble protein. UIP = undegradable protein. NSC = non-structural carbohydrate.

Table 7.16 HIGH FORAGE DIET FOR LACTATING DAIRY COWS* (LEAVER, 1993 UNPUBLISHED)

Diet		Diet specification (kg DM/day)		Performance (g/kg DM)	
Soyabean meal	1.8	CP	160	Milk yield (kg/day)	27.4
Rapeseed meal	1.8	NDF	438	Fat (g/kg)	43.7
Grass silage	4.9	ADF	271	Protein (g/kg)	33.1
Maize silage	11.4	NSC	171	LW gain (kg/day)	0.31
Total (kg/100 kg LW)	3.29				

*at week 20 of lactation

SUPPLEMENTATION FOR FARM PROFITABILITY

Nutritional advice to the farmer, whilst taking into account the implications for rumen microorganisms, and cow requirements, must be based on sound economics. What is optimal for the rumen microorganisms or for the individual cow, may not be optimal for farm profit. The resources of land, labour, capital and milk quota differ for each farm and therefore nutritional advice has to be tailored to each farm circumstance.

The optimum supplementation of maize silage and wholecrop cereal based diets will therefore be determined by a range of factors including the amount and quality of forages available and milk quota targets, as well as the needs of the rumen microorganisms and the potential of the cows.

Conclusions

Maize silage and wholecrop cereals are replacing grass silage in the diet of dairy cows in many areas of the UK. This trend seems likely to continue, but due to the complementary benefits between these forages (Phipps, 1994), inclusion rates (proportion of total forage) with grass silage will generally range from 25 to 75%.

These forage alternatives to grass silage are low in CP, minerals and vitamins and appropriate supplementation is required. Increasing the CP of the total diet to 160 to 190 g CP/kg DM (level depending on stage of lactation) increases DM intake, milk yield and milk constituent yield. Rumen degradable protein can contribute partially to the protein supplementation.

Supplementation with concentrates appears to give similar substitution rates to grass silage (generally 0.33 to 0.67) and therefore responses in milk yield are likely to be similar (0.7 to 1.2 kg milk/kg concentrate DM).

Maize starch has a lower degradability than wheat or barley starch, and this has implications for maize and wholecrop cereal forages as well as for types of cereal supplements. There are implications for FME supply, VFA proportions in the rumen, microbial protein production, feed intake and milk production. Future nutritional research will increasingly focus on attempting to synchronise the release of energy and protein substrates in the rumen to optimise rumen conditions for microbial growth.

For high genetic merit cows there is a trend towards diets which include maize silage or wholecrop cereals in which supplementation is targeted at producing much lower total diet NDF and higher NSC levels, than used previously. Whilst the objectives of improving rumen synchrony and meeting the requirements of high potential cows are logical nutritionally, an important objective of the farmer is to feed the herd profitably. There may be times when the three objectives are in conflict.

References

AFRC (1992) Technical Committee on Responses to Nutrients. Report No. 9. Nutritive Responses of Ruminant Animals: Protein. *Nutrition Abstracts and Reviews (Series B)*, **62**, 787-835.

Alderman, G. and Cottrill, B.R. (1993) *Energy and Protein Requirements of Ruminants*. Wallingford: CAB International.

Aston, K., Thomas, C., Daley, S.R. and Sutton, J.D. (1994) Milk production from grass silage diets: effects of the composition of supplementary concentrates. *Animal Production*, **59**, 335-344.

Broderick, G.A., Craig, W.M. and Ricker, D.B. (1993) Urea vs true protein as a supplement for lactating dairy cows fed grain plus mixtures of alfalfa and corn silages. *Journal of Dairy Science*, **76**, 2266-2274.

Campling, R.C. (1991) Processing cereal grains for cattle - a review. *Livestock Production Science*, **28**, 223-234.

Carroll, D.J., Barton, B.A., Anderson, G.W. and Smith, R.D. (1988) Influence of protein intake and feeding strategy on reproductive performance of dairy cows. *Journal of Dairy Science*, **71**, 3470-3481.

Castejon, M. and Leaver, J.D. (1994) Intake and digestibility of urea-treated wholecrop wheat and liveweight gain by dairy heifers. *Animal Feed Science and Technology*, **46**, 119-130.

De Visser, H. (1993) Characterisation of carbohydrates in concentrates for dairy cows. In *Recent Advances in Animal Nutrition - 1993*, pp 19-38. Edited by P.C. Garnsworthy and D.J.A. Cole. Nottingham: Nottingham University Press.

Egan, A.R. (1965) Nutritional status and intake regulation in sheep. II The influence of sustained duodenal infusions of casein or urea upon voluntary intake of low-protein roughages by sheep. *Australian Journal of Agricultural Research*, **16**, 451-462.

Ferguson, J.D. and Chalupa, W. (1989) Impact of protein nutrition on reproduction in dairy cows. *Journal of Dairy Science*, **72**, 746-766.

Garnsworthy, P.C. and Haresign, W. (1989) Fertility and nutrition. In *Dairy Cow Nutrition - The Veterinary Angles*, pp 23-34. Edited by A.T. Chamberlain. Reading: University of Reading.

Gibson, J.P. (1984) The effects of feeding frequency on milk production of dairy cattle: an analysis of published results. *Animal Production*, **38**, 181-189.

Givens, D.I., Moss, A.R. and Adamson, A.H. (1993) The digestion and energy value of wholecrop wheat treated with urea. *Animal Feed Science and Technology*, **43**, 51-64.

Givens, D.I., Cottyn, B.G., Dewey, P.J.S. and Steg, A. (1995). A comparison of the neutral detergent-cellulase method with other laboratory methods for predicting the digestibility *in vivo* of maize silages from three European countries. *Animal Feed Science and Technology*, **54**, 55-64.

Hargreaves, A. (1993) *Wholecrop barley silage as a supplementary feed for grazing dairy cows*. PhD thesis: Wye College, University of London.

Herrera-Saldana, R., Gomez-Alarcon, R., Torabi, M. and Huber, J.T. (1990) Influence of synchronizing protein and starch degradation in the rumen on nutrient utilisation and microbial protein synthesis. *Journal of Dairy Science*, **73**, 142-148.

Hill, J. and Leaver, J.D. (1999) Energy and protein supplementation of lactating dairy cows offered urea-treated whole-crop wheat as the sole forage. *Animal Feed Science and Technology*, **82,** 177-193

Hill, J. and Leaver, J.D. (1993) The intake, digestibility and rate of passage of wholecrop wheat and grass silage by growing heifers. *Animal Production*, **56**, 443.

Hoover, W.H. (1986) Chemical factors involved in ruminal fiber digestion. *Journal of Dairy Science*, **69**, 2755-2766.

Kelly, E.F. and Leaver, J.D. (1990) Lameness in dairy cattle and the type of concentrate given. *Animal Production*, **51**, 221-227.

Kristensen, V.F. (1992) The production and feeding of whole-crop cereals and legumes in Denmark. In *Whole-Crop Cereals*, pp 21-37. Edited by B.A. Stark and J.M. Wilkinson. Canterbury: Chalcombe Publications.

Kung, L. and Huber, J.T. (1983) Performance of high producing cows in early lactation fed protein of varying amounts, sources, and degradability. *Journal of Dairy Science*, **66**, 227-234.

Kung, L., Tung, R.S. and Carmean, B.R. (1992) Rumen fermentation and nutrient digestion in cattle fed diets varying in forage and energy source. *Animal Feed Science and Technology*, **39**, 1-12.

Leaver, J.D. (1988) Level and pattern of concentrate allocation to dairy cows. In *Nutrition and Lactation in the Dairy Cow*, pp 315-326. Edited by P.C. Garnsworthy. London: Butterworth.

Leaver, J.D. (1990) Effects of feed changes around calving on cattle lameness. In *Update in Cattle Lameness, Proceedings of the VIth International Symposium on Diseases of the Ruminant Digit*, pp 102-108. Neston: The British Cattle Veterinary Association.

Leaver, J.D. (1991) *Forage maize production for dairy cattle. A Farm Study.* Wye: Wye College.

Leaver, J.D. and Hill, J. (1992) Feeding cattle on whole-crop cereals. In *Whole-Crop Cereals*, pp 59-69. Edited by B.A. Stark and J.M. Wilkinson. Canterbury: Chalcombe Publications.

Leaver, J.D. and Hill, J. (1995) The performance of dairy cows offered ensiled whole-crop wheat, urea-treated whole-crop wheat or sodium hydroxide-treated wheat grain and wheat straw in a mixture with grass silage. *Animal Science*, **61**, 481-489.

Manson, F.J. and Leaver, J.D. (1988) The influence of dietary protein intake and of hoof trimming on lameness in dairy cattle. *Animal Production*, **47**, 191-199.

Mayne, C.S. and Gordon, F.J. (1984) The effect of type of concentrate and level of concentrate feeding on milk production. *Animal Production*, **39**, 65-76.

Newbold, J.R. (1994) Practical application of the metabolisable protein system. In *Recent Advances in Animal Nutrition - 1994*, pp 231-264. Edited by P.C. Garnsworthy and D.J.A. Cole. Nottingham: Nottingham University Press.

Nocek, J.E., Steele, R.L. and Braund, D.G. (1986) Performance of dairy cows fed forage and grain separately versus a total mixed ration. *Journal of Dairy Science*, **69**, 2140-2147.

Oldham, J.D. (1984) Protein-energy interrelationships in dairy cows. *Journal of Dairy Science*, **67**, 1090-1114.

Orskov, E.R. (1987) *The Feeding of Ruminants.* Marlow: Chalcombe Publications.

Overton, T.R., Cameron, M.R., Elliott, J.P., Clark, J.H. and Nelson, D.R. (1995) Ruminal fermentation and passage of nutrients to the duodenum of lactating cows fed mixtures of corn and barley. *Journal of Dairy Science*, **78**, 1981-1998.

Owens, F.N., Zinn, R.A. and Kim, Y.K. (1986) Limits to starch digestion in the ruminant small intestine. *Journal of Animal Science*, **63**, 1634-1648.

Palmquist, D. (1984) Use of fats in diets for lactating dairy cows. In *Fats in Animal Nutrition*, pp 357-381. Edited by J. Wiseman. London: Butterworths.

Phipps, R.H. (1994) Complementary forages for milk production. In *Recent Advances in Animal Nutrition - 1994*, pp 215-230. Edited by P.C. Garnsworthy and D.J.A. Cole. Nottingham: Nottingham University Press.

Phipps, R.H., Bines, J.A., Fulford, R.J. and Weller, R.F. (1984) Complete diets for dairy cows: a comparison between complete diets and separate ingredients. *Journal of Agricultural Science, Cambridge*, **103**, 171-180.

Phipps, R.H., Weller, R.F., Elliot, R.J. and Sutton, J.D. (1988) The effect of level and type of concentrate and type of conserved forage on dry matter intake and milk production of lactating dairy cows. *Journal of Agricultural Science, Cambridge*, **111**, 179-186.

Phipps, R.H., Sutton, J.D. and Jones, B.A. (1995) Forage mixtures for dairy cows: the effect on dry-matter intake and milk production of incorporating either fermented or urea-treated whole-crop wheat, brewers' grains, fodder beet or maize silage into diets based on grass silage. *Animal Science*, **61**, 491-496.

Pond, W.G., Church, D.C. and Pond, K.R. (1995) *Basic Animal Nutrition and Feeding. Fourth Edition*. New York: John Wiley and Sons.

Porter, J.W.G., Balch, C.C., Coates, M.E., Fuller, R., Latham, M.J. and Sharpe, M. (1972) The influence of gut flora on the digestion, absorption and metabolism of nutrients in animals. *Biennial Reviews*, pp 13-36. Reading: National Institute for Research in Dairying.

Sinclair, L.A., Garnsworthy, P.C., Newbold, J.R. and Buttery, P.J. (1993) Effect of synchronizing the rate of dietary energy and nitrogen release on rumen fermentation and microbial protein synthesis in sheep. *Journal of Agricultural Science, Cambridge*, **120**, 251-264.

Sloan, B.K., Rowlinson, P. and Armstrong, D.G. (1988) Milk production in early lactation by dairy cows given grass silage *ad libitum*: influence of concentrate energy source, crude protein content and level of concentrate allowance. *Animal Production*, **46**, 317-331.

Storry, J.E. and Brumby, P.E. (1980) Influence of nutritional factors on the yield and content of milk fat: protected non-polyunsaturated fat in the diet. In *Factors Affecting the Yields and Contents of Milk Constituents of Commercial Importance*, pp 105-120. International Dairy Federation, document no 125, Brussels: IDF.

Sutton, J.D., Morant, S.V., Bines, J.A., Napper, D.J. and Givens, D.I. (1993) Effect of altering the starch:fibre ratio in the concentrates on hay intake and milk production by Friesian cows. *Journal of Agricultural Science, Cambridge*, **120**, 379-390.

Sutton, J.D., Abdalla, A.L., Phipps, R.H., Cammell, S.B. and Humphries, D.J. (1995) Digestibility and nitrogen balance in dairy cows given diets of grass silage and wholecrop wheat. *Animal Science*, **60**, 510.

Terry, R.A., Tilley, J.M.A. and Outen, G.E. (1969) Effect of pH on the cellulose digestion under *in vitro* conditions. *Journal of the Science of Food and Agriculture*, **20**, 317-320.

Theurer, C.B. (1986) Grain processing effects on starch utilization by ruminants. *Journal of Animal Science*, **63**, 1649-1662.

Thomas, C. (1980) Conserved forages. In *Feeding Strategies for Dairy Cows*, pp 8.1-8.14. Edited by W.H. Broster, C.L. Johnson and J.C. Tayler. London: Agricultural Research Council.

Thomas, C. (1987) Factors affecting substitution rates in dairy cows on silage-based rations. In *Recent Advances in Animal Nutrition - 1987*, 205-218. Edited by W. Haresign. London: Butterworths.

Thomas, P.C. and Chamberlain, D.G. (1984) Manipulation of milk composition to meet market needs. In *Recent Advances in Animal Nutrition - 1984*, pp 219-245. Edited by W. Haresign and D.J.A. Cole. London: Butterworths.

Thomas, P.C. and Martin, P.A. (1988) The influence of nutrient balance on milk yield and composition. In *Nutrition and Lactation in the Dairy Cow*, pp 97-118. Edited by P.C. Garnsworthy. London: Butterworths.

Wilkinson, J.M. (1978) The ensiling of forage maize: effects on composition and nutritive value. In *Forage Maize*, pp 201-237. Edited by E.S. Bunting, B.F. Pain, R.H. Phipps, J.M. Wilkinson and R.E. Gunn. London: Agricultural Research Council.

This paper was first published in 1996

8

EFFECTS OF FEEDING STARCH TO DAIRY CATTLE ON NUTRIENT AVAILABILITY AND PRODUCTION

C. K. REYNOLDS, J. D. SUTTON and D. E. BEEVER
Centre for Dairy Research, Department of Agriculture, The University of Reading, Earley Gate, Reading, RG6 6AT, Berks, UK

Introduction

Sustained increases in the genetic potential for milk production by dairy cattle have stressed the need for rations formulated to provide maximal energy and protein availability for milk synthesis. High producing cows produce milk energy at the expense of body energy reserves in early lactation, but the yield achieved and the extent of body tissue mobilization are determined by energy intake relative to the propensity for milk synthesis. By maximizing net nutrient supply from the diet higher yields can be achieved and in the long term the extent of body fat and protein mobilization and associated metabolic and reproductive disturbances may be reduced. High yielding cows have a greater capacity for intake and use of absorbed nutrients and can only achieve their full productive potential through maximal nutrient intake. Maximum energy intake can be achieved by maximizing dry matter (DM) intake and by increasing energy concentration of the diet by adding fat or increasing the inclusion rate of energy concentrates. In practical terms this often means feeding more cereal grain starch. In addition, nutrient availability to the cow can be maximized by simultaneously optimizing rumen fermentation and amounts of protein and carbohydrate digested in the small intestine (Clark *et al.*, 1992). There have been a large number of reviews written on the effect of starch feeding, starch type and processing and starch digestion characteristics on production responses in ruminants (e.g. Nocek and Tamminga, 1991; De Visser, 1993; Sutton, 1979 and 1989; Ørskov, 1976 and 1986; Owens *et al.*, 1986; Theurer, 1986) and there is a large volume of literature available on the response of milk fat to starchy concentrate feeding, but there has also been recent interest in the effects of feeding starch on milk protein content. This chapter will review effects of starch supplementation and site of starch digestion on nutrient availability and milk production.

Starch analysis

In spite of the importance of starch as a feedstuff component for all sectors of the animal industry as well as for human diets, it is difficult to obtain precise and accurate estimates of the starch content of ration components. In a recent ring test (Beever *et al.*, 1996) 8 commercial laboratories reported starch content of maize silage samples ranging from 165 to 272 g/kg DM (mean ± sem: 228±36) for a low DM silage (276 g DM/kg) and from 194 to 311 g/kg DM (mean ± sem: 262±42) for a high DM silage (335 g DM/kg). For this test one laboratory refused to report starch concentrations because of their general dissatisfaction with the analytical methods available. Much of the variation between laboratories in the analysis of starch content of feedstuffs relates to differences in the procedures used. There is an official AOAC method approved for measuring the starch content of cereals (AOAC, 1995) which specifies the use of a purified glucoamylase from a specific source under very strict assay conditions, except for the temperature for glucoamylase hydrolysis which is given as 'optimal temperature of glucoamylase used'. Among laboratories using enzymatic assays the procedures published by MacRae and Armstrong (1968) are widely used. Variation between laboratories using assays requiring enzymatic hydrolysis for starch analysis can be attributed to differences in sample preparation, the source of the enzyme used and the conditions used for enzymatic hydrolysis. Sources of enzyme vary considerably in their activity, purity and sensitivity to assay conditions. In addition, batches of enzyme from the same source can vary as well (P. J. Van Soest, personal communication). Sample processing is important as well because gelatinization can destroy carbohydrate and Maillard products can inhibit complete digestion. There are also a number of assays available for total nonstructural carbohydrates (Nocek and Tamminga, 1991), but these measurements often include pectins, fructans, ß-glucans and sugars which have different digestive characteristics than starch. For these reasons, data describing starch digestion from different studies should be compared with caution. Improved methods of starch analysis (De Visser, 1993) or at least a strict standardization of starch analysis procedures are needed for ration formulation based on starch content and digestive characteristics to be justified.

Starch Supplementation, Fibre Digestion and Voluntary Feed Intake

In practice, feeding starchy concentrates often reduces intake of the forage component of the diet such that the forage to concentrate ratio is reduced. However, the response to starch supplementation varies considerably depending on the type of forages and concentrates fed, the method of concentrate inclusion, the physiological status of the cow and resulting effects on intake and production. In cows fed grass silage *ad libitum*, doubling the inclusion of 'standard' starchy concentrates decreased silage dry matter intake by about 0.4 kg/kg concentrate dry matter fed (Sutton *et al.*, 1994), which is similar to responses observed in other studies (Agnew *et al.*, 1996). In contrast, increasing concentrate crude protein content increased silage dry matter intake (Sutton *et al.*, 1994). Therefore any comparison of the digestive and production responses to supplementation of starch with different levels, types or processing characteristics must carefully consider the basal diet employed for the comparison. For example the response to grain fed within a total mixed ration (TMR) is likely to differ from the response achieved when forage is fed *ad libitum* and grain is only provided in large meals fed at milking. When grass silage was fed 2 or 4 times per day or in a TMR and concentrate was fed at 2, 4, 6 or 8 kg/d, concentrate feeding caused a linear decrease in silage intake, but higher silage intakes were achieved with the TMR (Agnew *et al.*, 1996). The substitution rate of silage for concentrate was approximately 0.5, 0.4 and 0.3 for twice daily, 4 times daily and TMR feeding, respectively. Decreases in silage intake with concentrate feeding are probably due to multiple factors such as the total capacity for organic matter digestion and metabolizable energy (ME) utilization as well as specific effects on rumen fermentation and the products of digestion (Forbes, 1995).

As observed by Agnew *et al.* (1996), forage intake is often greater when concentrates are fed in a TMR rather than as meals provided at milking. In addition to the obvious difference in the ability of the cow to discriminate against diet components, and thus alter diet forage to concentrate ratio and total forage intake by selection, changes in the pattern of rumen digestion also contribute to the reduction in forage intake with meal feeding of concentrates. When starchy concentrates are fed as meals the fermentation of large amounts of starch over short periods of time can lead to the production and absorption of large amounts of volatile fatty acids (VFA), with associated increases in ruminal VFA concentration. Even when as much as 90% of the diet is composed of rapidly degraded starchy concentrates, rumen pH concentrations remain fairly constant when the daily ration is provided in frequent (hourly) meals but fall dramatically when concentrates are only fed at milking (Sutton *et al.*, 1986). These differences in the pattern of rumen acid concentration were associated with differences in metabolic and production responses to meal frequency. Feeding at milking alone caused a greater nutrient and insulin elevation in jugular vein blood and a larger depression in milk fat concentration than when large amounts of starch were fed more frequently (Sutton *et al.*, 1985).

Accumulation of acid in the rumen when cereal starches are digested in the rumen can damage the rumen epithelium and inhibit the activity of celluloytic microorganisms (Ørskov, 1976) which can cause a depression in fibre digestion and may lead to reductions in forage and (or) total dry matter intake (Grant, 1994). In general, increasing the rate of starch digestion in the rumen by processing or by feeding more rapidly digested starch types such as barley or wheat causes a greater depression in rumen pH and fibre digestion than when more slowly digested starch types such as maize or sorghum are fed (Ørskov, 1976). In early lactation cows, feeding steam-rolled barley compared to ground maize increased ruminal digestion of starch, decreased dry matter intake and decreased neutral detergent fibre (NDF) digestibility in the rumen and total digestive tract (McCarthy *et al.*, 1989). Although in this study rumen pH, measured hourly, was not different across diets, concentrations of VFA were much higher and pH was numerically lower in rumen fluid when barley was fed. Thus a depression in cellulolytic activity of the rumen microflora may have contributed to the lower digestion of fibre when barley was fed, although rumen pH was very low (less than 6) and both rumen and total tract NDF digestibility were low for all treatments in this study (McCarthy *et al.*, 1989). The low fibre digestibilities measured in these cows may also be attributed to low diet crude protein concentrations, which were less than 150 g/kg DM, and resulting low rumen ammonia concentrations which may also have limited the growth of cellulolytic microbes. Rumen ammonia concentration in these cows was lowered by feeding barley compared with maize, presumably due to a greater use of ammonia for microbial protein synthesis in the rumen, which may also explain the depression in fibre digestion and intake when barley was fed. Similar responses were observed when barley was incrementally substituted for ground maize in TMRs containing over 160 g crude protein/ kg dry matter, except that depressive effects of increased barley inclusion on rumen pH and fibre digestion were more significant (Overton *et al.*, 1995). Starch source also may alter fibre digestibility via other factors, such as changes in microbial species and the efficiency of microbial growth, which also influences the efficiency of microbial protein synthesis. Total fibre digestion was also depressed when barley was substituted for maize in mid-lactation cows, but rumen pH and dry matter intake were not affected (DePeters and Taylor, 1985). In contrast, fibre digestion in the rumen and dry matter intake tended to be higher when ground barley was compared to ground maize in studies with lactating dairy cows (Herrera-Saldena *et al.*, 1990). The fibre in these diets was provided primarily by alfalfa hay and cotton seed hulls. In other studies at the same location, increasing rumen digestion of sorghum or maize starch by steam processing increased rumen fibre digestion and (or) dry matter intake (Poore *et al.*, 1993; Chen *et al.*, 1994). These responses may be explained by an enhancement of the digestion of grain fibre itself or a limited availability of rapidly fermentable organic matter for microbial growth when maize or sorghum grain-based diets are fed. It appears then that the intake response to starch supplementation of dairy cow rations is influenced by the method of feeding employed, the level and degradability of dietary protein, the type of forage and the type and amount of starch fed.

In addition to effects on fibre digestion, feeding additional starch may also reduce total dry matter and energy intake via increased ruminal production and absorption of propionate and subsequent metabolic and endocrine responses (Forbes, 1995). In early lactation, forage intake was higher when cows were supplemented with a high fibre concentrate compared to a starchy concentrate providing equal ME (Garnsworthy and Jones, 1993). Rumen fluid from steers fed these concentrates contained higher concentrations of propionate and less acetate when the starchy concentrate was fed. The effect of increased propionate absorption into the portal vein on intake in *ad libitum* fed, lactating dairy cows was clearly demonstrated by the mesenteric vein propionate infusion studies of Casse *et al.* (1994). Cows reduced their dry matter intake during propionate infusions such that the total amount of propionate removed by the liver was remarkably similar to the amount removed during control infusions, but the absorption of other nutrients such as lipogenic precursors was reduced. The reduction of acetate, butyrate and ß-hydroxybutyrate availability without a concomitant drop in glucose supply provides a likely explanation for the decrease in milk fat concentration observed (Casse *et al.*, 1994).

Milk fat responses to starch feeding

Decreased milk fat concentration is the most predictable production response to increased starchy concentrate supply (Sutton, 1989) and the response is generally associated with a shift in VFA production in the rumen away from acetate and towards propionate or perhaps more specifically a reduction in the relative availability of lipogenic versus glucogenic precursors. The reduction in milk fat concentration is generally associated with an increase in lipid deposition in body tissue. This shift in energy partition away from milk towards body tissue is often illustrated by data from calorimetry studies conducted by W. P. Flatt *et al.* in which lactating dairy cows were fed diets differing in the ratio of alfalfa hay to ground maize and soyabean meal (the mixture formulated to be isonitrogenous to the hay) and their energy balance measured (Tyrrell, 1980). As concentrate level increased dry matter intake decreased, total ME remained relatively constant and milk energy output decreased due primarily to reductions in milk fat concentration, but tissue energy retention was increased such that net energy balance (milk plus tissue energy) remained constant. This shift in energy retention from milk towards body fat was associated with a decrease in rumen acetate to propionate ratio and presumably an increase in glucose availability. Other studies have shown that feeding higher concentrate diets increases total glucose turnover and plasma insulin concentrations (Evans *et al.*, 1975). Higher insulin concentrations should depress lipolysis and promote lipogenesis at the expense of milk lipid production, but recent studies have questioned the role of insulin in milk fat depression (McGuire *et al.*, 1995). In lactating dairy cows infusion of large amounts of insulin and glucose for 4 days caused a nonsignificant decrease in milk fat concentration which was considered small relative to the severe milk fat depression often observed when high starch levels are fed. While elevated insulin may not be the sole cause of milk fat depression, a shift in tissue energy balance towards body fat deposition accompanies the depression in milk fat output and this response is associated with, and in part mediated by, an elevation in peripheral insulin concentration.

Recently the role of trans- geometric isomers of unsaturated fatty acids as a potential cause of milk fat depression when high concentrate diets are fed (Davis and Brown, 1970) have received renewed interest (Gaynor *et al.*, 1994; Wonsil *et al.*, 1994; Romo *et al.*, 1994; Griinari *et al*, 1995). Cereal grains contain oils of which a large proportion are often linoleic acid and many maize varieties can be particularly high in oil content (4.1% or more) compared with other cereal grains. Trans-isomers are a step in the microbial biohydrogenation of linoleic acid to stearic acid. If biohydrogenation of linoleic acid is incomplete, or rumen turnover is increased by high intakes, then large amounts of transoctadecanoates may reach the small intestine. Recent abomasal infusion studies have shown that increased intestinal supply of trans-fatty acids markedly reduces milk fat concentration, probably via direct effects on the mammary gland (Gaynor *et al.*, 1994; Romo *et al.*, 1994). Milk fat depression was caused by the addition of oil containing unsaturated fatty acids to a high (80%) concentrate diet, but not when the oil was added to a 40% concentrate diet (Griinari *et al.*, 1995). The addition of an oil high in saturated fatty acids had little effect on milk fat concentration when added to either basal diet, suggesting that trans-fatty acids cause milk fat depression as a consequence of incomplete biohydrogenation of unsaturated fatty acids when high starch diets are fed. It appears then that when large amounts of starchy concentrates are fed severe milk fat depression may to a large extent be a consequence of increased absorption of specific trans-isomers of unsaturated fatty acids.

Energetic efficiency

The energetic benefit of feeding starch versus cellulose as a dietary carbohydrate for ruminants has long been recognized (Armsby, 1903), but the reasons for the improved efficiency of metabolizable energy (ME) use for production (milk and body tissue synthesis) for concentrates compared to forages has long been the subject of scientific debate. As for milk fat depression, the response is often attributed to a shift in the proportions of acetate and propionate produced in the rumen and subsequent postabsorptive effects on lipogenic and glucogenic nutrient supply and metabolism, with higher efficiency thought to be a consequence of greater availability of glucose relative to acetate (Armstrong and Blaxter, 1961). There is a much larger data base available for comparing the energetic efficiency of concentrates versus forages in growing animals than in lactating dairy cows, but in early calorimetry studies at Beltsville increasing forage to concentrate ratio from 50:50 to 100:0 (by varying proportions of alfalfa hay versus maize and soyabean meal) reduced the efficiency of ME use for milk energy adjusted for tissue energy loss or gain (ie net energy corrected for tissue energy loss) from 0.65 to 0.54 when a constant maintenance requirement was assumed (Coppock *et al.*, 1964). In other work at Beltsville increasing the maize and soyabean meal content of a maize-silage based diet from 300 to 600 g/kg dry matter fed decreased estimated maintenance energy requirement, but the efficiency of ME use for milk energy corrected for tissue energy gain or loss, excess protein intake and pregnancy (ie net energy milk [NE_{milk}]) decreased from 0.61 to 0.54 (Tyrrell and Moe, 1972). This decrease in the use of ME for milk and body tissue energy was in part due to a decrease in milk yield and fat content, but also may have been a consequence of a low diet crude protein content for the high maize meal diet (140 g/kg DM) compared with the low maize meal diet (155 g/kg DM).

The difference in the efficiency of ME utilization between forages and concentrates may to a large extent be attributable to alterations in gut metabolism. In order to achieve equal ME intakes greater dry matter intakes are required for forages, therefore gut fill and the work of rumination and digestion are generally greater than for concentrates. In addition, greater amounts of acetate are produced in the rumen. Greater dry matter intake, gut fill and acetate absorption can all contribute to an increase in gut mass. Ultimately these differences in the mechanical and biochemical processes of carbohydrate digestion and nutrient absorption affect portal-drained visceral (PDV; the gut, spleen, pancreas and associated fat) heat production and the relative outputs of acetate versus glucose from the total splanchnic (PDV and liver combined) tissues (Reynolds *et al.*, 1994). In growing beef heifers fed diets similar to those used in previous Beltsville calorimetry studies (Coppock *et al.*, 1964) differing in forage:concentrate ratio (75:25 versus 25:75) and fed at two equal ME intakes, ME use for tissue energy was lower for the high forage diet due to greater heat production. This difference between diets in the loss of ME as heat was due almost totally to differences in PDV heat production (Reynolds and Beever, 1995). In addition, the PDV of heifers fed the high forage diet absorbed more acetate and used more glucose from arterial blood on a net basis. Liver glucose production was the same for the two diets, but due to differences in absorption the ratio of acetate:glucose released by the splanchnic tissues was reduced by half when the concentrate diet was fed. This difference in acetate availability relative to glucose may also contribute to differences in the efficiency of ME utilization for growth, but it is important to remember that at maintenance intakes as much as half of the acetate produced in the rumen is utilized by the PDV (Bergman and Wolff, 1971).

A number of studies with lactating dairy cows have determined the utilization of energy from diets containing varying types of concentrates. In many of these studies there is little difference between types of concentrates in terms of the efficiency of utilization of ME for NE (milk plus tissue energy), but substantial differences in the extent to which ME is partitioned between milk and tissue. For example, cows fed a fibrous concentrate, beet pulp, retained a greater proportion of ME for milk energy versus tissue energy compared with when they were fed a maize-based concentrate (Tyrrell, 1980). Similar results were obtained when fibrous (sugar beet and citrus pulp with cotton seed) and starchy (barley, wheat and maize gluten) concentrates were compared using grass-silage based diets (Gordon *et al.*, 1995). These differences probably reflect a difference in the relative absorption rate of lipogenic and glucogenic precursors. In addition, studies comparing genotype (Moe and Tyrrell, 1979), maturity (Wilkerson and Glenn, 1996) and processing (Moe *et al.*, 1973; Wilkerson and Glenn, 1996) of maize grain have found that differences in energy utilization are due primarily to effects on organic matter and energy digestibility, but that greater starch digestibility can shift energy partition away from milk and towards body tissue (Moe *et al.*, 1973). However, in studies where physical form or maturity increased grain digestibility and ration metabolizability there were concommitant increases in milk yield and protein content (Moe *et al.*, 1973; Wilkerson and Glenn, 1996).

It is well established that differences in the efficiency of energy utilization or nutrient partitioning between lactation and body tissue arising from the feeding of varying carbohydrate sources are associated with, and probably attributable to, differences in the proportions of glucogenic and lipogenic VFA produced in the rumen. However, data describing the production of any of the VFA in the rumen of lactating dairy cows at high levels of intake are scarce (Sutton, 1985). With one exception (Wiltrout and Satter, 1972) data describing the production of any of the VFA in cows producing more than 20 kg milk/day are nonexistent, yet VFA production rates are the basis of most current models of nutrient utilization in lactating dairy cows. In spite of the difficulties in obtaining these measurements, and the errors of measurement involved, they are sorely needed if for no other reason than to confirm or dispute the assumption that relative concentrations reflect relative production rates (Sutton, 1979). As part of a major effort conducted at the former National Institute for Research in Dairying at Shinfield to determine the effects of starchy concentrate feeding on digestive and production responses in lactating dairy cows (Sutton *et al.*, 1980), a study was conducted in 5 lactating rumen-fistulated Friesian cows fed twice daily diets containing either 60 or 90 % barley-based concentrates with grass hay and supplying equal intakes of digestible energy. Measurements of acetate, propionate and n-butyrate production in the rumen were measured by non-steady state isotope dilution using ^{14}C-acetate, ^{14}C-propionate and ^{14}C-n-butyrate on 3 separate days at the end of each dietary treatment period (Sutton *et al.*, unpublished observations; Table 8.1). The data clearly show a decrease in acetate production and increase in propionate production with increased concentrate intake, but the relative response of propionate production, which more than doubled, is much greater than the relative response of acetate production. These are the only measurements of ruminal production in lactating dairy cows which include all 3 major VFA in the same cows during more than one dietary treatment period. With the current limitations on the conduct of these types of intensive studies it is unlikely that similar measurements of VFA production from high yielding cows will be repeated. Without measurements of rumen production, measurements of net PDV absorption of VFA will provide insight into their availability to tissues other than the PDV, but these measurements underestimate true rates of absorption because PDV tissues utilize VFA.

Table 8.1 NET VFA PRODUCTION (MOL/DAY) IN LACTATING DAIRY COWS FED AT EQUAL DIGESTIBLE ENERGY INTAKE BARLEY-BASED CONCENTRATES AT 2 LEVELS OF INCLUSION WITH GRASS HAY (Sutton *et al.*, unpublished observations*; for ration details see Sutton *et al.*, 1980).

| | Concentrate inclusion | | | |
	60 % Barley	*90 % Barley*	*SEM*	*P<*
Acetate	56.8	48.3	3.3	0.10
Propionate	16.3	36.4	2.8	0.01
n-Butyrate	6.5	4.7	1.2	NS

*Subsequently published in *Journal of Dairy Science*, **84**, Supplement 1, 79 (Abstr) 2001

Site of starch digestion

Another consideration when feeding starch to lactating dairy cows is the extent to which starch escapes the rumen and is digested in the small intestine or the hindgut. This has been the subject of numerous reviews since the early work in Kentucky (Karr *et al.*, 1966) and the United Kingdom (Armstrong and Beever, 1969; Ørskov *et al.*, 1969). Chemical and structural characteristics affecting extent and site of starch digestion vary both with source (Waldo, 1973; Ørskov, 1986; Owens *et al.*, 1986) and processing (Hale, 1973; Ørskov, 1976; Theurer, 1986). Of the 4 cereal grains most commonly fed to lactating dairy cows in the United States and United Kingdom, wheat and barley provide more rapidly digested starch to the rumen than maize and sorghum because they have a higher proportion of soluble starch (65 vs 30 %) which is more rapidly digested (21 vs 4 %/h). Based on *in situ* disappearance rates and estimates of rumen outflow in lactating dairy cows, de Visser (1993) calculated that 42 % of insoluble starch in maize and sorghum escapes the rumen, compared to only 8 % for wheat and barley. A commonly held belief is that the energetic efficiency of starch digested in the intestines will be greater than for starch digested in the rumen because small intestinal starch digestion liberates glucose directly while ruminal starch digestion produces VFA, of which the propionate fraction can be converted to glucose in the liver. Although data from glucose infusion studies support this concept in sheep fed at maintenance (Armstrong *et al.*, 1960), production studies generally show a greater efficiency of utilisation for liveweight gain when grain is processed to increase ruminal digestion (Owens *et al.*, 1986). This is because total starch digestion and ME are increased as well. However, multiple regression analysis of data available suggested that starch digestion in the small intestine provides 42 % more energy than starch digested in the rumen of growing cattle. In addition, infusion studies suggest an improved rate of gain when glucose is provided to the abomasum rather than the rumen, but the additional gain was accounted for primarily as increased abdominal fat deposition (Owens *et al.*, 1986). In growing heifers, the partial efficiency of ME use for tissue energy was 0.47 for a barley-based ration and 0.53 for a maize-based ration (Tyrrell *et al.*, 1972).

There is little evidence in the literature that at equal rates of digestion starch digested postruminally is used for milk production more efficiently than starch digested in the rumen. When ground barley and maize were compared in maize silage-based diets fed to lactating dairy cows the proportional use of ME for NE_{milk} was 0.58 for barley-based diets and 0.63 for maize-based diets, but the difference was not significant (Tyrrell and Moe, 1974). A recent review of the effects of site of starch digestion on lactation performance in dairy cows concluded that "production studies provide no clear evidence that site of starch digestion enhances milk yield or changes composition" (Nocek and Tamminga, 1991). Comparisons of starch type and processing methods which alter site of starch digestion in production studies are often confounded by alterations in dry matter intake or changes in total tract starch digestibility (McCarthy *et al.*, 1989; Overton *et al.*, 1995; Khorasani *et al.*, 1994; Poore *et al.*, 1993). In lactating cows fed 65%

concentrates with alfalfa hay and cotton seed hulls, substituting sorghum for barley increased postruminal starch digestion by 1.4 kg/d but decreased total starch digestion by 0.8 kg/d (Herrera-Saldena *et al.*, 1990).   In a series of studies conducted at the University of Arizona, milk yield and milk protein composition have been increased by feeding steam flaked sorghum compared with dry rolled sorghum (eg Chen *et al.*, 1994; Poore *et al.*, 1993).   In one of these studies, steam flaking sorghum increased starch digestion in the rumen by 1.5 kg/d and decreased postruminal starch digestion by 0.6 kg/d, thus total tract digestion increased by 0.8 kg/d (Poore *et al.*, 1993).   In addition, microbial protein synthesis increased at the expense of undigested feed protein flow to the intestines, but the net effect was an increase in total protein availability for digestion. In general, sorghum starch is the least digestible starch source fed to dairy cattle in the United States and shows the most improvement in feeding value for fattening rations when processed to increase its digestibility (Hale, 1973; Ørskov, 1976). Similarly, lactation responses to steam flaking of maize grain are less than for sorghum (Chen *et al.*, 1994).

Numerous studies measuring duodenal starch flow and faecal starch output have shown that the capacity for postruminal starch digestion in the lactating dairy cow is large. In the study of Klusmeyer *et al.* (1991a) postruminal starch digestion reached 5.4 kg/d and averaged over 4 kg/d in a number of recent studies for which ground maize was fed to lactating dairy cows (Table 8.2), but few studies have measured the capacity for small-intestinal starch digestion in the lactating dairy cow. These measurements are needed in order to predict production responses to shifting the site of starch digestion. Total tract digestion of maize is often lower in cattle than sheep, due to differences in grain mastication and flow rate from the rumen, therefore feeding values determined in sheep should be applied to lactating cows with caution (Reynolds and Beever, 1995). In 11 trials with growing cattle fed on maize grain processed by various methods and encompassing 44 treatment means, starch digestibility in the small intestine was 530 g/kg (Owens *et al.*, 1986). In these same trials, total postruminal starch digestibility was 720 g/kg. For the additional starch digestion in the large intestine and caecum the average digestibility was 390 g/kg. Starch digestibility in the rumen for maize-based diets averaged 720 g/kg, thus the digestibility of maize starch in steers appears to decrease as it flows through the gastrointestinal tract. This is because within each successive site of digesion the more digestible starch fraction is removed first, leaving the fraction with lower rate and extent of potential digestion which is more likely to escape to the next site of digestion. With greater intake level and rate of passage for lactating dairy cows compared to steers starch digestibility in the rumen would be expected to be lower and in lactating dairy cows consuming from 3.8 to 10.6 kg ground maize starch/d ruminal starch digestibility averaged 460 g/kg (Table 8.2).

Short term infusion studies have suggested that as starch supply to the abomasum increases fractional digestion in the small intestine decreases (Kriekemeier *et al.*, 1991). However, in growing cattle which were adapted to their dietary treatments, regression of rate of starch digestion in the small intestine on rate of starch flow to the duodenum was linear and positive. This suggests that in these studies, where starch flow to the

Table 8.2 RECENTLY PUBLISHED MEASUREMENTS OF RUMINAL AND POSTRUMINAL STARCH DIGESTION IN LACTATING DAIRY COWS.

Diet	DM Intake	Milk yield	Starch passage, kg/d			Digestion, g/kg		Reference
			Intake	Duodenal	Faecal	Rumen	Postrumen	
Barley + CSM	18.3	20.0	5.8	1.2	0.3	800	709	Herrera-Saldena et al., 1990.
Barley + BDG	19.6	''	6.0	1.2	0.4	800	681	
Sorghum + CSM	20.2	''	6.3	3.2	0.6	498	800	
Sorghum + BDG	18.3	''	4.5	2.5	0.6	488	744	
Maize SBM - 14.5% CP	21.8	29.3	9.1	3.8	0.5	583	868	Klusmeyer et al., 1990.
Maize SBM - 11.0% CP	20.9	26.9	9.8	4.6	0.7	530	848	
Maize MGM - 14.5% CP	20.9	29.6	9.5	4.4	0.6	530	864	
Maize MGM - 11.0% CP	21.6	26.6	10.4	4.6	0.9	556	804	
Maize SBM	25.1	39.9	10.6	5.4	0.8	485	854	Klusmeyer et al., 1991a.
Maize SBM + CaLCFA	23.8	39.9	9.0	5.4	0.4	399	930	
Maize FM	23.4	41.7	9.8	5.3	0.5	460	879	
Maize FM + CaLCFA	22.3	40.5	8.9	5.2	0.4	417	925	
Low forage	25.5	36.0	9.3	4.7	0.4	499	917	Klusmeyer et al., 1991b.
Low forage + CaLCFA	24.0	37.4	8.0	4.4	0.3	434	922	
High forage	24.7	35.3	7.0	3.5	0.3	494	914	
High forage + CaLCFA	23.3	35.7	5.9	2.8	0.2	525	914	
Ground maize	23.1	31.2	7.6	4.2	0.2	455	943	Cameron et al., 1991.
Ground maize + urea	23.0	31.8	7.5	4.9	0.2	344	946	
Ground maize + starch	21.6	29.9	8.3	4.2	0.2	491	926	
Ground maize + both	21.0	31.4	8.0	3.8	0.1	524	954	

Table 8.2 Continued

Diet	DM Intake	Milk yield	Starch passage, kg/d			Digestion, g/kg		Reference
			Intake	Duodenal	Faecal	Rumen	Postrumen	
Ground maize	19.9	29.1	5.8	3.6	0.3	433	900	Lynch et al., 1991.
Ground maize + Met/Lys	19.4	27.9	5.5	3.3	0.2	432	926	
Ground maize + bST	20.0	33.3	5.8	4.1	0.2	306	933	
Ground maize + both	19.9	31.2	5.8	3.6	0.2	401	939	
Alfalfa + rolled sorghum	20.7	18.2	6.2	3.6	1.0	426	691	Poore et al., 1993.
Alfalfa + flaked sorghum	20.7	19.2	6.1	1.8	0.1	711	921	
Straw + rolled sorghum	21.3	18.6	7.2	3.3	1.4	535	565	
Straw + flaked sorghum	20.7	19.6	6.8	1.6	0.1	763	915	
Maize:Barley - 100:0	22.8	26.9	7.5	4.3	0.7	419	809	Overton et al., 1995.
75:25	22.1	27.8	7.3	2.8	0.5	606	804	
50:50	21.3	26.6	7.1	2.7	0.4	609	800	
25:75	19.5	25.2	6.6	1.7	0.3	744	801	
0:100	19.6	22.6	6.7	1.7	0.3	744	812	
Maize - dry rolled	16.5	22.9	3.9	2.0	0.9	470	488	Plascenia and Zinn, 1996.
Maize - flaked, .39 kg/l	17.8	25.5	4.3	2.3	0.3	453	834	
Maize - flaked, .32 kg/l	17.3	25.6	4.3	1.5	0.1	646	915	
Maize - flaked, .26 kg/l	17.8	25.5	4.8	1.5	0.1	691	958	

small intestine reached over 4 g/kg BW, the capacity of the small intestine for starch digestion was not exceeded (Owens *et al.*, 1986). For published studies in lactating dairy cattle a positive, linear relationship between starch flow to the intestines and total postruminal starch digestion has also been reported (Nocek and Tamminga, 1991). Their regression suggested that total postruminal starch digestibility was 730 g/kg and that the capacity for digestion was not reduced at duodenal flows of up to 4 kg/d, which agrees with the conclusions of Owens *et al.* (1986) for growing cattle. However, in more recent studies in lactating dairy cows (Table 8.2), total postruminal starch digestion averaged 860 g/kg. For the studies reported in Table 8.2, relationships between starch inputs and ruminal, postruminal and total tract starch digestion are shown in figures 8.1, 8.2 and 8.3, respectively. The linear regression for data from studies where ground maize was the primary starch source is also depicted. The slope of the regression for total postruminal starch digestion for all starch sources (0.945±0.037; r^2=0.95) suggests that the capacity for postruminal starch digestion in the lactating dairy cow is high. With one exception where ground maize was fed (Plascencia and Zinn, 1996), sorghum appeared to be the only source of starch resistant to postruminal digestion for the studies cited. Nocek and Tamminga (1991) implied that with increasing postruminal supply the digestibility of starch in the small intestine of the lactating dairy cow is decreased and an increasing proportion of postruminal digestion occurs in the hindgut, but rates of starch digestion in the small intestine appear to have been estimated using data from growing cattle (Owens *et al.*, 1986). Starch fermentation in the hindgut provides VFA which are available for absorption, but microbial protein synthesized in the hindgut is not digested and elevates endogenous faecal N (Ørskov, 1986), which decreases apparent N digestibility.

Available data describing small-intestinal starch digestion in lactating dairy cows are presented in Table 8.3. These data were all obtained using markers to estimate starch flow in the duodenum and ileum and in each case problems in obtaining representative digesta samples, or with the markers themselves, were reported. In the study of Knowlton *et al.* (1996) greater flow of starch in the ileum than in the duodenum for rolled maize was blamed on segregation of particles (maize grain) during sampling and processing. Similarly, problems encountered with measurements of duodenal flow using cannulae placed near the pylorus were attributed to segregation of digesta particles at the sampling site and therefore the data reported for starch flow were based on measurements obtained using a more distal cannulation site after the pancreatic duct (Palmquist *et al.*, 1993). The data of Knowlton *et al.* (1996) do suggest that although duodenal starch flow was lower for the less mature, fermented maize grain, due to more extensive digestion in the rumen, the starch reaching the duodenum was more digestible and therefore total starch digestion in the small intestine was greater for the high moisture than the more mature, dry grain. Thus, for the rations based on mature maize, a much greater proportion of total-tract starch digestion occurred in the hindgut.

The data of Sutton and Oldham (Table 8.3) are unpublished data from 4 lactating cows in a study for which the experimental design did not allow direct statistical

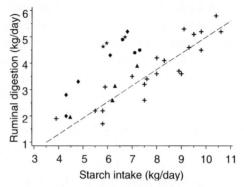

Figure 8.1. Relationship between ruminal starch digestion and starch intake in lactating dairy cows fed diets containing starch primarily from ground maize (+), barley (★), sorghum (▲), steam-flaked maize or sorghum (♦) or mixtures of ground maize and barley (●). The linear regression for ground maize based diets (y = -1.154 + 0.614(x), r²=0.837) is shown. Data from Table 8.2.

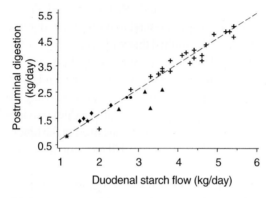

Figure 8.2 Relationship between postruminal starch digestion and duodenal starch flow in lactating dairy cows fed diets containing starch primarily from ground maize (+), barley (★), sorghum (▲), steam-flaked maize or sorghum (♦) or mixtures of ground maize and barley (●). The linear regression for ground maize based diets (y = -0.272 + 0.965(x), r²=0.918) is shown. Data from Table 8.2.

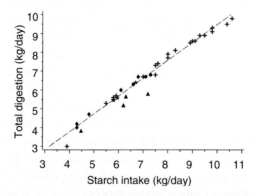

Figure 8.3 Relationship between total starch digestion and starch intake in lactating dairy cows fed diets containing starch primarily from ground maize (+), barley (★), sorghum (▲), steam-flaked maize or sorghum (♦) or mixtures of ground maize and barley (●). The linear regression for ground maize based diets (y = -0.025 + 0.950(x), r²=0.982) is shown. Data from Table 8.2.

Table 8.3 SITE OF STARCH DIGESTION IN LACTATING DAIRY COWS FITTED WITH RUMINAL, DUODENAL AND ILEAL CANNULAE

| | | Starch passage, kg/d | | | | Starch digestion, g/kg | | | |
	DMI	Milk yield	Intake	Duodenal	Ileal	Faecal	Rumen	S. Intestine	Hindgut	Reference
Control	17.9	28.5	4.2	0.5	0.12	0.03	887	745	750	a
+ Fat	16.2	29.0	2.4	0.2	0.06	0.02	901	750	667	
+ Protein	17.2	30.6	2.9	0.2	0.05	0.02	921	780	600	
+ Fat + Protein	16.0	28.8	1.6	0.2	0.03	0.01	893	824	667	
Dry maize - ground	23.4	35.2	7.9	3.1	2.7	0.9	609	132	674	b
Dry maize - rolled	23.4	33.4	7.9	2.5	2.9	2.0	692	-	696	
HM maize - ground	24.4	35.0	8.8	1.1	0.5	0.2	868	588	319	
HM maize - rolled	23.7	35.2	8.3	1.6	0.6	0.4	812	633	345	
Barley - 60%	12.9	14.6	4.0	0.6	0.1	0.1	843	773	562	c
Barley - 90%	11.0	14.5	5.5	0.8	0.2	0.1	857	715	663	
Maize - 60%	12.4	15.6	4.4	2.2	0.6	0.2	507	738	438	
Maize - 90%	12.0	17.5	6.4	3.5	1.1	0.7	454	676	368	

a - Palmquist et al., 1993
b - Knowlton et al., 1996
c - Sutton and Oldham, unpublished

comparisons, therefore the data presented are treatment means unadjusted for missing observations or period effects. In addition, problems were encountered with the use of the marker employed (Cr_2O_3) and therefore corrections have been applied. These flow rates were measured in cows fed either 60 or 90% concentrates based on rolled barley or ground maize in a 2 × 2 factorial design. Measurements of VFA production for the barley-based diets (Table 8.1) were obtained using different cows as a companion study to these measurements of site of starch digestion. Compared to barley, feeding maize decreased starch digestion in the rumen and increased starch digestion in both the small intestine and hindgut, but the digestibility of starch digested in the small intestine was not dramatically lower for maize (711 g/kg) than for barley (744 g/kg). In contrast, starch digestibility in the hindgut did appear to be lower for maize (408 g/kg) than for barley (612 g/kg), but the amount of starch reaching the hindgut was much lower for the barley-based diets. Across all these studies, the largest amount of starch digested in the small intestine of the lactating dairy cow was 2.4 kg/d (Table 8.3). Total postruminal starch digestibility was 909 and 855 g/kg for barley and maize starches, respectively. These values for maize starch digestion in the small intestine and postruminal tract are higher than the averages reported for growing cattle, but not outside the range (Owens *et al.*, 1986).

In a recent study in early lactation cows, a suspension of maize starch was infused into the duodenum of 4 cows at 0, 700, 1400 and 2100 g/d in a 4 x 4 Latin Square design with 2-week periods for adaptation to the infused starch (Reynolds *et al.*, 1996). Dry matter intake and faecal starch concentration were not affected by starch infusion, thus even at the highest level of infusion nearly all the starch supplied was digested. During the last 4 days of each infusion, milk yield was increased by starch infusion, but milk fat concentration was reduced, especially at the lower rates of infusion (Table 8.4). This reduction in milk fat concentration, although small, was probably caused by an increase in glucose availability and could not be attributed to an increase in trans-fatty acid absorption because trans-fatty acids produced in the hindgut would not be available for absorption. As a consequence of the reduction in milk fat concentration, milk energy output was only increased by the highest level of starch infusion, suggesting that much of ME from the starch infused was either oxidized or used for body tissue energy retention. At the highest level of starch infusion the recovery of infused gross energy as milk energy output was only 17.5%. Although nearly all the starch infused was digested, the proportion of infused starch digested in the small intestine to glucose versus the proportion digested in the hindgut is uncertain. Any carbon from starch fermented in the hindgut could be absorbed as VFA and utilized in the gut or postabsorptive tissues, emitted as gas, or excreted as microbial biomass in faeces.

Postruminal starch digestion and glucose absorption

Across a variety of rations, measurements of net PDV glucose flux in lactating cattle

Table 8.4 MILK COMPOSITION AND YIELD DURING THE LAST 4 DAYS OF 10-DAY DUODENAL INFUSION OF MAIZE STARCH IN 4 DAIRY COWS IN EARLY TO MID-LACTATION (REYNOLDS *et al.*, 1996).

| | *Starch, g/d* | | | | | |
	0	681	1374	2019	SEM	P<
DM intake, kg/d	18.0	18.2	18.4	18.4	0.2	0.521
Faecal starch, g/kg	6.8	7.5	11.3	14.5	3.4	0.412
Milk yield, kg/d	31.8	33.1	32.5	33.8	0.3	0.039
FCM, kg/d[1]	32.4	32.7	32.6	33.9	0.1	0.006
Milk energy, MJ/d[2]	97.8	98.8	98.4	102.9		
Protein content, g/kg	29.9	29.8	30.4	30.2	0.4	0.717
Protein yield, g/d	943	986	984	1012	19	0.264
Fat content, g/kg	41.6	39.3	40.1	40.7	0.4	0.071
Fat yield, g/d	1315	1298	1305	1361	4	0.005
Lactose content, g/kg	46.2	46.2	46.2	46.1	0.1	0.959
Lactose yield, g/d	1468	1529	1506	1559	14	0.065

[1] Fat corrected (4%) milk.
[2] Calculated as described by Tyrrell and Reid (1965).

vary around zero and in many cases are negative (Reynolds *et al.*, 1994). Even when large amounts of maize grain are fed, net PDV glucose absorption is low relative to the amount of starch estimated to be reaching the small intestine (Weighart *et al.*, 1986; Casse *et al.*, 1994). A negative PDV glucose flux does not mean that no glucose is absorbed, but that PDV use of arterial glucose exceeds glucose absorption into the portal vein. Numerous studies in growing cattle have found that increases in net glucose absorption by the PDV only account for roughly a third of the glucose in starch provided to the small intestine (Harmon, 1992), but this recovery assumes a complete digestion of starch to glucose. In studies where net PDV glucose absorption and changes in ileal flow of starch were measured simultaneously, the recovery of infused maize starch as increased net PDV glucose absorption ranged from 380 (Kreikemeier *et al.*, 1991) to 570 (Kreikemeier and Harmon, 1995) g/kg starch disappearing from the small intestine. The fate of the missing starch carbon is not certain, but a large part of the missing glucose must be utilized for triacylglyceride and fat synthesis or ATP generation in the PDV. The PDV includes mesenteric and omental fat deposits which account for up to 20% of total body fat. In addition, gut epithelial tissue and muscle use glucose as an energy substrate. Measurements of net glucose absorption do not account for any simultaneous increase in uptake of glucose from arterial blood by the PDV when glucose absorption increases the postabsorptive supply of glucose. Thus net PDV glucose absorption underestimates true glucose absorption to the extent that glucose is utilized both during absorption, before reaching venous blood, and from arterial blood. It should be remembered that the PDV receives roughly 40 to 50% of cardiac output in cattle (Huntington *et al.*, 1990), therefore a similar proportion of glucose reaching the heart is immediately returned to the PDV and available for metabolism there. In a recent study in sheep (Cappelli *et al.*, 1993) intraduodenal infusion of glucose increased body glucose turnover by 67% and PDV utilization of arterial glucose by 48%. These increases in body and PDV glucose utilization represented 78% and 20% of the glucose infused, respectively.

As discussed previously, increased PDV energy deposition will contribute to an overall improvement in energetic efficiency, but at the expense of milk energy output. Theoretically, increased glucose absorption does make more glucose available for milk synthesis if the propensity for milk synthesis is greater than the maximal capacity for glucose extraction by the mammary gland (less the gland's glucose requirement for maintenance and growth). One would expect however that except in very early lactation endogenous synthesis is capable of meeting the needs of the mammary gland and that additional glucose from the small intestine will to a large extent be used for tissue energy retention, cause a reduction in endogenous synthesis, or both. Indeed, postruminal or intravenous infusion of glucose in fed lactating dairy cows causes only a slight, if any, increase in milk yield relative to the amount infused (Reynolds *et al.*, 1994). When starch was infused into the duodenum (Table 8.4), increases in lactose yield accounted for only 25 to 81 g/kg glucose equivalents infused.

Although an increase in arterial glucose utilization by the PDV may in part explain the low recovery of abomasally infused starch as increased net PDV glucose absorption, the recovery of abomasally infused glucose as increased net PDV glucose flux is always higher than for infused starch, dextrin or partially hydrolyzed starch (Harmon, 1992). In steers equipped with ileal cannulae cited previously, increases in net PDV glucose absorption accounted for 900 (Kreikemeier *et al.*, 1991) and 733 (Kreikemeier and Harmon, 1995) g/kg of infused glucose not reaching the ileum. This is much higher than the recovery of abomasally infused starch in these steers, therefore either there are fates other than glucose absorption for starch disappearing from the small intestine or the glucose liberated by starch digestion is metabolized differently than infused glucose. This might be due to differences in the postabsorptive endocrine and metabolic response to the glucose absorbed. One major difference between the two routes of carbohydrate administration is the region of the small intestine in which glucose is available for absorption. In multicatheterized steers increases in net PDV glucose flux accounted for a much greater proportion of glucose infused into the duodenum than when glucose was infused into the mid-jejunum and in lambs the mRNA for glucose transporter is higher in the proximal 25% of the intestine (Krehbiel *et al.*, 1996). On the other hand, less than 10 % of starch digestion occurred prior to the mid-jejunum (first 40% of the small intestine) in steers abomasally infused with starch (Russell, 1979 as cited by Krehbiel *et al.*, 1996). Data from growing steers indicates that maltase and isomaltase activity is lowest in the duodenum and highest in the mid-jejunum and ileum in cattle (Kreikemeier *et al.*, 1990).

Thus ruminants appear to be efficient at absorbing glucose from the proximal small intestine, but inefficient at digesting starch to glucose prior to the mid-jejunal region where glucose absorption is severely limited. This increases the concentration of glucose and oligosaccharides in the ileum where increasing pH and back flush from the large intestine may allow a limited microbial population to survive and ferment small amounts of carbohydrate (Armstrong and Beever, 1969). In addition, the presence of undigested carbohydrate and VFA may stimulate release of ileal peptides (Taylor, 1993) which may also modulate metabolic responses to starch via signals which are distinct from those arising when abomasally infused glucose is absorbed prior to the ileum.

Limits to starch digestion in the small intestine

Although regression analysis has suggested that the digestibility of maize starch in the small intestine remains relatively constant across a broad range of duodenal inputs (Owens *et al.*, 1986), numerous studies in cattle have suggested that the capacity of the small intestine for starch digestion may be limited (Ørskov, 1986; Harmon, 1992). In some cases these limitations may be a consequence of limited treatment periods which do not allow time for adaptation to increased starch supply (Waldo, 1973). Limits to starch digestion may be a consequence of starch physical structure or the capacity of α-amylase, disaccharidases or glucose absorption (Kreikemeier and Harmon, 1995). Both physical processing and maturity of maize grain may alter the accessibility of maize grain starch to enzymatic hydrolysis in the small intestine (Hale, 1973; Knowlton *et al.*, 1996). Data of Krehbiel *et al.* (1996) suggest that glucose-transporter activity limits glucose absorption in the distal small intestine. A resulting increase in luminal glucose concentration may cause end-product inhibition of the activity of disaccharidases directly and α-amylase directly or indirectly via a build up of oligosaccharides (Kreikemeier and Harmon, 1995). The presence of large amounts of ethanol-soluble α-glucoside (amylose) and short-chain α-glucoside (oligosaccharide) in the ileal digesta of steers abomasally infused with starch suggests that the activity of both groups of enzymes may be limiting. Although a number of early infusion studies showed that increasing starch flow to the duodenum increased α-amylase secretion from the pancreas, these studies are confounded by effects of total ME supply (Harmon, 1992). Steers fed maize-based rations had less α-amylase capacity in the pancreas and intestine than steers fed alfalfa hay at equal ME, but α-amylase capacity increased with increasing ME for both rations (Kreikemeier *et al.*, 1990). This suggests that ME, rather than rumen escape starch *per se*, increases α-amylase capacity in the intestine of cattle; however, the positive effect of duodenal protein flow on pancreatic α-amylase secretion must also be considered in interpreting these studies. The presence of similar amounts of short-chain α-glucoside in the ileal digesta of steers abomasally infused with maize starch or maize dextrin suggests that the α-1,4 glucosidase (maltase) may be more limiting than α-1,6 glucosidase (isomaltase) because dextrin is highly branched (Kreikemeier and Harmon, 1995). If the α-1,6 glucosidase was limiting then one would expect more short-chain glucosidase to be present in the ileal digesta of steers infused with dextrin. The limited time for α-amylase action in the proximal small intestine, the limited availability of disaccharidases in the proximal small intestine, the limited capacity of glucose transporters in the distal small intestine and the negative effect of duodenal starch flow on pancreatic α-amylase secretion all contradict the concept that rumen-escape starch is a more efficient source of ME in cattle than rumen degradable starch. Thus, when considering site of starch digestion, we must also consider site of starch digestion within the small intestine.

Milk protein concentration

Recent articles in the popular press have reported that providing more rumen- escape starch by feeding maize will increase milk protein concentration, but on the same page reports from other studies suggest that feeding more rumen- fermentable carbohydrate will increase milk protein concentration (Farmer's Weekly, 1996). How can these conflicting results be resolved? The small, positive response of milk protein concentration to ME supply is well documented (Emery, 1978) and it is now dogma that increasing ME will increase milk protein concentration if the increased energy is provided via carbohydrate and not fat. This relationship has been found in other summarizations as well (Sutton, 1989), but is not necessarily predictable within individual studies. The response may be due to changes in rumen fermentation as well as changes in postabsorptive metabolic and endocrine responses, particularly changes in glucose and insulin status. With increasing ME from carbohydrate, rates of organic matter digestion in the rumen (fermentable ME [FME]) will in most cases increase as well. As long as sufficient quantities of rumen degradable protein and nonprotein N are available, this will increase microbial protein synthesis in the rumen and metabolizable protein supply to the small intestine (Waldo, 1973). This is due to effects of increased FME and not starch fermentation *per se*. Comparisons between barley and beet pulp have shown that both sources of FME are equally effective in increasing milk protein concentration (de Visser, 1993). Thus a part of the milk protein response to ME must be attributable to increases in FME and microbial protein synthesis, but this cannot explain a milk protein response to increased postruminal starch digestion.

In addition to increasing metabolizable protein supply, increasing ME and FME may also increase glucose supply via increased availability of propionate and other glucose precursors. Based on the rumen infusion studies of Rook and Balch (1961) the milk protein response to ME has often been attributed to an increase in propionate absorption, but few subsequent infusion studies have supported this view. This is in part due to the negative effects of propionate on intake which often confound interpretation of responses (Casse *et al.*, 1994). If increased ME does increase propionate absorption and/or glucose turnover then in most cases this may elicit an insulin response, especially in cows in positive energy balance, and there is evidence that milk protein concentration and yield may be increased with increased glucose and insulin turnover. In early lactation, cows fed rations containing either 20% or 60% maize-based concentrate at equal digestible energy, plasma glucose concentration and turnover during the postprandial period were nearly doubled by feeding the higher concentrate ration and this was associated with a dramatic increase in milk protein concentration (Evans *et al.*, 1975). This increase in glucose availability was associated with an increase in plasma concentrations of insulin. Recent data provide direct evidence that elevated insulin and glucose can increase milk protein concentration (McGuire *et al.*, 1994). Cows were infused intravenously with large amounts of insulin and glucose for 4 days using a euglycaemic insulin clamp technique in which the rate of glucose infusion was varied in order to maintain basal blood glucose concentration during the insulin infusion. Initial trials showed that this would increase milk protein concentration (McGuire *et al.*, 1995), therefore the study was repeated with the addition of an abomasal casein infusion to increase amino acid supply to the mammary gland. When additional metabolizable protein was combined with the insulin and glucose infusion there was a significant increase in milk yield, milk protein concentration and milk protein yield (McGuire *et al.*, 1994). The mechanisms behind this response are not certain and may involve other hormones in the somatrophic axis. Depending on the physiological status of the cow and her basal diet, ME supply and/or increased ruminal or postruminal starch digestion could all contribute to an increase in glucose and insulin turnover. Cows in early lactation may be resistant to effects of insulin and may use additional glucose for milk synthesis, therefore positive effects of increased glucose and insulin supply may be greater in cows in positive energy balance and with lower somatotropin:insulin ratios. However, any milk protein response will still require an adequate supply of amino acids to the mammary gland.

Based on these observations, elevated glucose supply represents one mechanism by which increased postruminal starch digestion might increase milk protein concentration. It has also been hypothesized that increased glucose absorption might spare amino acids from catabolism in the gut by supplying additional energy for gut metabolism (de Visser, 1993). To date this hypothesis has not been rigorously tested, but the principal amino acids providing energy for gut enterocytes are the nonessential amino acids glutamine, glutamate and aspartate. These are the amino acids present in the largest amount in microbial protein and any sparing of amino acid catabolism by absorbed glucose in the small intestine would probably provide more of these amino acids rather than essential amino acids limiting milk protein synthesis (Reynolds *et al.*, 1995). In cows at peak lactation fed a diet containing 180 g/kg crude protein, duodenal starch infusion had no affect on milk protein concentration or yield (Reynolds *et al.*, 1996), which does not support the concept that increased glucose supply from postruminal starch digestion increases milk protein concentration by changing gut metabolism of amino acids or insulin status.

Conclusions

In general, when lactating dairy cows are fed increasing amounts of cereal starch, ME supply will increase if dry matter intake is not reduced. This is often associated with a decrease in milk fat concentration and an increase in body tissue fat synthesis which may be due in part to a glucose and insulin response, but in more severe cases there is strong evidence that an increased supply of trans-fatty acids is the cause. At the same time it is generally accepted that increased ME from carbohydrate often increases milk protein concentration. This response may be due to an increase in microbial protein synthesis attributable to increased FME in the rumen, but there is evidence that the response may also be linked to an increase in glucose supply and associated changes in insulin status or other hormonal responses. Thus stage of lactation and genetic merit may affect the response. In terms of feeding supplemental starch *per se*, the milk protein concentration response varies considerably. If rapidly digested starch is fed the response may be negative due to depressions in dry matter and total ME intake and resulting decreases in microbial protein and glucose supply. Feeding rumen escape starch reduces rumen acid load and allows more total starch intake, but the recovery of starch reaching the intestines as net glucose absorption is low, in part due to limits to starch digestion in the small intestine and the use of glucose by the PDV, thus a portion of the starch reaching the intestines will be fermented in the hindgut. Fermentation in the hindgut will not benefit microbial protein supply. Therefore, although sources of rumen-escape starch also provide undegraded feed protein to the small intestine the overall effect is usually a decrease in metabolizable protein supply. Any increase in milk protein output will require a sufficient amino acid supply to support that response, and microbial protein may have advantages over many cereal grain proteins in terms of amino acid profile.

References

Agnew, K.W., Mayne, C.S. and Doherty, J.G. (1996) An examination of the effect of method and level of concentrate feeding on milk production in dairy cows offered a grass silage-based diet. *Animal Science*, **63**, 21–32.

AOAC (1995) AOAC Official method 979.10: Starch in Cereals. In *Official Methods of Analysis of AOAC International*, Chapter 32, p 25. Edited by P. Cunniff. AOAC International: Arlington, VA.

Armsby, H.P. (1903) *The Principles of Animal Nutrition*. John Wiley and Sons: New York, NY.

Armstrong, D.A., Blaxter, K.L. and N. McC. Graham (1960) Fat synthesis from glucose by sheep. *Proceedings of the Nutrition Society*, **19**, xxxi–xxxii.

Armstrong, D.A. and Blaxter, K.L. (1961) The utilization of the energy of carbohydrate by ruminants. In *Symposium on Energy Metabolism*, pp 187–199. Edited by E.

Brouwer and A.J.H. van Es, European Association for Animal Production Publication Number 10, Wageningen, The Netherlands.

Armstrong, D.A. and Beever, D.E. (1969) Post-abomasal digestion of carbohydrate in the adult ruminant. *Proceedings of the Nutrition Society*, **28**, 121–131.

Beever, D.E., Cammell, S.B. and Humphries, D.J. (1996) The effect of stage of maturity at the time of harvest on the subsequent nutritive value of maize silage fed to lactating dairy cows. CEDAR Report No 66.

Bergman, E.N., and Wolff, J.E. (1971) Metabolism of volatile fatty acids by liver and portal-drained viscera in sheep. *American Journal of Physiology*, **221**, 586–592.

Cameron, M.R., Klusmeyer, T.H., Lynch, G.L., Clark, J.H. and Nelson, D.R. (1991) Effects of urea and starch on rumen fermentation, nutrient passage to the duodenum, and performance of cows. *Journal of Dairy Science*, **74**, 1321–1336.

Cappelli, F.P., Seal, C.J. and Parker, D.S. (1993) Portal glucose absorption and utilization in sheep receiving exogenous glucose intravascularly or intraduodenally. *Journal of Animal Science*, **70 (Suppl. 1)**, 279.

Casse, E.A., Rulquin, H. and Huntington, G.B. (1994) Effect of mesenteric vein infusion of propionate on splanchnic metabolism in primiparous Holstein cows. *Journal of Dairy Science*, **77**, 3296–3303.

Chen, K.H., Huber, J.T., Theurer, C.B., Swingle, R.S., Simas, J., Chan, S.C., Wu, Z. and Sullivan, J.L. (1994) Effect of steam flaking of corn and sorghum grains on performance of lactating cows. *Journal of Dairy Science*, **77**, 1038–1043.

Clark, J.H., Klusmeyer, T.H. and Cameron, M.R. (1992) Microbial protein synthesis and flows of nitrogen fractions to the duodenum of dairy cows. *Journal of Dairy Science*, **75**, 2304–2323.

Coppock, C.E., Flatt, W.P. and Moore, L.A. (1964) Effect of hay to grain ratio on utilization of metabolizable energy for milk production by dairy cows. *Journal of Dairy Science*, **12**, 1330–1338.

Davis, C.L. and Brown, R.E. (1970) Low-fat milk syndrome. In *Physiology of Digestion and Metabolism in the Ruminant*, pp. 545–565. Edited by A.T. Phillipson. Oriel Press: England.

DePeters, E.J. and Taylor, S.J. (1985) Effects of feeding corn or barley on composition of milk and diet digestibility. *Journal of Dairy Science*, **68**, 2027–2032.

De Visser, H. (1993) Characterization of carbohydrates in concentrates for dairy cows. In *Recent Advances in Animal Nutrition - 1993*, pp 19–38. Edited by P.C. Garnsworthy and D.J.A. Cole. Nottingham University Press: Nottingham.

Evans, E., Buchanan-Smith, J.G., MacLeod, G.K. and Stone, J.B. (1975) Glucose metabolism in cows fed low- and high-roughage diets. *Journal of Dairy Science*, **58**, 672–677.

Emery, R.S. (1978) Feeding for increased milk protein. *Journal of Dairy Science*, **61**, 825–828.

Farmers Weekly. 1996. Milk special. Higher quality - by design. March 22 issue, p. 50.

Forbes, J.M. (1995) Voluntary intake: a limiting factor to production in high-yielding dairy cows? In *Breeding and Feeding the High Genetic Merit Dairy Cow*, pp 13–19. Edited by T.J.L. Lawrence, F.J. Gordon and A. Carson. British Society of Animal Production Occasional Publication No. 19.

Garnsworthy, P.C. and Jones, B.P. (1993) The effects of dietary fibre and starch concentrations on the response by dairy cows to body condition at calving. *Animal Science*, **57**, 15–22.

Gaynor, P. J., Erdman, R.A., Teter, B.B., Sampugna, J., Capuco, A.V., Waldo D.R.and Hamosh, M.(1994) Milk fat yield and composition during abomasal infusion of *cis* or *trans* octadecenoates in Holstein cows. *Journal of Dairy Science*, **77**, 157–165.

Gordon, F.J., Porter, M.G., Mayne, C.S., Unsworth, E.F. and Kilpatrick, D.J. (1995) Effect of forage digestibility and type of concentrate on nutrient utilization by lactating dairy cattle. *Journal of Dairy Research*, **62**, 15–27.

Griinari, J.M., Bauman, D.E. and Jones, L.R. (1995) Low milk fat in New York Holstein herds. In *Proceedings of the Cornell Nutrition Conference for Feed Manufacturers*. pp. 96–105.

Grant, J.J. (1994) Influence of corn and sorghum starch on the in vitro kinetics of forage fiber digestion. *Journal of Dairy Science*, **77**, 1563–1569.

Hale, W.H. (1973) Influence of processing on the utilization of grains (starch) by ruminants. *Journal of Animal Science*, **37**, 1075–1080.

Harmon, D.L. (1992) Dietary influences on carbohydrases and small intestinal starch hydrolysis capacity in ruminants. *Journal of Nutrition*, **122**, 203–210.

Herrera-Saldena, R., Gomez-Alarcon, R., Rorabi, M. and Huber, J.T. (1990) Influence of synchronizing protein and starch degradation in the rumen on nutrient utilization and microbial protein synthesis. *Journal of Dairy Science*, **73**, 142–148.

Huntington, G. B., J. H. Eisemann, and J. M. Whitt. 1990. Portal blood flow in beef steers: comparison of techniques and relation to hepatic blood flow, cardiac output and oxygen uptake. *Journal of Animal Science*, **68**, 1666–1673.

Karr, M.R., Little, C.O. and Mitchell, G.E. (1966) Starch disappearcnce from different segments of the digestive tract of steers. *Journal of Animal Science*, **25**, 652–654.

Khorasani, G.R., De Boer, G., Robinson, B. and Kennelly, J.J. (1994) Influence of dietary protein and starch on production and metabolic responses of dairy cows. *Journal of Dairy Science*, **77**, 813–824.

Klusmeyer, T.H., McCarthy, R.D.Jr., Clark, J.H. and Nelson, D.R. (1990) Effects of source and amount of protein on ruminal fermentation and passage of nutrients to the small intestine of lactating cows. *Journal of Dairy Science*, **73**, 3526–3537.

Klusmeyer, T.H., Lynch, G.L., Clark, J.H. and Nelson D.R. (1991a) Effects of calcium salts of fatty acids and protein source on ruminal fermentation and nutrient flow to duodenum of cows. *Journal of Dairy Science*, **74**, 2206–2219.

Klusmeyer, T.H., Lynch, G.L., Clark, J.H. and Nelson D.R. (1991b) Effects of calcium salts of fatty acids and proportion of forage in diet on ruminal fermentation and nutrient flow to duodenum of cows. *Journal of Dairy Science*, **74**, 2220–2232.

Knowlton, K.F., Glenn, B.P. and Erdman, R.A. (1996) Effect of corn grain maturity and processing on performance, rumen fermentation, and site of starch diegestion in early lactation diary cattle. *Journal of Dairy Science*, **79 (Suppl. 1)**, 138.

Krehbiel, C.R., Britton, R.A., Harmon, D.L., Peters, J.P., Stock R.A. and Grotjan, H.E. (1996) Effects of varying levels of duodenal or midjejunal glucose and 2-deoxyglucose infusion on small intestinal disappearance and net portal glucose flux in steers. *Journal of Animal Science*, **74**, 693–700.

Kreikemeier, K.K., Harmon, D.L., Peters, J.P., Gross, K.L., Armendariz, C.K. and Krehbiel, C.R. (1990) Influence of dietary forage and feed intake on carbohydrase activities and small intestinal morphology of calves. *Journal of Animal Science*, **68**, 2916–2929.

Kreikemeier, K.K., Harmon, D.L., Brandt, R.T., Avery, T.B. and Johnson, D.E. (1991) Small intestinal starch digestion in steers: effect of various levels of abomasal glucose, corn starch and corn dextrin infusion on small intestinal disappearance and net glucose absorption. *Journal of Animal Science*, **69**, 328–338.

Kreikemeier, K.K. and Harmon, D.L. (1995) Abomasal glucose, maize starch and maize dextrin infusions in cattle: Small intestinal disappearance, net portal glucose flux and ileal oligosaccharide flow. *British Journal of Nutrition*, **73**, 763–772.

Lynch, G.L., Klusmeyer, T.H., Cameron, M.R., Clark, J.H. and Nelson, D.R. (1991) Effects of somatotropin and duodenal infusion of amino acids on nutrient passage to duodenum and performance of dairy cows. *Journal of Dairy Science*, **74**, 3117–3127.

MacRae, J.C. and Armstrong, D.G. (1968) Enzyme method for determination of α-linked glucose polymers in biological materials. *Journal of the Science of Food and Agriculture*, **19**, 578–581.

McCarthy, R.D., Klusmeyer, T.H., Vicini, J.L., Clark, J.H. and Nelson, D.R. (1989) Effect of source of protein and carbohydrate on ruminal fermentation and passage of nutrients to the small intestine of lactating cows. *Journal of Dairy Science*, **72**, 2002–2016.

McGuire, M.A., Griinari, J.M., Dwyer, D.A. and Bauman, D.E. (1994) Potential to increase milk protein in well-fed cows. In *Proceedings of the Cornell Nutrition Conference for Feed Manufacturers*, pp 124–133.

McGuire, M.A., Griinari, J.M., Dwyer, D.A. and Bauman, D.E. (1995) Role of insulin in the regulation of mammary synthesis of fat and protein. *Journal of Dairy Science*, **78**, 816–824.

Moe, P.W., Tyrrell, H.F. and Hooven, N.W. (1973) Physical form and energy value of corn grain. *Journal of Dairy Science*, **56**, 1298–1304.

Moe, P.W. and Tyrrell, H.F. (1979) Effect of endosperm type on incremental energy value of corn grain for dairy cows. *Journal of Dairy Science*, **62**, 447–454.

Nocek, J.E. and Tamminga, S. (1991) Site of digestion of starch in the gastrointestinal tract of dairy cows and its effect on milk yield and composition. *Journal of Dairy Science*, **74**, 3598–3629.

Ørskov, E.R., Fraser, C. and Kay, R.N.B. (1969) Dietary factors influencing the digestion of starch in the rumen and small and large intestine of early weaned lambs. *British Journal of Nutrition*, **23**, 217–226.

Ørskov, E.R. (1976) The effect of processing on diegestion and utilization of cereals by ruminants. *Proceedings of the Nutrition Society*, **35**, 245–252.

Ørskov, E.R. (1986) Starch digestion and utilization in ruminants. *Journal of Animal Science*, **63**, 1624–1633.

Overton, T.R., Cameron, M.R., Elliot, J.P., Clark, J.H. and Nelson, D.R. (1995) Ruminal fermentation and passage of nutrients to the duodenum of lactating cows fed mixtures of corn and barley. *Journal of Dairy Science*, **78**, 1981–1998.

Owens, F.N., Zinn, R.A. and Kim, Y.K. (1986) Limits to starch digestion in the ruminant small intestine. *Journal of Animal Science*, **63**, 1634–1648.

Palmquist, D.L., Wesibjerg, M.R. and Hvelplund, T. (1993) Ruminal, intestinal, and total digestibilities of nutrients in cows fed diets high in fat and undegradable protein. *Journal of Dairy Science*, **76**, 1353–1364.

Plascencia, A. and Zinn, R.A. (1996) Influence of flake density on the feeding value of steam-processed corn in diets for lactating cows. *Journal of Animal Science*, **74**, 310–316.

Poore, M.H., Moore, J.A., Eck, T.P., Swingle, R.S. and Theurer, C.B. (1993) Effect of fiber source and ruminal starch degradability on site and extent of digestion in dairy cows. *Journal of Dairy Science*, **76**, 2244–2253.

Reynolds, C. K., D. L. Harmon and M. J. Cecava (1994) Absorption and delivery of nutrients for milk protein synthesis by portal-drained viscera. *Journal of Dairy Science*, **77**, 2787–2808.

Reynolds C.K. and Beever, D.E. (1995) Energy requirements and responses: a UK perspective. In *Breeding and Feeding the High Genetic Merit Dairy Cow*, Edited by T.J.L. Lawrence, F.J. Gordon and A. Carson, pp 31–41. British Society of Animal Production Occasional Publication No. 19.

Reynolds, C., Crompton, L., Firth, K., Beever, D., Sutton, J., Lomax, M., Wray-Cahen, D., Metcalf, J., Chettle, E., Bequette, B., Backwell, C., Lobley, G. and MacRae, J. 1995. Splanchnic and milk protein responses to mesenteric vein infusion of 3 mixtures of amino acids in lactating dairy cows. *Journal of Animal Science*, **73** (**Suppl. 1**), 274.

Reynolds, C.K., Beever, D. E., Sutton, J.D. and Newbold, J.R. (1996) Effects of incremental duodenal starch infusion on milk composition and yield in dairy cows. *Journal of Dairy Science*, **79 (Suppl. 1)**, 138. [Full paper published 2001. *Journal of Dairy Science*, **84**, 2250-2259.

Romo, G., Erdman, R., Teter, B. and Casper, D.P. (1994) Potential role of trans fatty acids in diet induced milk fat depression in dairy cows. *Proceedings of the Maryland Nutrition Conference for Feed Manufacturers.* pp 64–71.

Rook, J.A.F., and Balch, C.C. 1961. The effects of intraruminal infusions of acetic, propionic and butyric acids on the yield and composition of the milk of the cow. *British Journal of Nutrition*, **15**, 361–369.

Sutton, J.D. (1979) Carbohydrate fermentation in the rumen - variations on a theme.*Proceedings of the Nutrition Society*, **38**, 275–282.

Sutton, J.D., Oldham, J.D. and Hart, I.C. (1980) Products of digestion, hormones and energy utilization in milking cows given concentrates containing varying proportions of barley or maize. In *Energy Metabolism, Proceedings of the 8th Symposium*, pp 303–306 Edited by L.E. Mount. European Association of Animal Production Publication 26, Butterworths: London.

Sutton, J. D. (1985) Digestion and absorption of energy substrates in the lactating cow. *Journal of Dairy Science*, **68**, 3376–3393.

Sutton, J.D., Broster, W.H., Napper, D.J. and Siviter, J.W. (1985) Feeding frequency for lactating cows: Effects on digestion, milk production and energy utilisation. *British Journal of Nutrition*, **53**, 117–130.

Sutton, J.D., Hart, I.C., Broster, W.H., Elliott, R.J. and Schuller, E. (1986) Feeding frequency for lactating cows: effects on rumen fermentation and blood metabolites and hormones. *British Journal of Nutrition*, **56**, 181–192.

Sutton, J.D. (1989) Altering milk composition by feeding. *Journal of Dairy Science*, **72**, 2801–2814.

Sutton, J.D., Aston, K., Beever, D.E. and Fisher, W.J. (1994) Milk production from grass silage diets: the relative importance of the amounts of energy and crude protein in the concentrates. *Animal Science*, **59**, 327–334.

Taylor, I.L. (1993) Role of peptide YY in the endocrine control of digestion. *Journal of Dairy Science*, **76**, 2094–2101.

Theurer, C. B. (1986) Grain processing effects on starch utilization by ruminants. *Journal of Animal Science*, **63**, 1649–1662.

Tyrrell, H.F. and Reid, J.T. (1965) Prediction of the energy value of cow's milk. *Journal of Dairy Science*, **48**, 1–9.

Tyrrell, H.F., Moe, P.W. and Oltjen, R.R. (1972) Energetics of fattening heifers on a corn vs. barley ration. *Journal of Animal Science*, **35 (Suppl. 1)**, 277.

Tyrrell, H.F. and Moe, P.W. (1972) Net energy value for lactation of a high and low concentrate ration containing corn silage. *Journal of Dairy Science*, **55**, 1106–1112.

Tyrrell, H.F. and Moe, P.W. (1974) Net energy value of a corn and a barley ration for lactation. *Journal of Dairy Science*, **57**, 451–458.

Tyrrell, H.F. (1980) Limits to milk production efficiency by the dairy cow. *Journal of Animal Science*, **51**, 1441–1447.

Waldo, D.R. (1973) Extent and partition of cereal grain starch digestion in ruminants. *Journal of Animal Science*, **37**, 1062–1074.

Wieghart, M., R. Slepetis, J. M. Elliot, and D. F. Smith. 1986. Glucose absorption and hepatic gluconeogenesis in dairy cows fed diets varying in forage content. *Journal of Nutrition*, **116**, 839–850.

Wilkerson, V.W. and Glenn, B.P. (1996) Energy balance in early lactation Holstein cows fed corn grain harvested as dry or high moisture and ground or rolled. *Journal of Animal Science*, **74 (Suppl. 1)**, 270.

Wiltrout, D.W., and Satter, L.D. (1972) Contribution of propionate to glucose synthesis in the lactating and nonlactating cow. *Journal of Dairy Science*, **55**, 307–317.

Wonsil, B.J., Herbein, J.H. and Watkins, B.A. (1994) Dietary and ruminally derived *trans*-18:1 fatty acids alter bovine milk lipids. *Journal of Nutrition*, **124**, 556–565.

This paper was first published in 1997

9

PROBLEMS ASSOCIATED WITH FEEDING RAPESEED MEAL TO DAIRY COWS

M.EMANUELSON
Department of *Animal Nutrition* and *Management, Swedish University* of *Agricultural Sciences, Kungsiingen Research Station, S-75323 Uppsala, Sweden*

Introduction

Rapeseed products *(Brassica napus oleifera* and *Brassica campestris oleifera)* have been used in dairy cow rations for many years. It is not clear when the use of such products in animal feeds began; however, products from plants in the genus *Brassica* (Br.) have been important components of human diets since antiquity (Bell, 1984).

In temperate countries oilseed rape has become an important crop. The seed consists of about 40% oil, and after oil extraction, a protein supplement is obtained. Since the introduction of cultivars containing low levels of erucic acid in the oil, rapeseed oils have been extensively evaluated in terms of their safety and nutritional value when used as cooking oils. Metabolic studies in humans have shown that such oil is as effective as sunflower oil, safflower oil and soya-bean oil in improving the lipoprotein profiles of healthy subjects (McDonald, 1992; Nydahl, Gustafsson, Öhrvall and Vessby, 1992). The small amount of erucic acid remaining in today's double-zero cultivars appears to be harmless. They are therefore used extensively owing to their favourable fatty acid profile, i.e. low in saturated fatty acids but high in oleic acid.

The residue left after oil extraction is used as a high-protein feed for livestock. Rapeseed meal (RSM) was already a common ingredient in dairy cow rations at the turn of the century. In most of the experiments conducted around 50 years ago, the substitution of between 1 and 1.5 kg of RSM per day in the ration, for other protein feeds such as soya bean meal and coconut cakes, increased milk production but lowered milk fat content (e.g. Bünger, Schultz, Augustin, Schelper, Richter, Herbst and Stang, 1938; Jarl, 1951; Witt, Huth and Hartman, 1959).

However, the inclusion of rapeseed products from early varieties in dairy cow rations was limited to about 1 kg RSM/day. The restricted use can be ascribed to the occurrence of high levels of glucosinolates, a class of sulphur-containing glucosides which may reduce palatability and adversely affect thyroid function and fertility, among other aspects of animal health.

In 1974 the first double low (00 or LG) cultivar of *Br. napus* was licensed in Canada. The name "canola" was introduced in Canada in 1979 and applied to all double low cultivars; i.e. erucic acid less than 2% of the total fatty acids and glucosinolate content less than 30 μmol per g of fat-free meal dry matter (DM) (Shahidi, 1990). Since then, extensive breeding work has resulted in a dramatic lowering of the total glucosinolate content. At the same time, the effects of using rapeseed in dairy cow rations have been widely investigated.

The usefulness of rapeseed meal as an animal feedstuff in general (Mawson, Heaney, Piskula and Kozlowska, 1993a; Mawson, Heaney, Zdunczyk and Kozlowska, 1993b; Mawson, Heaney, Zdunczyk and Kozlowska, 1993c; Mawson, Heaney, Zdunczyk and Kozlowska, 1993d; Mawson, Heaney, Zdunczyk and Kozlowska, 1993e) and for ruminants in particular (Hill, 1991) has recently been extensively reviewed. This report focuses strictly on dairy cows. It covers the various properties of RSM that may limit its use and gives an up-to-date review of the effects of various levels of RSM on dairy cow performance and reproduction. Fat-rich products have attracted increasing attention as a useful source of energy for high producing cows. However, they have not been dealt with here since they are covered in a separate chapter (van Kempen and Jansman, 1994). Where relevant, comparisons with soya bean meal (SBM) are made since rapeseed and soya bean feeds have been compared in a number of studies.

Rapeseed production

Today rapeseed is produced all over the world. It ranks third among the world's oilseeds, with an annual production of 26 million tonnes (Mt). Soya beans (110 Mt) followed by cottonseed (35 Mt) rank first and second respectively (FAa, 1993). Rapeseed production for 1993/1994 has been predicted to be 27.5 Mt (Oil World Statistics Update, 1993). In 1992 the total production of oilseeds within Europe was 17.4 Mt. Rapeseed is the largest crop, amounting to approximately 8 Mt, followed by sunflower seed (6.7 Mt) and soya bean (2.0 Mt) (FAO, 1993). Within the countries of the European Community (EC), rapeseed and sunflower seed each account for approximately 45% of the oilseed-cultivated area. Almost all (99%) of the rapeseed in the EC-countries is produced from double low cultivars (Swedish Board of Agriculture, 1992).

The production of rapeseed in Europe has increased greatly during the last 10 years, from 3.2 Mt in 1980 to 8-9 Mt today (Table 9.1). This increase is a result of EC policies encouraging the production of oilseeds and leguminous protein crops. Most of this increase can be accounted for by expanded production in France, the former West Germany, the UK and Denmark. However, changes in regulations within the EC countries, expected in 1994, should lead to reduced production. Most probably, a quota system will be introduced; however, no details concerning the expected changes are yet available. Among European rapeseed producers outside the EC, Poland produces the most rapeseed (approximately 1 Mt), followed by Czechoslovakia (0.49 Mt) and Sweden (0.25 Mt) (FAO, 1993).

Table 9.1 RAPESEED PRODUCTION IN EUROPE AND WORLDWIDE IN 1979—81, 1991 AND 1992, IN 1,000 METRIC TONNES. COUNTRIES PRODUCING LESS THAN 1,000 TONNES ARE NOT SHOWN

	1979-81	*1991*	*1992*
Austria	7	121	115
Czechoslovakia	165	446	430
Denmark	204	726	430
Finland	68	95	102
France	871	2,270	1,819
Germany, former East	264 ⎫	2,973	2,590
Germany, former West	354 ⎭		
Hungary	71	120	100
Poland	434	1,043	750
Sweden	313	291	247 *
United Kingdom	274	1,276	1,200
EC-12	1,748	7,370	6,090
Europe	3,204	9,592	7,982
World	11,292	27,985	26,144

*From the Swedish Board of Agriculture (1993). (After FAO, 1993)

In Europe, production is almost exclusively based on *Br. napus*. In Canada, *Br. campestris* used to be the dominant oilseed crop, but today the two species are grown to a similar extent (Mawson, *et al.*, 1993a). In the following text rapeseed will be used as the common name for products from both *Br. napus* and *Br. campestris*.

Composition of rapeseed meal

The composition of RSM can vary quite extensively depending on the cultivar, region, growing conditions and processing methods. About 50% of the meal consists of crude fibre plus nitrogen-free extract fractions. There are relatively small quantities of monosaccharides and disaccharides and only trace amounts of starch (Bell, 1984). The crude fat content of RSM is 10 to 30 g/kg, depending on the processing method. The major components of RSM and the most important, from a nutritional standpoint, will be reviewed.

FIBRE

Rapeseed has a high fibre content owing to the thick seed coat. In the regular, brown-coated varieties the hull fraction makes up between 16.5 and 18.7% of the seed (Appelqvist and Ohlson, 1972) or from 28 to 30% of the rapeseed meal. Accordingly, the levels of NDF, ADF and lignin (Table 9.2) are high, being more than twice those in SBM. However, variation occurs in seed-coat thickness, with yellow-hulled strains containing less hull, and thus less fibre and lignin, compared with brown-hulled strains. The lower fibre content of the yellow strains is associated with higher digestibility, particularly in non-ruminants (Bell, 1984; Thomke, Björklund and Olsson, 1989). Yellow-hulled varieties are also slightly superior in terms of their content of digestible energy for ruminants, such as in sheep (Bush, Nicholson, MacIntyre, and McQueen, 1978) and in bull calves (Sharma, Ingalls, and Devlin, 1980).

Table 9.2 CHEMICAL COMPOSITION (% OF DRY MATTER) OF RAPESEED MEAL AND SOYA BEAN MEAL AND AVAILABLE ENERGY VALUES FOR CATTLE

	Rapeseed meal	*Soya bean meal*
Crude protein	37.7-42.8	49.5-51.0
Ether extract	2.0-4.8	1.0-2.2
Crude fiber	12.3-13.6	6.0-7.1
Ash	7.3-8.5	7.0-7.1
Starch	0.9-2.5	6.2
Neutral detergent fiber (NDF)	23.0-25.9	8.6-14.0
Acid detergent fiber (ADF)	17.2-18.0[1,2]	6.1-6.9[1,2]
Lignin	5.0[2]	0.9[2]
Nitrogen free extract	34.0-40.0	34.0-35.0
Effective protein degradation (EPD), %	46*-72	30*-64
Ca	0.7-0.8	0.3
P	1.2-1.3	0.7
Mg	0.5-0.7	0.3
K	1.4-1.5	2.3-2.4
Na	0.01-0.03	0.01-0.03
Cl	0.02	0.04
S	0.9[1]	0.5[1]
Metabolisable energy, MJ/kg	11.3-12.5	14.6
Digestible energy, MJ/kg	13.3-14.8	17.1-17.8

*Heat-treated meal
[1]Downey and Bell, 1990
[2]Emanuelson unpublished
(After Canola Council, 1985; Landsudvalget for kvaeg, 1992; Exab Foder AB, 1993; Spörndly, 1993)

ENERGY

The energy value of RSM for cattle, expressed as metabolisable energy (ME), varies widely. Hill (1991) summarized results from two different digestibility studies, where values ranging from 11.0 to 13.4 MJ/kg dry matter (DM) were reported. The mean value was 12.5 MJ/kg DM, which is close to the value used in the Swedish feed table (see Table 10.2). A lower value of 11.0 MJ/kg DM has been adopted by the National Research Council (NRC) (1989). The lipid content is a major factor influencing the energy value. Few direct comparisons of digestible energy (DE) or ME have been made between meals composed of high (HG) and low (LG) glucosinolate varieties (Ingalls and Sharma, 1975; Laarveld, Brockman and Christensen, 1981a) and no statistically significant differences have been found.

CRUDE PROTEIN (CP)

The crude protein (CP) content of rapeseed meal is 350-400 g/kg DM and is well balanced with regard to essential amino acids. The contents of the sulphur containing amino acids methionine and cysteine are higher in RSM than in the CP of SBM, whereas the lysine content is lower (Table 9.3). Such information can be valuable now that it is common to balance dairy cow rations for amino acids. In all new protein evaluation systems, protein degradability in the rumen is an important factor. The rumen degradability of CP from "regular" RSM is 5-10 percentage units higher than that of SBM, according to the Danish feed table (Landsudvalget for kvaeg, 1992) and to Lindberg (1986).

Table 9.3 ESSENTIAL AMINO ACID COMPOSITION OF RAPESEED MEAL AND SOYA BEAN MEAL (g/16 g N)

	Rapeseed meal	*Soyabean meal*
Crude protein, g/kg DM	390-410	490-510
Arginine	5.8-6.6	6.6-7.5
Histidine	2.9-3.5	1.9-2.8
Isoleucine	4.0-4.3	4.7-4.8
Leucine	6.1-7.6	7.0-7.8
Lysine	4.8-5.7	5.9-6.4
Methionine	1.8-2.0	0.7-1.5
Cystine	1.9-2.2	0.7-1.5
Tryptophan	0.9-1.0	1.2-1.6
Phenylalanine	3.8-4.3	4.9-5.0
Valine	4.6-5.7	4.7-5.1
Threonine	4.0-4.6	3.8-3.9

(After Canola Council, 1985; Kendall *et al.,* 1991; Exab Foder AB 1993; Spörndly, 1993)

There is large variation however and, according to Swedish (Emanuelson, unpublished data) as well as Finnish data (Touri, 1992), RSM and SBM have similar values. Effective protein degradation (EPD) values for RSM from 63 to 77% were obtained in nylon bag studies, according to the procedure used in the Nordic AAT/PBV system (Madsen and Hvelplund, 1985). The Agricultural Research Council (ARC) (1984) uses a value of 72% and, according to the Swedish and Danish feed tables, it can vary from 46 to 72% (Spörndly, 1993; Landsudvalget for kvaeg, 1992). In view of the large amount of variation in these values, there is good reason to regularly measure the rumen degradability of CP in RSM and other protein sources as well as the post-ruminal digestibility of rumen-undegradable protein. Variation in CP quality can be related to the method used at the processing plant, among other factors (Kendall, Ingalls and Boila, 1991).

Chemical and physical methods aimed at protecting RSM-protein from rumen degradation have been evaluated (Mir, MacLeod, Buchanan-Smith, Grieve and Grovum, 1984). Treatments with formaldehyde (e.g. Rooke, Brookes and Armstrong, 1983; Varvicco, Lindberg, Setiilii and Syrjiilii-Qvist, 1983) and acids (e.g. Khorasani, Robinson and Kennelly, 1989; Khorasani, Robinson and Kennelly, 1993) have been used with varying degrees of success. Physical methods have been based mainly on heat and moisture (e.g. Deacon, DeBoer and Kennelly, 1988; Dahlen, Lindh and Munter, 1989; Bertilsson, 1989; Tuori, 1992; Bertilsson, Gonda and Lindberg, 1993).

Heat-moisture treatment appears to be an effective method that is commonly used in Sweden and Finland. With this treatment, EPD-values can be reduced by up to 20 percentage units. Furthermore, if performed correctly, there will be no adverse effects on intestinal digestibility, quantified directly with the mobile nylon bag technique (Vanhatalo and Aronen, 1991) or as apparent total-tract digestibility (Gonda, Lindberg and Bertilsson, 1993).

In all systems, there is always a, risk that the intestinal digestibility of rumen- escape protein can be reduced. Such effects have been reported with formaldehyde (Rook *et al.*, 1983; Mir *et al.*, 1984) as well as with the heat-moisture treatment (Tuori, 1992). Chemical or heat treatment of feed protein can also affect the availability of amino acids, even though digestibility may not be impaired. According to Ashes, Mangan and Sidhu (1984) lysine, tyrosine and cystine are more sensitive to formaldehyde than are other amino acids. Regular estimation of protein quality is therefore warranted. The degradability of extruded RSM, another heat-treatment method, was evaluated in nylon bags (Deacon *et al.*, 1988), but instead of over-protection, almost no protection at all was obtained in that study.

MINERALS

The mineral content of RSM is shown in Table 9.2. In general, contents of the major minerals are higher in RSM than in SBM. For example, contents of Ca, P and Mg are almost twice as high in RSM. However, the K content is lower in RSM than in SBM. As is true for cereal grains and other oilseed meals, nearly two thirds of the phosphorus in RSM can be bound to phytin (Bell, 1984). However, in ruminants, phytate phosphorus is probably utilized as readily as other forms of phosphorus, owing to the presence of bacterial phytases in the rumen (McDonald, Edwards and Greenhalgh, 1988).

PHENOLIC COMPOUNDS

The content of phenolics in RSM is about 30 times that reported for soya bean meal (Kozlowska, Naczk, Shahidi and Zadernowski, 1990). These compounds may contribute to the dark colour and bitter taste. Sinapine is a bitter tasting choline ester of sinapic acid and choline. Its content in rapeseed varies between 7.8 and 13.3 g/kg (Appelqvist and Ohlson, 1972). The fishy smell in eggs from certain strains of laying hens producing brown-shelled eggs has been ascribed to this compound. Such hens have a genetic defect resulting in the incomplete degradation of trimethylamine in the liver and kidneys (Pearson, Butler, Curtis, Fenwick, Hobson-Frohock and Land, 1979). The presence of sinapine may also be responsible for the bad taste of butter from cows fed LG-RSM (Clausen, Eggum, Jacobsen, Larsen, Ploger and Srensen, 1986).

Tannins, found in the rapeseed hull, constitute another class of complex phenolics with a bitter taste. The tannin content of rapeseed meal ranges from 20 to 30 g/kg (Fenwick and Hoggan, 1976). Although few studies have been conducted with ruminants, antinutritional effects have been reported (Kumar and Singh, 1984). For example, tannins could adversely affect palatability; however, such effects would probably be difficult to distinguish from those of sinapine.

GLUCOSINOLATES

The usefulness of rapeseed products as feedstuffs has been limited, mainly owing to the presence of glucosinolates. These sulphur-containing glycosides are hydrophillic and strongly acidic, and occur as salts. More than 100 different glucosinolates are known today (Mawson *et al.*, 1993a), but only 9 or 10 occur in oilseed rape. The basic structure is as follows:

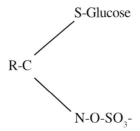

They can be divided up into alkenyl- and indolyl-glucosinolates on the basis of their side chain (R). The most significant glucosinolates in rapeseed are presented in Table 9.4. The alkenyl glucosinolates progoitrin and gluconapin predominate in the single-low or high-glucosinolate (HG) cultivars. Progoitrin predominates in *Br. napus,* while gluconapin is dominant in *Br. campestris.* Breeding for low glucosinolate content has resulted in a reduction in these glucosinolates, while the indolyl-glucosinolates have, so far, been more or less unaffected. The proportion of the indolyl-glucosinolates, in relation to the alkenyl glucosinolates, has therefore increased in the low glucosinolate (LG) cultivars and in some cases amounts to more than 50% of the total content of glucosinolates (Uppstrom, personal communication).

Table 9.4 MAJOR GLUCOSINOLATES IN RAPESEED MEAL FROM *BRASSICA NAPUS* AND *BR. CAMPESTRIS*

Trivial name	Glucosinolate
Gluconapin	3-butenyl-
Glucobrassicanapin	4-pentenyl-
Progoitrin	2-hydroxy-3-butenyl-
Napoleiferin	2-hydroxy-4-pentenyl-
Glucobrassicin	3-indolyl-methyl-
4- hydroxyglucobrassicin	4- hydroxy- 3- indolylmethyl-

(After Bell, 1984; Mawson *et al.,* 1993)

Glucosinolates are converted into toxic compounds as a result of enzymatic degradation. They are hydrolysed after any cell lesion of the seed by the endogenous enzyme myrosinase (thioglucoside glucohydrolase, EC 3.2.3.1). At neutral pH, glucose and sulphate are released in addition to free goitrogenic compounds (aglucones). Vinyl-thiooxazolidinethione (VTO or goitrin) is formed from progoitrin, and various isothiocyanates and thiocyanate are also formed. Indolyl-glucosinolates yield thiocyanate. Nitriles, which are not goitrogenic but do possess other antinutritional properties, can be produced at low pH or when coming into contact with ferrous ions. The pattern and amount of hydrolysis products formed during processing or after ingestion is therefore highly dependent on the nature of the glucosinolates present (the structure of their R-group) as well as on the environmental pH and any treatments carried out (Paik, Robblee and Clandinin, 1980; Fenwick, Heany and Mullin, 1983; Mawson *et al.,* 1993a). Also, several microbial species inhabiting the gastrointestinal tract of mammals have enzyme systems that can hydrolyse glucosinolates. This has been shown in several studies with rats (e.g. Greer and Deeney, 1959; Lo and Hill, 1972a,b) and in *in vitro* studies with rumen fluid (Lanzani, Piana, Piva, Cardillo, Rastelli and Jacini, 1974; Kamell, 1988). Hence, inactivating the endogenous myrosinase, e.g. by heating the rapeseed products, will not eliminate the harmful effects of glucosinolates. However, knowledge about how glucosinolates are metabolized within the gastrointestinal tract is still vague, especially in ruminants.

During the past decade, standards for the glucosinolate content of LG-cultivars have differed between countries, thereby complicating comparisons between trials. According to Canadian standards, glucosinolate concentrations in canola-cultivars may not exceed 30 μmol/g of fat-free meal DM. These standards only consider the four alkenyl glucosinolates (Shahidi, 1990). Since 1991, the maximum allowable total glucosinolate content of the LG-rapeseed cultivars produced in EC-countries has been 20 μmol/g air-dried seed, with the indolyl-glucosinolates included (Swedish Board of Agriculture, 1992). For the last two years (i.e. 91/92 and 92/93) Swedish, commercial LG-RSM has contained 9.0 (sd=2.0) and 7.5 (sd=1.1) μmol of total glucosinolates/g fat free DM, respectively (Exab Foder AB, 1993).

Feed intake and palatability

Glucosinolates are only one of several components of rapeseed that have been associated with impaired palatability. As mentioned earlier, the bitter taste could also be due to phenolic compounds such as tannins and sinapine. Since glucosinolates and phenolics are all present together in rapeseed, it is virtually impossible to separate their individual effects. Nevertheless, it has been concluded that the palatability problems that sometimes occur in connection with using rapeseed as a feedstuff are associated with a high glucosinolate content rather than the presence of sinapine or tannins. This conclusion is based on results from experiments with rats fed single glucosinolates (Bjerg, Eggum, Jacobsen, Otte and Srensen, 1989) as well as with pigs (Lee, Pittam and Hill, 1984) and lambs and calves (Stedman and Hill, 1987), among other species. The main focus has been on monogastric species, and the relationships were thoroughly reviewed recently (Mawson *et al.,* 1993b). Restrictions on the dietary inclusion levels of high-glucosinolate rapeseed products have been recommended for calves as well as for monogastrics. Tolerance levels for glucosinolates are difficult to set since they vary depending on factors such as the form in which the rapeseed is fed and the overall composition of the diet (Hill, 1991; Mawson *et al.,* 1993b).

For adult ruminants there does not seem to be a close relationship between glucosinolate intake and total feed consumption. However, no strict palatability or preference studies concerning rapeseed products have been conducted with dairy cows. Furthermore, no specific measurements of consumption rates have been made. Instead, effects on feed intake and palatability have been assessed indirectly, based on the results of regular production trials. Few direct comparisons have been made between HG- and LG-RSM in dairy cow rations. Papas, Ingalls and Campbell (1979) did not detect any differences in intake between RSM containing 20.5 μmol/g glucosinolates and RSM containing 36.2 μmol/g when 2 kg of both were supplied per day. On the other hand, a significantly lower intake of a grain mixture was reported when feed with a 12% LG-RSM content in the total ration was replaced by meal with the same proportion of HG-RSM, with an unknown glucosinolate content (Ingalls and Sharma, 1975).

Several short- as well as long-term studies were conducted during the 1970s in which comparisons were made between HG-RSM and SBM (Waldern, 1973; Ingalls and Sharma, 1975; Lindell, 1976; Laarveld and Christensen, 1976). In most cases no detrimental effect on feed intake was reported, although total intake tended to be lower when consumption of HG-RSM was more than 1.5 kg per day. Other factors, such as feeding strategy, method of processing and interactions with other components in the diet, are probably more important than the glucosinolates for regulating feed intake. However, the inclusion levels of HG-RSM, and thus the levels of glucosinolates, in most studies with dairy cows were lower than those used in many of the studies conducted on pigs and rats. Hill (1991) suggested that the glucosinolate contents of the whole diets used in studies with HG-RSM were all below 10.0 μmol/g. This is not necessarily true however, since glucosinolate contents were not measured in some of the older studies.

Results from experiments, in which LG-RSM has been compared with other protein sources are more consistent with regard to feed intake and palatability. Reports based on several short-term studies showed that LG-RSM can be substituted for SBM (Sharma, Ingalls and McKirdy, 1977; Papas, Ingalls and Cansfield, 1978; Laarveld *et al.,* 1981a) or cottonseed meal (Sanchez and Claypool, 1983; DePeters and Bath, 1985) without negatively affecting feed intake. This was confirmed in a long-term study, lasting over three lactations, in which up to 2.5 kg DM LG-RSM and 0.9 kg DM LG full-fat rapeseed were fed per day (Emanuelson, Ahlin and Wiktorsson, 1993). In one study (Fisher and Walsh, 1976) intake was reduced, but in that case the meal had a dark colour, probably due to overheating.

Dedenon (1985) showed that feed consumption by dairy cows was reduced when concentrates contained more than 40% RSM, irrespective of the glucosinolate content. Palatability problems were more pronounced when RSM was fed separately and when the feeding time was restricted, as is the case when feed is given in a milking parlour.

Based on these findings it can be concluded that the risk of encountering palatability problems when feeding RSM to adult dairy cattle is minimal, especially when LG-cultivars are used. For example, if 4 kg LG-RSM, containing 15 mmol glucosinolates/kg DM is included in a dairy cow ration of 25 kg DM, the total diet will contain 2.4 mmol glucosinolates/kg DM. This value is lower than the highest recommended glucosinolate concentration of 4.4 mmol/kg DM obtained from studies on rats (Vermorel, Davicco and Evrard, 1987) and pigs (Lee and Hill, 1983). In the latter study progoitrin levels below 2.3 mmol/kg DM had little effect on palatability, whereas palatability was impaired at levels between 2.3 and 4.65 mmol/kg diet DM, It should therefore be possible to feed dairy cows grain/concentrate mixes with a 20 to 30% LG- RSM content without impairing feed intake or palatability.

Milk yield and composition

MILK YIELD OF COWS FED UNTREATED RSM

Thomke (1981) summarized the results from almost all milk production experiments conducted in the 1970s with high as well as low glucosinolate RSM. Milk yield remained unchanged or increased in 15 out of 17 experiments in which RSM rations were compared with rations containing SBM or other protein supplements. In two trials milk yield was decreased (Ingalls and Sharma, 1975 (HG-RSM); Fisher and Walsh, 1976 (LG-RSM)). The most probable explanation for the reduction was the decreased feed intake. Milk yields were not negatively affected in any of the more recent (i.e. 1980 and later), short-term experiments, in which up to 4.1 kg LG-RSM was substituted for either SBM (e.g. Laarveld *et al.,* 1981a; Vincent and Hill, 1988; Vincent, Hill and Campling, 1990) or cottonseed meal (Sanchez and Claypool, 1983; DePeters and Bath, 1986). In a recent study, LG- RSM was substituted for corn gluten meal in high- as well as low-concentrate diets fed to cows in early lactation. Surprisingly, no differences were detected in milk yield or composition, despite a large difference in protein degradability between the two protein sources (Robinson and Kennelly, 1991a,b). Furthermore a high rate of milk production was sustained for three lactations, when up to 2.5 kg DM LG-RSM plus 0.9 kg DM LG full-fat rapeseed was substituted for SBM and tallow (Emanuelson *et al.,* 1993).

MILK YIELD OF COWS FED TREATED RSM

As mentioned above, both RSM and SBM contain proteins that are rapidly degraded in the rumen and various treatments aimed at lowering their degradability have been tested. Although several studies have been conducted to evaluate such treatments on animal performance the results have been inconsistent. Tuori (1992) found that although protein protection is a theoretically sound concept, only a few experiments have provided results supporting the theory. In a 12-week experiment with dairy cows, the inclusion of two different levels of formaldehyde- treated LG-RSM (13 or 23.5%) in the total diet, were evaluated (Rae, Ingalls and McKirdy, 1983). Formaldehyde treatment did not have any positive effect on milk production or composition, even though enhanced absorption of essential amino acids from the gut was observed. One reason for the lack of success was a limited absorption of those amino acids which were limiting milk production. Approximately 58% and 20% of the LG-RSM tyrosine and lysine, respectively were lost by the treatment. Touri (1992) reported that heat-treatment (Öpex® heat-moisture) enhanced milk production, but only in one of three experiments. In that experiment, the EPD-value of the LG-RSM was lowered by 20 percentage- units. In the other two, the difference in EPD obtained was rather small. However, the low inclusion level of RSM (1-1.7 kg/day), might also explain the lack of response.

Bertilsson *et al.* (1993) reported increased milk and protein production when LG-RSM (heat-treated according to the Expro®-method described by Dahlen *et al.,* 1989; EPD-value 52%) was substituted for untreated RSM (EPD-value 72%) in the concentrate mixture at levels of 8 and 25%. Milk production was highest with 25% Expro-treated LG-RSM in the concentrate. However, the most interesting result was that cows fed the concentrate with an 8% Expro®-treated LG-RSM content performed as well as those fed the concentrate with a 25% untreated LG-RSM content. Thus it was possible to reduce the input of nitrogen in the feed without sacrificing the performance. Furthermore, the nitrogen output via urine and faeces was reduced, thereby lowering the nitrogen load on the animal, as well as on the environment (Gonda *et al.,* 1993). In Sweden, almost all RSM used in commercial feeds for dairy cows today, has been heat-treated.

MILK FAT AND PROTEIN CONTENT

A review of the data from experiments with LG and HG cultivars, did not reveal any consistent relationship between feed glucosinolate content and milk fat or protein contents. However, in the long-term experiment referred to above, the milk protein content showed a clear positive association with the content of LG-RSM in the ration (Emanuelson *et al.,* 1993). The relation (rise in milk-protein content with increasing LG-RSM content) was significant during lactations 1 (p<0.05) and 3 (p<0.10) but not in lactation 2. There is no good explanation for this. One possibility is that the fat, in the form of full-fat rapeseed fed to the "rapeseed groups" was less detrimental to the rumen microbes than tallow, which was used in the control group. Evidence for such a difference was provided by Emanuelson, Murphy and Lindberg (1991). Rough calculations showed that the daily supply of methionine was about 10 g higher/day in the RSM diets, in early lactation, than in the control diet. There were no good evidence that methionine really played a role. Another explanation could be that microbial protein production in the rumen and/or the passage rate of undegraded protein to the duodenum were slightly higher in the RSM-groups. This difference was indicated by the fact that milk urea levels during all three lactations, were consistently lower in cows fed diets containing RSM than in those receiving the control diet, containing SBM.

Increases in milk protein content were also reported in two different experiments in which untreated or heat-treated LG-RSM (Öpex® or Expro® methods) was substituted for SBM (Bertilsson, 1989). Similar tendencies were also observed in the studies by Lindell (1976) and Lindell and Knutsson (1976). There are several possible reasons why the positive response was obtained only in the Swedish studies. The primary one is probably that most other studies have been shorter, e.g. changeover trials, in which the effects might have been masked somewhat. The use of low inclusion levels and other types of forages, such as corn silage, could also explain some of the differences in response. This is an area that requires further research.

Anti-nutritional substances and iodine in milk

By the use of feeds containing glucosinolates for cows, hydrolysis products, such as thiocyanate (SCN-), goitrin (vinyl thiooxazolidinethione) and unsaturated nitrites are also secreted in the milk. However, no clear relationship has been established between intake and output, partly because the metabolism of glucosinolates in ruminants is not very well understood. The hydrolysis products measured in the milk have, in most cases, not been determined in the feed, which further hinders relevant calculations. Differences in methodology also complicate comparisons between experiments. Nevertheless some general trends will be discussed.

THIOCYANATE

Thiocyanate has been measured in a number of experiments, often together with iodine. Iwarson (1973) suggested that there is an inverse relationship between concentrations of the two in milk. His hypothesis is based on the finding that ingested thiocyanate inhibits iodine absorption by the mammary gland in the same way as it inhibits iodine absorption in the thyroid gland. However, the mechanism of iodine uptake by the mammary gland seems to be much more sensitive to thiocyanate as compared with uptake by the thyroid gland (Reineke, 1961; Piironen and Virtanen, 1963). As a result, the presence of thiocyanate in the blood system induces the cow to save iodine instead of secreting it in the milk. Consequently, Emanuelson (1989) did not find a close relationship between the milk contents of total iodine and thiocyanate ions.

Hill (1991) summarized results from experiments in which levels of thiocyanate as well as iodide had been measured in milk. The thiocyanate level increased in every case where RSM was included, but the degree of increase varied greatly. The highest levels were obtained by Laarveld *et al.* (1981a). A daily intake of total glucosinolates of 314.2 mmol resulted in a thiocyanate concentration of 0.183 mmol/l milk, which is unusually high. Although levels as high as 0.200-0.250 mmol/l of thiocyanate have been reached (Virtanen and Gmelin, 1960), the daily supply of thiocyanate in that study was 6 g (105 mmol).

In a Swedish study covering three lactations, the thiocyanate concentration in milk was measured at different stages of the first two lactations (Emanuelson, 1989). The treatments were (1) no rapeseed (NR), (2) up to 1.2 kg DM LG-RSM plus 0.2 kg DM LG-full-fat rapeseed (MR) and (3) up to 2.5 kg DM LG-RSM plus 0.9 kg DM LG-full-fat rapeseed (HR). The concentration of thiocyanate in the milk was significantly elevated when LG-RSM was included in the diet at the expense of SBM (treatment NR). In lactation 1, the two different inclusion levels of RSM corresponded to an average total glucosinolate intake of 34 (MR) and 53 (HR) mmol/cow/day in early lactation and 24 and 33 mmol/day, respectively in late lactation. As can be seen from Table 9.5, there were no differences between the two inclusion levels of rapeseed in lactation 1 (MR and HR). Total amounts secreted/day in milk were also elevated and similar in the two groups fed rapeseed. There were no marked differences between the two lactations.

Table 9.5 LEAST-SQUARE MEANS OF THE CONCENTRATION OF THIOCYANATE IONS (mmol/l) IN MILK FOR EACH TREATMENT AND STAGE OF FIRST LACTATION IN AN EXPERIMENT WHERE TWO DIFFERENT INCLUSION LEVELS OF LG-RSM MEAL WERE TESTED (STANDARD ERRORS VARIED BETWEEN 0.003 AND 0.004)

		Treatment	
Days after calving	*NR[1]*	*MR[1]*	*HR[1]*
Number of cows	27	28	25
30	0.026[a]	0.077[b]	0.082[b]
60	0.025[a]	0.083[b]	0.088[b]
90	0.024[a]	0.085[b]	0.084[b]
150	0.038[a]	0.100[b]	0.105[b]
300	0.037[a]	0.141[b]	0.114[c]

[1]No rapeseed (NR), medium level (MR) and high level (HR) of low- glucosinolate rapeseed products included in the concentrate mixtures. See text for more information.
[a-c]Means in the same line with different superscript differ at $p < 0.05$. (After Emanuelson, 1989)

As stated above, concentrations of thiocyanate in the milk differed between studies. Laarveld *et al.* (1981a) reported higher concentrations of thiocyanate ions in milk (0.126-0.138 mmol/l) than did Emanuelson (1989), although the level of intake of glucosinolates in the two studies was the same. By contrast, Papas *et al.* (1978, 1979) reported much lower levels (0.041 and 0.035 mmol/l, respectively) for a similar level of intake. Total daily secretion also differed between the studies of Papas and Emanuelson: At a daily intake of 44 mmol of intact glucosinolates, for example, Papas *et al.* (1979) reported a total secretion of thiocyanate in milk of 0.82 mmol per day, whereas Emanuelson (1989) measured levels of 1.8-1.9 mmol. The reasons for these discrepancies between studies are not clear, but differences in methodology may be a contributing factor. Another possible source of variation was the intake of the thiocyanate-yielding glucosinolates, mainly the indolyl glucosinolates, which were not analysed in any of the studies presented above. However, this cannot explain why there were no differences in thiocyanate concentrations between the two groups fed different levels of LG-RSM in the study by Emanuelson (1989), even though there were differences in the intake of glucosinolates. Other factors that have to be considered include the source of forage and the experimental design. Changeover studies, with four to five week periods between shifts in diet, may in some cases be too short to induce an observable response.

IODINE

The iodide content of milk can be significantly decreased by including RSM in feed (reviewed by Hill, 1991). However, the concentration of thiocyanate causing the reduction in iodine varied greatly between experiments. The daily intake of iodine has been found to be the most important factor regulating iodine concentrations in milk (e.g. Miller, Swanson and Spalding, 1975). Differences in intake are probably also the main reason for the large variation between experiments.

Papas *et al.* (1979), Laarveld *et al.* (1981a) and Emanuelson (1989) showed that the amount of RSM-thiocyanate needed to exert maximum effects on milk iodine concentration is very small; i.e. within each of the experiments there were no differences in iodine content between groups receiving different levels of RSM. Moreover, it has been shown that it is almost impossible to totally compensate for a milk iodine depression caused by thiocyanate-producing glucosinolates by elevating iodine concentrations in the diet (e.g. Piironen and Virtanen, 1963). Brockman, Laarveld and Christensen (1980) added extra iodine (3 mg/kg DM) to a diet with a 7% content of LG-RSM in the concentrate. Nevertheless, the milk iodine concentration was still significantly lower, around 1.5 µmol/l, than that obtained in cows consuming concentrate lacking LG- RSM (4.7 µmol/l).

Although the relationships are not fully understood, it can be concluded that the milk iodine levels obtained in the rapeseed studies reviewed here were within the acceptable range, i.e. above 0.2 µmol/l. Lower values are, according to Iwarsson and Ekman (1975), indicative of iodine deficiency. It seems clear that the level of iodide in the milk can be increased to normal by adding extra iodine to the diet. However, the recommended addition rate of 2 mg iodine/kg DM for cruciferous feedstuffs (Agricultural Research Council (ARC), 1980) may be unnecessarily high if LG-cultivars are used.

GOITRIN

Goitrin, a hydrolysis product from progoitrin, has frequently been measured in milk in Finnish studies. Data concerning the proportion of progoitrin in the feed that is actually converted to goitrin and excreted into the milk are limited. According to Virtanen, Kreula and Kiesvaara (1963), about 0.05% of the goitrin fed ends up in the milk, whereas Bachmann, Theus, Lüthy and Schlatter (1985) stated that up to 0.1% can be transferred. Touri (1992) measured goitrin in milk in three different experiments. Goitrin levels ranging from 1 to 22.8µg/l were found in milk from cows fed LG-cultivars or heat-treated HG-cultivars. The percentage of the output of goitrin in the milk and the intake, in the form of progoitrin, viared between 0.009% and 0.064%. The highest goitrin content observed was 75.3µg/l, which was regarded as an outlier. Touri (1992) attributed the large variation in the amount transferred to differences in the amounts of progoitrin in feed as well as to differences in the efficiency of transfer from feed to milk. He also cited a recent study (Touri and Syrjälä-Qvist, 1992 unpublished) where 1.3-1.6 kg/day of LG-RSM (less than 10 µmol of glucosinolates/g fat-free meal) was fed to dairy cows. The goitrin content in that milk varied between 3.5 and 6.4µg/l.

With the exception of the extremely high concentrations (up to 700 µg/l milk) measured by Bachmann *et al.* (1985), levels of goitrin reported in milk have generally been very low and in some cases even non-detectable (e.g. Hoppe, Kozlowska and Rutkowski, 1971; Papas *et al.*, 1979). In the study by Emanuelson (1989) the goitrin level was estimated indirectly based on a study with growing rats consuming dried milk corresponding to 31-43 g fresh milk per day. If 2 µg goitrin/day is sufficient to cause enlargement of the rat thyroid gland, as was reported by Peltola (1965), it should have been possible to indirectly detect milk contents of about 40-65 µg goitrin/l based on the weights of their thyroid glands. Because the thyroids of the rats were unaffected, it was assumed that the goitrin levels in the milk were low.

Animal health and reproduction

GOITRONGENIC EFFECTS OF RAPESEED GLUCOSINOLATES

A great deal of information about the goitrogenic properties of different cultivars of rapeseed as well as various types of glucosinolates has been obtained from feeding studies in rats, poultry and pigs. By contrast, few such studies have been made with ruminants (reviewed by Mawson *et al.*, 1993d). Among the problems associated with glucosinolates (or more accurately, with their hydrolysis products), those affecting the thyroid gland have been studied in greatest detail. The intake of glucosinolates will lead to a hypothyroid condition, characterised by increased thyroid activity and reduced circulating levels of thyroid hormones (T3 and T4). Thyroid hormones inhibit anterior pituitary secretion of thyroid stimulating hormones (TSH) via the hypothalamus. However, in the case of hypothyroidism, induced by high levels of glucosinolates, for example, the lowered levels of T3 and T4 will result in an excessive secretion of TSH which in turn induces increased thyroid activity and gland hypertrophy. All of the break-down products from glucosinolates probably contribute to hypothyroidism (Mawson *et al.*, 1993d). In short, goitrin exerts its effect by interfering with the synthesis of thyroid hormones. This is a serious problem because it cannot be alleviated by iodine supplementation. Thiocyanate, on the other hand, competes with iodine for uptake by the thyroid gland. Thus, this condition can easily be corrected by adding extra iodine to the feed (Van Etten, 1969).

Hypothyroidism can lead to abnormalities in the internal organs (liver, kidneys and suprarenal glands), especially in non-ruminants. Thus, it is probable that goitrogenic substances also have adverse effects on animal health, in general. The relationship between hypothyroidism in cattle caused by iodine deficiency, sometimes in combination with goitrogenic agents, and reproductive disorders has also been described by Wilson (1975). The conditions are often expressed as increased prevalence of congenital goitre and stillborn calves. Furthermore, retained placentas tend to be more common, resistance to infections can be reduced, and susceptibility to ketonaemia in cows can increase.

There is, however, little information in the literature about the goitrogenic effects of rapeseed glucosinolates in ruminants. In those cases where it has been studied, no severe effects have been reported. One reason for the lack of serious effects could, of course, be low inclusion levels. The very low levels of gJucosinolate metabolites found in milk (see above) may also indicate that glucosinolates are metabolized *in vivo,* yielding unexpected products. Lanzani *et al.* (1974), for example, showed that several other aglucones besides goitrin were produced when progoitrin was incubated in sheep rumen fluid. Karnell (1988) also showed that glucosinolates were degraded rapidly *in vitro* in rumen fluid from cows. Approximately 90% had been degraded after 60 minutes of incubation. A faster rate of degradation, with the formation of more goitrin, was also seen *in vitro* when RSM was degraded in rumen fluid from cows fed rapeseed, compared with values obtained using rumen fluid from cows given a diet containing no rapeseed (Emanuelson and Petterson, unpublished data). Although this area requires more research, it is not considered to be important when rapeseed products with low levels of glucosinolates are used. It can be concluded that the dynamics of glucosinolate metabolism are determined more by the overall composition of the ration than by the level of RSM *per se.*

Few results from the literature support the hypothesis that thyroid enlargement in ruminants is directly related to the level of glucosinolate intake. In the few cases where increased thyroid weights have been reported, the studies dealt with calves and growing animals. In heifers, histological evidence of goitrogenicity (but no weight changes), significantly elevated plasma levels of thiocyanate and significantly depressed levels of plasma thyroxine (T4) were reported by Vincent, Hill and Williams (1988).

In a changeover study with 12 cows given feed with a 25% LG-RSM content for four weeks, T4 levels were depressed (Sharma *et al.,* 1977). Similar results were obtained by Papas *et al.* (1979) when LG- and HG-RSM (44.1 and 73.5 mmol glucosinolates/day, respectively) were fed to cows for 12 weeks. These investigators contended that T4 levels are not an accurate indicator of the size and histology of the thyroid gland. It is also uncertain whether their findings are representative of genuine hypothyroidism conditions or merely a subclinical hypothyroid state, which might even have been compensated.

In a changeover study, Laarveld, Brockman and Christensen (1981b) introduced a more sensitive method to evaluate the effects of the glucosinolates in rapeseed products. Their method involved measuring the change in plasma TSH concentrations in response to intravenous administration of thyrotropin releasing hormone (TRH). When thyroid hormone production is depressed, the pituitary increases its output of TSH, which is actually estimated with the method. Laarveld *et al.* (1981b) reported a significant depression in T4 and an elevated TSH-response (interpreted as mild impairment of thyroid activity) in cows fed diets with a 13 and 19% content of a HG-RSM (75 μmol glucosinolates/g DM), corresponding to a total glucosinolate intake of 225 and 314 mmol/ day, respectively. However, no such effects were found in animals fed diets with a 6% content of HG- RSM (118 mmol glucosinolates/day) or 6, 13 and 19% contents of LG-RSM (11.5 μmol/g DM), resulting in a daily intake of glucosinolates of between 14 and 47 mmol.

The same method was used in a study, covering three lactations, in which 85 cows were divided into three treatment groups (Emanuelson *et al.*, 1993; Ahlin, Emanuelson and Wiktorsson, 1993). The treatments were; no rapeseed (NR), medium levels (MR) and high levels (HR) of rapeseed products (details were given above). The average intakes of glucosinolates in the two groups fed rapeseed are shown in Table 9.6. Basal levels of TSH did not differ between treatments. The TRH test was performed 90 and 300 days after calving in all three lactations. In lactation one, 90 days after calving, the TSH-response was significantly higher for the HR-group than for the NR-group. By contrast, no such differences were seen when the TRH-test was made around 300 days after calving or at any time during the two subsequent lactations. No prolonged response, characteristic of a more serious hypothyroid condition, was observed. In accordance with Laarveld *et at.* (1981b), it was concluded that the first lactating cows in the HR-group suffered from a very mild, subclinical, and probably compensated, form of hypothyroidism induced by the depressed iodine and elevated thiocyanate levels (Emanuelson *et al.*, 1993).

Table 9.6 LEAST-SQUARE MEANS (WITH 95% CONFIDENCE INTERVAL) FOR THE AVERAGE DAILY TOTAL AMOUNT OF ALKENYL-GLUCOSINOLATES CONSUMED (mmol/cow/day) DURING LACTATION WEEKS 1-13 IN AN EXPERIMENT WITH DAIRY COWS

| | Treatment | |
Lactation	MR[1]	HR[1]
1	34 (32-36)	52 (50-55)
2	36 (33-38)	60 (57-63)
3	23 (21-26)	40 (37-43)

[1]Medium level (MR) and high level (HR) of low-glucosinolate rapeseed products included in the concentrate mixtures. See text for more details.
(After Ahlin *et al.*, 1993)

The same challenge test was used recently (McLean and Laarveld, 1991) when somatotropin (30 mg/day) was administered to cows on barley-based diets containing either SBM or LG-RSM meal (13.4 μmol glucosinolates/g, as fed). Levels of all hormones, as well as the response to the TRH-challenge test, were all normal, indicating that thyroid functions were normal for both protein sources.

HEALTH AND FERTILITY

The published data on rapeseed products in relation to health and fertility are limited owing to the small number of long-term studies. In earlier reports (Lindell, 1976; Lindell and Knutsson, 1976), where up to 1.39 kg HG-RSM were fed, increased numbers of artificial inseminations (AI) per pregnancy and slightly prolonged calving to conception (CC) and calving intervals were observed, suggesting that fertility may have been reduced. Similar responses were reported by Ahlstrom (1978), when 7.5% expeller-crushed fines, based on a HG-cultivar, was fed to a group of primiparous cows.

In the Swedish study (Ahlin *et al.*, 1993) reduced fertility was observed in first calvers given the HR diet; i.e. the CC-interval was significantly longer, and there was a tendency for the number of AI per pregnancy to increase with the amount of rapeseed fed. However, no such differences were seen in the two following lactations. Although the consumption of glucosinolates was significantly higher among the second calvers compared with all other cows (see Table 9.6), the fertility of this group was not significantly reduced. Finally, there was no significant difference in disease incidence or in the occurrence of any reproductive disorders between the three treatments. Independent environmental factors such as experimental year, calving age and calving season had a greater influence on fertility measures and thyroid function than did treatment group. Ahlin *et at.* (1993) asserted that the reduced fertility of the first calvers in the study lent further support to evidence suggesting that young, growing animals are most sensitive to glucosinolates. Thus there is good reason to believe that these compounds can negatively affect fertility.

In view of the continuous trend towards decreasing levels of glucosinolates in LG-RSM, all results, hitherto, indicate that it should be safe to feed LG-RSM to adult dairy cows, even when it serves as the only source of supplementary protein. However, rapeseed meal of unknown origin should not be fed to calves or first-lactation cows. Finally, it should be remembered that the concentration of glucosinolates at which no effect on health or fertility can be detected, has not yet been determined.

Human concerns related to goitrogenic substances in milk

As mentioned above, goitrin can cause enlargement of the thyroid in rats and probably in other animals as well. According to Arstila, Krusius and Peltola (1969) the quantity of goitrin needed to induce the same effect in man is unknown. For thiocyanate, 200 mg/day (3.5 mmol) is needed to induce goitrogenic symptoms (Vilkki, Kreula and Piironen, 1962). Swedish studies have also shown that a daily intake, during three months, of 400 ml milk containing 0.34 mmol thiocyanate/l by persons with a normal iodine status did not affect the thyroid status of the subjects (Dahlberg, Bergmark, Björck, Bruce, Hambraeus and Claesson, 1984), neither did the intake of 250 ml/day for four weeks, of milk containing 0.33 mmol thiocyanate/l by iodine-deficient persons have any such effect (Dahlberg,

Bergmark, Eltom, Björck and Claesson, 1985). From the standpoint of human health, it may therefore be concluded that the levels of hydrolysis products from glucosinolates occurring in milk as a result of feeding cows RSM, particularly LG-RSM, are of negligible importance. Moreover, levels of goitrogenic compounds found in milk are much lower than those found in various vegetables (Sones, Heaney and Fenwick, 1984).

Increased levels of thiocyanate ions in milk could actually have beneficial effects. Thiocyanate plays a role in the lactoperoxidase/thiocyanate/hydrogen peroxide system (LP-system) present in the milk, which has antibacterial action. The system, which is activated through the addition of thiocyanate and hydrogen peroxide (Björck, 1978), helps in preventing bacteria from spoiling raw milk (Björck, Claesson and Schulthess, 1979) and perhaps also provides some protection against invading mastitis organisms (Korhonen, 1980). According to Ahrné and Björck (1985), levels of 0.1 mmol/l thiocyanate ions in the milk would be sufficient, but not optimal, provided that the concentration of hydrogen peroxide is also raised to at least the same level. These thiocyanate levels are not much different from those obtained in milk from cows fed a diet including RSM.

MILK FLAVOUR

Few studies have been made on the flavour of milk products from cows fed rapeseed meal. The inclusion of HG-RSM (Nordfeldt, 1958) as well as LG-RSM (Sanchez and Claypool, 1983; Vincent and Hill, 1988; Emanuelson *et al.,* 1993) did not result in any unpleasant flavour. On the contrary, in a Danish study where concentrates containing 0,25,50 and 75% LG rapeseed expeller cake were tested, a significant off-flavour in both milk and butter was obtained with the two concentrates containing the highest rapeseed contents, which was equivalent to more than 1.2 kg DM per day (Frederiksen, Andersen, Mortensen and Jensen, 1979). No likely cause was given, although it seems conceivable that the high lipid content of the feed could have been responsible for the off-flavour. Later, Clausen *et al.* (1986) suggested that sinapine was a contributing factor. To date, there have been no reports of increased levels of either sinapine or trimethylamine in milk. Pinnell and Kennelly (1983) measured the levels of trimethylamine in milk from cows fed approximately 3 kg LG-RSM per day and found that they were similar to levels obtained when SBM was used.

Conclusion

Rapeseed meal is a protein feed of high nutritional quality for dairy cows. Although the protein content is lower than that of SBM, it is more balanced in terms of essential amino acids. The content of available energy is also lower in RSM than in SBM, owing to its high fibre content.

RSM contains certain anti-nutritional substances, of which the goitrogenic glucosinolates are the most potent. Because of the high levels of glucosinolates in old cultivars of rapeseed, the content of RSM in dairy cow rations had to be kept low to minimize risks of negative effects on animal performance and reproduction. In the early 1970s, new cultivars were introduced that contain low levels of glucosinolates. These cultivars have, subsequently, been extensively evaluated in feeding trials with dairy cows. In most cases, no adverse effects on feed intake, milk production, animal health or fertility were found.

Based on the present state of knowledge it is still not possible to determine the maximum amounts of glucosinolates that can be fed to cows without causing problems. It can be concluded that RSM from the low-glucosinolate cultivars grown today can be included as the sole protein feed in dairy cow rations without reducing milk production or reproductive performance. However, caution should be exercised with calves, first lactating cows and heifers, since they seem to be more sensitive to glucosinolates. It is unlikely that RSM contains other substances potentially detrimental to the health of dairy cows.

Hydrolysis products from glucosinolates do find their way into the milk, but in such small amounts that risks for humans consuming the milk are negligible.

Heat-treatment methods offer a promising way to lower protein degradation in the rumen, which may help to reduce environmental nitrogen pollution.

There are several reasons why a continued increase in the production of rapeseed can be anticipated: The oil has an ideal fatty acid profile, which has contributed to increasing use as a cooking oil. The protein meal is well balanced in terms of essential amino acids. Furthermore, it can be expected that in the near future rapeseed meal from new cultivars, with higher protein levels, lower fibre contents and perhaps even lower glucosinolate contents, will offer a viable alternative to SBM. This meal might be used at higher inclusion levels by non-ruminant species, and maybe even as an alternative protein source for humans.

Acknowledgements

Dr. J. Bertilsson and Professor S. Thomke critically reviewed the manuscript, and Exab Foder AB provided financial support.

References

Agricultural Research Council (ARC) (1980) *The Nutrient Requirements* of *Ruminant Livestock.* Slough, England: Commonwealth Agricultural Bureaux
Agricultural Research Council (ARC) (1984) *The Nutrient Requirements* of *Ruminant*

Livestock. Supplement No 1. Slough, England: Commonwealth Agricultural Bureaux

Ahlin, K.-Å., Emanuelson, M. and Wiktorsson, H. (1993) Rapeseed products from double-low cultivars as feed for dairy cows. Effects of long-term feeding on thyroid function, fertility and animal health. *Acta Veterinaria Scandinavica,* **35,** 37-53

Ahlström, B. (1978) By-products from rapeseed protein concentrate (RPC) processing as feedstuffs. I. Fines to dairy cows. *Proceedings* of *the 5th International Rapeseed Conference,* Malmo, 1978. **2,**235-239

Ahrné, L. and Björck, L. (1985) Effect of the lactoperoxidase system on lipoprotein lipase activity and lipolysis in milk. *Journal* of *Dairy Research,* **52,** 513-520

Appelqvist, L.-Å. and Ohlson, R. (1972) *Rapeseed.* Amsterdam: Elsevier Publishing Company

Arstila, A., Krusius, F.-E. and Peltola, P. 1969. Studies on the transfer of thio-oxazolidone-type goitrogens into cow's milk in goitre endemic districts of Finland and in experimental conditions. *Acta Endocrinology,* **60,** 712-718

Ashes, 1.R., Mangan, 1.L. and Sidhu, G.S. (1984) Nutritional availability of amino acids from protein cross-linked to protect against degradation in the rumen. *British Journal of Nutrition,* **52,** 239-247

Bachmann, M., Theus, R., Liithy, J. and Schlatter, C. 1985. Vorkommen von goitrogenen stoffen in milch. 1. Mitteilung: Ubergang von Goitrin in die Milch von Kiihen bei Verfiitterung von Rapsextraktionsschrot. *Zeitschrift far Lebensmittel-Untersuchung und Forschung,* **181,**375-378

Bell, J .M. (1984) Nutrients and toxicants in rapeseed meal: A review. *Journal of Animal Science,* **58,** 996-1010

Bertilsson, J. (1989) Feeding protein supplements with different rumen degrad- abilities to dairy cows. Paper presented at the *40th annual meeting* of *EAAP,* Dublin, 29 August, 1989. 8 p

Bertilsson, J., Gonda, H. and Lindberg, J.-E. (1994) Protein level and degrad- ability in rations for dairy cows. 1. Animal performance. *Acta Agricultura' Scandinavica, Section A, Animal Science.* Submitted

Bjerg, B., Eggum, B.O., Jacobsen, I., Otte, J. and Srensen, H. (1989) Antinutri- tional and toxic effects in rats of individual glucosinolates (myrosinases) added to a standard diet (2). *Journal* **of** *Animal Physiology and Animal Nutrition,* **61,** 227-244

Björck, L. (1978) Antibacterial effect of the lactoperoxidase system on psychrotrophic bacteria in milk. *Journal of Dairy Research,* **45,** 109-118

Björck, L., Claesson, O. and Schulthess, W. (1979) The lactoperoxidase/thiocyanate/ hydrogen peroxide system as a temporary preservative for raw milk in develop- ing countries. *Milchwissenschaft,* **34,** 726-729

Brockman, R.P., Laarveld, B. and Christensen, D.A. (1980). Some effects of the level of iodine in Canol a meal concentrate on milk iodine and thiocyanate content of cows' milk. In *Research on Canola seed, oil, meal and meal fractions, 6th progress report,* **57**, 203-206. Winnipeg: Canola Council of Canada

Bünger, H., Schultz, J., Augustin, H., Schelper, E., Richter, K., Herbst, J. and Stang, V. (1938) Vergleichender Fiitterungs-versuch mit extrahiertem Rapsschrot und Rapskuchen an Milchkiihen. *Landwirtschaftliche Versuchsstation,* **129**, 34-70

Bush, R.S., Nicholson, J.W.G., MacIntyre, T.M. and McQueen, R.E. (1978) A comparison of Candle and Tower rapeseed meals in lamb, sheep and beef steer rations. *Canadian Journal of Animal Science,* **58**, 369-376

Canola Council of Canada (1985) *Feeding with Canola Meal,* **85**. Winnipeg: Canola Council of Canada

Clausen, S., Eggum, B.O., Jacobsen, I.M., Larsen, L.M., Plöger, A. and Sørensen, H. (1986) Individuelle aromatiske cholinestere og deres bidrag til tannin: kvalitets og ernreringsmressige problemer ved rapsfroprodukter. *Med- delelse fra Statens Husdyrbrugsforsg,* 609, 4p. Copenhagen: Statens Husdyrbrugsforsøg

Dahlberg, P.-A., Bergmark, A., Björck, L., Bruce, Å., Hambraeus, L. and Claesson, O. (1984) Intake of thiocyanate by way of milk and its possible effect on thyroid function. *American Journal of Clinical Nutrition,* **39**, 416-420

Dahlberg, P.-A., Bergmark, A., Eltom, M., Björck, L. and Claesson, O. (1985) Effect of thiocyanate levels in milk on thyroid function in iodine deficient subjects. *American Journal of Clinical Nitrition,* **41**, 1010-1014

Dahlén, J.Å.H., Lindh, L.A. and Münter, C.G.S. (1989) A new process for protein protection. *Proceedings* of *the world congress on vegetable protein utilization in human feeds and animal feedstuffs.* pp. 573-575. Singapore, October 1988

Deacon, M.A., De Boer, G. and Kennelly, J.J. (1988) Influence of Jet-Sploding and extrusion on ruminal and intestinal disappearance of canol a and soybeans. *Journal of Dairy Science,* **71**, 745-753

Dedenon, N. (1985) Appétibilité du tourteau de colza. *Proceedings* of *Tourteau de Colza l'enjeu, Paris,* 1985,76-95

DePeters, E.J. and Bath, D.L. (1986) Canola meal versus cottonseed meal as the protein supplement in dairy diets. *Journal of Dairy Science,* **69**, 148-154

Emanuelson, M (1989) Rapeseed products of double low cultivars to dairy cows: effects of long-term feeding and studies on rumen metabolism. *Dissertation. Report* 189, *Swedish University* of *Agricultural science, Department of Animal Nutrition and Management,* Uppsala, 82 p

Emanuelson, M., Ahlin, K.-Å. and Wiktorsson, H. (1993) Long-term feeding of rapeseed meal and full-fat rapeseed of double low cultivars to dairy cows. *Livestock Production Science,* **33**, 199-214

Emanuelson, M., Murphy, M. and Lindberg, J.-E. (1991) Effects of heat-treated and untreated full-fat rapeseed and tallow on rumen metabolism, digestibility, milk composition and milk yield in lactating cows. *Animal Feed Science and Technology,* **34**, 291-309

Exab Foder AB (1993) *Chemical Composition of Rapeseed Meal,* 1 p, Karlshamn, Sweden: Exab Foder AB

FAO (1993) *FAO quarterly bulletin* of *statistics,* 6, no 1. Rome: Food and Agriculture Organization of the United Nations

Fenwick, R.G. and Hoggan, H.A. (1976) The tannin content of rapeseed meals. *British Poultry Science,* **17**, 59-62

Fenwick, G.R., Heany, R.K. and Mullin, W.J. (1983) Glucosinolates and their breakdown products in food and food plants. In: *Critical reviews in food science and nutrition,* **18**, pp. 123-201. Edited by T.E. Furia. Florida: CRC Press, Inc

Fisher, L.J. and Walsh, D.S. (1976) Substitution of rapeseed meal for soybean meal as a source of protein for lactating cows. *Canadian Journal of Animal Science,* **56**, 233-242

Frederiksen, J.H., Andersen, P.E., Mortensen, B.K. and Jensen, F. (1979) Erglu-rapsekspeller til malkeker. *Meddelelse fra Statens Husdyrbrugsforsg,* **280**, 4p. Copenhagen: Statens Husdyrbrugsforsg

Gonda, H., Lindberg, J.-E. and Bectilsson, J. (1994) Protein level and degrad- ability in rations for dairy cows. 2. Digestibility and nitrogen metabolism. *Acta Agriculturre Scandinavica, Section A, Animal Science.* Submitted

Greer, M.A. and Deeney, J .M. (1959) Antithyroid activity elicited by the ingestion of pure progoitrin, a naturally occurring thioglycoside of the turnip family. *Journal of Clinical Investigations,* **38**, 1465-1474

Hill, R. (1991) Rapeseed meal in the diets of ruminants. *Nutrition Abstracts and Reviews, Series B,* 61, 139-155

Hoppe, K., Kozlowska, H. and Rutkowski, A. (1971) Rapeseed meal: XVII. Penetration of thioglucoside derivates from fodder into milk. *Milchwissenschaft,* **26**, 19-23

Ingalls, J .R. and Sharma, H.R. 1975. Feeding of bronowski, span and commercial rapeseed meals with or without addition of molasses or flavour in rations of lactating cows. *Canadian Journal of Animal Science,* **55**, 721-729

Iwarsson, K. 1973. Rapeseed meal as a protein supplement for dairy cows. 1. The influence of certain blood and milk parameters. *Acta Veterinaria Scandinavica,* **14**, 570-594

Iwarsson, K. and Ekman, L. (1975) Jodhalten i svensk mjolk under 1971-1974. (English summary). *Svensk Veteriniirtidning,* **27**, 393-399

Jarl, F. (1951) Utfodringsforsok med svenskt rapsmjol till mjolkkor. [Experiments on the Feeding of Swedish Rapeseed Oil Meal to Dairy Cows] *Bulletin* 45, *Statens Husdjursforsok,* 4p. Uppsala: Swedish University of Agricultural Science

Kärnell, R. (1988) *Degradation* of *glucosinolates in vitro in rumen fluid. Comparison between untreated rapeseed, heat-treated rapeseed and rapeseed meal.* Mimeo, English summary. Uppsala: Swedish University of Agricultural Sciences, Department of Animal Nutrition and Management, 35 p

Kendall, E.M., Ingalls, J.R. and Boila, R.J. (1991) Variability in the rumen degradability and postruminal digestion of the dry matter, nitrogen and amino acids of canola meal. *Canadian Journal of Animal Science,* **71**, 739-754

Khorasani, G.R., Robinson, P.R. and Kennelly, J.J. (1989) Effect of chemical treatment on *in vitro* and *in situ* degradation of canola meal crude protein. *Journal of Dairy Science,* **72**, 2074-2080

Khorasani, G.R., Robinson, P.H. and Kennelly, J.J. (1993) Effects of canola meal treated with acetic acid on rumen degradation and intestinal digestibility in lactating dairy cows. *Journal of Dairy Science,* **76**, 1607-1616

Korhonen, H. (1980) Potential role of the lactoperoxidase system (LP/SCN-/H2O2) in mastitis resistance. *Proceedings* of *Conference on Resistance Factors and Genetic Aspects of Mastitis Control,* Jablona, October 2-5 1980, 323-339

Kozlowska, H., Naczk, J., Shahidi, F. and Zademowski, R. (1990) Phenolic acids and tannins in rapeseed and canola. In *Canola and Rapeseed. Production, Chemistry, Nutrition and Processing Technology,* pp. 193-210. Edited by F. Shahidi. New York: Van Nostrand Reinhold

Kumar, R. and Singh, M. (1984) Tannins: Their Adverse Role in Ruminant Nutrition. Review. *Journal of Agriculture and Food Chemistry,* **32**, 447-453

Laarveld, B. and Christensen, B. (1976) Rapeseed meal in complete feeds for dairy cows. *Journal of Dairy Science,* **59**,1929-1935

Laarveld, B., Brockman, R.P. and Christensen, D.A. (1981a) The effects of Tower and Midas rapeseed meals on milk production and concentrations of goitrogens and iodide in milk. *Canadian Journal of Animal Science,* **61**, 131-139

Laarveld, B., Brockman, R.P. and Christensen, D.A. (1981b) The goitrogenic potential of tower and midas rapeseed meal in dairy cows determined by thyrotropinreleasing hormone test. *Canadian Journal of Animal Science,* **61**, 141-149

Landsudvalget for kvæg (1992) Fodermiddeltabel. Sammensretning og foder vrerdi af fodermidler til kvreg. *Landsudvalget for kvteg, rapport* 16. Århus: Landbrugets Radgivningscenter

Lanzani, A., Piana, G., Piva, G., Cardillo, M., Rastelli, A. and Jacini, G. (1974) Changes in Brassica napus progoitrin induced by sheep rumen fluid. *Journal of American Oil Chemists Society,* **51**, 517-518

Lee, P.A. and Hill, R. (1983) Voluntary feed intake of growing pigs given diets containing rapeseed meal, from different types and varieties of rape, as the only protein supplement. *British Journal of Nutrition,* **50**, 661-671

Lee, P.A., Pittam, S. and Hill, R. (1984) The voluntary food intake by growing pigs of diets containing 'treated' rapeseed meals or extracts of rapeseed meal. *British Journal of Nutrition,* **52**, 159-164

Lindberg, J.-E. 1986. Buffer solubility and rumen degradability of crude protein and rumen degradability of organic matter-nylon bag technique. *Report* 158, *Swedish University* of *Agricultural Sciences, Department* of *Animal Nutrition and Management,* Uppsala, 45 p

Lindell, L. (1976). Rapeseed meal in rations for dairy cows. 2. Comparison of two, levels of rapeseed meal. *Swedish Journal of Agricultural Research,* **6**, 65-71

Lindell, L. and Knutsson, P.-G. (1976) Rapeseed meal in rations for dairy cows. 1. Comparison of three levels of rapeseed meal. *Swedish Journal of Agricultural Research,* **6,** 55-63

Lo, M.T. and Hill, D.C. (1972a) Cyano compounds and goitrin in rapeseed meal. *Canadian Journal of Physiology and Pharmacology,* **50,** 373-377

Lo, M.T. and Hill, D.C. (1972b) Glucosinolates and their hydrolytic products in intestinal contents, feces, blood and urine of rats dosed with rape- seed meals. *Canadian Journal of Physiology and Pharmacology,* **50,** 962-966

Madsen, J. and Hvelplund, T. (1985) Protein degradation in the rumen. A comparison between *in vitro* nylon bag, *in vitro* and buffer measurements. *Acta Agriculturæ Scandinavica,* **Supplement 25,** 103-124

Mawson, R., Heaney, R.K., Piskula, M. and Kozlowska, H. (1993a) Rapeseed meal- glucosinolates and their anti nutritional effects Part 1. Rapeseed production and chemistry of glucosinolates. *Die Nahrung,* **37,**131-140

Mawson, R., Heaney, R.K., Zdunczyk, Z. and Kozlowska, H. (1993b) Rapeseed meal- glucosinolates and their antinutritional effects. Part II. Flavour and palatability. *Die Nahrung,* **37,** 336-344

Mawson, R., Heaney, R.K., Zdunczyk, Z. and Kozlowska, H. (1993c) Rapeseed meal- glucosinolates and their antinutritional effects. Part III. Animal growth and performance. *Die Nahrung,* in press

Mawson, R., Heaney, R.K., Zdunczyk, Z. and Kozlowska, H. (1993d) Rapeseed meal- glucosinolates and their anti nutritional effects. Part IV. Goitrogenicity and internal organs abnormalities in animals. *Die Nahrung,* in press

Mawson, R., Heaney, R.K., Zdunczyk, Z. and Kozlowska, H. (1993e). Rapeseed meal- glucosinolates and their antinutritional effects. Part V. *Animal Reproduction,* submitted

McDonald, B.E. (1992) Canol a oil in human nutrition-Physiological effects. *Proceedings* of *First International Symposium on Rapeseed Oil in Human Nutrition,* 12- 13 November 1992, 16 (Abstract)

McDonald, P., Edwards, R.A. and Greenhalgh, J.F.D. (1988) *Animal Nutrition.* 4th edition. New York: Longman Inc

McLean, C. and Laarveld, B. (1991) Effect of somatotropin and protein supple- ment on thyroid function of dairy cattle. *Canadian Journal of Animal Science,* **71,** 1053-1061

Miller, J.K., Swanson, E.W. and Spalding, G.E. (1975) Iodine absorption, excretion, recycling, and tissue distribution in the dairy cow. *Journal of Dairy Science,* **58,** 1578-1593

Mir, Z., MacLeod, G.K., Buchanan-Smith, J.G., Grieve, D.G. and Grovum, W.L. (1984) Methods for protecting soybean and canola proteins from degradation in the rumen. *Canadian Journal of Animal Science,* **64,** 853-865

National Research Council (NRC) (1989) *Nutrient Requirements of Dairy Cattle. Sixth Revised Edition.* Washington D.C.: National Academy Press

Nordfeldt, S. (1958) Smältbarhetsförsök och utfodringsförsök med rapsmjöl och senapsmjöl med läg resp. hög fetthalt till mjölkkor. Thesis, English summary. *Meddelande* nr. 66. 38 p. Uppsala: Statens husdjursförsök

Nydahl, M., Gustafsson, I.-B., Öhrvall, M. & Vessby, B. (1992) Comparison of the effects of dietary fats based on rapeseed oil and sunflower oil in healthy subjects. Proceedings from *First International Symposium on Rapeseed Oil in Human Nutrition*, 12-13 November 1992, 28 (Abstract)

Oil World Statistics Update (1993) In *Oil World*. Edited by T. Milke. Hamburg: ISTA

Paik, I.K., Robblee, A.R. and Clandinin, D.R. (1980) Products of the hydrolysis of rapeseed glucosinolates. *Canadian Journal of Animal Science*, **60**, 481-493

Papas, A., Ingalls, J.R. and Campbell, L.D. (1979) Studies on the effects of rapeseed meal on thyroid status of cattle, glucosinolate and iodine content of milk and other parameters. *Journal of Nutrition*, **109**, 1129-1139

Papas, A., Ingalls, J.R. and Cansfield, P. (1978) Effects of tower and 1821 rapeseed meals and tower gums on milk yield, milk composition and blood parameters of lactating dairy cows. *Canadian Journal of Animal Science*, **58**, 671-679

Pearson, A.W., Butler, E.J., Curtis, R.F., Fenwick, G.R., Hobson-Frohock, A. and Land, D.G. (1979) Effect of rapeseed meal on trimethyl amine metabolism in the domestic fowl in relation to egg taint. *Journal of the Science of Food and Agriculture*, **30**, 799-804

Peltola, P. (1965) The role of 1-5-vinyl-2-thio-oxazolidone in the genesis of endemic goiter in Finland. In *Current Topics in Thyroid Research. Proceedings of 5 th International Thyroid Conference*, 871-876. New York: Academic Press

Piironen, E. and Virtanen, A.I. (1963) The effect of thiocyanate in nutrition on the iodine content of cow's milk. *Zeitschrift Erniihrungswissennschaft*, **3**, 140-147

Pinnell, K. and Kennelly, J.J. (1983) Effect of dietary canola meal and choline on the incidence of fishy odour (trimethylamine) in cows milk. 62nd annual feeders' day report. *Agriculture and Forestry Bulletin* (special issue), 90-92. Edmonton: University of Alberta

Rae, R.C., Ingalls, J.R. and McKirdy, J.A. (1983) Response of dairy cows to formaldehyde-treated canola meal during early lactation. *Canadian Journal of Animal Science*, **63**, 905-915

Reineke, E.P. (1961) Factors affecting the secretion of iodine131 into milk of lactating goats. *Journal of Dairy Science*, **44**, 937-942

Robinson, P.H. and Kennelly, J.J. (1991a) Influence of degradability of supple- mental protein and time post-partum in early lactation dairy cows. 1. Rumen fermentation and milk production. *Livestock Production Science*, **28**, 121-138

Robinson, P.H. and Kennelly, J.J. (1991b) Influence of degradability of supple- mental protein and time post-partum in early lactation dairy cows. 2. Kinetics of rumen ingesta turnover and whole tract digestibility. *Livestock Production Science*, **29**, 167-180

Rooke, J.A., Brookes, I.M. and Armstrong, D.G. (1983) The digestion of untreated and formaldehyde-treated soya-bean and rapeseed meals by cattle fed a basal silage diet. *Journal of Agricultural Science (Cambridge),* **100**, 329-342

Sanchez, J .M. and Claypool, D. W. (1983) Canola meal as a protein supplement in dairy rations. *Journal of Dairy Science,* **66**, 80-85

Shahidi, F. (1990) Rapeseed and canola: Global production and distribution. In *Canola and Rapeseed. Production, Chemistry, Nutrition and Processing Technology,* pp. 3-13. Edited by F. Shahidi. New York: Van Nostrand Reinhold

Sharma, H.R., Ingalls, J.R. and Devlin, T.J. (1980) Apparent digestibility of Tower and Candle rapeseed meals in Holstein bull calves. *Canadian Journal of Animal Science,* **60**, 915-918

Sharma, H.R., Ingalls, J.R. and McKirdy, J.A. (1977) Effects of feeding high level of Tower rapeseed meal in dairy rations on feed intake and milk production. *Canadian Journal of Animal Science,* **57**, 653-662

Sones, K., Heaney, R.K. and Fenwick, G.R. (1984) An estimate of the mean daily intake of glucosinolates from cruciferous vegetables in the UK. *Journal of the Science of Food and Agriculture,* **35**, 712-720

Spörndly, R. (1993) *Fodertabeller för idisslare.* Speciella skrifter, 52. Swedish University of Agricultural Sciences. Uppsala. Edited by R. Spörndly

Stedman, J.A. and Hill, R. (1987) Voluntary food intake in a limited time of lambs and calves given diets containing rapeseed meal from different types and varieties of rape, and rapeseed meal treated to reduce the glucosinolate concentration. *Animal Production,* **44**, 75-82

Swedish Board of Agriculture (1992) *Jämförelse mellan oljeväxtsektorn i Sverige och EG.* Rapport 26, 55 P

Thomke, S. (1981) Review of rapeseed meal in animal nutrition: Ruminant animals. *Journal of the American Oil Chemists Society,* **58**, 805-810

Thomke, S., Björklund, K. and Olsson, A.C. (1989) *Nutritive evaluation with pigs of rapeseed, expeller prepressed rapeseed and rapeseed meals of dark (00-) and yellow (000-) type.* Paper presented at the 46th annual meeting of EAAP, commission of pig production. 29 August 1989, Dublin. 1 p

Tuori, M. (1992) Rapeseed meal as a supplementary protein for dairy cows on grass silage diets with the emphasis on the Nordic AA T -PBV feed protein evaluation system. *Agricultural Science in Finland,* **1**, 369-439

VanEtten, C.H. 1969. Glucosinolates. In *Toxic constituents of Plant Foodstuffs,* 4, pp. 103-136. Edited by I.E. Liener. New York: Acad. Press

Vanhatalo, A. and Aronen, I. (1991) The ruminal and intestinal degradation estimates of either untreated or physically treated rapeseed meals measured by nylon bag techniques. *Proceedings of the 8th International rapeseed congress "Rapeseed in a changing world",* Saskatoon, Canada. pp. 424-424

van Kempen, G.J.M. and Jansman, A.J.M. (1994) Use of EC produced oil seeds in animal feeds. In *Recent Advances in Animal Nutrition-1994,* pp. 31-56. Edited by P.C. Garnsworthy and D.J.A. Cole. Nottingham: Nottingham University Press

Varvikko, T., Lindberg, J.E., Setälä, J. and Syrjälä-Qvist, L. (1983) The effects of formaldehyde treatment of soya-bean meal and rapeseed meal on the amino acid profile and acid-pepsin solubility of rumen undegraded protein. *Journal of Agricultural Science, Cambridge,* **101**, 603-612

Vermorel, M., Davicco, M.-J. and Evrard, J. (1987) Valorization of rapeseed meal. 3. Effects of glucosinolate content on food intake, weight gain, liver weight and plasma thyroid hormone levels in growing rats. *Reproduction, Nutrition, Developpement,* **27**, 57-66

Vilkki, P., Kreula, M. and Piironen, E. (1962) Studies on the goitrogenic influence of cow's milk on man. *Annales Academiae Scientiarum Fennicae,* (series A, II. Chemica), **110**, 1-13

Vincent, I.C. and Hill, R. (1988) Low glucosinolate rapeseed meal as a protein source for milk production. *Animal Production,* **46**, 505

Vincent, I.C., Hill, R. and Campling, R.C. (1990) A note on the use of rapeseed, sunflower and soyabean meals as protein sources in compound foods for milking cattle. *Animal Production,* **50**, 541-543

Vincent, I.C., Hill, R. and Williams, H.L. (1988) Rapeseed meal in the diet of pubertal heifers during early pregnancy. *Animal Production,* 47, 39-44 Virtanen, A.I. and Gmelin, R. (1960) On the transfer of thiocyanate from fodder to milk. *Acta Chemica Scandinavica,* **14,** 941-945

Virtanen, A.I., Kreula, M. and Kiesvaara, M. (1963) Investigations on the alleged goitrogenic properties of milk. *Zeitschrift Erniihrungswissenschaft,* **3**, 185-206

Waldern, D. E. (1973) Rapeseed meal versus soybean meal as the only protein supplement for lactating cows fed corn silage rations. *Canadian Journal of Animal Science,* **53**, 107-112

Wilson, J.G. (1975) Hypothyroidism in ruminants with special reference to foetal goitre. *Veterinary Record,* **97**, 161-164

Witt, M., Huth, Fr.-W. and Hartmann, W. (1959) Rapsschrot ein wertvolles Futter fur Milchvieh. *Zeitschrift für Tierphysiologie, Tierernährung und Futtermittelkunde,* **14,** 175-185

This paper was first published in 1994

10

MEETING THE COPPER REQUIREMENTS OF RUMINANTS

N.F. SUTTLE
Moredun Research Institute, Pentlands Science Park, Penicuik, EH26 0AP

Introduction

Research on copper-responsive conditions in ruminants in the UK and in most developed countries has entered what can at best be described as a 'quiescent' period. There are no major recent developments to report. Therefore, the current state of knowledge will be reviewed, avoiding temptations to oversimplify and thereby create notional problems that have no bearing on animal production. The main points to be made are these:

1. The tabulated copper requirements of ruminants give only an approximate measure of dietary needs.
2. The conventional indices of copper status in the animal give only an approximate measure of dietary adequacy.
3. The best diagnosis of deficiency is provided by an improvement in health or production following supplementation.
4. Copper chelates possess no superiority over $CuSO_4$ as a dietary supplement.
5. Copper deficiency constrains animal production less than is commonly believed and is less important than copper poisoning in sheep.

Copper requirements of ruminants

The most sophisticated attempt to define copper requirements for ruminants was by the ARC (1980) and its imperfections have been noted by Suttle (1983; 1986). It must be emphasised that they represent broad guidelines. The requirements given for a particular class of stock (e.g. Table 10.1) depend heavily on the figures chosen for copper availability within a band which ranges ominously from 1 to 12%. The major determinants of availability are dietary sulphur and molybdenum concentrations and their influence is now routinely allowed for, with nutritional value expressed as available, rather than total,

Table 10.1 EFFECT OF AVAILABILITY ON DIETARY REQUIREMENTS FOR COPPER IN CATTLE FROM WEANING TO MATURITY

	Live weight (kg)	Growth rate or milk yield (kg/d)	Dry matter intake (kg/d)	Requirement (mg/kg DM) Availability (%)		
				1	3	6
Calf	200	1	5.3	21.9	7.3	3.7
Cow	500	0	6.1	27.9	9.3	4.7
		30	17.2	27.3	9.1	4.6

*Availability of 3% is probably the norm for grazing livestock; 6% the norm for housed animals and 1 % applies only to cattle grazing pastures with> 5mg Mo/kg DM

copper. However, the equations used to predict copper availability in forages (Suttle, 1986) have not yet been validated and contain substantial error components. Furthermore, different foodstuffs with the same molybdenum and sulphur concentration differ in availability (cereals, brassicas > hay > silage > pasture), for reasons that are not fully understood, but may reflect the inhibitory effects of fibre, sulphide and protozoa in the rumen (Suttle, 1991). No studies have been made of what happens when foodstuffs of contrasting availability are mixed in the same ration. Thus, fattening cattle given silage and whole-barley, or high yielding, grazing cows given concentrates in the parlour, might be presented with dietary copper of availability anywhere between 2 and 6% and their copper requirements would vary accordingly. Although the prediction of availability represented a major advance, it cannot be said that a diet will fail to meet the actual copper requirements of ruminants simply because there is a deficit between the predicted requirement and predicted supply - both are uncertain.

Copper is required at particular places for particular purposes, rather than in daily amounts (Suttle, 1988). An example is antioxidant defence via the cuproenzyme superoxide dismutase (SOD). SOD counters the cytotoxic threat from superoxide (O_2-), a by-product of everyday O_2 transfer, which can vary widely in intensity. Exercise and infection are two factors that stimulate O_2 transfer and O_2- production, probably enhancing SOD and therefore copper requirements at the front line(s) (e.g. erythrocyte, alveolar macrophage and enterocyte). Deficits between tables of copper requirement and copper concentrations in feeds probably overestimate the risks of copper deficiency occurring at these functional sites because they have a priority for limited copper supplies (Suttle, 1988).

Biochemical criteria for dietary copper deficiency

There have been no major improvements in the diagnostic tools available for assessing whether ruminants have a sufficient dietary copper supply. Awareness of the need to focus on critical sites and functions has led to research on SOD in erythrocytes and leucocytes, cytochrome oxidase and copper in leucocytes in various species. As yet these techniques are at the experimental stage and they may never be suitable for routine diagnostic use. There is, however, substantial room for improvement in the way the established tools are used.

PHYSIOLOGICAL UNCERTAINTIES

Since copper deficiency was first reported in the 1930s, liver and blood copper analysis have been used to assess the copper status of ruminants, but too little attention has been given to the relationship between the two indices (Figure 10.1) Although the data are new, the patterns are long-established (e.g. Hartmans, 1984 for cattle; Wiener and Field, 1969 for sheep) and the important feature is the lack of a close fit. Thus a plasma copper value of 9μmol/l (a common 'diagnostic threshold' value) is associated with liver copper concentrations of 300-600μmol/kg DM, while a liver value of 315μmol/kg DM (another commonly used threshold) is associated with plasma values of 3-12μmol/l. Either one or both of these commonly used 'diagnostic' criteria must give the wrong diagnosis on occasions; unfortunately, they both do! What each says via the other is that at either threshold copper status is in fact marginal; each is a nutritional rather than a diagnostic threshold, providing a warning sign that it would do no harm and might subsequently do some good if copper status were increased.

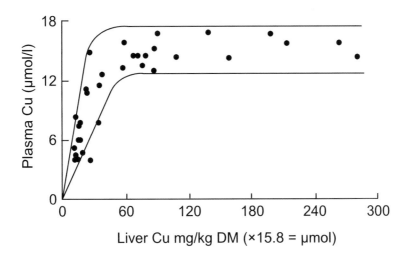

Figure 10.1 Relationship between plasma and liver biopsy copper concentrations in grazing Finnish Landrace Lambs

The vast majority of experimental and field studies suggest that health is unlikely to be compromised unless blood and liver copper values are substantially lower than those thresholds. This includes studies in which moderately increased molybdenum intakes have been associated with infertility (Phillippo, Humphries and Lawrence, 1982; Phillippo, Humphries, Atkinson, Henderson and Garthwaite, 1987) and lowered resistance to infection (e.g. Jones and Suttle, 1987). The use of additional thresholds of 4μmol copper/l for plasma and 158μmol copper/kg DM for liver delineate the lower limit of 'marginal' status and create a three-tier system (i.e. 'normal', 'marginal', 'deficient'), would concentrate the minds of veterinary practitioners, nutrition advisers and farmers wonderfully, improving the differential diagnosis of disease.

PATHOPHYSIOLOGICAL UNCERTAINTIES

The usefulness of liver and blood copper for predicting copper-responsiveness in ruminants will ultimately depend on how accurately they predict function-limiting deficits at performance-limiting sites. On two occasions it has been found that dietary molybdenum can deplete SOD activity in the gut mucosa while failing to hasten the depletion of liver or plasma copper (Suttle, 1991). Mucosal SOD may modulate the inflammatory response to worm infection (e.g. Suttle, Knox, Angus, Jackson, and Coop, 1992) and mucosal, rather than blood or liver, copper status may determine whether health is improved by copper supplementation. Local mucosal depletion of SOD (and other cuproenzymes) may occur in cattle grazing teart pastures of very high molybdenum content where diarrhoea develops in animals with normal liver and blood copper concentrations but responds to copper supplementation. Just how widespread such anomalies are in the field is a matter for conjecture.

The relationship between liver and blood copper changes dramatically following a challenge to the immune system. The effect on plasma copper of administering three multi-component vaccines to sheep is shown in Figure 10.2. The response was repeated after a second vaccination one month later, despite the 'marginal' copper status of some lambs. Even severely hypocupraemic lambs can show a sufficiently large increase in plasma copper for individuals to pass briefly from the deficient to adequate category, bypassing the 'marginal' status altogether. Peak responses occur 3-7 days after vaccination but the return to baseline values can take about three weeks. Natural infections such as pneumonia cause similar upheavals in plasma copper (N.F. Suttle, unpublished data) and they are part of the inflammatory or acute phase response to trauma. Caeruloplasmin is one of several proteins the synthesis of which increases during the acute phase response: caeruloplasmin normally provides 80% or more of the plasma copper but 100% of the increases shown in Figure 10.2. Studies with small laboratory animals suggest that changes occur concurrently in the liver (Kishore, Latman, Roberts, Barnett and Sorenson, 1984) as the distribution of copper in the body changes to meet local requirements and to

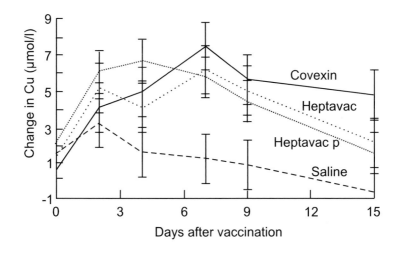

Figure 10.2 Changes in plasma copper concentrations in sheep receiving multi-component vaccines or saline

enhance the recovery from injury. It has yet to be established if daily copper requirements, and therefore the risk of deficiency, are invariably, or even occasionally, increased when the immune system is stimulated. In chronic parasitic infections of the abomasum, the rate of depletion of liver copper reserves can be increased (Bang, Familton and Sykes, 1990; Ortolani, Knox, Jackson, Coop and Suttle, 1993), but such infections are not accompanied by an acute phase response of the kind illustrated in Figure 10.2.

ANALYTICAL UNCERTAINTIES

All sampling and analytical procedures are accompanied by errors that make nonsense of a rigid separation of the diseased from the healthy on the basis of a 0.2 µmol/l difference in blood copper or a 5 µmol/kg DM difference in liver copper. The values reported by different laboratories for the same sample during quality control checks can vary substantially. The results obtained by atomic absorption spectrophotometry for plasma or serum from the same sheep with two pre-treatments in common use (dilution, 1:5) with water or removal of plasma proteins by precipitation with 8% trichloracetic acid (TCA, 1:4) are compared in Figure 10.3. Choice of sample type had a major influence on the result, the discrepancy increasing as copper concentrations increased. Serum gives low values because caeruloplasmin-copper is partially trapped during clot formation (Paynter, 1982). Sample pre-treatment has a smaller but still significant effect: dilution with water probably fails to release all the copper for atomisation, causing a slight underestimation that may vary from instrument to instrument, depending on nebulizer and burner design.

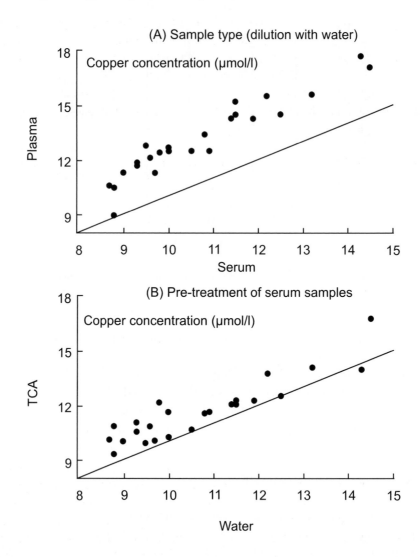

Figure 10.3 Effects of sample type (plasma and serum, A) and pre-treatment of samples (TCA precipitation of proteins or water dilution, B) on the copper concentration of ovine samples. Solid line equals line of equality.

Normal ranges have been derived largely for plasma from experimental studies but it is serum samples that are usually submitted from the field. Table 10.2 shows the serum values equivalent to the lower and upper limits of the proposed marginal range for plasma copper, for the two methods. Interpretation is clearly dependent on the sample and the chosen method but these are of far less diagnostic importance when a lower threshold of 4 µmol/l is used to characterise 'deficiency'. The conclusion on whether animals are at risk from toxicity is also greatly influenced by the sample chosen, serum samples requiring a 25% lower threshold. Pre-treatment with TCA does not invariably give maximum copper values because acidification leads to 'loss' (i.e. co-precipitation) of copper in ruminants on high molybdenum intakes, i.e. the very conditions under which copper requirements are least likely to be met. Furthermore, TCA-insoluble copper may become available (Suttle and Small, 1993) and a method that ignores its contribution may overestimate the risk of deficiency.

Table 10.2 ASSESSMENT OF BLOOD COPPER STATUS IS INFLUENCED BY THE SAMPLE TAKEN AND ITS METHOD OF TREATMENT, DILUTION WITH WATER (W) OR DEPROTEINATION WITH TRICHLORACETIC ACID (TCA)

	Observed value	*Predicted values**		
Sample	*Plasma*	*Plasma*	*Serum*	*Serum*
Pre-treatment	*W*	*TCA*	*W*	*TCA*
Toxicity	>25	24	19.7	19.6
Diagnosis adequacy	>9.4	10.6	7.9	9.2
Deficiency	<4	5.9	3.8	5.6

*Equivalent values for the diagnostic thresholds for water-diluted plasma and serum samples were predicted from equations underlying Figure 10.3

There are two further alternatives for assessing copper status in the blood, assays of caeruloplasmin (via its diamine oxidase or ferroxidase activity) and SOD, the principal copper constituent in erythrocytes. Caeruloplasmin is so highly correlated with TCA-soluble copper that it offers no diagnostic advantage, only quality control complications, beyond the few localities where pasture molybdenum concentrates are high enough (> 8 mg/kg DM for sheep; > 16 (?) for cattle) to cause TCA-insoluble copper to accumulate. SOD assays avoid complications associated with the acute phase response but present substantial quality control problems and tentative criteria of 'deficiency' proposed for sheep and cattle (Herbert, Small, Jones and Suttle, 1991) have yet to be validated.

Dose-response criteria as the ultimate test of dietary adequacy

A response to copper supplementation is the most reliable indicator of dietary inadequacy but recent field trials show how easily they too can be flawed. The trials were intended to establish how often lambs on improved hill pastures would benefit from copper supplementation and were prompted by consistent growth responses following dosage with copper particles (CuOp) on experimental sites (Whitelaw, Russel, Armstrong, Evans,

Fawcett and MacDonald, 1983; Woolliams, Woolliams, Suttle, Jones and Weiner, 1986). The outcome was surprising since only two out of 20 farms showed a significant and unequivocal benefit from administering copper. This was largely because the median herbage molybdenum concentration was only 1.8 mg/kg DM, much lower than that on the experimental sites and too low to impair copper absorption. However, the most surprising feature was the failure to obtain growth responses even with herbage molybdenum greater than 10 mg/kg DM.This may have been due to naive analysis of live-weight changes.

The standard way of analysing growth data is to deduct initial (I) from final (F) live weight (LW) but if ILW has been variably constrained either by a deficiency in the lamb of the element to be tested or by another factor (e.g. maternal milk yield, subsequent growth could be proportional to ILW and better handled by covariance analysis. If the supplemented element is needed, it should change the relationship between FLW and ILW and Table 10.3 indicates that it did so on a high molybdenum farm where there was no significant improvement in FLW between groups. The regression equations indicate that the heaviest (20 kg) lambs given CuOp gained 4.2 kg more than their untreated counterparts over the first six weeks.One possibility is that the lighter lambs had been held back by severe copper deficiency in the ewe that reduced her milk yield: giving CuOp to the lamb would not then alleviate the primary constraint on growth. As milk became less important as a source of nutrients in weeks 6-12, the maternal effect would diminish. Failure of CuOp to improve late LWG may have been partly due to failure to sustain a sufficient (12 weeks) dietary copper supply from a single dose of 1.3g CuOp or to the fact that growth had slowed with the approach to mature body size. On other farms, failure to obtain responses to CuOp may have been due to other design faults, such as failure to alleviate a concurrent deficiency of Co despite two injections of vitamin B12, occasional but substantial errors in recording live weight or curtailment of the trial at weaning, when copper was about to become limiting.

Table 10.3 LINEAR REGRESSIONS BETWEEN FINAL (F, 12 WEEK), MID-POINT (MP, 6 WEEK) OR INITIAL (I) LIVE WEIGHT (LW, kg) IN LAMBS CHANGE WITH COPPER SUPPLEMENTATION (CU) AND TIME ON A MOLYBDIFEROUS FARM (HERBAGE Mo 50—60 mg/kg DM)

Regression	Interval	Cu	Intercept (SD)		Coefficient (SD)	
MP on I	0-6	0	8.1[a]	(±2.19)	0.95[x]	(±0.162)
		+	1.1[b]	(±2.27)	1.51[y]	(±0.168)
F on MP	6-12	0	6.9	(±1.68)	0.88	(±0.080)
		+	5.38	(±1.06)	0.98	(±0.049)

a,b,x,y Different superscripts within columns denote significant effects of supplementation with cupric oxide needles at week 0: comparisons of mean LWG between groups were not significant after 6 or 12 weeks

Problems encountered in the above trials suggest the following primary requirements for a successful dose-response trial in addition to the obvious ones of using large groups (at least 20 replicates) and untreated controls.

1. Information on prior performance.
2. Use of (1.) by covariate analysis in assessing subsequent response to supplementation.
3. Sustained alleviation of deficiency by the chosen method of supplementation.
4. Assessment of responses over short intervals, but with observations made over the entire risk period.
5. Removal of as many other identifiable constraints as possible.

Implementation of such trials will facilitate not only diagnosis, but also the definition of minimum dietary requirements and diagnostic thresholds for copper. The minimum mineral intake needed to eliminate a response to supplementation in the field is a better measure of mineral requirement than factorial models based on experimental data and numerous major assumptions: plasma copper concentrations associated with the emergence of a growth response confirm a diagnostic threshold for this parameter.

Copper chelates as dietary supplements

The principal reason for copper deficiency occurring in ruminants is the poor absorption of copper from the diet. With other elements and species, chelating agents have sometimes overcome availability problems. For example, addition of ethylene diamine tetracetate (EDTA) to phytate-rich diets for pigs and poultry can enhance the absorption of zinc by reducing the formation of unabsorbable zinc-phytate complexes in the gut. Success is achieved because the chelate is strong enough to overcome competing ligands in the gut, small enough to be absorbed but weak enough to discharge its 'cargo' to trace element-dependent processes in the tissues. Because some trace elements can be highly toxic to tissues, chelates are also employed parenterally to reduce excessive body burdens (e.g. triethylamine tetramine (TETA) to treat copper overload) or to raise them without causing cytotoxicity (parenteral treatment of copper deficiency with CuCa-EDTA). Chelating agents with different properties are obviously required for these contrasting purposes; for oral supplementation, the chelator must be absorbable; for chelation therapy of overload, the complex must be poorly available but readily excretable; for parenteral supplementation, it must be poorly excreted and ultimately available for tissue uptake. TETA given parenterally will enhance urinary excretion of copper, but when given orally it is ineffective in sheep, possibly because it is not absorbed (Botha, Naude, Swan, Dauth, Dryer and Williams, 1993).

The characteristics of a copper chelate to be given in the diet to overcome problems of low dietary availability for ruminants can be set out. Low copper is determined principally in the rumen by formation of insoluble CuS and irreversible binding of copper to the solid phase of the digesta by thiomolybdates (Suttle 1991). To be effective, the copper chelate must have a stability constant that exceeds that of CuS and the thiomolybdate complexes. The latter is a particularly stringent requirement because thiomolybdates have such a strong affinity for copper that they can remove it from metallothionein, the body's natural 'copper-chelator' and protection agent (Gawthorne 1985). Thiomolybdates have been used as a de-coppering agent in sheep (Gooneratne, Howell and Gawthorne,1981; Humphries, Morrice and Bremner, 1988). Not only must the chelate resist the rival 'chelators', it must also resist displacement by competing elements. Such a complex has yet to be found.

MacPherson and Hemingway (1968) gave grazing lambs 70 mg copper/week as oral drenches of sulphate, glycinate or EDTA chelate for 45 weeks and found that the sources were equally effective in raising liver copper stores. This suggests either that the complexes were broken down or that 70 mg copper in a single dose as $CuSO_4$ overwhelmed the binding properties of any antagonists. The following experiment involving small copper supplements (N.F. Suttle, unpublished data) suggests that such chelates are broken down. Five groups of four Scottish Blackface ewes were used in a repletion experiment (c.f. Suttle, 1974) to compare the availability of copper from $CuSO_4$, CuEDTA, CuDTPA (diethylenetriamine pentacetate), CuTETA and CuDOS (diethylamine oxyquinoline sulphonate). Each source was added to a copper-deficient diet (containing 1 mg copper/kg DM) supplemented with molybdenum (3 mg) and sulphur (3 g/kg DM) to lower the availability of any 'unprotected' copper source: the sources provided firstly an additional 3 and secondly an additional 9 mg copper/kg DM, each repletion period lasting 21 days, with a week of copper depletion in between when no copper supplement was fed. The low copper diet had been fed before treatment to induce an initial state of hypocupraemia (mean plasma copper 3.4 µmol/l) so that any marked difference in copper availability should have been reflected by different rates of repletion in plasma copper. No source repleted the sheep at the lower level while all were equally effective at the second level, raising plasma copper from 2.4 to 4.2 0.27 µmol/l (Figure 10.4). Thus, using a model in which dietary copper availability was low (0.019) and animals were sensitive to a 2.5-fold increase in dietary copper concentration, no differences in copper availability were apparent. Although group size was small, major differences in availability should have been detectable.

Currently, interest is focused on another class of 'chelate' -the proteinate -a complex of copper with amino acids or peptides. Efficacy for copper- proteinates was expected and explored because *in vitro* and *in vivo'* studies involving small laboratory animals show that the absorption and membrane transport of trace elements can be enhanced by the presence of amino-acids, but results with ruminants have been disappointing. Hemingway (1991) included 10 mg supplementary copper/day in the pelleted grass diet of groups of 12 wether lambs as $CuSO_4$ or copper-proteinate for 14 days. Half the lambs were given molybdenum (as molybdate) and sulphur (as sulphate) in daily drenches providing 5 mg and 5 g, respectively. Balance studies showed no difference in the apparent availability, or urinary excretion, of copper. Studies with cattle have also failed

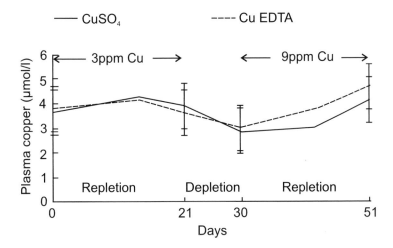

Figure 10.4 Repletion of hypocupraemic ewes was achieved with 9 but not with 3 mg Cu/kg DM added to a diet supplemented with Mo + S yet responses were similar with Cu added as CuSO₄ and CuEDTA

to show any advantage of copper-proteinate (Wittenberg, Boila and Shariff, 1990) or a copper-lysine complex (Ward, Spears and Kegley, 1993) over CuSO4 in the presence or absence of supplementary molybdenum (Figure 10.5). Kincaid, Blauwiekel and Gonrath (1986) reported higher liver and plasma copper levels in copper-proteinate treated versus CuSO₄-treated calves (n=12) after 12 weeks on a molybdenum-rich hay/concentrate diet: each source raised copper intake from 11 to 37 mg/day and the copper:molybdenum ratio from 0.8 to 2.8. However, the copper-proteinate did not prevent a reduction in liver copper or give a significant improvement when compared with an untreated group.

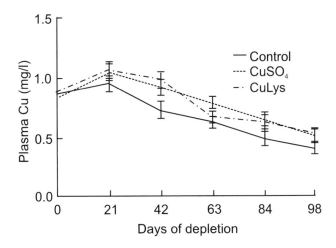

Figure 10.5 Effect of copper-lysine and copper sulphate administration on plasma Cu in cattle (from Ward *et al.*, 1993)

Furthermore, the difference between the two treated groups in plasma copper was as large on the day of treatment as it was after 12 weeks! There is no evidence of enhanced availability of copper from proteinates in 'unstressed' ruminants and no physicochemical reason why they should succeed where stronger chelates have failed. Under normal feeding conditions, there will always be an abundance of amino acids to form complexes with copper given in cheap inorganic forms such as $CuSO_4$. False hopes were probably raised for copper-proteinates because tests were conducted with *milieu* artificially low in amino acids (e.g. fasted rats, isolated loops of intestine, isolated membrane preparations). Nockels, DeBonis and Torrent (1993) have recently reported enhanced copper retention for copper given as Cu-lysine in steers after 36 hours starvation and an injection of adrenocorticotrophic hormone.

'By-pass' copper for cattle

For cattle, there remains a need for copper that is protected from rumen-based antagonisms but highly available for absorption beyond the rumen. Protection might be achieved by choice of copper source or manipulation of rumen fermentation. Although CuOp by-pass the rumen, they are of limited success because they contain copper that is of intrinsically low availability, i.e. their copper is largely 'protected' throughout their sojourn in the gastro-intestinal tract. Mineral- (e.g. Ca) containing soaps are widely used to enable energy-rich fatty acids to 'by-pass' the rumen. The inclusion of inorganic copper in non-rumen degradable micelles such as Cu-soaps may provide an efficient means of delivering copper to the sites of absorption where excessive dietary copper levels are otherwise necessary (on the molybdenum-rich 'teart' pastures). For intensively fed beef cattle, where the risks of copper deficiency are remote, copper should not be added to fat- supplemented diets until the extent and consequences of Cu-soap formation *in vivo* have been explored. Manipulation of rumen fermentation by administering a bolus that slowly releases an anti-protozoal agent (e.g. monensin) might protect normal dietary sources of copper for reasons given in the next section.

Avoiding chronic copper poisoning in sheep

For housed sheep, copper toxicity is a problem and the need is to expose copper to rumen-based and other antagonisms so that as little as possible is absorbed and the ever-present risk is reduced. The customary practice is for large feed compounders to add a cocktail of antagonists (molybdenum, sulphur, zinc and iron) to their products, but the reduction in copper retention can be less than expected (Suttle, 1993b) and few guarantee their products for susceptible breeds such as the Texel (Woolliams, Suttle, Wiener, Field, and Woolliams, 1982). It is possible that some antagonists do not produce additive effects because they compete for the same pool of absorbable copper. Another possibility is that an acid rumen environment, produced by the rapid ingestion of antagonists in a pelleted feed, is unfavourable to the formation of CuS and copper-thiomolybdate complexes. Once-daily feeding of a pelleted diet can increase copper availability by one fifth when compared with continuous feeding (Suttle and Peter, 1985). Antagonists may be of greater efficacy when fed in a loose or complete diet several times per day.

Compounders should be exceedingly wary of adding anti-protozoal agents such as monensin, on veterinary prescription, to feeds for vulnerable breeds. Liver copper concentrations are increased substantially by monensin supplementation (Van Ryssen and Barrowman, 1987) and this may be because of the elimination of sulphide-generating protozoa that normally lower copper availability (Ivan, 1988). Monensin will reduce the efficacy of molybdenum, sulphur and iron that rely on rumen sulphide to potentiate their respective antagonisms. It is in the feed industry's interests to encourage farmers to take their own steps to minimise the risk of chronic copper poisoning by administering antagonists via the roughage component of the diet, where they may be more effective. For example, addition of a slowly degradable sulphur source to the roughage (e.g. $CaSO_4$ at 375 g/25 kg bale of hay) can reduce subclinical liver damage due to copper poisoning (D. Cotton, personal communication).

Conclusions

Most 'copper-problems' that affect the livestock industry and its feed suppliers are artefacts of simplistic interpretations of dietary copper requirements and biochemical indices of copper status in the animal. Natural selection has produced livestock that afford priority of copper-supply to life-dependent processes, creating tolerance of copper supplies that fail to meet textbook requirements. Under rare conditions, such as molybdenum overload in cattle, tolerance may be broken and there are lessons still to be learnt. Elsewhere, the use of lower biochemical thresholds for separating animals of 'deficient' from those of a 'marginal' status will restore a proper perspective. By avoiding unnecessary supplementation, risks of chronic copper poisoning in sheep -which now exceed those of swayback - may be reduced.

References

Agricultural Research Council (1980) *The Nutrient Requirements of Ruminant Livestock.* Slough: Commonwealth Agricultural Bureaux

Bang, K.S., Familton, A.S. and Sykes, A.R. (1990) Effect of ostertagiasis on copper status of sheep: a study involving use of cupric oxide wire particles. *Research in Veterinary Science,* **49,** 306-314

Botha, C.J., Naude, T.W., Swan, G.E., Dauth, J., Dryer, M.J. and Williams, M.C. (1993) The cupruretic effect of two chelators following copper loading in sheep.

Onderstepoort Journal of Veterinary Reserch, **59**, 191-195

Gawthorne, J .M. (1985) Trace element interactions with special reference to copper. In *Ruminant Physiology: Concepts and Consequences,* pp.357-371. University of Western Australia

Gooneratne, S.R., Howell, J.McC. and Gawthorne, J.M. (1981) An investigation of the effects of intravenous administration of thiomolybdate on copper metabolism in chronic copper-poisoned sheep. *British Journal of Nutrition,* **46,** 457-480

Hartmans, J. (1974) Tracing and treating mineral disorders in cattle under field conditions. In *Proceedings of the Second International Symposium on Trace Element Metabolism in Animals,* pp. 261-273. Edited by W.G. Hockstra, J.W. Suttie, H.E. Ganther and W. Mertz. Baltimore: University Park Press

Hemingway, R.G. (1991) Retention by growing lambs of dietary copper given as either copper sulphate or a copper proteinate. In *Proceedings of the Seventh International Symposium on Trace Elements in Man and Animals,* pp. 15-9 to 15-10. Edited by B. Momcilovic. Dubrovnik

Herbert, E., Small, J.N. W., Jones, D.G. and Suttle, N.F. (1991) Evaluation of superoxide dismutase assays for the routine diagnostic assessment of copper status in blood samples. In *Proceedings of the Seventh International Symposium on Trace Elements in Man and Animals,* pp. 5-15 to 5-16. Edited by B. Momcilovic. Dubrovnik

Humphries, W .R., Morrice, P .C. and Bremner, I. (1988) A convenient method for treating chronic copper poisoning using subcutaneous ammonium tetrathio-molybdate. *Veterinary Record,* **123**, 41-53

Ivan, M.M. (1988) The effect of faunation on rumen solubility and liver content of copper in sheep fed low or high copper diets. *Journal of Animal Science,* **66**, 1496-1501

Jones, D.G. and Suttle, N.F. (1987) Copper and disease resistance. In *Proceedings of the 21st Annual Conference on Trace Substances in Environmental health,* pp. 514-525. Edited by D.D. Hemphill. Columbia: University of Missouri

Kincaid, R.L., Blauwiekel, R.M. and Gonrath, J.D. (1986) Supplementation of copper as copper sulphate or copper proteinate for growing calves fed forages containing molybdenum. *Journal of Dairy Science,* **693**, 160-163

Kishore, Y., Latman, N., Roberts, D. W., Barnett, J.B. and Sorenson, J.R.J. (1984) Effects of nutritional copper deficiency on adjuvant arthritis and immuno-competence in the rat. *Agents and Actions,* **14**, 274-282

MacPherson, A. and Hemingway, R.G. (1968) Effects of liming and various forms of oral copper supplementation on the copper status of growing sheep. *Journal of Science, Food and Agriculture,* **19**, 53-58

Nockels, C.F., DeBonis, J. and Torrent, J. (1993) Stress induction affects copper and zinc balance in calves fed organic and inorganic copper and zinc sources. *Journal of Animal Science,* **71**, 2539-2545

Ortolani, E., Knox, D.P., Jackson, F., Coop, R.L. and Suttle, N.F. (1993) Abomasal parasitism lowers liver copper status and influences the Cu x Mo x S antagonism in lambs. In *Proceedings of the Eighth International Symposium on Trace Elements in Man and Animals, Dresden.* Edited by M. Anke, D. Mersner and C.F. Mills. pp. 331-332. Verlag Media Touristik

Paynter, D.I. (1982) Differences between serum and plasma caeruloplasmin activities and copper concentrations: investigation of possible contributing factors. *Australian Journal of Biological Science,* **35**, 353-360

Phillippo, M., Humphries, W.R., Atkinson, T., Henderson G.D. and Garthwaite, P .H. (1987) The effect of dietary molybdenum and iron on copper status, puberty, fertility and oestrus cycles in cattle. *Journal of Agricultural Science, Cambridge,* **109**, 321-336

Phillippo, M., Humphries, W.R. and Lawrence, C.B. (1982) Investigation of the effect of copper status and therapy on fertility in beef suckler herds. *Journal of Agricultural Science, Cambridge,* **99**, 359-364

Suttle, N.F. (1974) A technique for measuring the biological availability of copper to sheep, using hypocupraemic ewes. *British Journal of Nutrition,* **32**, 395-405

Suttle, N.F. (1983) Bovine hypocuprosis. In *The Veterinary Annual,* 23rd issue, pp. 96-103. Edited by C.S.G. Grunsell and F. W.G. Hill. Bristol: Scientechnia

Suttle, N.F. (1986) Copper deficiency in ruminants: recent developments. *Veterinary Record,* **119**, 519-522

Suttle, N.F. (1988) The nutritional requirement for copper in animals and man. In *Copper in Man and Animals,* Volume I, pp. 21-43. Boca Raton, Florida: CRC Press

Suttle, N.F. (1991) The interactions between copper, molybdenum and sulphur in ruminant nutrition. *Annual Review of Nutrition,* **11**, 121-140

Suttle, N.F. (1993a) Overestimation of copper deficiency. *Veterinary Record,* **133**, 123-124

Suttle, N.F. (1993b) Control of copper poisoning and macro mineral imbalances in ruminants. *Journal of Science in Food and Agriculture,* **63**, 103

Suttle, N.F., Knox, D.P., Angus, K.W., Jackson, F. and Coop, R.L. (1992) Effects of dietary molybdenum on nematode and host during Haemonchus contortus infection in lambs. *Research in Veterinary Science,* **52**, 230-235

Suttle, N.F. and Peter, D.W. (1985) Rumen sulphide metabolism as a major determinant of copper availability in the diets of sheep. In *Proceedings of the Fifth International Symposium on Trace Elements in Man and Animals,* pp. 367-370. Edited by C.F. Mills, I. Bremner and J.K. Chesters. Slough: Commonwealth Agricultural Bureaux

Suttle, N.F. and Small, J.N.W. (1993) Delayed availability of copper: a new concept in the copper:molybdenum antagonism. In *Proceedings of the Sheep Veterinary Society,* **17**, 241

Van Ryssen, M. and Barrowman, T. (1987) Effect of ionophores on the accumula- tion of copper in the livers of sheep. *Animal Production,* **44**, 255-261

Ward, J.D., Spears, J.W. and Kegley, E.B. (1993) Effect of copper level and source (copper lysine vs copper sulphate) on copper status, performance and immune responses in growing steers fed diets with or without supplemental molybdenum and sulphur. *Journal of Animal Science,* **71**, 2748-2755

Whitelaw, A.G., Russel, A.J.F., Armstrong, R.H., Evans, C.C., Fawcett, A.R. and MacDonald, A.J. (1983) Use of cupric oxide needles in the prophylaxis of induced copper deficiency in lambs grazing improved hill pastures. *Veterinary Record,* **112**, 382-384

Wiener, G. and Field, A.C. (1969) Copper concentrations in the liver and blood of sheep of different breeds in relation to swayback history. *Journal of Comparative Pathology,* **79**, 7-14

Wittenberg, K.M., Boila, R.J. and Shariff, M.A. (1990) Comparison of copper sulphate and copper proteinate as copper sources for copper-depleted steers fed high molybdenum diets. *Canadian Journal of Animal Science,* **70**, 895-904

Woolliams, J.A., Suttle, N.F., Wiener, G., Field, A.C. and Woolliams, C. (1982) The effect of breed of sire on the accumulation of copper in lambs with particular reference to copper toxicity. *Animal Production,* **35**, 299-307

Woolliams, J.A., Woolliams, C., Suttle, N.F., Jones, D.G. and Wiener, G. (1986) Studies on lambs from lines genetically selected for low and high copper status. II Incidence of hypocuprosis on improved hill pastures. *Animal Production,* **43**, 303-317

This paper was first published in 1994

11

A NEW LOOK AT THE REQUIREMENTS OF HIGH-PRODUCING DAIRY COWS FOR B-COMPLEX VITAMINS

C.L. GIRARD

Dairy and Swine Research and Development Centre, Agriculture and Agri-Food Canada, Lennoxville, Québec, J1M 1Z3, Canada

Introduction

Historically, requirements for B-complex vitamins were defined as the smallest amount to include in the diet in order to avoid deficiency symptoms. According to this "minimalist" definition, under most conditions, there is no need for dietary supplements of B-complex vitamins because, in dairy cows, these vitamins are synthesized by ruminal microorganisms in amounts sufficient to avoid the appearance of deficiency symptoms. Most studies on ruminant requirements for B-complex vitamins were conducted half a century ago. However, during the past few decades, milk production has increased drastically. For example, in Québec, Canada, during the last 20 years, average milk production increased from 4 992 kg per cow for a 305-day lactation in 1978 to 7 599 kg in 1998 (Lefevre, Allard, Block and Sanchez, 1999). In order to sustain current production levels, the needs for nutrients increased as well as the demand on the major metabolic pathways. Therefore, what would be the requirements for these vitamins if the goal is to maintain maximum animal performance in these high-producing cows rather than to avoid deficiency?

This chapter will not deal with all B-complex vitamins. Even if there are many advantages in considering the B-complex vitamins as a group, from a nutritional point of view it should be borne in mind that most of them are unrelated chemically and that the group name has no chemical or metabolic significance. The present paper will focus on two B-complex vitamins sharing one common metabolic pathway, folic acid and vitamin B_{12}, as well as on two factors closely linked to them, methionine and choline. Experimental data will be reported in order to support a revision of the definition of requirements for B-complex vitamins for high-producing dairy cows.

Folic acid

ROLES OF FOLIC ACID

The molecule of folic acid (pteroylmonoglutamic acid), the synthetic form of the vitamin, is composed of three different parts: 1) a pteridine nucleus, 2) a para aminobenzoic moiety and 3) one molecule of glutamic acid. However, due to changes in the level of reduction of the pteridine nucleus (dihydro- or tetrahydrofolate), the addition of different one-carbon radicals (methyl, formyl, methenyl, etc.), and the presence of a variable number of glutamic acid molecules, more than 100 biologically active forms of this vitamin have been identified. The biologically active forms of the vitamin are called folates (Le Grusse and Watier, 1993; McDowell, 1989).

The main function of folate coenzymes is to accept or donate one-carbon units. Folate coenzymes are involved in protein metabolism, where they donate a one-carbon unit for the methionine formylation; the presence of a formylmethionine on a t-RNA is essential to the induction of protein synthesis. Folic acid is also necessary for purine and pyrimidine synthesis, essential constituents of RNA and DNA, ATP and cyclic AMP, playing a major role in tissue formation and metabolism. It is also involved in the formation of the primary methylating agent, S-adenosylmethionine and in amino acid metabolism: 1) glycine catabolism, this reaction is also vitamin B_6-dependent 2) histidine catabolism, 3) glycine-serine interconversion, one of the major sources of one-carbon units, also vitamin B_6-dependent and 4) methionine regeneration, vitamin B_{12}-dependent (Le Grusse and Watier, 1993; Weil, 1972).

METABOLIC NEEDS FOR FOLIC ACID

Given its metabolic roles, folic acid is critical for cell division and protein metabolism. Therefore, it seems to be an ideal candidate to begin with while reviewing B-vitamin requirements for a maximal production. Utilization of folic acid is increased by the synthesis of new tissues, foetus, foetal membranes, mammary gland, and by milk protein synthesis. It is logical to believe that requirements for folic acid are high in dairy cows because, under usual management conditions, most lactating cows are also in gestation during several months per year. Moreover, Zinn, Owens, Stuart, Dunbar and Norman (1987) observed that, compared with B-vitamin requirements of swine, pantothenic acid and folic acid supplies, evaluated from the amounts reaching the duodenum, are marginal in growing steers.

Some observations seem to substantiate the choice of this vitamin. Non-gestating cows have serum concentrations of folates superior to those of gestating cows (Arbeiter and Winding, 1973; Tremblay, Girard, Bernier-Cardou and Matte, 1991). Total serum folates of dairy cows decrease by 40 % from two months after calving to next calving (Girard, Matte and Tremblay, 1989). This dramatic fall in serum folates could reflect a huge uptake of folic acid by the animal's tissues as it was demonstrated in multiparous cows, in which uptake of folic acid by tissues is greater two months before calving than three weeks after calving (Girard and Matte, 1995).

IMPACT OF SUPPLEMENTARY FOLIC ACID ON MILK PRODUCTION AND COMPOSITION

In order to define the significance of these changes in folic acid uptake by cows' tissues, a series of trials was conducted to examine the effects of supplementary folic acid on lactational performance of dairy cows.

In a first trial, intramuscular injections of 0 or 160 mg of folic acid (pteroyl-monoglutamic acid) were given weekly from 45 days of gestation until six weeks after calving. This mode of administration of supplementary folic acid was chosen because neither the extent of destruction of folic acid by the ruminal microflora nor the impacts of these supplements on the microflora were known. The objective of the trial was to evaluate the metabolic effects of supplementary folic acid without any interference of ruminal microflora. The cows were fed a diet of more than 67 % forages (grass silage and hay) on a dry matter basis. Supplementary folic acid increased placental and colostral transfer of folates to the calf by 24 % and 54 %, respectively. Blood haemoglobin and packed cell volume were not modified by supplementary folic acid. Between 45 days of gestation and drying off, supplementary folic acid increased milk production by 1.5 kg/d and transfer of folic acid in milk and tended to increase milk protein concentration. After calving, injections of folic acid had no effect on milk production. Supplementary folic acid had no effect on milk protein concentration in primiparous cows, 33.2 and 33.7 g/kg for cows injected or not with folic acid. However, for cows in their second lactation or more, milk protein concentration was 35.1 and 32.3 g/kg for cows injected or not with folic acid, respectively. In spite of the increased milk and milk protein yields, dry matter intake of cows was not influenced by injections of folic acid (Girard, Matte and Tremblay, 1995). In view of the results obtained using parenteral supplements of folic acid, the amount of folic acid needed to reproduce the effects of intramuscular injections on serum concentrations of folates was determined (Girard, Matte and Lévesque, 1992).

Dietary supplements of 0, 2 or 4 mg of folic acid per kilogram of body weight were given daily to dairy cows from four weeks before the expected time of calving until 305 days of lactation. In this second production trial, forages contributed only to 40 % of the diet on a dry matter basis. Dietary supplements of folic acid increased serum folates, indicating that folic acid was efficiently absorbed. Milk folates were also increased, although there was no difference between the two doses of folic acid; this augmentation was larger in multiparous than in primiparous cows. During a 305 day lactation, there was no statistically significant effect of dietary folic acid on milk production of primiparous cows, although it was numerically lower for cows fed dietary supplements of folic acid.

In multiparous cows, milk production increased linearly with the quantity of folic acid ingested (Table 11.1; Girard and Matte, 1998).

Table 11.1 AVERAGE MILK PRODUCTION (KG/D) OF DAIRY COWS FED DIETARY SUPPLEMENTS OF FOLIC ACID DURING A 305-DAY LACTATION PERIOD

	Dietary supplements of folic acid (mg/kg BW/day)		
	0	2	4
Primiparous cows	26.9	25.1	25.2
Multiparous cows	27.2	28.0	29.4

(after Girard and Matte, 1998)

Milk casein content was not modified by the dietary supplements of folic acid, but casein yield was increased by folic acid supplements in multiparous dairy cows. Non-protein nitrogen content of milk was decreased during the first 100 days of lactation in multiparous cows fed supplementary folic acid, suggesting that nitrogen was used more efficiently. Moreover, dry matter intake was similar for all treatments. The effects of folic acid on feed intake, non-protein nitrogen in milk and milk production of multiparous cows indicate that folic acid might improve the efficiency of nutrient utilization.

Interactions between the metabolism of methionine and folic acid

According to these two studies, parenteral and oral supplements of folic acid increased milk and milk protein yields in dairy cows in their second lactation or more but the metabolic pathways involved were still unidentified. In these studies, the calculated supply of methionine was less than the recommended level (Rulquin, Pisulewski, Vérité and Guinard, 1993; Schwabb, Bozak, Whitehouse and Meshah, 1992). Folic acid is known to promote regeneration of methionine in mammalian tissues in a reaction in which the 5-methyltetrahydrofolate ($5\text{-}CH_3\text{-}THF$) gives a methyl group to homocysteine to form methionine (Le Grusse and Watier, 1993). Therefore, it is possible that an increased supply of folic acid, in presence of a sufficient supply of one-carbon units, could have augmented the amount of methionine available for milk protein synthesis. A third study was conducted to investigate the relationship between methionine and folic acid and its effects on lactational performance of dairy cows.

During a 305-day lactation, 54 multiparous cows were fed a diet calculated to provide the requirements for essential amino acids but only 0.80 of the methionine requirements. Half the cows received a supplement of rumen-protected methionine (Smartamine M[TM], 18 g/day). Within each level of methionine supplementation, dietary supplements of 0, 3 or 6 mg of folic acid per kilogram of body weight were given daily. None of the treatments changed milk production during the 305-day lactation (10818 ± 75 kg). Supplementary methionine increased total solids (121 vs 126 g/kg), fat (35 vs 37 g/kg), total protein (32.5 vs 34.6 g/kg) and casein (21.1 vs 22.8 g/kg) contents of milk. With the diet low in methionine, milk casein content was increased in cows fed 3 mg of folic acid per kilogram body weight compared with controls (21 vs 23 g/kg) whereas with the diet supplemented with methionine, folic acid had no effect (Girard, Lapierre, Matte and Lobley, 1998). According to these preliminary results, some of the effects of folic acid on milk protein synthesis seem to be mediated through an increased supply of methionine but it seems overly simplified to reduce the role of folic acid to an increased regeneration of methionine. Some other factors are likely to be involved.

Relationships among folic acid, vitamin B_{12} and vitamin B_6

Metabolic reactions requiring folates, often called one-carbon metabolism, are influenced by folate intake and also by intake of other essential nutrients such as vitamins B_6 and B_{12}. On one hand, after ingestion, the major part of the synthetic form of folic acid, pteroylmonoglutamic acid, is reduced and methylated during the absorption process and its passage in the liver; this reaction is irreversible (Cooper, 1977; Bhandari and Gregory, 1992). In cow serum, all folates are present as 5-CH_3-THF (Guay, Girard and Matte, unpublished data). The methyl group of the 5-CH_3-THF can be used only in the following reaction:

$$5\text{-}CH_3\text{-}THF + \mathbf{B_{12}}\text{-methionine synthase} \rightarrow CH_3\text{-}\mathbf{B_{12}}\text{-methionine synthase} + THF$$

$$CH_3\text{-}\mathbf{B_{12}}\text{-methionine synthase} + \text{homocysteine} \rightarrow \text{methionine} + \mathbf{B_{12}}\text{-methionine synthase}$$

In this reaction, the 5-CH_3-THF acts as a substrate, it donates its methyl group to homocysteine, a non-protein forming sulphur amino acid, to form methionine and regenerates THF (Bailey and Gregory, 1999, Le Grusse and Watier, 1993; Weil, 1972). The 5-CH_3-THF cannot be retained in cells or transformed into a pteroylpolyglutamate (Bässler, 1997); only the reduced form of folates conjugated to a polyglutamate chain is active in the cell (Scott, 1999). Moreover, regeneration of THF through this reaction is absolutely essential before conversion to 5-10-methylene-THF, a form of folates required for thymidylate synthesis and, thus, DNA synthesis (Bailey and Gregory, 1999, Le Grusse and Watier, 1993; Weil, 1972).

On the other hand, homocysteine can be condensed with serine, catalyzed by cystathionine ß-synthase, to form an intermediate compound, cystathionine. Cystathionine is subsequently cleaved to cysteine and homoserine by the enzyme γ-cystathionase. These two reactions are pyridoxal phosphate-dependent (Allen, Stabler and Lindenbaum, 1993; Stabler, Lindenbaum, Savage and Allen, 1993). When the quantity of methyl groups (one-carbon units) available is marginal, the methylation of homocysteine to methionine is favoured whereas, in the presence of an abundant supply of methyl groups, homocysteine will enter the pathway of degradation via cystathionine (Krebs, Hems and Tyler, 1976). Consequently, different levels of supply of methyl groups could change the demand for vitamin B_{12} or pyridoxal-phosphate (vitamin B_6) in relation with the metabolic pathways involved, methylation or degradation of homocysteine (Krebs, Hems and Tyler, 1976) (Figure 11.1).

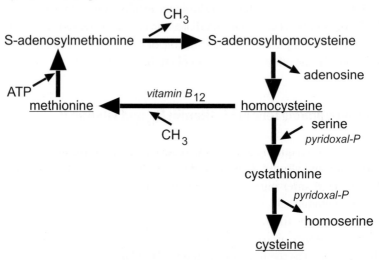

Figure 11.1 Metabolism of sulphur amino acids (after Bässler, 1997; Weil, 1972)

In the production trial previously described and looking at the effect of dietary supplements of folic acid on lactational performance of primiparous and multiparous dairy cows, changes in serum concentrations of vitamin B_6 and vitamin B_{12} were observed from four weeks before calving until the end of a 305-day lactation period. During this period, the major changes in serum concentrations of pyridoxal and pyridoxal-5-phosphate (two vitamers of vitamin B_6) appear during the peripartum period (four weeks before to four weeks after parturition); the concentrations of these vitamers were relatively stable thereafter during lactation. These data gave no indication of large changes in the supply and/or demand for vitamin B_6 during lactation (Girard and Matte, 1999). However, in this study, in spite of a sufficient dietary supply in cobalt, in early lactation, serum concentrations of vitamin B_{12} were low and serum concentrations of folates increased, especially in cows fed dietary supplements of folic acid. Later, after 8 to 12 weeks of lactation, serum concentrations of vitamin B_{12} increased whereas serum concentrations of folates fell in supplemented cows (Figure 11.2). Moreover, serum concentrations of vitamin B_{12} were lower in primiparous than in multiparous cows (Girard and Matte, 1999). Blood haemoglobin and packed cell volume of multiparous cows were not affected by supplementary folic acid whereas, in primiparous cows fed the highest level of folic acid, they were higher from the 16th week of lactation until the end of the lactation.

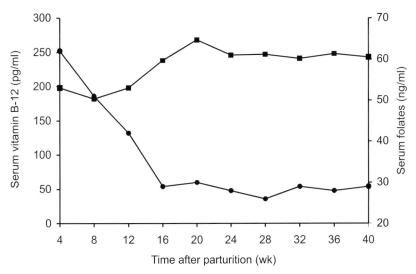

Figure 11.2 Serum concentrations of vitamin B$_{12}$ (■) and folates (●) in cows fed 4 mg of folic acid per kilogram of body weight from 4 weeks before calving until 305 days of lactation (after Girard and Matte, 1999).

Vitamin B$_{12}$ might be a limiting factor for the action of folic acid in primiparous cows; such hypothesis is in agreement with production data (Girard and Matte 1998) which showed that supplementary folic acid had no major effect on productivity of primiparous cows but increased milk production as well as the total amount of milk casein produced in multiparous cows.

These observations indicate that utilization of supplementary folic acid by the cow's tissues was reduced in early lactation, folic acid being "trapped" in serum under its methylated form by a lack of vitamin B$_{12}$ as described previously. In fact, a lack of vitamin B$_{12}$ inhibits methionine and *S*-adenosylmethionine synthesis. The cell "reaction" is then to direct all one-carbon units available towards synthesis of 5-CH$_3$-THF. This reaction is irreversible and the demethylation is blocked by the lack of vitamin B$_{12}$. Purine and DNA synthesis are therefore deprived of one-carbon units, proliferation of rapidly dividing cells is slowed down and protein incorporation of methionine is reduced in favor of more urgent methylation functions. Moreover, accumulation of 5-CH$_3$-THF leads to a lack of folates at the cell level. This is the explanation of anaemia observed during severe folic acid and/or vitamin B$_{12}$ deficiencies (Bässler, 1997). In the present experiment, responses of blood haemoglobin and packed cell volume of primiparous cows to supplementary folic acid when serum concentrations of vitamin B$_{12}$ increased give an indication that in this case, vitamin B$_{12}$ status was low enough to "create a severe methyl trap" situation.

In the study on the interactions between folic acid and methionine, a similar fall in serum concentrations of vitamin B$_{12}$ appeared in early lactation (Figure 11.3a); serum concentrations were even lower than those observed in primiparous cows during the previous study. As previously observed, serum folates increased in early lactation in cows fed dietary supplements of folic acid and decreased thereafter (Figure 11.3b). Moreover, in early lactation, serum concentrations of homocysteine were similar for cows fed 0 or 6 mg of folic acid per kilogram body weight. However, as lactation progressed and vitamin B_{12} increased, serum concentrations of homocysteine stayed low in cows fed supplementary folic acid but increased steadily in control cows (Figure 11.3c; Girard, Lapierre, Matte and Lobley, unpublished data). In other species, high levels of homocysteine are a better indicator of folic acid and/or vitamin B_{12} deficiency than circulating concentrations of these vitamins (Hall and Chu, 1990; Ueland, Refsum, Stabler, Malinow, Andersson and Allen, 1993). The amount of homocysteine in plasma is the result of a cellular export mechanism that complements the catabolism of homocysteine (Selhub, 1999). Moreover, serum concentrations of homocysteine decrease in response to dietary supplementation of folic acid and vitamin B_{12} (Brönstrup, Hages, Prinz-Langenohl and Pietrzik, 1998). However, supplementary folic acid is more efficient in reducing serum levels of homocysteine than vitamin B_{12} (Mason and Miller, 1992). In the present case, it is difficult to interpret serum concentrations of homocysteine without any doubt as an indication of folic acid and vitamin B_{12} status because the normal range of concentrations of homocysteine in cow's serum is not defined. However, there was no effect of supplementary folic acid on serum homocysteine in early lactation when serum vitamin B_{12} was low. Later in lactation, when vitamin B_{12} increased, serum homocysteine increased in control cows but not in those fed supplementary folic acid. It could then be hypothesized that in dairy cows, in early lactation, low supply of vitamin B_{12} could interfere with the methylation of homocysteine to form methionine and folate utilization.

The effects of supplementary folic acid on lactational performance of dairy cows do not seem to be only due to an increased supply of methionine because its effects are not completely mimiced by addition of rumen-protected methionine to the dairy cow diet. Therefore, it is possible that the effects of supplementary folic acid were due to an increased supply in folate cofactors and one-carbon units available for purine and DNA synthesis when the supply in vitamin B_{12} was sufficient to allow for the full utilization of supplementary folic acid.

The case for vitamin B_{12} in dairy cows

Unlike other B-complex vitamins, vitamin B_{12} is not synthesized by plants, the vitamin is produced only by bacterial synthesis. As one atom of cobalt is part of the molecule, it is assumed that ruminant requirements for vitamin B_{12} are equal to ruminal bacteria requirements for cobalt. The fact that this vitamin can only result from bacterial synthesis also explains the presence of several molecules with a chemical structure close to that of vitamin B_{12} but without its biological activity. Those molecules are called "vitamin B_{12}

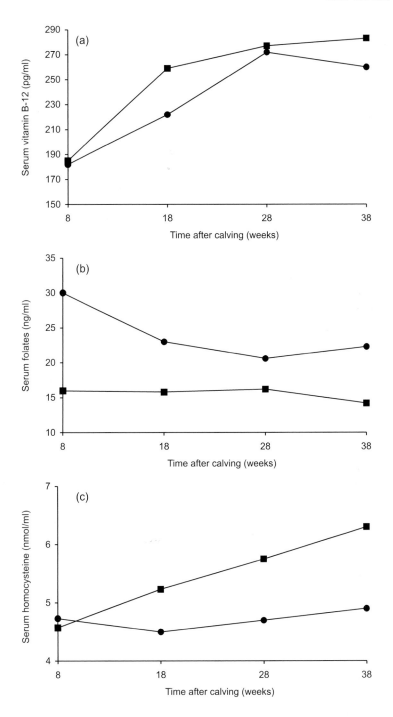

Figure 11.3 Changes in serum concentrations of a) vitamin B$_{12}$, b) folates and c) homocysteine in dairy cows fed 0 (■) or 6 mg (●) of folic acid per kilogram of body weight from 4 weeks before calving until 305 days of lactation (Girard, Lapierre, Matte and Lobley, unpublished data).

analogues, pseudo-vitamin B_{12} or vitamin B_{12}-like factors". They are probably intermediate molecules formed during vitamin B_{12} biosynthesis. They are present in substantial amounts in sewage, manure, ruminal contents and residues from fermentation (McDowell, 1989). Diet composition could change the ability of rumen microorganisms to synthesize the vitamin; high-concentrate diets stimulate synthesis by rumen microflora of vitamin B_{12} analogues at the expense of the biologically active forms of the vitamin (Walker and Elliot, 1972; Halpin, Harris, Caple and Peterson, 1984). Moreover, increasing concentrations of cobalt augments the *in vitro* ruminal production of vitamin B_{12} analogues (Kawashima, Henry, Bates, Ammerman, Littell and Price, 1997).

In dairy cows, only two enzymes are vitamin B_{12}-dependent. The first one is methionine synthase, essential to the transfer of a one-carbon unit from the methylated form of folic acid to an amino acid, homocysteine to form methionine. This reaction was described in the previous section. The second vitamin B_{12}-dependent enzyme is methylmalonyl-CoA mutase. This enzyme transforms methylmalonyl-CoA into succinyl-CoA which will enter the Krebs cycle. Methylmalonyl-CoA is the result of degradation of odd-chain fatty acids, some amino acids (valine, isoleucine, methionine, threonine) and propionate. In dairy cows, the role of the methylmalonyl-CoA mutase is very important in the metabolism of propionate (McDowell, 1989; Le Grusse and Watier, 1993).

The high-producing dairy cow requires a large supply of energy and glucose. Huge amounts of glucose are required by the lactating mammary gland to synthesize lactose, which is the primary osmotic controller of milk volume (Overton, 1998); a cow producing 40 kg of milk per day requires approximately 3 kg of glucose per day (Elliot, 1979). The nature of the ruminant digestive system imposes a huge dependence on gluconeogenesis, as very little glucose is absorbed. In ruminants, the rate of gluconeogenesis increases with feed intake, the opposite to the situation in monogastric animals (Hocquette and Bauchart, 1999), and the major substrates for gluconeogenesis are propionate, glucogenic amino acids and lactate. Lactate metabolism is tightly related to propionate metabolism because lactate is formed during catabolism of glucose by peripheral tissues or by degradation of propionate by the ruminal epithelium (Overton, 1998). The other major source of glucose is the gluconeogenic amino acids absorbed from the gastrointestinal tract. Additional amino acids for gluconeogenesis could be supplied by substantial degradation of skeletal muscle protein in early postpartum (Overton, 1998). However, taking into account the concomitant huge increase in requirements for amino acids for milk protein synthesis, a large proportion of glucose needs by the lactating cow is likely to be provided by propionate. Seal, Parker and Avery (1992) observed that 83% of propionate was transformed to glucose in steers, representing about 53% of the whole-body glucose.

The importance of propionate metabolism explains the higher ruminant requirements for vitamin B_{12} as compared with monogastric animals. Cattle are less sensitive to a lack of vitamin B_{12} than sheep (Kennedy, Young, Kennedy, Scott, Molloy, Weir and Price, 1995) but this study was conducted with steers from 6 to 22 months of age and no data for growth rate or feed intake were reported for these animals. However, it is likely that, even if these steers achieved a rapid growth rate, the metabolic demand for growth was largely inferior to that of high-producing dairy cow.

On one hand, high-concentrate diets stimulate synthesis of vitamin B_{12} analogues by rumen microflora at the expense of the biologically active forms of the vitamin (Walker and Elliot, 1972; Halpin *et al.*, 1984). On the other hand, these diets increase propionate production (Bauman, Davis and Bucholtz, 1971) also increasing the demand for vitamin B_{12} for conversion of propionate to succinate (McDowell, 1989). Moreover, low feed intake promotes synthesis of vitamin B_{12} analogues (Sutton and Elliot, 1972). Therefore, it is likely that, with high-concentrate diets, the production of vitamin B_{12} by rumen microflora is suboptimal to meet requirements of high-producing cows. This situation can be exacerbated in primiparous cows and in early lactation when feed intake is not optimal and high-concentrate diets fed in an attempt to fulfill energy requirements.

Most studies of the effects of vitamin B_{12} on dairy cow performance are in relation to a theory to explain the "low milk fat syndrome" observed in cows fed high-concentrate diets. According to this theory, methylmalonic acid might accumulate as a consequence of the increased propionate production and decreased vitamin B_{12} status due to high-concentrate diets. High concentrations of methylmalonic acid might inhibit fatty acid synthesis (Frobish and Davis, 1977). Unfortunately, subsequent studies failed to observe an increase in milk fat after supplementation in vitamin B_{12} (Croom, Rakes, Linnerud, Ducharme and Elliot, 1981; Elliot, Barton and Williams, 1979; Frobish and Davis, 1977). However, some of these studies reported a relation between an improvement of vitamin B_{12} status and an increased milk yield in early lactation (Elliot, 1979; Elliot, Barton and Williams, 1979).

Results from a preliminary study conducted on a small number of primiparous cows in early lactation seem to support the hypothesis that, in early lactation, the demand for vitamin B_{12} is not fulfilled. The primiparous cows were fed a diet identical to the one used in the previous experiment studying the interactions between folic acid and methionine; they also received dietary supplements of folic acid and rumen-protected methionine and weekly intramuscular injections of 0 or 10 mg of vitamin B_{12} (cyanocobalamin). Intramuscular injections of vitamin B_{12} increased, although not significantly, milk production (Figure 11.4); cows supplemented with vitamin B_{12} produced 2.5 kg/day more milk from 25 to 125 day of lactation, 28.4 vs 30.9 kg/day. Injections of vitamin B_{12} increased yields of milk solids by 12 % (3.4 vs 3.8 kg/day), milk fat by 16 % (847 vs 983 g/day) and milk non-fat solids by 12 % (2.5 vs 2.8 kg/day) (Girard and Matte, 1997).

Stangl, Schwarz and Kirchgessner (1999) observed in calves with a high growth rate that a moderately low cobalt intake reduced plasma vitamin B_{12} and induced many changes in lipid metabolism. They observed decreased phosphatidylcholine concentrations and phosphatidylcholine (PC):phosphatidylethanolamine (PE) ratio in liver as well as lipids in plasma very low density lipoproteins (VLDL). The decrease in the amounts of phospholipids in VLDL of moderately deficient calves is particularly marked. A

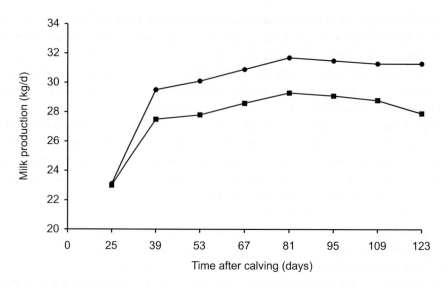

Figure 11.4   Milk production of primiparous cows given weekly intramuscular injections of 0 (■) or 10 mg (●) of vitamin B$_{12}$ from 25 to 125 days of lactation (after Girard and Matte, 1997)

decrease in the PC:PE ratio confirms a reduced methylation of phosphatidylethanolamine to phosphatidylcholine. Kennedy *et al.* (1995) found no effect of a cobalt-vitamin B$_{12}$ deficiency on liver concentrations of phosphatidylcholine and phosphatidylethanolamine, but the severity of the deficiency was difficult to assess because, although dietary concentrations of cobalt were reported, feed intake was not given nor growth rate.

Choline: its importance as a methyl donor

Choline is sometimes classified as a B-complex vitamin although it can be synthesized in the liver. Choline plays a role in the regulation of some metabolic processes but, unlike B-complex vitamins, it also functions as a structural constituent. As phosphatidylcholine, it is a structural constituent of membranes, sphyngomyelins and some plasmogens, it also promotes lipid transport. As acetylcholine, it is a neurotransmitter. Moreover, after its irreversible oxidation to betaine, it is a source of methyl groups (Combs, 1998).

   This latter function links choline to folate metabolism. During its degradation to betaine, choline can give a one-carbon unit for methylation of homocysteine to methionine (Figure 11.5). However, unlike the reaction of methylation of homocysteine described previously, which occurs in all tissues, this reaction does not require folates or vitamin B$_{12}$ and is confined mainly to the liver (Selhub, 1999). The reaction regenerates methionine but does not allow for demethylation of 5-CH$_3$-THF in THF. Both choline and methionine act as methyl donors. Both are very important in hepatic lipid metabolism due to their role in the provision of phosphatidycholine, essential to VLDL synthesis (Overton and Piepenbrink, 1999).

Dietary supplements of choline are extensively destroyed by rumen micro-organisms (Atkins, Erdman and Vandersall, 1988; Sharma and Erdman, 1988b). However, when given in relatively large amounts or infused in the abomasum, supplementary choline is frequently reported to increase milk fat content, milk fat yield as well as in some experiments, milk yield (Erdman, Shaver and Vandersall, 1984; Sharma and Erdman, 1989; Siciliano-Jones, Seymour, Nocek and English, 1990).

Dietary supply of both methionine and choline directly affects requirements for each other. Methionine can give methyl groups to ethanolamine to form choline whereas methyl groups provided by choline (and betaine) degradation can methylate homocysteine to methionine (Figure 11.5; McDowell, 1989). A decreased supply in folates and/or vitamin B_{12} alters methionine regeneration and increases choline requirements because a large proportion of choline is used for methionine production. The opposite is also true, an increased supply in methionine due to the diet or regeneration through the pathway involving 5-CH$_3$-THF and vitamin B_{12} decreases choline requirements. The link between methionine and choline requirements has been demonstrated in dairy cows (Sharma and Erdman, 1988a) although these authors also demonstrated that choline *per se* is also essential.

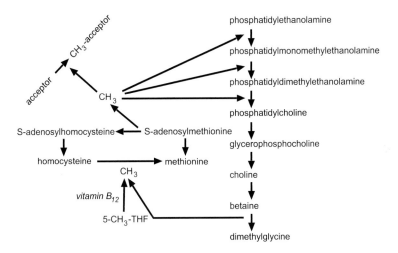

Figure 11.5 Relationships between metabolism of methionine, choline, folic acid and vitamin B_{12} (after Weil, 1972; McDowell, 1989; Selhub and Miller, 1992; Selhub, 1999)

Conclusion

The roles of folic acid and vitamin B_{12} in metabolism of high-producing cows are not yet clearly understood. Utilization of folic acid and vitamin B_{12} seems to be closely related to protein and energy metabolism, but a more in-depth investigation of the metabolic pathways involved is still to be conducted. Experimental data reported in the present paper give some indications that the supply in folic acid and vitamin B_{12} is not always optimal to maximise lactational performance of high-producing dairy cows. For multiparous dairy cows, when the supply in vitamin B_{12} is adequate, a daily dietary supplement of 2 to 4 mg of folic acid per kilogram body weight, to take account of destruction by the rumen microflora, could have a beneficial effect on milk production and composition. Nevertheless, other substances could interfere with folate utilization, such as vitamin B_{12}, or modify its requirement, such as choline and methionine.

Results reported in the present paper are only one example describing the impact of revised B-complex vitamin requirements on milk production and composition of high-producing dairy cows. The "best" diet for high-producing dairy cows should aim to establish an equilibrium among high milk production, good health and good reproductive performance. This diet should also decrease feeding costs by improving feed efficiency and reducing environmental wastes. To reach this equilibrium, it is essential to adjust precisely cow requirements and nutrient supply. While doing that, it is important not to neglect minor nutrients, such as B-complex vitamins because, even if given in small amounts, their impact on the major metabolic pathways could be huge.

The long-term goal in defining dairy cow requirements for B-complex vitamins involves identifying the amounts that, first, minimize deleterious processes associated with inadequate intake (the most dramatic ones already avoided by the amounts produced by the rumen microflora) and, second, optimize B-complex vitamin-dependent reactions in metabolism and cellular development. However, given that B-complex vitamins act generally as cofactors and/or coenzymes in metabolic reactions, determination of dairy cow requirements for maximal productivity is not easy because the need for each vitamin is largely influenced by the supply of major nutrients as well as other micronutrients.

References

Allen, R. H., Stabler, S. P. and Lindenbaum, J. (1993) Serum betaine, N, N-dimethylglycine and N-methylglycine levels in patients with cobalamin and folate deficiency and related inborn errors of metabolism. *Metabolism*, **42**, 1448-1460.

Arbeiter, V. K. and Winding, W. (1973) Folatbestimmungen im Serum von Rindern mit besonderem Bezug auf die Fruchtbarkeit. *Wienier Tierärztliche Monatsschrift*, **60**, 323-326.

Atkins, K. B., Erdman, R. A. and Vandersall, J. H. (1988) Dietary choline effects on milk yield and duodenal choline flow in dairy cattle. *Journal of Dairy Science*, **71**, 109-116.

Bailey, L. B. and J. F. Gregory (1999) Folate metabolism and requirements. *Journal of Nutrition*, **129**, 779-782.

Bässler, K. H. (1997) Enzymatic effects of folic acid and vitamin B_{12}. *International Journal of Vitamin and Nutrition Research*, **67**, 385-388.

Bauman, D. E., Davis, C. L. and Bucholtz, H. F. (1971) Propionate production in the rumen of cows fed either a control or high-grain, low-fiber diet. *Journal of Dairy Science*, **54**,1282-1287.

Bhandari, S. D. and Gregory, J. F. (1992) 5-methyl-tetrahydrofolate and 5-formyl-tetrahydrofolate exhibit equivalent absorption, metabolism and in vivo kinetics in rats. *Journal of Nutrition*, **122**,1847-1854.

Brönstrup, A., Hages, M., Prinz-Langenohl, R. and Pietrzik, K. (1998) Effects of folic acid and combinations of folic acid and vitamin B-12 on plasma homocysteine concentrations in healthy, young women. *American Journal of Clinical Nutrition*, **68**, 1104-1110.

Combs, G. F., jr. (1998) *The Vitamins. Fundamental Aspects In Nutrition And Health.* 2nd edition. Academic Press. San Diego.

Cooper, B. A. (1977) Physiology of absorption of monoglutamyl folates from the gastrointestinal tract. In *Folic Acid. Biochemistry and Physiology in Relation to the Human Nutrition Requirement*, pp 188-197. National Academy of Science. Washington, D.C.

Croom, W. J., jr., Rakes, A. H., Linnerud, A. C., Ducharme, G. A. and Elliot, J. M. (1981) Vitamin B_{12} administration for milk fat synthesis in lactating dairy cows fed a low fiber diet. *Journal of Dairy Science*, **64**, 1555-1560.

Elliot, J. M. (1979) Propionate metabolism and vitamin B_{12}. In *Digestive Physiology and Metabolism in Ruminants*, pp. 485-503. Edited by Y. Ruckebush and P. Thivend. AVI Publishing Co., Inc. Westport, Co.

Elliot, J. M., Barton, E. P. and Williams, J. A. (1979) Milk fat as related to vitamin B_{12} status. *Journal of Dairy Science*, **62**, 642-645.

Erdman, R. A., Shaver, R. D. and Vandersall, J. H. (1984) Dietary choline for the lactating cow: Possible effects on milk fat synthesis. *Journal of Dairy Science*, **67**, 410-415.

Frobish, R. A. and Davis, C. L. (1977) Theory involving propionate and vitamin B_{12} in the low-milk fat syndrome. *Journal of Dairy Science*, **60**, 268-273.

Girard, C. L. and Matte, J. J. (1995) Serum clearance and urinary excretion of pteroylmonoglutamic acid in gestating and lactating dairy cows. *British Journal of Nutrition*, **74**, 857-865.

Girard, C. L. and Matte, J. J. (1997) Parenteral supplements of vitamin B_{12} and milk performances of dairy cows. *Journal of Dairy Science*, **80** (Suppl.1), 240.

Girard, C. L. and Matte, J. J. (1998) Dietary supplements of folic acid during lactation: Effects on the performance of dairy cows. *Journal of Dairy Science*, **81**, 1412-1419.

Girard, C. L. and Matte, J. J. (1999) Changes in serum concentrations of folates, pyridoxal, pyridoxal-5-phosphate and vitamin B_{12} during lactation of dairy cows fed dietary supplements of folic acid. *Canadian Journal of Animal Science*, **79**, 107-113.

Girard, C. L., Matte, J. J. and Tremblay, G. F. (1989) Serum folates in gestating and lactating dairy cows. *Journal of Dairy Science*, **72**, 3240-3246.

Girard, C. L., Matte, J. J. and Lévesque, J. (1992) Responses of serum folates of preruminant and ruminant calves to a dietary supplement of folic acid. *Journal of Animal Science*, **70**, 2847-2851.

Girard, C. L., Matte, J. J. and Tremblay, G. F. (1995) Gestation and lactation of dairy cows: A role for folic acid? *Journal of Dairy Science*, **78**, 404-411.

Girard, C. L., Lapierre, H., Matte, J. J. and Lobley, G. E. (1998) Effects of dietary supplements of rumen-protected methionine and folic acid on lactational performance of dairy cows. *Journal of Dairy Science*, **81** (Suppl. 1), 295.

Hall, C. A. and Chu, R. C. (1990) Serum homocysteine in routine evaluation of potential vitamin B_{12} and folate deficiency. *European Journal of Haematology*, **45**, 143-149.

Halpin, C. G., Harris, D. J., Caple, I. W. and Peterson, D. S. (1984) Contribution of cobalamin analogues to plasma vitamin B_{12} concentrations in cattle. *Research in Veterinary Science*, **37**, 249-251.

Hocquette, J. F. and Bauchart, D. (1999) Intestinal absorption, blood transport and hepatic and muscle metabolism of fatty acids in preruminant and ruminant animals. *Reproduction Nutrition and Development*, **39**, 27-48.

Kawashima, T., Henry, P. R., Bates, D. G., Ammerman, C. B., Littell, R. C. and Price, J. (1997) Bioavailability of cobalt sources for ruminants. 3. In vitro ruminal production of vitamin B_{12} and total corrinoids in response to different cobalt sources and concentrations. *Nutrition Research*, **17**, 975-987.

Kennedy, D. G., Young, P. B., Kennedy, S., Scott, J. M., Molloy, A. M., Weir, D. G. and Price, J. (1995) Cobalt - vitamin B_{12} deficiency and the activity of methylmalonyl CoA mutase and methionine synthase in cattle. *International Journal of Vitamin and Nutrition Research*, **65**, 241-247.

Krebs, H. A., Hems, R. and Tyler, B. (1976) The regulation of folate and methionine metabolism. *Biochemical Journal*, **158**, 341-353.

Lefebvre, D., Allard, B., Block, E. and Sanchez, W. K. (1999) L'alimentation en période de transition: la clé d'une lactation profitable. In *23e Symposium sur les bovins laitiers, St-Hyacinthe, 21 octobre 1999*, pp 23-68. Conseil des productions animales du Québec inc.

Le Grusse, J. and Watier, B. (1993) *Les vitamines. Données biochimiques, nutritionnelles et cliniques*. Centre d'étude et d'information sur les vitamines. Neuilly-sur-Seine.

Mason, J. B. and Miller, J. W. (1992) The effects of vitamin B_{12}, B_6, and folate on blood homocysteine levels. In *Beyond deficiency*. Edited by H. E. Sauberlich and J. J. Machlin. Annals of the New York Academy of Sciences, **669**, 197-203.

McDowell, L. R. (1989) *Vitamins in Animal nutrition. Comparative Aspects to Human nutrition*. Academic Press, Inc. San Diego.

Overton, T. (1998) Substrate utilization for hepatic gluconeogenesis in the transition dairy cow In *Proceedings 1998 Cornell Nutrition Conference For Feed Manufacturers,* pp 237-246. Cornell University, Ithaca, NY.

Overton, T. R. and Piepenbrink, M. S. (1999) Liver metabolism and the transition cow

In *Proceedings 1999 Cornell Nutrition Conference for Feed Manufacturers,* pp.118-127. Cornell University, Ithaca, NY.

Rulquin, H., Pisulewski, P. M., Vérité, R. and Guinard, J. (1993) Milk production and composition as a function of postruminal lysine and methionine supply: a nutrient-response approach. *Livestock Production Science,* **37**, 69-90.

Schwabb, C. G., Bozak, C. K., Whitehouse, N. L. and Mesbah, M. M. A. (1992) Amino acid limitation and flow to duodenum at four stages of lactation. 1. Sequence of lysine and methionine limitation. *Journal of Dairy Science,* **75**, 3486-3502.

Scott, J. M. (1999) Folate and vitamin B_{12}. *Proceedings of the Nutrition Society,* **58**, 441-448.

Seal, C. J., Parker, D. S. and Avery, P. J. (1992) The effect of forage and forage-concentrate diets on rumen fermentation and metabolism of nutrients by the mesenteric- and portal-drained viscera in growing steers. *British Journal of Nutrition,* **67**, 355-370.

Selhub, J. (1999) Homocysteine metabolism. *Annual Reviews in Nutrition,* **19**, 217-246.

Selhub, J. and Miller, J. W. (1992) The pathogenesis of homocysteinemia: interruption of the coordinate regulation by *S*-adenosylmethionine of the remethylation and transsulfuration of homocysteine. *American Journal of Clinical Nutrition,* **55**, 131-138.

Sharma, B. K. and Erdman, R. A. (1988a) Abomasal infusion of choline and methionine with or without 2-amino-2-methyl-1-propanol for lactating dairy cows. *Journal of Dairy Science,* **71**, 2406-2411.

Sharma, B. K. and Erdman, R. A. (1988b) Effects of high amounts of dietary choline supplementation on duodenal choline flow and production responses of dairy cows. *Journal of Dairy Science,* **71**, 2670-2676.

Sharma, B. K. and Erdman, R. A. (1989) Effects of dietary and abomasally infused choline on milk production responses of lactating dairy cows. *Journal of Nutrition,* **119**, 248-254.

Siciliano-Jones, J., Seymour, W. M., Nocek, J. E. and English, J. E. (1990) Choline supplementation to first-calf heifers. *Journal of Dairy Science,* **73** (Suppl. 1), 167.

Stabler, S. P., Lindenbaum, J., Savage, D. G. and Allen, R. H. (1993) Elevation of serum cystathionine levels in patients with cobalamin and folate deficiency. *Blood,* **81**, 3404-3413.

Stangl, G. I., Schwarz, F. J. and Kirchgessner, M. (1999) Moderate long-term cobalt deficiency affects liver, brain and erythrocyte lipids and lipoproteins of cattle. *Nutrition Research,* **19**, 415-427.

Sutton, A. L. and Elliot, J. M. (1972) Effect of ratio of roughage to concentrate and level of feed intake on ovine ruminal vitamin B_{12} production. *Journal of Nutrition,* **102**, 1341-1346.

Tremblay, G. F., Girard, C. L., Bernier-Cardou, M. and Matte, J. J. (1991)

Nycterohemeral variations of concentration of serum folates in dairy cows. *Canadian Journal of Animal Science*, **71**, 919-923.

Ueland, P. M., Refsum, H., Stabler, S. P., Malinow, M. R., Andersson, A. and Allen, R. H. (1993) Total homocysteine in plasma or serum: Methods and clinical applications. *Clinical Chemistry*, **39**, 1764-1779.

Walker, C. K. and Elliot, J. M. (1972) Lactational trends in vitamin B_{12} status on conventional and restricted-roughage rations. *Journal of Dairy Science*, **55**, 474-479.

Weil, J. H. (1972) *Biochimie générale*. Masson et Cie, ed. Paris.

Zinn, R. A., Owens, F. N., Stuart, R. L., Dunbar, J. R. and Norman, B. B. (1987) B-vitamin supplementation of diets for feedlot calves. *Journal of Animal Science*, **65**, 267-277.

This paper was first published in 2000

12

NUTRITION OF THE HIGH GENETIC MERIT DAIRY COW – ENERGY METABOLISM STUDIES

R.E. AGNEW[1 2 3], T. YAN[1] and F.J. GORDON[1 2 3]
[1] *Agricultural Research Institute of Northern Ireland, Hillsborough, Co Down*
[2] *The Department of Agriculture for Northern Ireland*
[3] *The Queen's University of Belfast*

Introduction

The rate of genetic improvement in the dairy herd in the British Isles up to 1985 was relatively slow, approximately 0 to 0.005 per year. This is in contrast to that achieved during the same period in North America, where genetic merit for milk production increased by proportionately 0.015, equivalent to over 150 kg of milk, per year (Funk, 1993). More recently, however, there has been a marked increase in the rate of genetic improvement within the British Isles, with Coffey (1992) reporting current rates of genetic gain of proportionately 0.013 per year, in milk fat plus protein yield, for the indexed populations in the United Kingdom and Republic of Ireland. The increased rate of genetic progress can be attributed to relaxation of regulations which previously prevented importation of semen from North America and Europe, coupled with advances in progeny testing schemes and the introduction of advanced statistical techniques to evaluate progeny test data from different countries. As these trends continue there is a need to understand how they will influence the nutritional requirements of dairy cows. In addition, feed rationing systems must be appropriate for the high levels of performance that can now be achieved. The objective of this paper is to review the implications of increasing genetic merit and reassess the present energy feeding standards.

Genetic merit and its implications

ASSESSING GENETIC MERIT

The current system used to assess genetic merit of dairy cattle in the British Isles is the Individual Animal Model (IAM). Through this a genetic index is produced that is a measure of an animal's ability to transmit its genes to the next generation. Thus a genetic index is not a measure of a physical trait, such as milk production, but a reflection of the animal's genotype (genetic make up) and hence makes an estimate of its ability to transmit genes by discounting the effects of management regimes and other environmental factors.

As indicated earlier rapid increases have occurred in the genetic merit of the Holstein-Friesian cow population since the mid 1980s. The data presented in Figure 12.1 (M. Coffey, personal communication) illustrate the increases in Predicted Transmitting Ability (PTA_{95}) for female calves registered with the Holstein Friesian Society over the period 1989—1995. A marked increase in PTA_{95} values has occurred, with the current rate of increase in PTA_{95} fat + protein values being approximately 4.5 kg per year. Assuming milk of standard composition, this suggests that genetic merit for milk yield is increasing by approximately 62 litres/lactation per year.

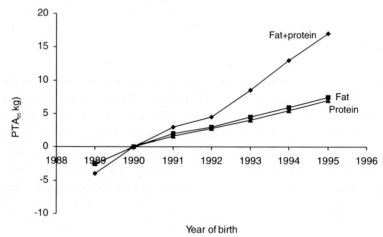

Figure 12.1 Trends in pedigree index PTA_{95} (kg) of UK Holstein-Friesian females born 1989-1995 (M. Coffey, personal communication)

Whilst the data in Figure 12.1 represent the average genetic merit of the registered Holstein Friesian population, there are many animals with very much higher values than those presented. For example, the highest genetic index heifer registered up to September 1997 had PTA_{95} values of + 1087 kg milk, + 36.8 kg butterfat and + 36.6 kg protein, and a Profit Index (PIN_{95}) value of £137. This compares with the average PIN_{95} value of £40 for all calves registered during the same period. At the present time there is no indication that the rate of genetic progress will slow down in the foreseeable future. However, genetic merit is only a measure of the animal's ability to transmit its genes to the next generation and the actual production of the animal will depend not only on the genotype but also the nutrition and management which the animal receives.

IMPACT OF GENETIC MERIT ON BIOLOGICAL EFFICIENCY

The impact of large differences in genetic merit on biological efficiency have been assessed in recent studies at Hillsborough. In the first study (Gordon, Patterson, Yan, Porter, Mayne and Unsworth, 1995a) a grass silage based diet was offered to cows of three differing genetic merits over a 150-day feeding period. In the second study (Ferris, Gordon, Patterson, Mayne and Kilpatrick, 1998a and Ferris, Gordon, Patterson and Porter, 1998b) animals of two genetic merits were offered similar complete diets for an 84-day period. The data presented in Table 12.1 indicate consistent increases in overall efficiency of conversion of feed metabolizable energy (ME) to milk energy output as cow genetic merit is increased, with proportionately 0.250 and 0.125 increases in efficiency being obtained in studies 1 and 2 respectively. However, results of detailed digestibility, metabolizability and energy exchange measurements undertaken on a proportion of the cows in these studies indicated that genetic merit had no effect on the digestibility or metabolizability of energy. Furthermore it did not influence the efficiency with which ME potentially available for milk was converted into milk energy output (adjusted to zero tissue change), (k_l), assuming ME requirement for maintenance (ME_m) is as given by AFRC (1990). These data therefore support the view that whilst increasing genetic merit improves overall efficiency of ME use for milk production, it does not alter the individual components of energy digestion and utilization. Hence, given the relatively small increases that occur in food intake as genetic merit increases, the increased milk production in high-merit animals is largely attributable to changes in the partitioning of nutrients between milk output and tissue gain. Consequently, on a given feeding regime, high-merit animals will sustain higher levels of milk production partly by increased mobilization of body reserves and/or reduced rates of tissue deposition (Table 12.1).

Table 12.1 EFFECT OF DAIRY COW GENETIC MERIT ON ANIMAL PERFORMANCE AND GROSS (MILK ENERGY OUTPUT/ME INTAKE) AND PARTIAL (k_L) ENERGETIC EFFICIENCY OF MILK PRODUCTION

	Genetic Merit[a]	DM intake (kg/d)	Milk yield (kg/d)	Energy Digest- ibility	ME/GE	Gross energetic efficiency	k_l^b	Condition score change
Gordon *et al.* (1995a)	45	20.2	37.2	0.77	0.67	0.45	0.58	-0.18
	15	19.4	30.6	0.76	0.67	0.40	0.58	0.54
	5	19.0	29.0	0.78	0.68	0.36	0.59	0.52
Ferris *et al.* (1998a and b)	53	21.4	37.0	0.79	0.68	0.45	0.55	-0.03
	11	20.2	33.0	0.79	0.67	0.40	0.52	0.23

[a] PTA_{90} fat + protein (kg)
[b] k_l was calculated using the equation of AFRC (1990) to predict ME_m

This highlights one of the key issues which arises in the feeding of high genetic merit cows, namely that the small responses in food intake associated with increasing genetic merit will not support the increased nutrient demands of lactation. As a consequence the long term production, health and welfare implications associated with a potential loss of body condition obviously presents a major challenge in dairying systems. This could be particularly important in systems with a high reliance on either grazed or conserved grass.

HORMONAL CONTROL OF MILK PRODUCTION

The metabolic status of the high yielding dairy cow was studied by Bauman and Currie (1980). They examined the relationship between energy intake and requirements for lactation in high yielding cows (average 9534 kg milk in a 305 d lactation). As expected, they found that peak milk yield preceded maximum dietary intake by several weeks and throughout the first third of lactation the cows were in negative energy balance and mobilizing body tissue. In fact the cows did not consume sufficient energy to meet their daily requirements until approximately the 16th week of lactation, when milk yield had fallen to less than 0.80 of peak production. These workers highlighted this aspect by calculating that during the first month of lactation the energetic equivalent to 0.33 of total milk output was produced by mobilizing body reserves. These data indicate that at peak lactation, and for several weeks thereafter, the metabolism of the high yielding dairy cow is directed towards satisfying the considerable demands of the udder. During this period changes occur in most areas of intermediary metabolism and all these changes are, to a greater or lesser extent, coordinated and integrated by the cow's endocrine system.

To consider this integration in terms of the individual hormones is an over simplification. Hormonal control is a function of several processes including the concentration of hormones in the body and the number and affinity of hormone receptors; both of these processes may themselves be hormonally regulated. Furthermore, certain hormones can play both catabolic and anabolic roles (e.g. growth hormone, glucocorticoids and thyroid hormones) depending upon the metabolic status of the animal and the process considered. Figure 12.2 (from Bines and Hart, 1986) is a diagrammatic summary, derived from ruminant and non ruminant data, of the hormones most likely to be concerned with three important aspects of supplying the mammary gland with nutrients i.e. (i) mobilizing body fat and protein reserves; (ii) increasing the rate of gluconeogenesis, particularly in the liver; and (iii) diverting the products of digestion and intermediary metabolism away from tissue deposition thus making them available for milk synthesis. From both a hormonal and metabolic standpoint these processes are interdependent.

Mechanisms have been established (Bines and Hart, 1986) by which a satisfactory supply of metabolites is available for milk synthesis. The partition between the mammary gland and body tissue is governed, to a considerable extent, by the influence of insulin relative to that of those hormones which chronically inhibit aspects of tissue deposition, notably growth hormone, glucagon and glucocorticoids. Although there may be differences

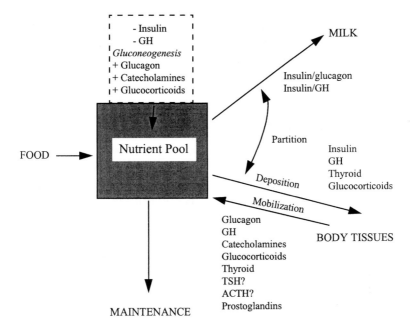

Figure 12.2 Hormones probably involved in lactation control (from Bines and Hart, 1986)

in emphasis, to comply with the ruminant mode of digestion and intermediary metabolism (Bauman, 1976; Bassett, 1981), insulin exerts the same anabolic actions in ruminants as in non ruminants, i.e. it stimulates the incorporation of glucose, amino acids and fatty acids into body tissue.

It has been known for some years that treatment of lactating cows with insulin causes an immediate reduction in milk yield that can be reversed by infusing glucose (Kronfield, Mayer, Robertson, and Raggi, 1963). Comparison of circulating insulin levels in high and low yielding cattle (Hart, Bines, Morant and Ridley, 1978; Hart, Bines and Morant, 1979; Hart, 1983) revealed that during lactation the concentration of this hormone was significantly higher in the plasma of low yielding cows, that were in energy surplus and gaining body weight, than in high yielding animals that were in energy deficit and losing weight during the early part of lactation. The difference in insulin concentration disappeared when the animals stopped lactating.

The foregoing evidence suggests that when high yielding cows are in energy deficit insulin secretion is suppressed, thus reducing the removal of metabolites by body tissues and increasing the rates of gluconeogenesis, lipolysis and proteolysis. This contention is supported by the results of a study carried out by Hart (1983) in which high and low yielding cows were fed to give similar changes in live weight. Under these same metabolic conditions the differences in insulin response were no longer apparent. However, attempts to manipulate energy metabolism by changing insulin secretion are less likely to be successful than attempts to vary growth hormone. The wide ranging effects of this latter hormone on protein, carbohydrate, fat and mineral metabolism have been set out by Machlin (1976). It was proposed by Raben (1973) that the primary metabolic role of growth hormone is to preserve body protein, particularly during periods of energy deficit, by inhibiting proteolysis and stimulating the incorporation of amino acids into muscle, whilst diverting glucose and fatty acids away from tissue deposition thus making them available as sources of energy. It therefore seems likely that growth hormone plays an important role in partitioning nutrients away from tissue deposition towards milk production. This view is supported by several facts (i) plasma growth hormone is higher in high than in low yielding cows (Sartin, Kemppainen, Cummins and Williams, 1988) and this difference is not evident when the cows are in similar metabolic states (Hart, 1983; Hart *et al.*, 1978; Hart, Bines, Balch and Cowie, 1975); (ii) changes in growth hormone are positively correlated with changes in milk yield (Hart *et al.*, 1979), and (iii) treatment with growth hormone appears to increase the efficiency with which cows convert food into milk (Machlin, 1973; Bines, Hart and Morant, 1980).

The cow's diet mainly consists of carbohydrates, proteins and fats containing approximately 17, 24 and 40 MJ gross energy per kg respectively. These components undergo anaerobic fermentation in the rumen resulting in the formation of volatile fatty acids (VFA; mainly acetic, propionic and butyric acid), microbial and ammonia N, some microbial lipid, methane, CO_2 and fermentation heat. This fermentation process supplies the microbes with energy in the form of ATP required for their maintenance and growth. The major part of this ATP comes from the conversion of carbohydrates to VFA with the yield of ATP being 3.5—4.5 moles per mole of glucose fermented. Since fermentation of amino acids yields considerably less ATP than the fermentation of a similar amount of energy as glucose, fermented dietary protein contributes little ATP.

Appropriate feeding of these high producing animals can only be achieved if:

(a)   accurate information is available on the cow's requirements for nutrients (energy and protein) for various body processes, such as maintenance, milk production, liveweight gain etc.

(b)   information is available on the extent of, and variation in, the partitioning of nutrients between milk output and body tissue gain, and

(c)   diets can be accurately characterized in relation to the contribution that they can make to meeting requirements and influencing nutrient partitioning.

This paper addresses the first two of these issues in relation to energy.

Within the United Kingdom, the amount of dietary energy required to support the maintenance and productive demands of ruminant livestock is estimated in terms of metabolizable energy (ME), with diets being formulated to meet these requirements according to the ME content of the individual components. The ME rather than Net Energy system is therefore the baseline for this chapter.

Energy requirements

Feed energy use by the dairy cow is represented schematically in Figure 12.3. Whilst there is considerable debate about the simplistic approach of attributing energy requirements into specific components (e.g. ME_m, k_l), in reality there is no more useful approach to formulating diets. The key components therefore necessary in ration formulation are the maintenance requirement (ME_m) and the efficiencies with which the remaining energy is converted to milk energy (k_l) or body gain (k_g).

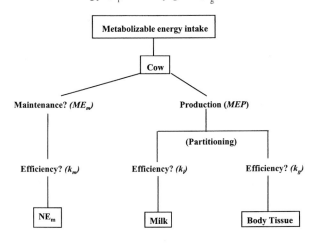

Figure 12.3 Schematic representation of dietary ME use in the dairy cow

HIGHLIGHTING PRESENT PROBLEMS

The estimates of ME_m, k_l and k_g used in today's ME feed rationing systems (AFRC, 1990 and 1993) were based on classical energy metabolism studies undertaken 30—50 years ago using very different animals and diets to those in use today. However there is an increasing body of evidence to suggest that total energy requirements derived by this factorial route are not relevant to many of the situations which presently exist. An example of this was the recent conflict which arose when scientists adopted the actual ME values for grass silages, determined *in vivo,* and found that realistic feeding options were not obtained. It was necessary to reduce k_l in order to produce more practical feed rationing predictions.

However, there is other much more substantiated evidence of this problem. Recent data have been presented from a number of calorimetric studies on lactating cows undertaken in the UK, which have highlighted the major differences between actual and predicted (AFRC, 1990) performances. For example the data given in Table 12.2 are taken from 4 recently published studies from two centres. From these data it can be

Table 12.2 A COMPARISON OF OBSERVED AND PREDICTED (AFRC, 1990) PERFORMANCE FROM DAIRY CATTLE IN RECENT CALORIMETRIC STUDIES

References	Forages (forage/diet)	ME/GE	ME intake (MJ/d) Observed	Predicted	Difference MJ/d	Prop
Beever *et al.*(1997)	Maize silage (0.60)	0.593	239	220	20	0.082
Ferris *et al.*(1998b)	Grass silage (0.46)	0.676	238	203	35	0.147
Sutton *et al.*(1997)	Crop wheat (0.61)	0.565	207	190	17	0.082
Yan *et al.*(1996)	Grass silage (0.61)	0.634	176	150	26	0.173
Mean		0.617	215	191	25	0.121

seen that adopting the present ME system of ME_m, k_l and k_g (AFRC, 1990) considerably underestimates the total ME requirement of dairy cows in today's environment, mean underestimation of 25 MJ/d (range 17-35). This effect can be further demonstrated through a more comprehensive examination of all the data from published calorimetric studies from around the world over the last 30 years. The sources of these data are given in Table 12.3. Figure 12.4 presents the results from these 31 calorimetric studies by setting predicted ME requirements for the level of performance achieved in the studies (AFRC, 1990) against the actual observed ME intakes. As all but five of the 31 studies fall on, or below, the $y = x$ line this again highlights the major degree of underprediction by AFRC (1990). A summary of this degree of underprediction is presented in Table 12.3 and shows AFRC (1990) to underpredict requirements by approximately 10 MJ/d (s.d. 11.6) from a mean of more than 1200 dairy-cow calorimetric measurements.

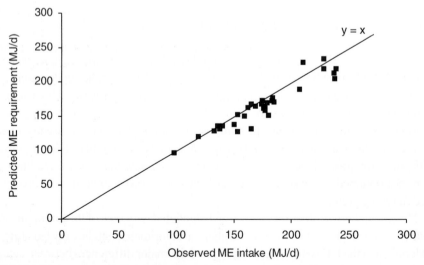

Figure 12.4 The relationship between observed ME intake and predicted ME requirement (AFRC, 1990) using calorimetric data (n=31) published since 1969

Table 12.3 CALORIMETRIC DATA PUBLISHED SINCE 1969

References	Forages	No.	ME (MJ/d) Obs.[a]	Pred.[b]	Obs.-Pred. (MJ/d)
Beever *et al.*, 1997	Maize silage	32	239	220	20
Ferris *et al.*, 1998b	Grass silage	24	238	203	35
Sutton *et al.*, 1997	Whole crop wheat	16	207	190	17
Carrick *et al.*, 1996	Grass silage	48	237	213	24
Cushnahan *et al.*, 1995	Grass silage	36	165	132	33
Birkelo *et al.*, 1994	Maize silage/alfalfa hay	36	228	234	-7
Hayasaka *et al.*, 1995					
Early lactation	Grass hay/silage	39	228	220	8
Mid-late lactation	Grass hay/silage	14	159	151	8
Terada & Muraoka, 1994	Alfalfa/grass hay	32	162	163	-1
Gädeken *et al.*, 1991	Dried grass	23	136	136	0
Münger, 1991					
Holst./Friesian	Maize silage/grass	49	177	165	12
Jersey	Maize silage/grass	50	133	129	4
Simmental	Maize silage/grass	50	169	165	4
Sutter *et al.*, 1991	Roughage	20	176	162	14
Sutton *et al.*, 1991	Grass silage	48	184	177	7
Unsworth, 1991	Grass silage	108	177	159	18
Windisch *et al.*, 1991	Maize silage/hay	60	140	136	3
Kirchgeßner *et al.*, 1989	Maize silage/hay	32	138	132	6
Jilg *et al.*, 1987	Grass hay	20	183	173	10
Tyrrell & Varga, 1987	Maize/alfalfa silage	47	185	171	13
Janicki *et al.*, 1985	Maize/grass silage	102	210	229	-19
Kirchgeßner *et al.*, 1982	Grass hay		165	168	-3
Tyrrell *et al.*, 1982	Maize silage	12	179	170	9
Tyrrell & Moe, 1980	Alfalfa hay/maize silage	36	175	173	2
Patle & Mudgal, 1977	Oat silage/grass hay	24	119	121	-2
Van Es & Van der Honing, 1976	Fresh grass	36	174	168	6
Tyrrell & Moe, 1972	Maize silage	46	153	153	0
Flatt *et al.*, 1969a	Alfalfa hay	72	150	138	12
Flatt *et al.*, 1969b	Purified food	42	98	97	1
Keady, personal comm.	Grass silage	18	180	152	28
Mayne, personal comm.	Grass silage	12	164	128	25
Mean		40	175	165	10
s.d.		23.2	35.2	33.7	11.6

[a]   Obs. - Observed ME intake
[b]   Pred. - Predicted ME requirement using the equations of AFRC (1990)

Whilst calorimetric studies provide accurate measurements on animals under controlled conditions, it is not known whether the discrepancies discussed above are carried through into the practical environment. To examine this, it is necessary to determine the ME (or DE) concentration of the experimental diet using cows in calorimeters and to record individual animal intake and performance data over periods of reasonable length. A total of 637 such individual-animal data are available from a series of production studies, with a minimum feeding period of 8 weeks, from the Agricultural Research Institute of Northern Ireland (Ferris, Gordon, Patterson, Mayne and McCoy, 1997; Ferris *et al.*, 1998a; C. P. Ferris, personal communication; Gordon *et al.*, 1995a; Keady, Mayne and Marsden, 1997 and 1998; Patterson, Yan and Gordon, 1996). The live-weight gain of the cows was obtained by linear regression of live weight against time (weeks). These data have been used to predict ME requirements for the performance achieved (AFRC, 1990) and compared with the actual levels of ME intake achieved. The results of this analysis are shown in Figure 12.5 along with the $y = x$ line. Again this figure demonstrates that proportionately 0.79 of the data points fall below the $y = x$ line indicating considerable underprediction. A summary of the mean data and the deviations between predicted and actual ME intakes are given in Table 12.4 and show a mean underprediction of 19 MJ/d (s.d. 28.2). These performance data support the evidence from the calorimetric studies that ME intakes predicted for animals achieving a given level of performance using AFRC (1990) are considerably below those necessary to meet that level of performance.

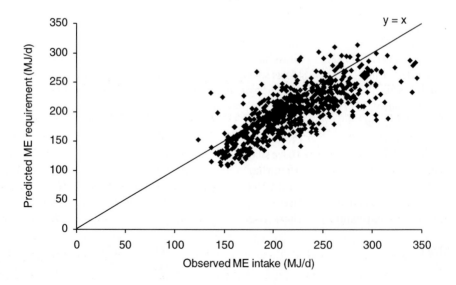

Figure 12.5 The relationship between observed ME intake and predicted ME requirement (AFRC, 1990) using data (n=637) from long term production studies at Hillsborough

Table 12.4 A COMBINATION OF CALORIMETRIC AND PRODUCTION STUDIES - OBSERVED VERSUS PREDICTED (AFRC, 1990) PERFORMANCE FROM DAIRY CATTLE

	ME intake (MJ/d)				Difference			
Source (No)	*Observed*		*Predicted*		*MJ/d*		*Proportion*	
	Mean	*s.d.*	*Mean*	*s.d.*	*Mean*	*s.d.*	*Mean*	*s.d.*
Calorimetry (>1200)	175	35.2	165	33.7	10	11.6	0.061	0.061
Production (637)	221	41.1	202	40.7	19	28.2	0.080	0.126

In the light of this evidence there is a need to reconsider the whole question of energy requirements for lactating cows. While it could be argued that some improvement could be pragmatically achieved by increasing the overall AFRC (1990) requirements by a proportion of around 0.05, as in AFRC (1993), this approach is extremely simplistic and does not identify which component of the factorial estimates of requirements is in error. Instead, it assumes that all components are equally in error. It has also been argued that it is counterproductive to debate whether the errors lie in the estimates of ME_m or k_l or k_g. Such debate fails to recognize that diets must be formulated for cows across an ever increasing range of milk outputs and whether the error lies in ME_m or k_l therefore has major implications for feeding animals at extremes of the production scale. For these reasons, it is important that a more accurate factorial approach to providing estimates of requirements is developed. Only when this is achieved can the whole question of safety margins to minimize the proportion of animals which are underfed in a given situation be logically addressed.

METABOLIZABLE ENERGY REQUIREMENT FOR MAINTENANCE

The classical studies used to develop the present maintenance energy requirements adopted for dairy and beef cattle were based on measuring the fasting metabolism of non-lactating cattle (mainly steers). For example ARC (1980) used this type of data to develop an equation to calculate the Net Energy (NE) requirement for maintenance (NE_m) of dairy cattle. The ME_m is calculated from NE_m using the efficiency of utilization of ME for maintenance (k_m), which is related to the metabolizability (q) of the diet for dairy cattle. This approach was adopted again in the more recent review by AFRC (1990), which suggested an ME_m of 0.48 MJ/kg$^{0.75}$ for an adult Holstein-Friesian cow given a diet with a metabolizability of 0.65. This represents today's accepted ME_m of 58 MJ/d for a 600 kg dairy cow given a diet with a q of 0.65. However, a series of fasting metabolism studies carried out recently at Hillsborough, using forage-based diets, offered at near-*ad libitum* prior to fasting, and currently available dairy cow genotypes, indicated a mean ME_m of 0.62 MJ/kg$^{0.75}$ (Yan, Gordon, Ferris, Agnew, Porter and Patterson,

1997b) representing a ME_m of 75 MJ/d for a 600 kg cow given a diet with a q of 0.65. This is some 0.29 above the figure widely used today. However, in both these studies (ARC, 1980; Yan *et al.*, 1997b), energy metabolism of animals was measured after 4 - 5 days fasting (post-absorptive state) and this inevitably means non-lactating animals. In addition, concerns have been expressed about the validity of measuring metabolism following fasting and it has been suggested that such studies should be undertaken with animals receiving one third of their energy requirement for maintenance (Chowdhury and Ørskov, 1994).

An alternative approach for determining ME_m is to use regression methods on large data sets to relate ME intake to milk energy output adjusted to zero body energy change. Between 1992 and 1995 a number of experiments were carried out at the Agricultural Research Institute of Northern Ireland in which lactating dairy cows (n = 221) were offered diets based on grass silage and subjected to gaseous exchange measurements in indirect open-circuit respiration calorimeters. Each animal in these studies was subjected to a 6-day diet digestibility and nitrogen (N) balance study prior to being transferred to the calorimeters (Carrick, Patterson, Gordon and Mayne 1996; Cushnahan, Mayne and Unsworth, 1995; Ferris *et al.*, 1998b; Gordon *et al.*, 1995a; Gordon, Porter, Mayne, Unsworth and Kilpatrick, 1995b; Gordon, personal communication; Yan, Patterson, Gordon and Porter, 1996; C.S. Mayne, personal communication). The cows remained in the calorimeters for 3 days with measurements of gaseous exchange being made over the final 48 h period. All equipment, procedures, analytical methods and calculations used in the calorimetric studies were described by Gordon *et al.* (1995b). The animals were at a range of lactation stages and of varied genetic merit. The mean values, and standard deviations (s.d.), for lactation number, milk yield, days of pregnancy and live weight of the animals during the calorimetric measurements, are presented in Table 12.5, together with data on the composition of the feeds used. A total of 21 perennial ryegrass silages were offered and these were spread over primary growth and first and second regrowth. All silages were well preserved. Thirty six of the 221 cows were offered silage as the sole diet, but in all other experiments the cows (n=185) were offered silages with proportions of concentrate ranging from 0.18 to 0.70. The concentrate portion of the diet was offered either in a complete diet (mixed with the grass silage), or as a separate feed from the silage. All cows were offered either silage or the complete diet *ad libitum*.

With pregnant cows the ME required for pregnancy was subtracted from the ME intake (AFRC, 1990). The milk energy output adjusted to zero energy balance ($E_{l(0)}$) was calculated from milk energy output (E_l) plus positive energy balance (E_g) or E_l minus 0.84 x negative E_g (AFRC, 1990). Using varying combinations of these data the ME_m and k_l were estimated using the following range of regression techniques.

Table 12.5 DATA ON ANIMAL, FEED AND ENERGY UTILIZATION (n = 221) FOR ANIMALS USED IN REGRESSION ANALYSIS (FROM YAN *et al.,* 1997a)

	Minimum	*Maximum*	*Mean*	*s.d.*
Cows				
Milk yield (kg/d)	3.2	49.1	23.7	8.25
Live weight (kg)	385	733	573	61.4
Days of pregnancy	0	138	13	26.5
Lactation No.	1	9	3.2	1.72
Silage composition				
Dry matter (g/kg)	168	398	226	60.8
pH	3.60	4.19	3.86	0.176
NH_3-N/Total-N (g/kg)	44	120	79	18.5
Crude protein (g/kg DM)	106	193	146	26.5
Gross energy (MJ/kg DM)	17.8	20.0	18.7	0.56
Ash (g/kg DM)	66	105	85	11.0
Acid detergent fibre (g/kg DM)	301	435	357	35.5
Energy utilization				
Gross energy intake (MJ/d)	137.3	460.3	316.1	65.43
Energy output (MJ/d)				
Faeces	25.6	133.3	75.8	18.52
Urine	5.1	27.6	13.5	4.02
Methane	7.6	29.9	21.0	3.83
Heat production	79.5	182.8	125.1	20.84
Milk	11.1	141.2	76.0	26.39
Energy retained (MJ/d)	-88.2	70.6	4.6	25.54

$$E_{l(0)} = a\ MEI + b \tag{1}$$
$$E_{l(0)} = a\ MEI + b\ (q - 0.65) + c \qquad \textit{(Van Es et al., 1970)} \tag{2}$$
$$E_{l(0)} = P_3\ [1 - \exp\ (-P_1\ (MEI - P_2))] \qquad \textit{(Cammell et al., 1986)} \tag{3}$$
$$MEI = a\ MW + b\ E_l + c\ (+E_g) + d\ (-E_g) \qquad \textit{(Moe et al., 1970)} \tag{4}$$
$$E_{l(0)} = a\ ME_p + b \tag{5}$$

Where MW, $(+E_g)$ and $(-E_g)$ are respectively metabolic liveweight, positive E_g and negative E_g, MEI is ME intake, and ME_p is energy available for production (ME_p = MEI - ME_m). The value of 0.65 in equation (2) was the mean q of the diets for the 221 cows. Equation (2) (Van Es, Nijkamp and Vogt, 1970) is intended to eliminate the effect of q. Equation (3) was developed by Cammell, Thomson, Beever, Haines, Dhanoa and Spooner (1986), in which the P_2 is taken as ME_m. Equation (4) (Moe, Tyrrell and Flatt, 1970) divides energy balance into two components, positive and negative.

The linear and multiple regression equations developed using these techniques, and the derived estimates of the ME_m and k_l are presented in Table 12.6 (from Yan, Gordon, Agnew, Porter and Patterson, 1997a). For all equations the proportion of variation accounted for by the variables is very high, ranging from 0.87 to 0.90, and all relationships are highly significant (P<0.001). Using the linear regression equation (Equation 1) developed from these data as an example of the methodology indicates estimates of ME_m of 0.67 MJ/kg$^{0.75}$ and k_l of 0.65. This relationship is shown diagrammatically in Figure 12.6 (from Yan *et al.*, 1997a).

Table 12.6 THE LINEAR AND MULTIPLE REGRESSION EQUATIONS, AND THE DERIVED ME REQUIREMENT FOR MAINTENANCE (ME_M) AND THE EFFICIENCY OF ME UTILIZATION FOR LACTATION (K_L) OBTAINED FROM STUDIES AT HILLSBOROUGH (n = 221) (FROM YAN *et al.*, 1997a)

Equations		R^2	ME_m MJ/kg$^{0.75}$	k_l	
$E_{l(0)} = 0.65\, MEI - 0.435$		0.90	0.67	0.65	(1)
$E_{l(0)} = 0.61\, MEI + 0.93 \times (q_m - 0.65) - 0.372$		0.90	0.61	0.61	(2)
$E_{l(0)} = -6.94\,[1 - EXP\,(-(-0.088)\,(MEI - 0.66))]$		0.89	0.66		(3)
$MEI = 0.75\, MW + 1.48\, E_l + 1.11\, (+E_g) + 1.08\, (-E_g)$		0.92	0.75	0.68	(4)
$E_{l(0)} = 0.65\, ME_p$		0.88		0.65	(5)

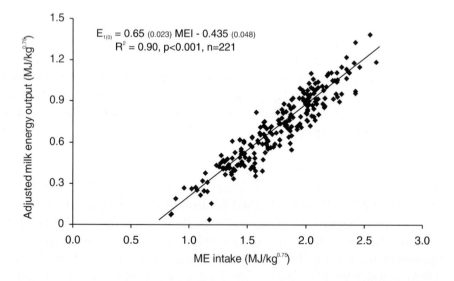

Figure 12.6 The relationship between ME intake and milk energy output adjusted to zero energy balance using calorimetric data of lactating dairy cows at Hillsborough

The mean ME_m derived from the range of regression techniques adopted was 0.67 MJ/ $kg^{0.75}$. This is relatively close to that obtained in the fasting metabolism studies reported earlier (0.62) but is again considerably higher than that widely used across the industry at present. This high ME_m value obtained in the Hillsborough calorimetric studies could reflect a number of issues. It is probable that the lactating cows in the present study had higher metabolic rates than the steers and dry cows used by ARC (1980) to establish the equations from which ME_m is calculated. The cows in the present study were lactating, often at high levels, and always offered diets *ad libitum*, whereas the steers and dry cows used by ARC (1980) were offered diets at maintenance levels, or at low planes of nutrition prior to fasting. In a comparison of ME_m for lactating and non lactating dairy cows, Moe *et al.*, (1970) statistically analysed the energy metabolism data obtained in their laboratory using multiple regression of MEI against metabolic live weight, milk energy output and energy balance, and reported that the ME_m for the lactating dairy cow (n=350) was proportionately 0.21 higher than that for the dry dairy cow (n=193). In addition, with fasting-metabolism studies, plane of nutrition offered to cattle before fasting has been reported to influence fasting metabolism and hence ME_m. For example, Birkelo, Johnson and Phetteplace (1991), in a study over 5 seasons, recorded proportionately 0.07 and 0.14 higher fasting heat production and ME_m respectively for steers offered diets at 2.27 rather than 1.20 x maintenance level prior to fasting. Similar results have been reported by Marston (1948) and Thorbek and Henkel (1976).

The high proportions of grass silage offered in the present study could be a further reason for the high estimated ME_m value. Grass silage varied from 0.18 to 1.00 of the total diets. To examine the influence of silage proportion on ME_m the present data set was divided into three, according to silage GE intake as a proportion of total GE intake (<0.50, 0.51—0.99 and 1.00). The linear regressions of $E_{l(0)}$ against MEI within each of these three categories are given in Table 12.7 along with the derived estimates of ME_m and k_l. These data indicate that the ME_m values significantly increase with increasing proportion of silage in the diet. This positive relationship could reflect an increased oxygen consumption attributable to the larger gastrointestinal tract normally associated with silage-based diets. It is therefore possible that much greater allowances should be made for dietary influences on ME_m, particularly the nature of the energy substrates within the diet.

The data from Hillsborough suggesting higher ME_m values than those adopted by AFRC (1990 and 1993) are supported by linear regression of the mean data from the 26 non-Hillsborough calorimetric studies reported since 1969 (Table 12.3). Subjecting these mean data to linear and multiple regression analysis produced the following equations:

$$E_{l(0)} = 0.64 \text{ (s.e. 0.041) MEI} - 0.37 \text{ (s.e. 0.060)} \qquad R^2 = 0.91 \quad (9)$$

$$\begin{aligned} MEI &= 0.60 \text{ (s.e. 0.048) MW} + 1.52 \text{ (s.e. 0.081) } E_l \\ &\quad + 0.98 \text{ (s.e. 0.121) } E_g \qquad\qquad\qquad R^2 = 0.96 \quad (10) \end{aligned}$$

Table 12.7 EFFECT OF SILAGE GE INTAKE AS A PROPORTION OF TOTAL GE INTAKE ON THE LINEAR RELATIONSHIP BETWEEN ADJUSTED MILK ENERGY OUTPUT ($E_{L(0)}$) (MJ/KG$^{0.75}$) AND ME INTAKE (MEI) (MJ/KG$^{0.75}$) AND THE DERIVED ME REQUIREMENT FOR MAINTENANCE (ME_M) AND THE EFFICIENCY OF ME UTILIZATION FOR LACTATION (K_L) (FROM YAN *et al.*, 1998)

Silage GE/Total GE	n	Equations	R^2	ME_m MJ/kg$^{0.75}$	k_l	
<0.50	99	$E_{l(0)} = 0.62\,MEI - 0.365$	0.80	0.59	0.62	(6)
0.51-0.99	86	$E_{l(0)} = 0.64\,MEI - 0.434$	0.85	0.68	0.64	(7)
1.00	36	$E_{l(0)} = 0.63\,MEI - 0.465$	0.89	0.74	0.63	(8)

Where MEI is ME intake and MW is metabolic live weight (kg$^{0.75}$) of cows. Equation 9 is shown illustrated in Figure 12.7. These relationships resulted in estimates of ME_m of 0.58 and 0.60 MJ/kg W$^{0.75}$ for the linear and multiple regression methods respectively, and k_l values of 0.64 and 0.66 respectively. All these values are relatively close to those obtained at Hillsborough and support the present hypothesis that maintenance rather than k_l (discussed later) is the component which is underestimated in AFRC (1990 and 1993).

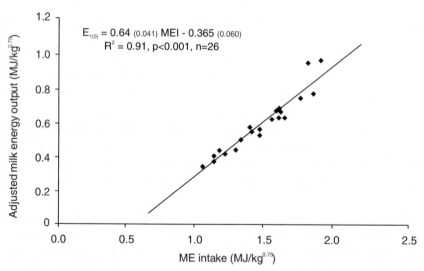

Figure 12.7 The relationship between ME intake and milk energy output adjusted to zero energy balance (AFRC, 1990) using calorimetric data of dairy cows published since 1969 (excluding Hillsborough data)

A number of other authors have estimated ME_m and k_l using a range of regression techniques using large sets of calorimetric data from lactating cows. A summary of ME_m and k_l values derived by these authors is given in Table 12.8. The analysis by Moe

Table 12.8 SUMMARY OF THE ME REQUIREMENT FOR MAINTENANCE (ME_M) AND THE EFFICIENCY OF ME UTILIZATION FOR LACTATION (K_L) BY LACTATING DAIRY CATTLE, CALCULATED BY A RANGE OF AUTHORS USING REGRESSION TECHNIQUES AND POOLED CALORIMETRIC DATA (FROM YAN *et al.*, 1997a)

Reference	*Scale*	*Forage*	*Method*	ME_m $(MJ/kg^{0.75})$	k_l
Moe *et al* (1970)	350 trials	Lucerne hay/ grass hay	Multiple regression	0.51	0.64
Van Es *et al* (1970)	198 trials	Hay/silage	Linear regression	0.49	0.62
Van Es (1975)	1148 cattle	A range of roughages	Linear regression	0.49	0.60
Unsworth *et al* (1994)	13 trials	Grass/silage	Linear regression	0.64	0.67
Hayasaka *et al* (1995)	53 trials	Hay/silage	Multiple regression	0.59	0.64
Mean				0.54	0.63
s.d.				0.067	0.026

et al. (1970), Van Es *et al.* (1970) and Van Es (1975) resulted in ME_m values relatively close to those calculated by the method of AFRC (1990) (range 0.49-0.51 MJ/kg$^{0.75}$). However, two of the most recent studies (Unsworth, Mayne, Cushnahan and Gordon, 1994; Hayasaka, Takasuri and Yamagishi, 1995), resulted in much higher values of 0.64 and 0.59 MJ/kg$^{0.75}$ respectively - values which are close to those found in the analysis reported here.

The weight of evidence from recent calorimetric studies is therefore suggesting that ME_m is considerably underestimated by AFRC (1990 and 1993). The degree of underestimation appears to be related to the nature of the diet being offered, with the present analysis suggesting that this could vary from around 0.60 to 0.74 depending upon diet type. The fasting-metabolism studies indicate a value of around 0.62, which lies within this range. It is therefore suggested that AFRC (1990 and 1993) underestimate ME_m by proportionately 0.30-0.40.

EFFICIENCY OF UTILIZATION OF ME FOR LACTATION (K_L)

When calculating the estimates of ME_m discussed above, estimates of k_l were also obtained. The regression techniques used on the total calorimetric data set from Hillsborough (Table 12.6) indicated a range in k_l values from 0.61 to 0.68 with a mean of 0.65 (from Yan *et al.*, 1997a). The same figure was obtained from Equation 5 (Table

12.6) by using the mean ME_m estimated from the present data set (0.67 MJ/kg$^{0.75}$) to calculate ME_p and then relating this to $E_{l(0)}$. This overall mean of 0.65 is very similar to those of 0.66 and 0.67 obtained by regression of the 26 sets of calorimetric data published since 1969 (Equations 9 and 10). Equally, the sets of calorimetric data examined by a number of other authors (Moe *et al.*, 1970; Van Es *et al.*, 1970; Van Es, 1975; Unsworth *et al.*, 1994 and Hayasaka *et al.*, 1995), as shown in Table 12.8, have indicated a range of k_l values between 0.60 and 0.67, with a mean of 0.63. All these k_l values are very similar to those predicted by ARC (1980) from the equation of $k_l = 0.35\ q_m + 0.42$. Indeed using this equation the mean k_l value predicted for the Hillsborough data set is 0.65 which is identical to the mean of those determined across the range of regression analysis. It is also interesting to note that, as indicated in Table 12.7, the proportion of GE intake derived from silage had no effect on k_l (range from 0.62 to 0.64).

All these k_l values developed by regression techniques are much higher than those from studies where ME_m has been calculated from AFRC (1990) and then used to calculate ME available for production. For example using this approach Gordon *et al.* (1995a) reported average k_l values of 0.58, Unsworth *et al.* (1994) of 0.56 and Beever, Cammell, Sutton and Humphries (1997) of 0.54, all of which are considerably lower than the predicted AFRC (1990) values. These low k_l values are however a direct reflection of the value chosen for ME_m. For example if AFRC (1990) ME_m is adopted for the present set of data ($n = 221$) then the calculated k_l is 0.53, but this increases to 0.65 if the ME_m of 0.67, as determined in this review, is used. This would therefore support the view that the low k_l values reported by many authors may have been a direct reflection of the ME_m used in the calculations and that this value may have been in error.

RELATIONSHIP BETWEEN K_L AND K_G

It is generally accepted that the utilization of ME for milk secretion is a more efficient process than for tissue retention by non-lactating cows (ARC, 1980). However, there is doubt about the extent of this difference. There is also concern about the efficiency with which energy is retained in tissue when retention occurs simultaneously with lactation. In a recent study at Hillsborough a forced drying-off procedure was adopted to study how the efficiency of ME changed with physiological state of the animal (Yan *et al.*, 1997b). These data indicated that the efficiency of ME utilization for lactation was proportionately 0.07 higher than that for tissue retention in dry cows. However, the efficiency of ME utilization for concomitant tissue retention during lactation would appear to be similar to that for lactation.

The partitioning of energy between tissue and milk

The previous discussion concentrates on ideas for developing energy feeding standards that will enable the most accurate rationing of dairy cows when there is either zero tissue energy retention or a given tissue energy change. However, such approaches are of limited practical value in commercial situations where optimum feeding levels and strategies have to be predicted for animals of differing milk yield potential, producing in a range of physical and economic environments. In this context the key factor is how the animal responds to additional increments of feed. This is primarily driven by how the animal partitions the additional feed between milk output and body tissue gain. Sensible feeding approaches can only be developed when this partitioning relationship, and how it is influenced by both animal and feed factors, are understood. This has been recognized for many years, and the concepts were well set out by Blaxter (1966). Unfortunately there have been few attempts to really address this issue, so a number of key questions remain unanswered. For example, how is the partitioning of additional increments of nutrients influenced by the cow (e.g. genetic parameters, milk yield, body state, previous nutritional history and stage of lactation) and the feed (e.g. plane of nutrition, diet composition and method of feeding) and even interactions between the cow and its feed?

The most fundamental element of this concept is the influence of plane of nutrition on energy partitioning. A number of workers have clearly demonstrated the curvilinear nature of the relationship between feed input and milk output (e.g. Gordon, 1984; Ferris *et al.*, 1997) when using groups of cows offered differing levels of input. The validity of such data is not in question, but it has been argued that such a diminishing response curve for a group of animals does not necessarily imply a similar curvilinear relationship for individual animals within a group. This was clearly demonstrated by Curnow (1973), who showed that it could equally reflect the summation of a series of 'broken stick' relationships for individual animals. In this case there would be a linear response in milk output to changes in feed input up to a maximum and above this there would be no further response. Whilst this debate may seem academic it directly affects future development of dynamic feeding models. It would certainly have major implications when using such models to determine optimum economic feed inputs for individual animals differing in genetic merit or stage of lactation.

This key uncertainty of the response of the dairy cow to plane of nutrition has not been resolved. Blaxter (1966) obtained production data from individual animals and proposed that a curvilinear response existed for each animal. However, Friggens, Emmans, Robertson, Chamberlain, Whittemore and Oldham (1995) could not confirm this. Both these research programmes attempted to disentangle the issue by measuring responses in yield and live-weight gain in production studies. However, measuring production response, and tissue gain, for individual cows is extremely difficult, mainly due to the inherent inaccuracies of measuring changes in tissue energy. The use of indirect calorimetry offers an opportunity to explore these aspects with much greater precision and this approach has recently been adopted at Hillsborough. In this study four dairy cows in mid-lactation were each offered sequentially four levels of ME intake, (ranging from approximately 240-120 MJ ME/day), from a single total mixed ration. At each level of ME intake individual animals were subjected to energy balance measurements and from these data the relationships between ME intake and milk energy output (E_l) and tissue energy gain (E_g) were calculated for each animal. The data from this study have conclusively demonstrated that each individual animal follows a curvilinear response between ME intake and E_l output, and in addition the converse response is obtained for E_g. The mean relationships for the four cows in ME partition between E_l and E_g are shown in Figure 12.8. Using these two relationships, and their differentials, it has been computed that where E_g = zero (i.e. requirements are met) the marginal response in milk to additional ME intake is 0.27 MJ E_l/MJ ME intake. This marginal response may appear low but must not be confused with the theoretical response inherent within traditional feeding standards (e.g. representing an efficiency of proportionately 0.27 in comparison with the theoretical value of 0.62). The present response is very close to that of 0.25 MJ E_l/MJ ME intake reported by Friggens *et al.* (1995) and is directly in line with earlier studies in which responses have been quoted in milk yield (e.g. Steen and Gordon, 1980). All these responses reflect the considerable partitioning of additional ME intake towards tissue gain. For example, in the present study at zero E_g a unit increase in ME intake (MJ/d) produced a response in E_g of 0.24 MJ, in addition to the 0.27 MJ response in E_l. Using the data of Yan *et al.* (1997b), which indicate that the efficiency of ME use for E_g during lactation is 0.95 of the efficiency of use for E_l, the present results would suggest that when animals were fed to meet requirements then an additional increment of ME intake was partitioned approximately equally between E_l and E_g.

The relationship between responses in E_l and E_g for incremental changes in ME intake alters considerably with feeding level (Figure 12.8). At low ME intake there is a high response in E_l and little response in E_g yet at high ME intake the opposite effect is obtained. In practical terms the whole concept of optimum feeding level therefore hinges upon the cost of feed relative to milk value and how nutrients are partitioned within the cow. The objective for researchers is therefore to quantify those animal and feed factors which influence these partitioning relationships and to build these into a feeding system along with any new estimates of maintenance, k_l and k_g which may become available.

Conclusions

Since the mid-1980s there have been major increases in the rate of genetic improvement in the dairy herd in the British Isles. Studies have shown that the higher milk production of high-merit cows and their higher overall efficiency of converting ME intake into milk is largely attributable to increases in partitioning of nutrients towards milk production rather than to tissue gain. Increased genetic merit has only a small effect on food intake and there is no effect on digestive or energetic efficiency.

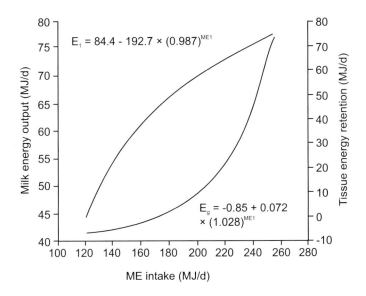

Figure 12.8 Effect of level of ME intake (MEI) on milk energy output (E_l) and tissue energy retention (E_g)

Within the United Kingdom, energy is rationed according to the ME system. From the review presented here, these feeding standards underestimate feed requirements.

This would appear to relate to ME_m rather than k_l. Data from Hillsborough indicate that the ME_m for lactating dairy cows offered grass silage based diets, with a q of 0.65, is 0.67 MJ/kg$^{0.75}$ and that this figure is influenced by the proportion of concentrates in the diet. These data also demonstrate that k_l is in line with that quoted by AFRC (1990 and 1993).

Deficiencies in the ME system also relate to the inability to predict both animal response and the composition of milk. Further areas of concern include the provision of estimates of not only the ME content but also characterisation of the composition of the ME. The importance of nutrient interactions must also be addressed, as well as an improved understanding of hormonal regulation of the processes. Genetic differences among animals may exist in the extent of digestion and absorption of nutrients to the various body tissues, and in the interrelationship of nutrient utilization and regulation of intake. Variation in regulation of nutrient partitioning could involve inherited differences in circulating hormones, in cellular recognition of these signals and in cellular expression of these signals.

In the future, feeding cows of high genetic merit will depend upon accurately knowing the animals' energy and nutrient requirements for differing functions; utilising information on what influences the partitioning of nutrients between tissue and milk; using dynamic models dealing with requirements and responses and having effective laboratory methods for predicting the characteristics of feeds. The essential issue is that milk production must be recognised as a dynamic system, as distinct from a stable predetermined cycle of daily output through lactation, supported by appropriate inputs proportional to yield and based on an assumption of a standard rate of intake proportional to yield.

Acknowledgement

The authors acknowledge partial funding from 'MAFF LINK: Feed into Milk. The development of an improved system of characterising ruminant feeds leading to the development of a nutritional model for dairy cows'

References

AFRC, Agricultural and Food Research Council (1990) Technical Committee on Responses to Nutrients, Report No 5, Nutritive Requirements of Farm Animals: Energy. *Nutrition Abstracts and Reviews (Series B),* **60,** 729-804

AFRC, Agricultural and Food Research Council (1993) *Energy and Protein Requirements of Ruminants.* CAB International, Wallingford, Oxon, England.

ARC, Agricultural Research Council (1980) *The Nutrient Requirements of Ruminant Livestock, Technical Review.* Farnham Royal, CAB.

Bassett, J. M. (1981) Regulation of insulin and glucagon secretion in nutrients. In *Hormones and Metabolism in Ruminants (Workshop of University of Leeds 1980),* pp. 65-79. Edited by J. M. Forbes. Agricultural Research Council, London.

Bauman, D. E. and Currie, W. B. (1980) Partitioning of nutrients during pregnancy and lactation: a review of mechanisms involving homeostasis and homeorhesis. *Journal of Dairy Science,* **63,** 1514-1529.

Bauman, D. E. (1976) Intermediary metabolism of adipose tissue. *Federation Proceedings,* **35,** 2308-2313.

Beever, D. E., Cammell, S. B., Sutton, J. D. and Humphries, D. J. (1997) The effect of stage of harvest of maize silage on the concentration and efficiency of utilization of metabolizable energy by lactating dairy cows. In *Proceedings of the 14th Symposium on Energy Metabolism of Farm Animals.* Newcastle, Northern Ireland.

Bines, J. A. and Hart, I. C. (1986) Control and manipulation of nutrient partition. In *Principles and Practice of Feeding Dairy Cows.* Edited by W. H. Broster, R. H. Phipps and C. L. Johnson. Technical Bulletin 8, NIRD.

Bines, J. A., Hart, I. C. and Morant, S. V. (1980) Endocrine control of energy metabolism in the cow: the effect on milk yield and levels of some blood constituent of injecting growth hormone and growth hormone fragments. *British Journal of Nutrition,* **43,** 179-188.

Birkelo, C. P., Brouk, M. J. and Schingoethe, D. J. (1994) The effect of wet corn distillers grain on energetic efficiency of lactating cows. In *Energy Metabolism of Farm Animals*, pp 183-186. Edited by J. F. Aguilera. European Association for Animal Production Publication No 76, Mojácar, Spain.

Birkelo, C.P., Johnson, D.E. and Phetteplace, H.P.(1991) Maintenance requirements of beef cattle as affected by season on different planes of nutrition. *Journal of Animal Science*, **69**, 1214-1222.

Blaxter, K. L. (1966) The feeding of dairy cows for optimal production. *The George Scott Robertson Memorial Lecture*, The Queen's University of Belfast, Belfast.

Cammell, S.B., Thomson, D.J., Beever, D.E., Haines, M.J., Dhanoa, M.S. and Spooner, M.C. (1986) The efficiency of energy utilization in growing cattle consuming fresh perennial ryegrass (*Lolium perenne* cv. Melle) or white clover (Trifolium repens cv. Blanca). *British Journal of Nutrition*, **55**, 669-680.

Carrick, I. M., Patterson, D. C., Gordon, F. J. and Mayne, C. S. (1996) The effect of quality and level of protein on the performance of dairy cattle of differing genetic merits. *Animal Science*, **62**, 642 (Abstract).

Chowdhury, S. A. and Ørskov, E. R. (1994) Implications of fasting on the energy metabolism and feed evaluation in ruminants. *Journal of Animal and Feed Sciences*, **3**, 161-169.

Coffey, M. (1992) Genetic trends - Has progress been made in the last six years? *Holstein Friesian Journal*, **74**, 62-63.

Curnow, R. N. (1973) A smooth population response curve based on an abrupt threshold and plateau model for individuals. *Biometrics*, **29**, 1.

Cushnahan, A., Mayne, C. S. and Unsworth, E. F. (1995) Effects of ensilage of grass on performance and nutrient utilization by dairy cattle. 2. Nutrient metabolism and rumen fermentation. *Animal Science*, **60**, 347-360.

Ferris, C. P., Gordon, F. J., Patterson, D. C., Mayne, C. S. and McCoy, M. (1997) The response of high genetic merit dairy cows to changes in silage quality and level of supplementary concentrate. In: *Proceedings of the British Society of Animal Science*, Winter Meeting, Scarborough. Page 40.

Ferris, C. P., Gordon, F. J., Patterson, D. C., Mayne, C. S. and Kilpatrick, D. J. (1998a) The influence of dairy cow genetic merit on the direct and residual responses to level of concentrate supplementation. *Journal of Agricultural Science, Cambridge* (In Press).

Ferris, C. P., Gordon, F. J., Patterson, D. C. and Porter, M. G. (1998b) The effect of genetic index and concentrate proportion in the diet on nutrient utilization by lactating dairy cows. Submitted to *Journal of Agricultural Science, Cambridge*.

Flatt, W. P., Moe, P. W., Munson, A. W. and Cooper, T. (1969a) Energy utilization by high producing dairy cows. 2. Summary of energy balance experiments with lactating Holstein cows. In *Energy Metabolism of Farm Animals*, pp 235-251. Edited by K. L. Blaxter, J. Kielanowski and G. Thorbek. European Association for Animal Production Publication No 12, Warsaw, Poland.

Flatt, W. P., Moe, P. W., Oltjen, R. R., Putnam, P. A. and Hooven, N. W., Jr. (1969b) Energy metabolism studies with dairy cows receiving purified diets. In *Energy*

Metabolism of Farm Animals, pp 109-121. Edited by K. L. Blaxter, J. Kielanowski and G. Thorbek. European Association for Animal Production Publication No 12, Warsaw, Poland.

Friggens, N., Emmans, G. C., Robertson, S., Chamberlain, D. G., Whittemore, C. T. and Oldham. J. D. (1995) The lactational responses of dairy cows to amount of feed and to the source of carbohydrate energy. *Journal of Dairy Science, 78,* 1734-1744.

Funk, D. A. (1993) Optimal genetic improvement for the high producing herd. *Journal of Dairy Science, 76,* 3278-3286.

Gädeken, D., Rohr, K. and Lebzien, P. (1991) Effects of nitrogen fertilizing and of harvest season on net energy values of hay in dairy cows. In *Energy Metabolism of Farm Animals*, pp 321-324. Edited by A. Schürch and C. Wenk. European Association for Animal Production Publication No. 13, Vitznau, Switzerland.

Gordon, F.J. (1984) The effect of concentrate supplementation given with grass silage during the winter on the total lactating performance of autumn-calving dairy cows. *Journal of Agricultural Science, 102,* 163-179.

Gordon, F. J., Patterson, D. C., Yan, T., Porter, M. G., Mayne, C. S. and Unsworth, E. F. (1995a) The influence of genetic index for milk production on the response to complete diet feeding and the utilization of energy and nitrogen. *Animal Science, 61,* 199-210.

Gordon, F. J., Porter, M. G., Mayne, C. S., Unsworth E. F. and Kilpatrick, D. J. (1995b). The effect of forage digestibility and type of concentrate on nutrient utilization for lactating dairy cattle. *Journal of Dairy Research, 62,* 15-27.

Hart, I. C. (1983) Endocrine control of nutrient partition in lactating ruminants. *Proceedings of Nutrition Society, 42,* 181-194.

Hart, I. C., Bines, J. A., Balch, C. C. and Lowie, A. T. (1975) Hormone and metabolite differences between lactating beef and dairy cattle. *Life Science, 16,* 1285-1292.

Hart, I. C., Bines, J. A., Morant, S. V. and Ridley, J. L. (1978) Endocrine control of energy metabolism in the cow: comparison of levels of hormones (prolactin, growth hormone, insulin and thyroxin) and metabolites in the plasma of high and low yielding cattle at various stages of lactation. *Journal of Endocrinology, 77,* 333-345.

Hart, I. C., Bines, J. A. and Morant, S. V. (1979) Endocrine control of energy metabolism in the cow: correlations of hormones and metabolites in the plasma of high and low yielding cattle at various stages of lactation. *Journal of Dairy Science, 62,* 270-277.

Hayasaka, K., Takasuri, N. and Yamagishi, N., (1995) Energy metabolism in lactating Holstein cows (in Japanese, with English abstract). *Animal Science and Technology, 66,* 374-382.

Janicki, F. J., Holter, J. B. and Hayes, H. H. (1985) Varying protein content and nitrogen solubility for pluriparous, lactating Holstein cows: Digestive performance during early lactation. *Journal of Dairy Science,* **68,** 1995-2008.

Jilg, T., Susenbeth, A., Ehrensvärd, U. and Henke, K. H. (1987) Effect of treatment of soya beans on energy and protein metabolism of lactating dairy cows. In *Energy Metabolism of Farm Animals*, pp 354-357. Edited by P. W. Moe, H. F. Tyrrell and P. J. Reynolds. European Association for Animal Production, Publication No. 32, Airlie, Virginia, USA.

Keady, T. W. J., Mayne, C. S. and Marsden, M., (1997) An examination of the effect of concentrate energy source and changes in ERDP:DUP ration on milk composition of dairy cows offered grass silages differing in digestibility and intake characteristics. Proceedings *British Society of Animal Science*, Scarborough, p9.

Keady, T. W. J., Mayne, C. S. and Marsden, M., (1998) The effects of concentrate energy source on silage intake and animal performance with lactating dairy cows offered a range of grass silages. *Animal Science,* **66,** 21-34.

Kirchgeßner, M., Müller, H. L. and Schwab, W. (1982) Experimental studies on the feeding frequency of dairy cows. In *Energy Metabolism of Farm Animals*, pp. 30-33. Edited by A. Ekern and F. Sundstøl. European Association for Animal Production Publication No 29, Agricultural University of Norway, Norway.

Kirchgeßner, M., Schwab, W. and Müller, H. L. (1989) Effect of bovine growth hormone on energy metabolism in lactating cows in long-term administration. In *Energy Metabolism of Farm Animals*, pp 143-146. Edited by Y. Van der Honing and W. H. Close. European Association for Animal Production Publication No 43, Pudoc, Wageningen, The Netherlands.

Kronfield, D. S., Mayer, G. P., Robertson, J. McD. and Raggi, F. (1963) Depression of milk secretion during insulin administration. *Journal of Dairy Science,* **46,** 559-563.

Machlin, L. J. (1973) Effect of growth hormone on milk production and feed utilization in dairy cows. *Journal of Dairy Science,* **56,** 575-580.

Machlin, L. J. (1976) Role of growth hormone in improving animal production. In *Anabolic Agents in Animal Production 43*. Edited by F. C. Luard and J. Rendel. (FAO/WHO Symposium, 1975, Rome), Thiene, Stuttgart.

Marston, H. R. (1948) Energy transactions in sheep. 1. The basal heat production and heat increment. *Australian Journal of Scientific Research* (B), **1,** 93-129.

Moe, P. W., Tyrrell, H. F. and Flatt, W. P. (1970) Partial efficiency of energy use for maintenance, lactation, body gain and gestation in the dairy cows. In *Energy Metabolism of Farm Animals*, pp 65-68. Edited by A. Schürch and C. Wenk. European Association for Animal Production Publication No 13. Vitznau, Switzerland.

Münger, A. (1991) Milk production efficiency in dairy cows of different breeds. In *Energy Metabolism of Farm Animals*, pp 292-295. Edited by C. Wenk and M.

Boessinger. European Association for Animal Production Publication No 58, Kartause Ittingen, Switzerland.

Patle, B. R. and Mudgal, V. D. (1977) Utilization of dietary energy for maintenance, milk production and lipogenesis by lactating crossbred cows during their midstage of lactation. *British Journal of Nutrition,* **37,** 23-33.

Patterson, D. C., Yan, T. and Gordon, F. J. (1996) The effects of wilting of grass prior to ensiling on the response to bacterial inoculation. 2 . Intake and performance by dairy cattle over three harvests. *Animal Science,* **62,** 419-430.

Raben, M. S. (1973) In *Methods in Investigative and Diagnostic Endocrinology,* p. 261. Edited by S. A. Benson and R. I. Yalow. Amsterdam, The Netherlands.

Sartin, J. L., Kemppainen, R. J., Cummins, K. A. and Williams, J. C. (1988) Plasma concentrations of metabolic hormones in high and low producing dairy cows. *Journal of Dairy Science,* **71,** 650-657.

Steen, R. W. J. and Gordon, F. J. (1980) The effect of level and system of concentrate allocation to January/February calving cows on total lactation performance. *Animal Production,* **30,** 39-51.

Sutter, F., Bickel, H. and Wenk, C. (1991) Energy and protein metabolism at the onset of lactation in dairy cows. In *Energy Metabolism of Farm Animals,* pp 337-340. Edited by C. Wenk and M. Boessinger. European Association for Animal Production Publication No 58, Kartause Ittingen, Switzerland.

Sutton, J. D., Cammell, S. B., Beever, D. E., Haines, M. J., Spooner, M. C. and Harland, J. I. (1991) The effect of energy and protein sources on energy and protein balances in Friesian cows in early lactation. In *Energy Metabolism of Farm Animals,* pp 288-291. Edited by C. Wenk and M. Boessinger. European Association for Animal Production Publication No 58, Kartause Ittingen, Switzerland.

Sutton, J. D., Cammell, S. B., Beever, D. E., Humphries, D. J. and Phipps, R. (1997) Treatment of urea-treated whole crop wheat to improve its energy value for lactating dairy cows. In *Proceedings of the 14th Symposium on Energy Metabolism of Farm Animals.* Newcastle, Northern Ireland.

Terada, F. and Muraoka, M. (1994) Effect of heat stress on the efficiency of utilization of metabolizable energy for lactation. In *Energy Metabolism of Farm Animals,* pp 323-326. Edited by J. F. Aguilera. European Association for Animal Production Publication No 76, Mojácar, Spain.

Thorbek, G. and Henkel, S. (1976) Studies on energy requirement for maintenance in farm animals. In *Energy Metabolism of Farm Animals,* p 117. Edited by M. Vermorel. European Association for Animal Production Publication No. 19, de Bussac, Clermont-Ferrand, France.

Tyrrell, H. F., Brown, A. C. G., Reynolds, P. J. and Haaland, G. L. (1982) Effect of growth hormone on utilization of energy by lactating Holstein cows. In *Energy Metabolism of Farm Animals,* pp 46-49. Edited by A. Ekern and F. Sundstøl.

European Association for Animal Production Publication No 29, Agricultural University of Norway, Norway.

Tyrrell, H. F. and Moe, P. W. (1972) Net energy value for lactation of a high and low concentrate ration containing corn silage. *Journal of Dairy Science,* **55,** 1106-1112.

Tyrrell, H. F. and Moe, P. W. (1980) Effect of protein level and buffering capacity on energy value of feeds for lactating dairy cows. In *Energy Metabolism of Farm Animals*, pp 311-313. Edited by L. Mount. European Association for Animal Production Publication No 26, Cambridge, England.

Tyrrell, H. F. and Varga, G. A. (1987) Energy value for lactation of rations containing ground whole ear maize or maize meal both conserved dry or ensiled at high moisture. In *Energy Metabolism of Farm Animals*, pp 306-309. Edited by P. W. Moe, H. F. Tyrrell and P. J. Reynolds. European Association for Animal Production Publication No. 32, Airlie, Virginia, USA.

Unsworth, E. F. (1991) The efficiency of utilization of metabolizable energy for lactation from grass silage-based diets. In *Energy Metabolism of Farm Animals*, pp 329-332. Edited by C. Wenk and M. Boessinger. European Association for Animal Production Publication No. 58, Kartause Ittingen, Switzerland.

Unsworth, E. F., Mayne, C. S., Cushnahan, A. and Gordon, F. J. (1994) The energy utilization of grass silage diets by lactating dairy cows. In *Energy Metabolism of Farm Animals,* pp 179-181. Edited by J. F. Aguilera. European Association for Animal Production Publication No. 76, Mojacar, Spain.

Van Es, A. J. H. (1975) Feed evaluation for dairy cows. *Livestock Production Science,* **2,** 95-107.

Van Es, A. J. H. and Van der Honing, Y. (1976) Energy and nitrogen balances of lactating cows fed fresh or frozen grass. In *Energy Metabolism of Farm Animals*, pp 237-240. Edited by M. Vermorel. European Association for Animal Production Publication No 19, Vichy, France.

Van Es, A. J. H., Nijkamp, H. J. and Vogt, J. E. (1970) Feed evaluation for dairy cows. In *Energy Metabolism of Farm Animals*, pp 61-64. Edited by A. Schürch and C. Wenk. European Association for Animal Production Publication No 13. Vitznau, Switzerland.

Windisch, W., Kirchgeßner, M. and Müller, H. L. (1991) Effect of different energy supply on energy metabolism in lactating dairy cows after a period of energy restriction. In *Energy Metabolism of Farm Animals*, pp. 304-307. Edited by C. Wenk and M. Boessinger. European Association for Animal Production Publication No 58, Kartause Ittingen, Switzerland.

Yan, T., Patterson, D. C., Gordon, F. J. and Porter, M. G. (1996) The effects of wilting of grass prior to ensiling on the response to bacterial inoculation. 1. Silage fermentation and nutrient utilization over three harvests. *Animal Science,* **62,** 405-418.

Yan, T., Gordon, F. J., Agnew, R. E., Porter, M. G. and Patterson, D. C. (1997a) The metabolizable energy requirement for maintenance and the efficiency of utilization of metabolizable energy for lactation by dairy cows offered grass silage-based diets. *Livestock Production Science,* **51,** 143-153.

Yan, T., Gordon, F. J., Ferris, C. P., Agnew, R. E., Porter, M. G. and Patterson, D. C. (1997b) The fasting heat production and effect of lactation on energy utilization by dairy cows offered forage-based diets. *Livestock Production Science,* **52,** 177-186.

Yan, T., Gordon, F. J., Agnew, R. E. and Porter, M. G. (1998) The metabolizable energy requirement for maintenance and the efficiencies of utilization of metabolizable energy for lactation and tissue retention in dairy cows. In: *Energy Metabolism of Farm Animals* (eds. K. McCraken, E.F. Unsworth and A.R.G. Wylie) Proceedings of the 14th Symposium on Energy Metabolism of Farm Animals. Newcastle, Northern Ireland, pp.97-100.

This paper was first published in 1998

13

PRACTICAL APPLICATION OF THE METABOLISABLE PROTEIN SYSTEM

J.R. NEWBOLD
Provimi Research and Technology Centre, Lenneke Marelaan 2, B-1932 Sint-Stevens-Woluwe, Belgium

Introduction

The Metabolisable Protein (MP) system was published in November 1992 (AFRC, 1992). Since then, a plethora of papers has appeared in which the scheme has been dissected and debated, culminating in the 'user's manual' of AFRC (1993). To describe the system, to review it's antecedents or to compare and contrast the various analogues proposed around the world would be to repeat information given by AFRC (1992), Webster (1992) and Beever and Cottrill (1994), amongst others.

The MP system was designed to be useful to nutritionists and farm advisors. In this context, it is important to define what exactly is meant by the term 'useful'. Nutritionists seek common currencies -nutrients -with which to express, in quantitative terms, the value of foods and the responses of animals to those foods. The demand for ever more accuracy has led to the use of complex derived nutrients, whose calculation involves so many steps and interactions as to merit use of the term 'system'. In the case of the 'MP system', MP is simply a nutrient used to describe the protein value of foods, and the 'system' refers to the web of calculations required to quantify MP. Nutrients -measured and derived -involved in the MP system are summarised in Figure 13.1.

Feed evaluation systems are used to answer two basic questions; what ration is *required* to support a defined animal response, and what is the *response* to a specified ration? Schiere and de Wit (1993) provided a similar classification: high input systems, where feeds are adapted to the animal (i.e requirement systems) and low input systems, where the animal is adapted to the feed (i.e. response systems). For European Union dairy farmers, working within strict quotas, the greatest need is for accurate requirement systems, although response models help evaluate prospective feeding and management strategies. The MP system (AFRC, 1992) was designed as a requirement model, and its success or failure must be judged accordingly. However, MP, as a nutrient, may be of use in predicting various animal responses to food, not described formally by the MP system. Some responses of major economic importance to the dairy farmer are listed in Figure 13.1.

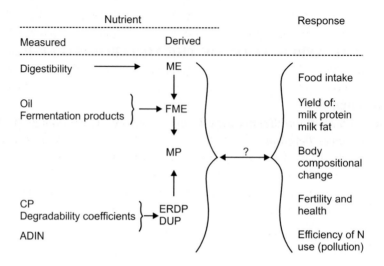

Figure 13.1 Nutrients defined within the ME/MP system (AFRC, 1990, 1992) and some important responses of dairy cows to diet

The response of groups of lactating cows to increased intakes of protein is likely to be curvilinear (Figure 13.2). The perfect 'broken-stick' response, implied by requirement models such as AFRC (1992), with no effect of protein supplied in excess of requirement, is never observed in practice, not least because responses are plotted through means of several individuals, an ever diminishing proportion of which are capable, genotypically, of further response to the next increment of protein supply (Curnow, 1973). Farmers are often concerned with responses of groups of animals, rather than individuals.

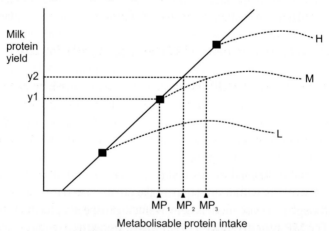

Figure 13.2. Theoretical milk protein yield response to energy and protein intake. Solid lines denote response when protein is limiting, dashed lines show responses when protein ceases to be limiting at low (L), medium (M) or high (H) intakes of ME. .= optimal MP:ME ratio for given milk protein yield (protein requirement). Adapted from ARC (1980). Also shown are alternative strategies for increasing milk protein yield from yl to y2.

These distinctions between nutrients (e.g. MP) and systems (e.g. the MP system of AFRC (1992)), between requirements and responses, and between individual animals and groups, form the structure of this paper, and define the term 'useful'. Feed evaluation systems are only useful if the nutrients they define can predict the food requirements, or responses to food, of individuals and groups of animals, and if computation of those nutrients is practicable.

The paper begins with a consideration of how well the MP system performs as a requirement model; predicting MP requirement, when protein is limiting to performance, and MP supply. This is followed by discussion of various factors used in the calculation of MP requirement and supply. The value of MP as a predictor of animal response to protein is then considered, with a final comment on the application of the system to groups of animals, rather than individuals. Throughout, attention is focused on the dairy cow.

Evaluation of the MP system

AFRC (1992) made only two claims on behalf of the MP system; firstly, that MP supply can be calculated satisfactorily and, secondly, that the requirement for MP at any given level of ME supply (i.e. the optimal MP:ME ratio) can be predicted. (In effect, the system claims to predict the slope of the response to MP, when protein is limiting to performance, Figure 13.2). The success of the system, as published by AFRC (1992), must be judged solely by evaluating these two claims.

AFRC (1992) applied the MP system to a large dataset collated by AFRC (1991), having taken care to select data where protein, rather than energy, was likely to be limiting to performance. Within this restricted dataset:

MP requirement (g/d) = 161 + 0.849 (MP supply, g/d) (r^2=0.83)

When MP supply = 1600 g/d (i.e. milk yield around 30 kg/d), MP requirement = 1519 g/d, a discrepancy of 81 g/d, or 5%. Thus, high-yielding cows yield less milk protein than predicted by the MP system (MP supply> MP requirement). For low-yielding cows (MP requirement below 1060 g/d), estimates of MP requirement exceed those of MP supply.

The relationship found by AFRC (1992) is given support by studies of Newbold, Cottrill, Mansbridge and Blake (1994). In production experiments at AD AS Bridgets, in dietary treatments where ME balance calculations suggested that MP was limiting to performance, MP supply in early lactation (calculated by applying equations of AFRC (1992) to measured feed intakes, CP concentrations and *in situ* protein degradability figures) was approximately 100gid greater than MP requirement (calculated from net protein requirement for maintenance, observed liveweight change and milk protein yield, using efficiencies of utilisation of AFRC (1992)). Relationships between calculated MP requirement and supply are compared with the equation of AFRC (1992) in Figure 13.3.

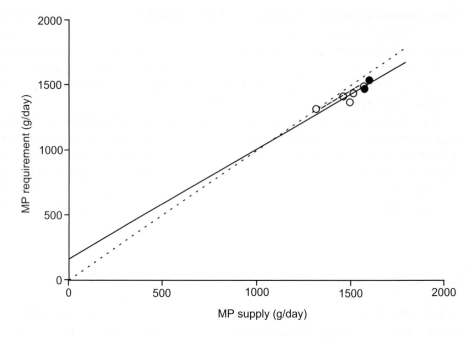

Figure 13.3 MP requirement versus MP supply. Dotted line is line of equality. Solid line represents equation of AFRC (1992) (MP requirement (g/d) = 161 + 0.85 (MP supply, g/d)). Dashed line represents data of Newbold *et al.* (1994): symbols represent treatment means for a four-week period in early lactation from Experiment 1 (●; n=10) or Experiment 2 (○; n=12). Only treatment means where MP supply was judged limiting to performance are included.

Although both datasets are encouraging in the close overall fit between MP supply and requirement, some small modification may be justified when the system is used in practice. For most cows likely to be rationed using the MP system (milk yields of 20 kg/d or above), estimates of MP supply exceed - slightly -those of requirement (Figure 13.3). Any such adjustment (increase in requirement or diminution of supply) would be a 'bias correction', rather than a safety factor used to translate a requirement, calculated for an individual, into an allowance for a group or herd: this issue should be addressed separately. It is worth noting that there is evidence of biases of similar or greater magnitude within the ME system, which are not currently accommodated within the AFRC recommendations (AFRC, 1990). Relationships shown in Figure 13.3 imply that the size of the modification should increase as MP supply rises beyond 1060 g/d. At present, evaluation of the MP system at very high milk yields is limited and experiments are needed to compare diets formulated at optimal MP:ME ratio for different milk yields.

It is impossible, from production data alone, to determine whether any discrepancy between MP requirement and supply arises from underestimation of the former, overestimation of the latter, or some combination of the two.

Estimation of MP requirement

Underestimation of MP requirement could be due to underestimation of net protein (NP) needs (for maintenance, growth, lactation or pregnancy) or over-estimation of efficiencies of utilisation. For the high-yielding cow, the efficiency of utilisation of MP for lactation (k_l) has a major impact on MP requirement.

AFRC (1992) pointed out the difficulties of testing the veracity of the 0.68 estimate of k_l, since accurate estimates of MP supply are, frustratingly, difficult to obtain. Webster (1992) concluded that this figure was a valid coefficient to predict MP requirement from NP requirement, but doubted whether it had any sacrosanct biological meaning. In the data of Newbold *et al.* (1994), MP supply and requirement could have been brought into balance by reducing the estimate of k_l from 0.68 to 0.62. A figure of 0.64 is used in France (INRA, 1988) and 0.65 in the USA (NRC, 1989).

Just as MP requirement is a function of two factors (NP requirement and *k)*, so k_l is defined as the product of the efficiency of utilisation of the ideal amino acid mixture for lactation $(k_{AAl}, 0.85)$, and the relative value (RV) of amino acids in the MP supplied (estimated as 0.80, as a default value, AFRC (1992). Progress towards a system based on metabolisable essential amino acids (MEAA) requires that two principal issues be addressed: the 'requirement side' issue of the adequacy of 0.85 as an estimate of k_{AAl} and the 'supply side' issue of the calculation of MEAA supply (in order to estimate RV). Issues of requirement only are discussed here.

The adoption of 0.85 as an estimate of k_{AAl} followed a review by Oldham (1987) of data from a range of species. Postruminal infusion of amino acids (e.g. Schwab, Satter and Clay, 1976) or casein (Choung and Chamberlain, 1992) gives efficiencies of utilisation of MP for lactation reasonably close to this ideal. Mepham (1982) concluded that efficiency of utilisation varied widely among individual EAA. The recently-proposed amino acid sub-model of the Cornell Net Carbohydrate and Protein System (CNCPS, O'Connor, Sniffen, Fox and Chalupa, 1993) uses a value of 1.0 to describe the utilisation of phenylalanine, with values for other EAA ranging from 0.42 (arginine) to 0.98 (methionine). O'Connor *et al.* (1993) and Ainslie, Fox, Perry, Ketchen and Barry (1993) both highlighted the limiting efficiency of utilisation of individual EAA as a major uncertainty within the CNCPS amino acid sub-model. Differences between amino acids in their efficiency of use are discussed further by Oldham (1994). Translating an understanding of the biochemistry of protein utilisation in the mammary gland into appropriate coefficients to convert net EAA requirements into MEA A requirements thus remains a significant challenge; as important, perhaps, as further refinements of estimates of MEAA supply.

Reports of production benefits from formulating rations on the basis of EAA supply must be interpreted with caution. Frequently, responses to amino acid balance *per se* are difficult to distinguish from responses to MP, especially in comparisons of conventional protein supplements such as fishmeal and soya bean meal, or postruminal infusions of casein, which usually lack an iso-MP control. Rulquin and Verite (1993) provided a comprehensive summary of the production benefits of increasing the essential amino acid content of feed proteins and reviewed responses to protected amino acids.

Ainslie *et al.* (1993) applied the CNCPS, and the CNCPS extended to include the amino acid sub-model of O'Connor *et al.* (1993), to four data sets describing the live-weight gain of Holstein steers offered a variety of protein sources. The bias of prediction of observed live-weight gain was reduced from 8% to 5% when predictions were made on the basis of MP and MEAA, rather than MP alone. Evaluation of the Cornell amino acid sub-model in lactating cows is required.

Strachan, Wilson and Kelly (1987) developed an amino acid sub-model for the ARC (1980) protein system, using the amino acid composition of *in situ* nylon bag residues to predict MEA A supply. Milk protein yield tended to be greater when the diet was formulated to meet MEAA requirements (Table 13.1).

Table 13.1 RESPONSE OF DAIRY COWS TO COMPOUNDS VARYING IN LEVEL AND PROFILE OF UNDEGRADABLE ESSENTIAL AMINO ACIDS

	Treatment	
	1	*2*
CP (kg/d)	3.07	3.06
Undegradable essential amino acids (g/d)	250	280
Milk protein (g/kg)	27.3[a]	31.0[b]
Milk protein (g/d)	880	940

[a,b]Means with different superscripts are significantly different (P<0.01) (From Strachan et *al.,* 1987)

Adoption of systems based on requirements for MEAA, rather than MP (whether explicitly as MEAA or implicitly via dynamic estimates of RV) should improve the predictability of animal performance when MP:ME ratio is sub-optimal (protein limiting). Exploiting this potential depends, obviously, on our ability to quantify MEAA supply.

ESTIMATION OF MP SUPPLY

Most of the equations within the MP system of AFRC (1992) are concerned with issues of MP supply, rather than requirement, and with ruminal, rather than post-ruminal, metabolism.

Webster (1992). confessed himself a heretic by stating that 'measurements of the efficiency of utilisation of amino acids based only on the entry of amino acid N to the duodenum are, in ruminants, an expensive irrelevance'. This remark highlights an important imbalance within the MP system (and its many analogues) between the detailed quantification of ruminal N metabolism and the superficial quantification of post-ruminal metabolism. With the development of reliable multicatheterization techniques allowing measurement of net nutrient flux across the liver and splanchnic bed (Huntington, Reynolds and Stroud, 1989), this imbalance is beginning to be addressed. Models such as the MP system are, inevitably, partly 'technique driven'. Data describing the post-absorptive metabolism of amino acids were, for the most part, unavailable during the development of the MP system, and are not discussed in detail here. Up-to-date reviews of progress in this field are given by Lindsay (1993) and Seal and Reynolds (1994).

Various steps in the calculation of MP supply within the MP system are highlighted below, focusing on areas in which new data have become available since the publication of AFRC (1992). It is not intended as a comprehensive review.

Protein degradability and ERDP

The way the MP system calculates N supply to rumen microorganisms raises several issues. Many of these were reviewed by Cottrill (1993) and a few points only are made here. Firstly, it is simplistic to assume that the requirement is simply for N: source is also important (Argyle and Baldwin, 1989). Assimilation of ammonia, amino acids and peptides has been reviewed recently by Nolan (1993). Understanding the complex N needs of rumen microorganisms is of particular importance in rations which rely on grass silages, which contain significant amounts of non-protein N. The low efficiency of microbial protein synthesis on such silages (ARC, 1984) is often attributed to asynchrony between rates of N and energy supply: effects of N source may be more important.

Defining the N sources required is but the first step: the second is to describe the rate of N supply. The key reference remains Ørskov and McDonald (1979), who used exponential curves to describe protein loss from nylon bags incubated in the rumen. In the intervening years, modified curves, incorporating lag times, have been suggested (Dhanoa, 1988) and a whole literature has accumulated in which variations on this technique are debated (Nocek, 1988). Being linked inextricably to the Ørskov/McDonald approach, the MP system cannot easily accommodate foods exhibiting more complex patterns of degradation.

One point which has received increased attention since the MP system began to be implemented in practice, is the use of '0 hour' nylon bag degradability measurements in the estimation of quickly-degraded protein. Across five compound foods used by Newbold *et al.* (1994), the solubility of N in cold water was only 0.44 of the '0 hour' N degradability figure. Cockburn, Dhanoa, France and Lopez (1993) found that a significant proportion of the quickly-degraded fraction comprised small particle insoluble material. A correction for the washout of small particles was outlined by Madsen and Hvelplund (1994), but further work is required to determine rates of degradation and passage.

Despite these reservations, the *in situ* technique remains the method of choice, and can give good prediction of UDP supply. Recently, Arieli, Mabjeesh, Tagari, Bruckental and Zamwell (1993) showed good correlation between measured and predicted duodenal flow of UDP, with the former determined by standard marker techniques and the latter estimated from *in situ* degradability curves. The success of alternative techniques, notably enzyme methods and near infra-red spectroscopy (NIR, Cottrill, 1993) is hard to judge, since they are compared, almost invariably, with *in situ* data.

One further point is relevant to the use of degradability coefficients. The MP system involves calculation of ERDP and DUP contributions from individual raw materials. These values are then summed to give the ERDP and DUP supply from the total ration. The alternative -to average *a,* band c coefficients prior to computation of ERDP and DUP -is invalidated by the non-additivity of the rate constant c. However, this procedure must be followed to obtain estimates of *a,* band c for premixes, blends and compounds, which are then used as feedstuffs when formulating the ration. For simple blends or premixes, consisting of large amounts of a few diverse raw materials, this could lead to substantial errors in the estimation of ERDP and DUP (Table 13.2).

Table 13.2 CALCULATION OF ERDP, DUP AND MP FOR MIX OF GRASS SILAGE AND SIMPLE CONCENTRATE SUPPLEMENT. FEED COMPOSMON DATA TAKEN FROM MAFF (1992). RUMEN OUTFLOW RATE = 0.08/h. FME NOT LIMMNG TO MICROBIAL GROWTH. ADIN ASSUMED = 2g/kg DM FOR ALL FOODS

	Proportion in total ration	*a*	*b*	*c*	*g/kg DM*		
					CP	ERDP	DUP
(a) Calculation from ERDP and DUP of individual ingredients							
Silage	0.5	0.619	0.268	0.130	168	56	31
Supplement	0.5						
Sugar beet pulp	0.11	0.324	0.883	0.031	121	6.7	4.9
Barley	0.22	0.245	0.697	0.350	129	21.6	4.4
Maize gluten feed	0.10	0.609	0.357	0.090	220	14.9	3.8
Rapeseed meal	0.07	0.323	0.608	0.160	400	18.6	4.7
MP from ERDP or DUP							
(g/kg DM)						75	49
MP (g/kg DM)							124
(b) Calculation from average degradability coefficients for supplement							
Silage:	0.5	0.619	0.268	0.130	168	56	31
Supplement:	0.5	0.346	0.657	0.201	183	69	29
MP from ERDP or DUP							
(g/kg DM)						80	60
MP (g/kg DM)							140

In conclusion, it is the author's view that accurate description of the pattern of degradation is more important than force-fitting of equations which have little biological justification. The MP system is insufficiently flexible in this regard.

Energy availability and FME

The approach used by AFRC (1992) to describe the energy available to sustain microbial growth can be criticised on several grounds. A reminder of our objective may be worthwhile. An analogy can be drawn with the prediction of milk protein yield, where we need to know the requirement and supply of both energy and protein, which we choose to define in terms of ME and MP. Similarly, when predicting microbial protein yield, we need to define requirements for both available energy and available protein. Two points may be made regarding the requirement for energy.

Firstly, there is an upper limit to the supply of available energy, a ceiling above which rumen dysfunction is likely. This point will vary according to levels of acids, bases and buffers in the ration. Considerable effort has been devoted to quantifying this limit (e.g. Mertens, 1992; De Visser, 1993). Nocek and Russell (1988) suggested that an optimal diet for a high-yielding cow should contain 0.78 total carbohydrate, of which 0.53 should be rumen-available carbohydrate (RAC, see Nocek and Russell (1988) for definition). Aldrich, Muller, Varga and Griel (1993) stated that 'exact amounts of RAC and [rumen-available] protein that maximise microbial yields are not known'. They formulated diets based on maize and lucerne silage, to supply either 240 or 300 g of rum in ally available non-structural carbohydrate per kg DM. Intake of DM tended to be lower at the higher level of available carbohydrate. Such figures have limited relevance for diets based on grass silage. AFRC (1992) did not define an upper limit for FME, the supply of which cannot, by definition, exceed ME supply.

Secondly, there is a requirement for available energy dictated by the rate of microbial growth, just as there is a requirement for ME dictated by the desired level of milk yield. AFRC (1992) made a real advance by linking the efficiency of utilisation of available energy to the level of animal performance (multiples of maintenance). Thus, FME requirement was predicted to fall from 0.11 MJ/g microbial crude protein at an outflow rate of 0.02/h, to 0.09 MJ/g when outflow rate was 0.08/h, reflecting dilution of the maintenance requirement. However, any praise for the approach used by AFRC (1992) to define the energy requirements of rumen micro-organisms must be tempered by criticisms of the estimations of supply.

The MP system involves a sophisticated description of the rate of N supply to rumen microorganisms, but no attempt is made to account for effects of intake on rumen outflow of FME or to describe the rate of fermentation of FME. For example, increased rates of passage can decrease the extent of starch digestion in the rumen by 10-30% (Mertens, 1992). Tamminga, van Vuuren, van der Koelan, Ketelaar and von der Togt (1990) tabulated rates of fermentation of a variety of carbohydrates. Otherwise, there is a general paucity of data, which limits our ability to formulate rations to ensure synchrony between N and energy supply to rumen microorganisms. This pre-supposes, of course, that benefits will result from improved synchrony.

Rumen synchrony can be defined as 'ensuring the optimal ratio between N and energy supply to rumen microorganisms throughout the 24 hours of the day'. Experiments purporting to examine the concept of rumen synchrony often confound differences in rate of degradation or fermentation with differences in extent. Treatment effects are then ascribed erroneously to improved or reduced synchrony, when they could simply reflect differences in total daily nutrient supply, or in the ratio of daily N supply to daily energy supply (e.g. Herrera-Saldana, Gomez-Alarcon, Torabi and Huber, 1990).

Newbold and Rust (unpublished) proposed a simple model which used patterns of fermentation and degradation of OM and CP to formulate diets to provide the same total daily supply of degraded N and fermented OM, in either synchronous or asynchronous patterns. Sinclair, Garnsworthy, Newbold and Buttery (1993) developed this model and offered sheep complete diets formulated for high or low degrees of synchrony (represented by a 'Synchrony Index', where 0=low, 1=high). The efficiency of microbial protein growth (g N/kg OM apparently digested in the rumen) was 33.8 at a Synchrony Index of 0.58 rising to 41.6 at a Synchrony Index of 0.93. These data illustrate the benefits possible by formulating diets according to the rate at which energy, as well as protein, becomes available to rumen micro-organisms.

The choice of FME as the index of ruminally-available energy is not helpful, for a number of reasons. The first difficulty is philosophical. How can an index of the energy metabolisable by the animal (absorbed, but not yet utilised) provide the basis for an index of the energy metabolisable by rumen microorganisms (pre-absorption)? In order to obtain estimates of ME, losses of energy in faeces, urine and (in ruminants) methane, are deducted from GE. Some of the energy in faeces is in the form of rumen microorganisms (i.e. microbial NE), while energy in methane represents an inefficiency in microbial energy utilisation (logically, part of the difference between microbial ME and microbial NE): deduction of these components from GE in order to obtain an estimate of energy available to rumen micro-organisms (FME) is nonsensical. On these grounds, estimation of fermentable gross energy (FGE, or effective FGE, by analagy with ERDP) would seem preferable. However, this point is entirely academic if requirements for both FGE and FME are derived by empirical extrapolation from earlier estimates of microbial protein yield per unit organic matter digested (ARC, 1984). In such circumstances, estimates of requirements for FGE and FME would be correlated perfectly.

A second criticism of the term FME concerns its definition, by AFRC (1992), as 'ME -ME in oil -ME in fermentation end-products'. It is surprising that no attempts were made to discount undegradable protein, starch and cell wall when calculating FME. Beever and Cottrill (1994) pointed out that the published estimate (AFRC, 1992) of FME of fishmeal is 85% of the ME value (i.e. only 15% non-fermentable), even though approximately 56% of ME is in the form of undegradable protein. The concentration of FME in high-protein compound foods and supplements will overestimate the supply of energy to rumen microorganisms. Alternatives to FME (or FGE) are to revert to ruminally digestible organic matter (ARC, 1980) or to use RAC (Nocek and Russell, 1988). It is easy to formulate compound diets isoenergetic in terms of ME which contain similar concentrations of oil and protein, but widely different levels of sugar, fermentable starch and degradable cell wall. Such diets would be expected to drive different rates of microbial growth. These differences are reflected in RAC, but not in FME (Figure 13.4). Harstad and VikMo (1985) showed that the efficiency of microbial protein synthesis was related more closely to RAC than to apparently digested OM.

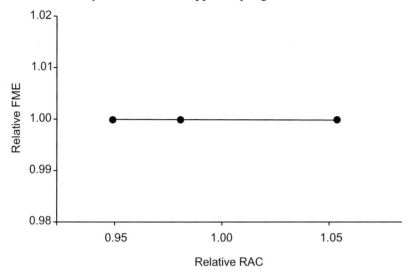

Figure 13.4 Concentrations of FME and ruminally-available carbohydrate (RAC) in three commercial iso-energetic compound feeds

A third criticism of the term FME relates to problems of measurement. A jumble of chemical entities are represented in FME, the estimation of which pools the errors of several analytical techniques. Routine determination of fermentation end-products, such as VFA in silages, to provide FME values for advisory purposes, is not practicable using traditional chromatographic methods. The development of NIR techniques applicable to undried silages (Givens, 1993; Morris, Newbold, Fisher, Wilson, Reece and Ashby, 1994) solves this problem, and values can also be deduced from the titration curve of silage juice (Moisio and Heikonen, 1989).

In conclusion, the term FME is not satisfactory as an index of energy supply to rumen micro-organisms. Alternatives include effective FME or effective FGE, but terms based on defined substrates (i.e. rates of fermentation of defined carbohydrate fractions) offer additional potential advantages as predictors of animal performance (see later). Adoption of such terms would necessitate a re-examination of microbial growth responses to carbohydrate source (and, thus, of carbohydrate requirement for specified rates of microbial growth).

Composition of microbial crude protein

ARC (1980, 1984) assumed that true protein constituted 0.8 of microbial CP. AFRC

(1992) noted evidence from an EAAP ring test which found a mean value of 0.722 across six laboratories, and adopted a value of 0.75. Interestingly, use of 0.72 rather than 0.75 reduces MP supply by approximately 80-100 g/d: broadly equivalent to the discrepancy between MP requirement and supply reported by Newbold *et al.* (1994).

The large standard error (0.072) found in the ring-test suggests that the composition of microbial CP is highly variable. From the review of Clark, Klusmeyer and Cameron (1992) it is evident that, in the long-term, it may be necessary to predict variation in the amino acid composition of microbial CP, according to dietary conditions and rumen ecology. Consequences for methionine flow to the small intestine, using the extremes of the Clark data, are shown in Table 13.3.

Table 13.3 POTENL1AL EFFECT OF VARIATIONS IN METHIONINE CONCENTRATION IN RUMEN MICRO-ORGANISMS ON METHIONINE FLOW TO THE DUODENUM

	Mean	*Min*	*Max*
Methionine in ruminal bacteria (g/l00g amino acids)	2.6	1.1	4.9
Flow of microbial methionine to duodenum (g/d)	29	6	142

(From Clark *et al.,* 1992)

Acid-detergent insoluble nitrogen (ADIN)

The use of ADIN in the calculation of DUP has been criticised by Waters, Kitcherside and Webster (1992) on the grounds that for certain feeds, notably distillery by-products, up to half the AD IN is, in fact, digestible. On the other hand, tannins in feedstuffs such as dried coffee residues may lead to an apparent increase in ADIN through the digestive tract.

Nakamura, Klopfenstein and Britton (1994) pointed out that use of ADIN as an index of intestinal N indigestibility is based on work with heat damaged forage proteins, rather than the unheated, non-forage proteins to which it is now applied so readily. Their data confirm that ADIN is an unreliable index of digestibility in both unheated and heat-treated proteins (Figure 13.5). In a separate experiment, the same authors reported that AD IN accounted for only 0.24 of the variation in true N digestibility among seven dried maize distillers grains sourced from different distilleries. Pass (personal communication) found that the true digestibility of ADIN in rats was 0.85 and 0.75 for distillers dark grains from wheat and barley, respectively. Conversely, true N digestibility was higher for barley than wheat dark grains, implying the existence of other, non- ADIN, indigestible N components in the wheat by-product. Better description of indigestible N fractions is required if sources of UDP are to be differentiated according to efficiency of absorption.

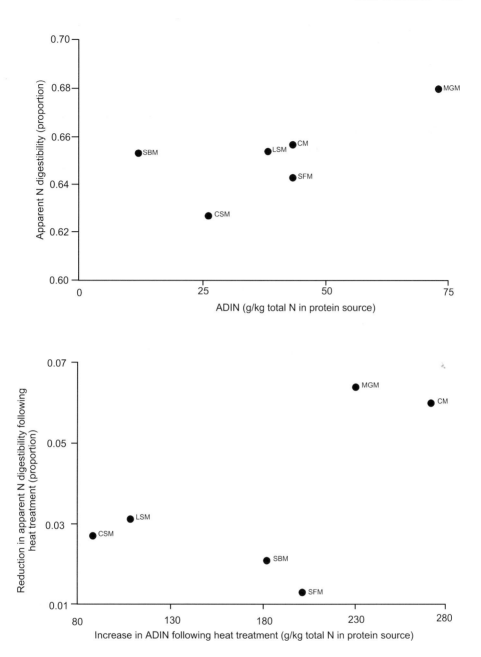

Figure 13.5 Relationships between ADIN and N digestibility. (a) Apparent N digestibility versus ADIN for a variety of unheated non-forage protein sources. (b) Increased ADIN following heat treatment (Maillard reaction) is a poor predictor of change in digestibility. (CM, canola meal; CSM, cottonseed meal; LSM, linseed meal; MGM, maize gluten meal; SBM, soya bean meal; SFM, sunflower meal)

Protein composition of live-weight loss in dairy cows

Estimates of MP supply (or requirement) are sensitive to the protein composition of live-weight loss or gain (AFRC, 1992). The MP system retained data from ARC (1980), which appear to be based on re-calculations of carcass specific gravity data obtained in the mid-1960s. A new set of serial slaughter data is now available (Gibb, Ivings, Dhanoa and Sutton, 1992).

ARC (1980) suggested that the CP composition of empty-body weight change was approximately 150 g/kg, and AFRC (1992) converted this to a live weight basis assuming that liveweight change = 1.09 × empty-body weight change. This ignores variations in gut fill during lactation; in the data of Gibb *et al.* (1992), empty-body weight change (loss) *exceeded* live-weight change (loss) in early lactation, reflecting increasing gut-fill (Figure 13.6). From their data it can be calculated that CP mobilisation represents 99 g/kg empty-body weight loss (during first eight weeks of lactation). Converting to a live weight basis, using reported ratios between empty-body weight change and live-weight change, gives a contribution to MP supply of 130 g CP/kg live-weight loss, very close to the figure of 138 g CP/kg used by AFRC (1992).

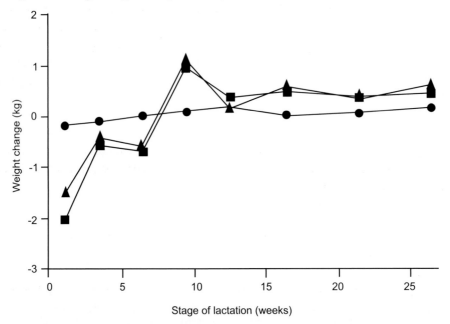

Figure 13.6 Change in live weight (▲), empty-body weight (■) and weight of crude protein in empty body (•) during weeks 0-29 of lactation (Calculated from Gibb *et al.,* 1992)

Estimates of the size of the labile protein reserve in early lactation were reviewed by Journet, Champredon, Pion and Verite (1983), who suggested that between 7 and 13 kg body protein could be mobilised within two to four weeks in early lactation. In the study of Gibb *et al.* (1992), 5.6 kg of body protein were mobilised during the first eight weeks of lactation. Van Saun, Idleman and Sniffen (1993) attempted to manipulate the level of body protein reserves via nutrition of heifers in the three weeks before calving. Heifers fed a high DUP supplement tended to lose less weight and condition in early lactation and gave higher concentrations of milk protein during the first six weeks of lactation, compared with heifers offered a low DUP supplement. Effects on intake post-partum were not determined. A similar study by Hook, Odde, Aguilar and Olson (1989) reported an effect on milk yield, but not composition. Further data on the amino acid composition of mobilised protein are required; it is possible that this complements the pattern of amino acids supplied directly in dietary MP.

Clearly, it is simplistic to describe the cow's physiological state (as the MP system does) simply according to live weight and potential milk yield, without knowing her nutritional history. Changes in protein content of empty body weight in the dataset of Gibb *et al.* (1992) appear predictable from live weight and ultrasound measurements (Ivings, Gibb, Dhanoa and Fisher, 1993). However, routine prediction of MP supply from mobilised reserves (as an alternative to use of current or revised static estimates) will remain problematic for the foreseeable future.

Results of Gibb *et al.* (1992) highlight one further point. The size of the cow's metabolic apparatus changes markedly during lactation. For example, in the first eight weeks, a further 5 m were added to small intestinal length and liver weight increased from 0.016 to 0.021 of empty body weight. Such changes will influence both MP requirement and supply. Absorption of nutrients, including amino acids, may become more efficient as the gut develops, due to a greater flow of blood to a larger absorptive surface area (Oldham, 1984).

In conclusion, better definition of the physiological state of the cow will be central to future 'improved' MP systems. An ideal model would operate over a range of time scales; minute-by-minute, perhaps, in terms of nutrient supply to rumen micro-organisms, and week-by-week, or lactation-by-lactation, in terms of repletion and depletion of labile body amino acid reserves.

THE MP SYSTEM AS A PREDICTOR OF MP REQUIREMENT AND SUPPLY - CONCLUSION

Despite a raft of concerns over the estimation of both MP requirement and supply, available production data suggest that the MP system is sufficiently robust for use in practical dairy farming -although a small increase in MP requirement (or optimal MP:ME ratio) may be advisable. MP offers significant advantages over CP as a predictor of milk protein yield. Across two experiments reported by Newbold *et al.* (1994), MP intake accounted for 0.89 of the variation in milk protein yield: CP intake, by comparison, accounted for only 0.78 (Figure 13.7).

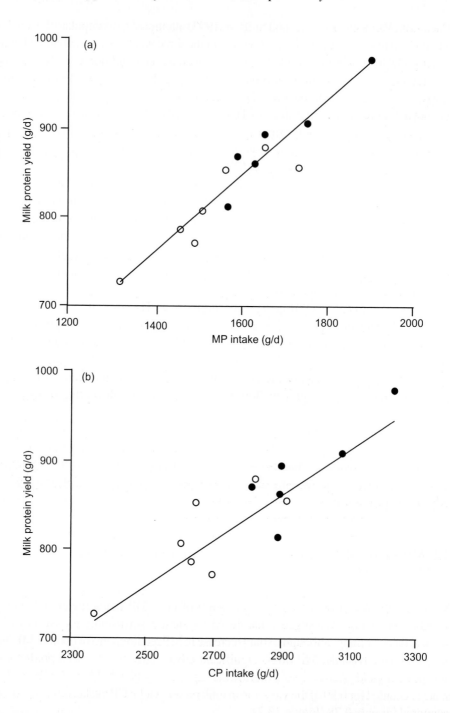

Figure 13.7 Prediction of milk protein yield of multiparous cows from (a) MP intake and (b) CP intake. Each point represents one treatment mean for a four-week period in early lactation from Experiment 1 (●; n=l0) or Experiment 2 (○; n=12) of Newbold *et al.* (1994)

MP, ERDP and FME as predictors of animal response

A clear distinction should be drawn between the MP system of AFRC (1992) and MP. The MP system makes no formal claims regarding the value of MP as a predictor of animal response, other than as a predictor of MP output at or below the optimal MP:ME ratio (Figure 13.2).

Metabolisable protein and other terms defined within the MP system, such as ERDP and FME, could be of use in predicting a range of cow responses to food, all of which are of economic importance (Figure 13.1).

DRY MATTER INTAKE

Positive responses in dry matter intake (DMI) of cows to increased dietary crude protein (CP) concentration are well documented (Oldham and Alderman, 1982). For example, across several studies, Murphy, Gleeson and Morgan (1985) found an average response of 81 g silage DM/d per 10 g/kg DM increase in supplement CP concentration.

These responses could be due partly to effects of protein on digestibility in the rumen, and partly to improved amino acid supply to the animal (Egan, 1965). In the current nomenclature, intake could be a function of both effective rumen degradable protein (ERDP, influencing digestibility) and MP (influencing amino acid supply). Oldham (1984), summarising data collated by Oldham and Alderman (1982) calculated that increases in DMI (per 10 g CP/kg DM) were 420 g/d for maize silage-based diets, and 190 g/d for diets based on grass silage. In high-yielding dairy cows, the ERDP:FME ratio is around 6 g/MJ in maize silage, and 14 g/MJ in grass silage (AFRC, 1992), against a predicted optimum of approximately 11 g/MJ. The implication is that intake responses on grass silage diets are due to MP supply, and responses on maize silage diets due to effects of both MP and ERDP.

Dry matter intake response to MP

Intake responses to MP are often plagued by confounding factors such as ERDP supply and energy source, and may depend upon the MP:ME ratio and the amino acid composition of MP. Experiments in which proteins or amino acids are infused post-ruminally are particularly useful in this respect, since many of these confounding factors can be controlled.

Choung and Chamberlain (1992) infused 230 g casein/d into the abomasa of cows offered grass silage *ad libitum* and 5 kg/d of a barley/soya based concentrate (184 g CP/kg DM). Silage DMI increased by 600 g/d or, assuming casein digestibility is 0.95, 2.7 g DM/g MP. Intake responses to MP are better expressed as a response to MEAA: in the study of Choung and Chamberlain (1992) infusion of soya protein failed to boost intake. Schwab *et al.* (1976) infused caseinate or a variety of amino acid mixtures and observed no response in intake when maize silage was available *ad libitum.* Schwab *et al.* (1976) designed their basal rations to supply 0.70-0.75 of the prevailing NRC CP requirements, while estimates of ME and MP balance suggest the basal diet used by Choung and Chamberlain (1992) was limiting in energy.

These data lead to the suggestion that intake responses to MP (or, rather, MEAA) occur only when energy rather than protein limits animal performance. Supplying more MP in these circumstances creates potential for increased production if the fuel can be found. Consumption of more energy is accompanied invariably by consumption of protein, so that the incremental efficiency of MP use for milk protein synthesis will be less than the theoretical value of 0.68 (AFRC, 1992).

According to Smith (1988), in most of the production experiments reviewed by Oldham (1984), energy supply rather than protein supply, was limiting to performance. Oldham (1984) estimated that, with grass silage diets (ERDP presumed not limiting), each percentage (10 g/kg) increase in dietary CP resulted in extra feed intake, worth 4MJ ME/d, or approximately 23 g/d extra milk protein. From these data, the marginal efficiency of the milk protein yield response to extra MP -mediated through increased ME supply due, in turn, to increased DMI -is approximately 0.2-0.3, depending on the assumptions made (Table 13.4). This is similar to the figure of 0.2 deduced by AFRC (1992) from data from the joint ADAS/GRI/NIRD evaluation of the ARC (1980) proposals and data of Mayne and Gordon (1985).

Experimental reports are available in which feed composition is defined in sufficient detail to allow intake responses to dietary protein to be interpreted in terms of MP. One difficulty, however, is the choice of descriptor of MP supply. Considerable autocorrelation exists when plotting intake as a response to MP 'concentration' which, strictly speaking, does not exist except in association with defined levels of intake. Nor can the amount of supplemental MP be calculated; this, too, depends on intake, and on the characteristics of the rest of the ration. These problems arise because both protein degradability and the efficiency of microbial protein synthesis are linked to level of feeding (ME intake) within the MP system. One solution -adopted in Table 13.4 -is to assume a potential level of intake *a priori,* and use this, within an experiment, to calculate MP supply for all diets.

Newbold *et al.* (1994) defined intake responses to a series of diets differing in MP supply, in which ERDP:FME ratio was constant. Across experimental treatments which were estimated to supply MP in excess of requirement, silage intake increased by approximately 5 g/g MP (calculated from *in situ* degradability measurements and a constant silage intake typical of the herd, Table 13.4). The incremental efficiency of use of this extra MP for milk protein synthesis was approximately 0.4 (Table 13.4).

Various experiments reporting responses to supplemental CP, rather than MP, were selected according to the following criteria: MP and ERDP are estimable from published details of diet composition, ME (rather than MP) appears limiting to performance, grass silage is offered *ad libitum,* and variations in ERDP supply and energy source do not confound seriously responses to MP. A few examples of such studies are shown in

Table 13.4 EXAMPLES OF RESPONSES OF GRASS SILAGE INTAKE AND MILK PROTEIN
YIELD TO INCREASED MP SUPPLY, WHEN MILK PRODUCTION IS LIMITED BY ENERGY
SUPPLY, WITH SILAGE OFFERED *AD LIBITUM*

Reference	Silage intake[1] (g DM/d per g MP)	Milk protein yield[2] (g/d per g MP)
Oldham (1984)	2.2[3]	0.28[4]
Choung and Chamberlain (1992)		
Experiment 1[5]	2.9	0.32
Experiment 2[6,7]	1.8	0.14
Newbold *et al.* (1994)	5.0	0.40
Sutton *et al.* (1993)[7]	1.7	0.26
Davies *et al.* (1992)[8]	1.9	0.25
Cody *et al.* (1990)[9]	1.6	0.19
Small and Gordon (1990)[10]	1.1	0.12

[1]For production experiments (Choung and Chamberlain (1992); Experiment 2, Newbold *et al.* (1994); Sutton *et al.* (1993); Davies *et al.* (1992); Cody *et al.* (1990); Small and Gordon (1980)), the predictor of silage intake is MP supply calculated assuming constant food intake within each experiment

[2]MP supply calculated using reported food intakes

[3]Calculated from reported response of 190 g silage DM/d per 10 g CP/kg DM, assuming total intake = 17 kg DM/d and MP = CP x 0.5

[4]Assuming MP intake = 1500 g/d, total intake = 17 kg DM/d. Then, MP concentration = 88 g/kg DM. MP concentration x 1.1 = 98 g/kg DM x 17 = 1666 g/d.
This increase is associated with 46 g milk protein (assuming milk composition of 40 g/kg fat, 32 g/kg protein, with all additional ME from silage used for milk production). Then, 46/166 = 0.28

[5]Casein infused per abomasum. MP from casein assumed = casein infused x 0.95

[6]Supplementary protein offered via diet

[7]MP supply estimated from published diet composition

[8]MP calculations provided by Alderman (1993)

[9]MP supply estimated from reported degradability coefficients and FME estimated from diet composition

[10]MP supply calculated according to ARC (1980) by Small and Gordon (1990)

Table 13.4. The response of silage intake to MP supply (calculated *a priori* at constant intake) is approximately 1-3 g/g MP, leading to efficiencies of MP use for milk protein synthesis of 0.2-0.3 (Small and Gordon, 1990; Davies, 1992; Sutton, Beever, Aston and Daley, 1993; Table 13.4). Other experiments are more difficult to interpret, with possible confounding effects of energy source or ERDP supply. Choung and Chamberlain (1992) reported a second experiment in which cows were fed concentrates containing 176 or 334 g CP/kg DM. In order to maintain a constant energy concentration, the source of energy varied: starch concentration was 539 g/kg DM in the low protein food and 275 g/kg DM in the high protein food. Apparent effects of protein on intake of silage (which contained 116 g/kg lactic acid) may have been partly due to stabilisation of rumen pH, and thus fibre digestion, consequent upon lower starch supply.

Where MP rather than ME is limiting to performance, intake responses to MP are less apparent, supporting results of infusion experiments such as Schwab *et al.* (1976). In a second experiment, Newbold *et al.* (1994) found no significant response of intake to MP across treatments where MP was predicted to be limiting. At first sight, results of Cody, Murphy and Morgan (1990) appear to contradict this, as intake of grass silage rose from 7.77 kg/d to 8.35 kg/d as MP supply (estimated at silage intake of 7.77 kg/d) rose from 0.86 to 1.11 of requirement. However, this response was not linear, and it could be argued that most of the response of intake to MP occurred between 1.00 and 1.11 of requirement (Figure 13.8).

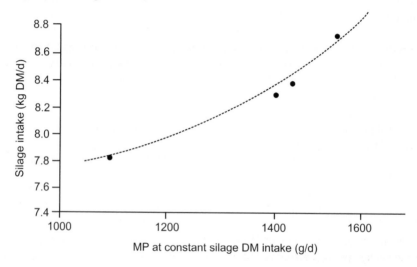

Figure 13.8 Response of silage dry matter intake to MP supply (Estimated from data of Cody *et al.*. 1990)

Increased intake provides one explanation for the continued response of milk protein yield to increments of MP in energy-limited diets (Figure 13.2). The mean incremental efficiency of MP use, consequent upon extra intake of grass silage, in Table 13.4 is 0.25. The range of estimates is quite large (0.12 to 0.41), even allowing for the inaccuracies and assumptions involved in compiling the Table. Webster (1992) stated that the mechanism of the incremental response to MP above requirement was of little relevance in practice, provided that the effect could be quantified. However, an understanding of the mechanism helps decide whether the incremental response is worth exploiting in practice. If forage supplies are limited, it may make more sense to 'buy-in' concentrates to provide ME, rather than boost MP to increase forage intake, as an alternative strategy to raise milk protein yield (Figure 13.2). One would expect little response to MP where intake was under predominantly physical, rather than physiological, control. The extent and efficiency of the intake response to an increment of MP would be expected to vary according to the MP:ME ratio of both the basal diet (i.e. how big is the MP excess?) and the extra food consumed, the amino acid composition of MP, and other changes in nutrient supply associated with a change in MP supply.

ARC (1980) hypothesized that with very high protein:energy ratios, performance may in fact be reduced (Figure 13.2). Negative metabolic effects of excess protein (whether from RDP or MP) are discussed further below, but one possible explanation is reduced intake at very high levels of protein feeding. If silage intake is variable and concentrate intake restricted (a common situation) and if the ERDP:FME ratio in silage is high (e.g. grass silage), one simple way for the cow to control plasma urea and ammonia would be to reduce silage intake. Limited evidence for this is provided by the highest protein treatment (6 kg/d of compound containing 400 g CP/kg DM) in the experiment of Sutton *et al.* (1993): there was no additional increment in silage intake compared with 6 kg/d containing 300 g CP/kg DM. Newbold, Morris and Haggis (unpublished) observed a similar effect in cows fed beyond 1.3 times their estimated MP requirement.

Dry matter intake response to ERDP

Intake responses to ERDP are often observed with straw-based rations, where intake is limited by rate of fibre digestion (Campling, Freer and Balch, 1962; Dias-da-Silva and Sundstol, 1986). Various estimates have been made of minimal ruminal ammonia concentrations required to maximise microbial growth (e.g. Madsen and Hvelplund, 1988). An equation relating minimum ammonia-N concentration to potential digestibility, developed by Erdman, Proctor and Vandersall (1986) predicts a requirement of approximately 140 mg ammonia-N/l for good quality silage, a level exceeded frequently with grass silage-based rations. However, responses to source of ERDP cannot be ruled out (Argyle and Baldwin, 1989).

Evidence for intake responses to ERDP (unconfounded by possible responses to MP) on grass silage diets is, not surprisingly, hard to find. Cody *et al.* (1990) supplemented grass silage with ground barley, such that CP concentration in the total ration was only 142 g/kg DM. Nevertheless, estimates of ERDP supply (using measured degradability coefficients and estimates of fermentable ME) indicate that a small surplus of ERDP was provided.

AFRC (1992) recognised that ERDP requirements (per unit available energy) rise as level of intake increases (efficiency of microbial protein synthesis is a function of level of feeding), but did not formally predict a response of DMI to ERDP:FME ratio. Newbold (1987) outlined an iterative model to account for interactions between RDP supply (ARC, 1980), microbial protein yield and intake.

Dry matter intake response to MP and ERDP -conclusion

While the ERDP:FME ratio has potential value as a predictor of feed intake, responses to MP are likely to be of greater practical significance, at least with diets based on *ad libitum* grass silage. Sufficient data are accumulating to permit empirical, semi-quantitative models of this response, and prediction of the circumstances in which it is likely. This mechanism could account for a large part of the incremental response of milk protein yield to supplemental MP above the optimal MP:ME ratio. It should be noted that neither the MP system nor current methods of predicting intake (AFRC, 1991) were designed to account for intake responses to MP.

BODY COMPOSITION CHANGE

Ørskov, Hughes-Jones and McDonald (1981) suggested that high-DUP supplements could be used as a tool to mobilise body fat in early lactation, depending upon the level of available fat reserves. Support comes from experiments with sheep (Cowan, Robinson, McHattie and Pennie, 1981), although fewer data are available with cows. Ørskov *et al.* (1977) infused casein into the abomasum of cows and reported a doubling of the calculated negative energy balance. Both Garnsworthy and Jones (1987) and Jones and Garnsworthy (1988) found that DUP stimulated fat mobilisation and negative energy balance in fat, but not thin, cows (as judged by changes in Condition Score). Thin cows might be expected to increase intake in response to improved MP status: in fact, the opposite was observed. This could reflect a confounding reduction in ERDP supply when extra DUP was supplied, and limitations imposed on intake by physical bulk of the food (low ME hay).

Mobilisation of body lipid could provide a further explanation of the continued response of milk protein yield to MP above the optimum dietary MP:ME ratio. Whitelaw, Milne, Ørskov and Smith (1986) infused casein *per abomasum* to give a range of MP:ME ratios both above, and slightly below, the predicted optimum for the prevailing milk yield. Calculated fat mobilisation responded to increased MP:ME ratio in a curvilinear manner (Figure 13.9). They argued that at high MP:ME ratios, diversion of amino acids towards gluconeogenesis could increase insulin and partition energy away from milk production towards body deposition. This suggests that the supply of glucogenic precursors will influence the extent of the body fat mobilisation response to increments of MP.

Classically, the balance of VFA generated during rumen fermentation is thought to influence the partition of energy between milk yield and body gain, with the latter favoured when the proportion of propionate is high (Sutton, 1981). Silage fermentation characteristics exert important effects on molar proportions of rumen VFA, with elevated propionate in animals fed extensively-fermented silages rich in lactic acid, and increased butyrate with high sugar, restricted-fermentation silages (Chamberlain and Choung, 1993). Rumen VFA proportions are also influenced by the type of supplemental carbohydrate

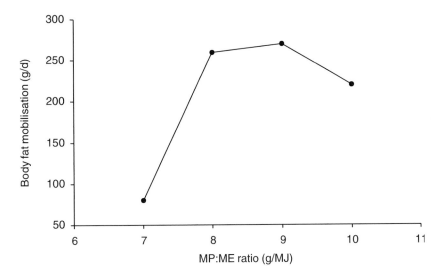

Figure 13.9 Response of estimated body fat mobilisation to MP:ME ratio. MP:ME ratio was manipulated by abomasal infusion of casein at a fixed intake of a mixture of ammonia-treated straw, unmolassed sugar beet pulp, rolled barley, molasses and urea (source Whitelaw *et al.,* 1986)

(Sutton, 1981). FME offers no potential to predict rumen VFA pattern and is not, therefore, a useful nutrient when trying to predict body fat mobilisation.

The effect of rumen VFA pattern, determined by both silage and concentrate composition, on the response of energy-partitioning to MP merits closer study (Lees, Oldham, Haresign and Garnsworthy, 1990). It is possible that the 'choice' between extra intake and more extensive fat mobilisation faced by a cow given MP in excess of requirement is dictated partly by the supply of glucogenic precursors. Studies of Newbold *et al.* (1994), Sutton *et al.* (1993) and Davies (1992), in which marked responses of intake to MP were observed, and in which cows were slowly gaining weight, all involved well-preserved, extensively-fermented silages.

Finally, the energy cost of detoxifying high levels of ammonia may itself worsen the energy status of cows already in negative energy balance. Twigge and van Gils (1984) estimated that 100 g surplus protein could cost 0.8 MJ to process and excrete, equivalent to the ME provided by approximately 50 g liveweight loss (AFRC, 1991). At very high dietary MP:ME ratios, this mechanism could prevent further milk protein yield responses to MP, as energy is diverted towards the detoxification process.

In summary, responses of body fat mobilisation to MP are quantified poorly in cows. Inadequate understanding of interactions between MP supply and level of tissue energy reserves, and between MP and products of carbohydrate digestion, limits our ability to predict fat mobilisation.

MILK PROTEIN YIELD RESPONSE

Milk protein yield response to MP above optimal MP:ME ratio

Two mechanisms by which increments of MP above requirement may support additional milk protein production have already been identified -increased dry matter intake and body fat mobilisation. There may be others.

It is possible that milk protein production could be limited by amino acid supply in a diet that appears adequate in MP. Additional MP will elicit a further response in milk protein production, with an efficiency dependent upon the concentration of the limiting amino acid within the extra MP supplied.

The use made of k_{AA1} within the MP system implies, firstly, that EAA are used only as precursors for milk protein synthesis, and, secondly, that non-essential amino acids are of no value. When MP is limiting, oxidation of EAA would be expected to be minimal (but dependent upon RV), to conserve a scarce resource. However, when MP is not limiting, and assuming no additional ME supply from extra intake or from body tissue mobilisation, use of a proportion of additional MP as ME (with the remainder used for milk protein synthesis) could support continued milk protein production, with an efficiency of MP use of around 0.2 (Oldham, 1994).

Bruckental, Oldham and Sutton (1980) concluded that only 0.02-0.03 of the glucose requirement for lactogenesis was met by amino acids, when protein was limiting. In contrast Dado, Mertens and Shook (1993) have argued, in a recent modelling exercise, that approximately 10% of glucose is derived from amino acids, even when protein is limiting to performance. This led them to estimate that, for milk containing 48 g/kg lactose, 35 g/kg fat and 33 g/kg protein, MP was used mainly for milk protein synthesis (0.763 of MP supply), but with significant amounts used for lactose and fat synthesis (0.141 and 0.096 of MP supply, respectively, mainly due to metabolism of amino acid-derived glucose). Dado *et al.* (1993) calculated that k_l (for MP, not MEAA) *rose* from 0.68 when no amino acids were used for glucose synthesis, to 0.90 when 0.1 of glucose supply was derived from amino acids, reflecting constructive use of non-essential amino acids which would otherwise be wasted. Interestingly, from data of Schwab *et al.* (1976), the efficiency of use of MP (from abomasal infusions of amino acids) for milk protein synthesis was greater (approximately 0.75) for a mixture of essential and non-essential amino acids than for EAA alone (0.67). If the ideal amino acid mixture is defined empirically as in ARC (1984) as 'that which leads to the highest utilisation of [metabolisable] protein', that mixture must include non-essential amino acids used for glucose synthesis, in addition to EAA. The estimate of 0.90 for k_{AA1} by Dado *et al.* (1993) compares reasonably well with the figure of 0.85 of AFRC (1992).

When protein is not limiting to milk protein synthesis, and amino acids do not limit the supply of glucose precursors (i.e. both MP:ME ratio and aminogenic:glucogenic precursor ratio supra-optimal), Oldham (1994) has argued that the efficiency of utilisation of additional MP could be around 0.25, due to use of glucogenic amino acids to generate lactose.

Milk protein yield response to FME

The impact of quantity and source of carbohydrate on milk component yield has been reviewed by De Visser (1993). The relationship between ruminal VFA pattern and milk protein concentration is contentious; Rook and Balch (1961) reported milk protein concentration responses to increased propionate supply, while more recent studies have indicated little or no effect (Hurtaud, Rulquin and Verite, 1992). Seal and Reynolds (1993) suggested that elevated propionate production could spare amino acids which would otherwise have been used for glucose production within intestinal tissues, thereby promoting MP supply at the mammary level.

Description of fermentable dietary components in terms of sugar, starch, cell walls and protein offers the potential to predict ruminal VF A pattern (Murphy, Baldwin and Koong, 1981), although factors affecting the stoichiometry remain poorly understood. Description of fermentable dietary components in terms of FME offers no such potential: FME is only useful in predicting milk protein yield through its use as an intermediate in the calculation of MP supply.

Milk protein yield response to MP and FME -summary

Milk protein yield responds to MP supplied above the optimal dietary MP:ME ratio, with a low and probably diminishing efficiency (approximately 0.2-0.3). Most of this response is, in fact, due to increased supply of energy, and the animal may be seeking, within restrictions imposed by her physiological state, diet and environment, to maintain an optimal protein:energy ratio at the metabolisable level. Faced with excess MP, the cow can pursue a number of strategies to obtain extra energy, and push the MP:ME ratio down towards the optimum. Options of increasing intake and mobilising body fat may be mutually exclusive (Figure 13.10). Increasing intake of a food in which the MP:ME ratio is sub-optimal (e.g. grass or maize silage) will frequently be an option in UK dairy farming systems, especially if cows carry low fat reserves or factors such as hormonal status inhibit fat mobilisation. If extra food intake is not possible - due, for example, to physical bulk of food, excessive body fat or managerial inadequacies on farm - then selective mobilisation of body fat is an alternative way of supporting a continued milk protein yield response to MP. Even if neither food intake nor body fat mobilisation can respond to MP, oxidation of a proportion of the surplus MP might maintain a constant MP:ME ratio in nutrients supplied to animal tissues.

The hypothesis could be widened to state that the cow seeks an optimum balance between oxidative, aminogenic, lipogenic and glucogenic substrates. Thus, even at optimal dietary MP:ME ratio, an imbalance between aminogenic and glucogenic precursors could promote gluconeogenesis from amino acids, leading to continued, relatively inefficient, milk protein yield responses to MP.

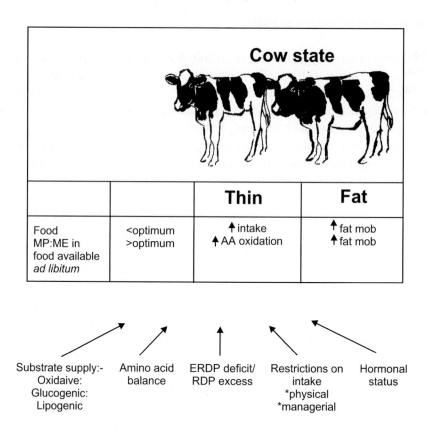

Figure 13.10 Some factors which may affect the strategy chosen by a cow to optimise MP:ME ratio when fed surplus MP

Responses to MP above the optimum dietary MP:ME ratio are of major practical importance. With the unit cost of dietary MP low, in relation to that of ME, in recent years, farmers and advisors have become accustomed to high protein diets and may, subconsciously, routinely be exploiting responses to MP above the optimal MP:ME ratio (i.e. obtaining y2, Figure 13.2, by feeding cows ME commensurate with y1, and MP3, rather than ME commensurate with y2, and MP2). Consequently, adoption of the MP system as published by AFRC (1992), without any allowance for the incremental response to MP above requirement, could in many cases lead to low silage intake and disappointing milk protein yields, albeit with a higher efficiency of protein use, relative to past experience on that farm. The decision to exploit responses of intake, body fat mobilisation, amino acid oxidation or gluconeogenesis to MP in energy limiting rations will depend upon farm circumstances, relative costs of MP and ME, and, perhaps, external restrictions on the efficiency of N use in order to control pollution.

MILK FAT YIELD

Increased dietary CP can result in reduced milk fat concentration, due to increased milk volume, with little effect on fat yield. Variations in milk fat concentration following delivery of amino acids into the small intestine (via infusion or rumen protection technology) are small, ranging from -4.3 to +5.6 g/kg in studies reviewed by Rulquin and Verite (1993), with an average response of +0.1g/kg.

Direct mechanisms could include increased production of microbial lipid due to enhanced methionine supply or direct effects of methionine on milk fat synthesis in the mammary gland (Chamberlain and Thomas, 1982). Dado *et at.* (1993) rationalised the contribution of amino acids to milk fat synthesis partly by assuming a requirement of 10 g MP/kg milk fat for synthesis of the alveolar apical membrane enveloping milk fat globules. Use of MP for milk fat synthesis, as a proportion of use for protein, was predicted to rise from 0.015 when glucose was synthesised entirely from propionate to 0.13 when 0.1 of glucose was derived from amino acids, reflecting use of A TP generated from amino acids. Such considerations provide one explanation for the positive response in milk fat concentration to MP (duodenal casein infusion) observed in early lactation when cows were in severe negative energy balance (Ørskov, Grubb and Kay, 1977).

Effects of carbohydrate supply, via ruminal VFA pattern, on milk fat are much clearer than effects on milk protein: according to Sutton (1993) variation in ruminal VF A proportions between low and high starch diets can account for more than 70% of the variation in milk fat concentration. Once again, FME is of little value in predicting such effects, compared with alternative indices such as RAC.

In conclusion, MP may be of some use in predicting the supply of lipogenic, as well as glucogenic and aminogenic, precursors for milk synthesis. Prediction of these substrates is essential to the development of feed evaluation systems capable of predicting milk component concentrations ('designer milks') as well as yields.

FERTILITY AND HEALTH

The extent of body compositional change in early lactation is often cited as the most important link between nutrition and fertility (Garnsworthy and Haresign, 1989). In light of links between MP supply and body composition, this could help explain responses of fertility to dietary protein, although there may be more direct effects.

Staples, Thatcher, Garcia-Bojalil and Lucy (1992) reviewed eight studies in which conception rate was monitored in cows fed diets with moderate or high percentages of dietary crude protein. On average, there was a 12 percentage point reduction in conception rate as dietary CP increased from 130-160 g/kg DM to 190-210 g/kg DM. Carroll, Barton, Anderson and Smith (1988) reported a higher incidence of assisted calvings, dystocia, cystic ovaries and metritis in cows fed rations of 200g CP/kg compared with those fed 130g CP/kg.

The explanation for these responses is probably multi-factorial. Effects on the pituitary-ovarian axis appear minor, at least over the range of dietary protein levels found in practice (Jordan and Swanson, 1979). High blood urea leads to high urea in vaginal mucus, and urea is a known toxin for both ova and sperm (Ferguson and Chalupa, 1989). Ferguson, Blanchard, Galligan, Hoshall and Chalupa (1988) found conception rates falling when serum urea rose above approximately 20 mg/l. Such North American studies may have limited direct relevance where irregular feeding may accentuate diurnal variations in blood urea (Jordan *et al.*, 1983). Staples *et al.* (1992) proposed that, if progesterone is depressed by high urea or ammonia, the immunosuppressive effect of progesterone may be depressed, leading a failure of maternal recognition and rejection of the embryo.

Sub-toxic effects of ammonia affect aspects of metabolism other than fertility, largely via effects on liver metabolism (Visek, 1984; Chamberlain and Choung, 1993). Liver damage due to ammonia may account, in part, for adverse effects of increased dietary crude protein on lameness reported by Manson and Leaver (1988).

In terms of predicting responses of lameness, fertility and, possibly, other metabolic disorders, all of which are traceable to sub-toxic plasma ammonia and urea levels, ERDP may be a more useful nutrient than MP. Ferguson and Chalupa (1989) re-interpreted seven experiments reporting effects of dietary CP on fertility in terms of the NRC (1989) 'absorbable protein' system (an analogue of ARC, 1980) with RDP calculated from tables of protein degradability. Most of the response of fertility to CP could be explained by RDP. Similar models could be developed using the nutrients ERDP and MP, as defined by AFRC (1992).

In fact, ERDP may not be the most useful nutrient: 0.2 of quickly-degraded protein may be ineffective as a source of N for microbial protein, but highly effective in raising plasma urea and ammonia concentrations. Similarly, FME may not be the best way to predict how much degradable N is captured by rumen microorganisms, and how much remains uncaptured.

In practice there would seem to be no conflict between optimising the diet for maximum milk production, according to AFRC (1992), and optimising the diet for fertility and health. Rations which precisely meet needs for MP and ERDP should provide little excess N to boost plasma urea and ammonia. Further work is required to improve predictions of fertility from ERDP (and/or quickly-degraded protein), using diets based on grass silage.

Animal responses versus group responses

One reason for formulating rations using nutrient requirements plus a safety margin (to give an allowance) is to ensure that the nutrient needs of a reasonable majority of individuals within a group are satisfied. Some insight into the variability within the group (e.g. in milk yield) permits calculation of the safety margin required, although this is beyond the scope of this chapter.

Rations are formulated for individuals (e.g. a standard cow yielding a defined amount of milk) but are often fed to groups. Alternatively, cows may be allocated an amount of concentrate individually, and allowed *ad libitum* access to forage.

Using the MP system, rations can be formulated which satisfy a requirement for MP at any level of ME intake. However, this MP:ME ratio will only be optimal for the particular animal rationed. The ratio of MP requirement:ME requirement increases as level of production rises (Figure 13.11), so that, within a group, cows yielding less than the individual being rationed will receive excess MP. Overall efficiency of MP utilisation within the group will be less than that predicted for the individual.

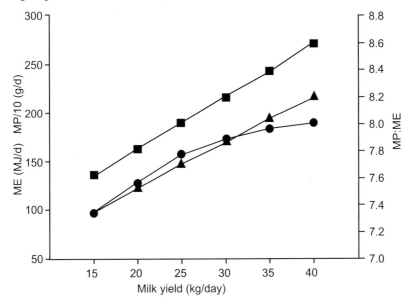

Figure 13.11 Effect of milk yield on requirements for ME (■) and MP (▲) calculated from AFRC (1990) and AFRC (1992). (● = MP:ME ratio). Assumptions: milk fat 40 g/kg; milk protein 32 g/kg; live weight 600 kg; live-weight change 0; no safety allowance used

This effect is mitigated against where restricted concentrate is offered alongside *ad libitum* forage, if (as is likely) the MP:ME ratio in the concentrate exceeds that in the forage. Reducing the allocation of concentrate will tend to reduce the ratio of MP:ME in the total diet, following the curve of optimal MP:ME ratio as yield declines. Of couse, the MP:ME ratio in a specific feedstuff depends upon other ration components, and the extent of this fall in MP:ME will depend upon composition of both concentrate and forage.

Further development of the MP system

Two conclusions seem "de rigueur" with this kind of chapter. Firstly, the author almost always says that 'further research is required on...' and proceeds to give a long list of topics and projects, without much thought to the practicality of the work proposed.

Because, as seems likely, dairy cows are often fed diets containing excess MP, research to clarify, quantify and predict different responses (e.g. intake, body fat mobilisation) to MP when MP:ME ratio is above optimum could be of as much practical value as further efforts to refine estimates of MP supply.

Continued effort is required to improve estimates of MP requirement and supply (Table 13.5). Oldham (1993) concluded that the MP system was fundamentally untestable, since methodologies for measuring MP supply are so unreliable. However, it is on such methodologies that the MP system was built. Techniques such as the use of the urinary excretion of purine derivatives to monitor microbial protein production (Dewhurst and Webster, 1992) may offer alternatives.

Table 13.5 METABOLISABLE PROTEIN: SOME PRIORITIES FOR FUTURE RESEARCH

---

1   *Responses to MP*

Limiting efficiency of utilisation of individual amino acids
Food intake and fat mobilisation responses to MP
   quantification and limits
   factors affecting
      animal state (level of fat reserves)
      composition of increments of food intake
Milk protein yield response to MP
   factors determining whether response due to enhanced milk yield or enhanced milk
   protein concentration
      supply of aminogenic and glucogenic precursors

---

2   *Ruminal responses to protein and energy*

Upper limits to supply of fermentable energy
Optimum ratio between degradable N and fermentable energy
Quantification of responses to N source
Synchrony between rate of supply of N and energy

---

3   *Estimation of MP, ERDP, FME*

Prediction of amino acid composition of microbial protein
Replacement of FME by term descriptive of carbohydrate quality and responsive to
  rumen outflow rate
Alternative methodologies for estimating rate of protein degradation
Quantification and composition of mobilised tissue protein

The second obligatory conclusion seems to be a plea for more mechanistic modelling to account for biochemical interactions affecting protein use. An intellectually satisfying predictive model combining accuracy with generality seems as elusive as ever. However, sharper focus on ME and MEAA as dietary components, and the introduction of the MP system as a means of estimating MP and MEAA supply, makes the development of a semi-empirical model encompassing a range of responses of animals of defined physiological state to supply of glucogenic, oxidative, amino genic and lipogenic substrates, a more realistic goal.

References

Agricultural and Food Research Council (1990) Technical Committee on Responses to Nutrients, Report No.5. Nutritive Requirements of Ruminant Animals: Energy. *Nutrition Abstracts and Reviews (Series B)*, **60,** 729-804

Agricultural and Food Research Council (1991) Technical Committee on Responses to Nutrients, Report No.8. Voluntary Intake of Cattle. *Nutrition Abstracts and Reviews (Series B)*, **61,** 815-823

Agricultural and Food Research Council (1992) Technical Committee on Responses to Nutrients, Report No.9. Nutritive Requirements of Ruminant Animals: Protein. *Nutrition Abstracts and Reviews (Series B)*, **62**, 787-835

Agricultural and Food Research Council (1993) *Energy and Protein Requirements of Ruminants.* Edited by G. Alderman in collaboration with B.R. Cottrill. Wallingford: CAB International

Agricultural Research Council (1980) *The Nutrient Requirements of Ruminant Livestock, No.2, Ruminants.* Farnham Royal: Commonwealth Agricultural Bureaux

Agricultural Research Council (1984) *The Nutrient Requirements of Ruminant Livestock, Supplement No.1.* Farnham Royal: Commonwealth Agricultural Bureaux

Ainslie, S.J., Fox, D.G., Perry, T.C., Ketchen, D.J. and Barry, M.C. (1993) Predicting amino acid adequacy of diets fed to Holstein steers. *Journal of Animal Science,* **71**, 1312-1319

Alderman, G. (1993) ADAS Pwllpeiran Experiment. *CEDAR Update,* 1 (4), 7-8

Aldrich, J.M., Muller, L.D., Varga, G.A. and Griel, L.C. (1993) Non-structural carbohydrate and protein effects on rumen fermentation, nutrient flow, and performance of dairy cows. *Journal of Dairy Science,* **76**, 1091-1105

Argyle, J.L. and Baldwin, R.L. (1989) Effects of amino acids and peptides on rumen microbial growth yields. *Journal of Dairy Science,* **72**, 2017-2027

Arieli, A., Mabjeesh. S., Tagari, H., Bruckental, I. and Zamwel, S. (1993) Evaluation of protein flow to the duodenum in dairy cattle by the *in sacco* method. *Livestock Production Science,* **35**, 283-292

Beever, D.E. and Cottrill, B.R. (1994) Protein systems for feeding ruminant livestock: an international perspective. *Journal of Dairy Science,* **77**, 2031-2043

Bruckental, I. Oldham, J.D. and Sutton, J.D. (1980) Glucose and urea kinetics in cows in early lactation. *British Journal of Nutrition,* **44**, 33-45

Campling, R.C., Freer, M. and Balch, C.C. (1962) Factors affecting the voluntary intake of food by cows. 3: The effect of urea on the voluntary intake of oat straw. *British Journal of Nutrition,* **16**, 115-124

Carroll, D.J., Barton, B.A., Anderson, G.W. and Smith, R.D. (1988) Influence of protein intake and feeding strategy on reproductive performance of dairy cows. *Journal of Dairy Science,* **71**, 3470-3481

Chamberlain, D.G. and Thomas, P.C. (1982) Effect of intravenous supplements of L-methionine on milk yield and composition in cows given silage-cereal diets. *Journal of Dairy Research,* **49**, 25-28

Chamberlain, D.G. and Choung, J.J. (1993) The nutritional value of grass silage. In *Proceedings of the 10th International Conference on Silage Research,* pp. 131-136. Edited by P.O'Kiely, M.O'Connell and J.Murphy. Dublin: Dublin City University

Choung, J.J. and Chamberlain, D.G. (1992) Protein nutrition of dairy cows receiving grass silage diets. Effects of silage intake and milk production of postruminal supplements of casein or soya-protein isolate and the effects of intravenous infusions of a mixture of methionine, phenylalanine and tryptophan. *Journal of the Science of Food and Agriculture,* **58**, 307-314

Clark, J.H., Klusmeyer, T.H. and Cameron, M.R. (1992) Microbial protein synthesis and flows of nitrogen fractions to the duodenum of dairy cows. *Journal of Dairy Science,* **75**, 2304-2323

Cockburn, J.E., Dhanoa, M.S, France, J. and Lopez, S. (1993) Overestimation of solubility by polyester bag methodology. *Animal Production,* **56**, 466-467

Cody, R.F., Murphy, J.J. and Morgan, D.J. (1990) Effect of supplementary crude protein level and degradability in grass silage-based diets on performance of dairy cows, and digestibility and abomasal nitrogen flow in sheep. *Animal Production,* **51**, 235-244

Cottrill, B.R. (1993) Characterisation of nitrogen in ruminant feeds. In *Recent Advances in Animal Nutrition* -1993, pp. 39-54. Edited by P.C. Garnsworthy and D.J.A. Cole. Nottingham: Nottingham University Press

Cowan, R.T., Robinson, J.J., McHattie, I. and Pennie, K. (1981) Effects of protein concentration in the diet on milk yield, change in body composition and the efficiency of utilisation of body tissue for milk production in ewes. *Animal Production,* **33**, 111-120

Curnow, R.N. (1973) A smooth population response curve based on an abrupt threshold and plateau model for individuals. *Biometrics,* **29**, 1-10

Dado, R.G., Mertens, D.R. and Shook, G.E. (1993) Metabolisable energy and absorbed protein requirements for milk component production. *Journal of Dairy Science,* **76**, 1575-1588

Davies, O.D. (1992) The effects of protein and energy content of compound supplements offered at low levels to October-calving dairy cows given grass silage *ad libitum*. *Animal Production,* **55**, 169-176

De Visser, H. (1993) Characterisation of carbohydrates in compound feeds. In *Recent Advances in Animal Nutrition* -1993, pp. 19-38. Edited by P.C. Garnsworthy and D.J.A. Cole. Nottingham: Nottingham University Press

Dewhurst, R.J. and Webster, A.J.F. (1992) Effects of diet, level of intake, sodium bicarbonate and monensin on urinary allantoin excretion in sheep. *British Journal of Nutrition,* **67**, 345-353

Dhanoa, M.S. (1988) On the analysis of dacron bag data for low degradability feeds. *Grass and Forage Science,* **43**, 441-444

Dias-da-Silva, A.A. and Sundstol, F. (1986) Urea as a source of ammonia for improving the nutritive value of wheat straw. *Animal Feed Science and Technology,* **14**, 67-79

Egan, A.R. (1965) Nutritional status and intake regulation in sheep. II. The influence of sustained duodenal infusions of casein or urea upon voluntary intake of non-protein roughages by sheep. *Australian Journal of Agricultural Research,* **16**, 451-462

Erdman, R.A., Proctor, G.H. and Vandersall, J.H. (1986) Effects of rumen ammonia concentration on *in situ* rate and extent of digestion of feedstuffs. *Journal of Dairy Science,* **69**, 2312-2320

Ferguson, J.D. and Chalupa, W. (1989) Impact of protein nutrition on reproduction in dairy cows. *Journal of Dairy Science,* **72**, 746-766

Ferguson, J.D., Blanchard, T., Galligan, D.T., Hoshall, D.C. and Chalupa, W. (1988) Infertility in dairy cattle fed a high percentage of protein degradable in the rumen. *Journal of the American Veterinary Medicine Association,* **192**, 659

Garnsworthy, P .C. and Haresign, W. (1989) Fertility and Nutrition. In *Dairy Cow Nutrition - The Veterinary Angles,* pp. 23-34. Edited by A.T.Chamberlain. Reading: University of Reading

Garnsworthy, P.C. and Jones, G.P. (1987) The influence of body condition at calving and dietary protein supply on voluntary food intake and performance in dairy cows. *Animal Production,* **44**, 347-353

Gibb, M.J., Ivings, W.E., Dhanoa, M.S. and Sutton, J.D. (1992) Changes in body components of autumn-calving Holstein-Friesian cows over the first 29 weeks of lactation. *Animal Production,* **55**, 339-360

Givens, D.I. (1993) The role of NIRS for forage evaluation -the present and future. In 'NIR Spectroscopy -Developments in Agriculture and Food', Proceedings of an International Conference, ADAS Drayton Feed Evaluation Unit

Harstad, O.M. and VikMo, L. (1985) Estimation of microbial and undegraded protein in sheep on grass silage based diets. *Acta Agriculturae Scandinavica,* Supplement 25, 37

Herrera-Saldana, R., Gomez-Alarcon, R., Torabi, M. and Huber, J.T. (1990) Influence of sunchronizing protein and starch degradation in the rumen on nutrient utilisation and microbial protein synthesis. *Journal of Dairy Science,* **73**, 142-148

Hook, T.E., Odde, K.G., Aguilar, A.A. and Olson, J.D. (1989) Protein effects on fetal growth, clostrum and calf immunoglobulins and lactation in dairy heifers. *Journal of Animal Science,* 67 (Supplement 1), 539

Huntington, G.B., Reynolds, C.K. and Stroud, B. (1989) Techniques for measuring blood flow in the splanchnic tissues of cattle. *Journal of Dairy Science,* **72**, 1583-1595

Hurtaud, C., Rulquin, H. and Verite, R. (1992) Effects on milk yield and composition of infusions of different levels and natures of energy into the digestive tract of dairy cows. *Annales Zootechnologie,* **41**, 105

Institut Nationale Recherche Agronomique (1988) *Alimentation des Bovins, Ovins et Caprins.* Edited by R.Jarrige. Paris: INRA

Ivings, W .E., Gibb, M.J., Dhanoa, M.S. and Fisher, A. V. (1993) Relationships between velocity of ultrasound in live lactating dairy cows and some post- slaughter measurements of body composition. *Animal Production,* **56**, 9-16

Jones, G.P. and Garnsworthy, P.C. (1988) The effects of body condition at calving and dietary protein content on dry matter intake and performance in lactating dairy cows given diets of low energy content. *Animal Production,* **47**, 321-333

Jordan, E.R. and Swanson, L. V. (1979) Serum progesterone and luteinizing hormone in dairy cattle fed varying levels of crude protein. *Journal of Animal Science,* **48**, 1154-1158

Jordan, E.R., Chapman, T.E., Holtan, D.E. and Swanson, L.V. (1983) Relationships of dietary crude protein to composition of uterine secretions and blood in high-producing dairy cows. *Journal of Dairy Science,* **66**, 1854-1862

Journet, M., Champredon, C., Pion, R. and Verite, R. (1983) Physiological basis of the protein nutrition of high producing cows. In *Protein Metabolism and Nutrition, Proceedings of the Fourth International Symposium,* pp. 433-447. Edited by M.Arnal, R.Pion and D.Bonin. Paris: INRA

Lees, J.A., Oldham, J.D., Haresign, W. and Garnsworthy, P.C. (1990) The effect of patterns of rumen fermentation on the response by dairy cows to dietary protein concentration. *British Journal of Nutrition,* **63**, 177-186

Lindsay, D.B. (1993) Metabolism of the portal-drained viscera. In *Quantitative Aspects of Ruminant Digestion and Metabolism,* pp. 268-289. Edited by J.M. Forbes and J. France. Wallingford: CAB International

Madsen, J. and Hvelplund, T. (1988) The influence of different protein supply and feeding level on pH, ammonia concentration and microbial protein synthesis in the rumen of cows. *Acta Agriculturae Scandinavica,* **38**, 115-125

Madsen, J. and Hvelplund, T. (1994) Prediction of *in situ* protein degradability in the rumen. Results of a European ringtest. *Livestock Production Science,* **39**, 201-212

Manson, F.J. and Leaver, J.D. (1988) The influence of dietary protein intake and of hoof trimming on lameness in dairy cattle. *Animal Production,* **47**, 191-199

Mayne, C.S. and Gordon, F.J. (1985) The effect of concentrate-to-forage ratio on the milk yield response to supplementary protein. *Animal Production,* **41,** 269-280

Mepham, T .B. (1982) Amino acid utilization by the lactating mammary gland. *Journal of Dairy Science,* **65**, 287-298

Mertens, D.R. (1992) Nonstructural and structural carbohydrates. In *Large Dairy Herd Management,* pp.219-235. Edited by H.H.Van Horn and C.J.Wilcox. Champaign, IL.: ADSA

Moisio, T. and Heikonen, M. (1989) A titration method for silage assessment. *Animal Feed Science and Technology,* **22**, 341-353

Morris, H. W., Newbold, J.R., Fisher, S.P., Reece, M.N., Wilson, S. and Ashby, C. W. (1994) Analysis of undried silage by near-infrared spectroscopy. *Animal Production,* **58,** 475 (Abst)

Murphy, J.J., Gleeson, P.A. and Morgan, D.J. (1985) Effect of protein source in the concentrate on the performance of cows offered grass silage ad libitum. *Irish Journal of Agricultural Research,* **24**, 151-159

Murphy, M.R., Baldwin, R.L. and Koong, L.J. (1982) Estimation of stoichiometric parameters for rumen fermentation of roughage and concentrate diets. *Journal of Animal Science,* **55**, 411-421

Nakamura, T., Klopfenstein, T.J. and Britton, R.A. (1994) Evaluation of acid detergent insoluble nitrogen as an indicator of protein quality in nonforage. *Journal of Animal Science,* **72**, 1043-1048

National Research Council (1989) *Nutrient Requirements of Dairy Cattle.* Washington DC: National Academy Press

Newbold, J .R. (1987) Nutrient requirements of intensively-reared beef cattle. In *Recent Advances in Animal Nutrition* -1987, pp. 143-172. Edited by W. Haresign and D.J.A. Cole. London: Butterworths

Newbold, J.R., Cottrill, B.R., Mansbridge, R.M. and Blake, J.S. (1994) Effect of Metabolisable Protein on silage intake and milk protein yield in dairy cows. *Animal Production,* **58**, 455 (Abst)

Nocek, J .E. (1988) *In situ* and other methods to estimate ruminal protein ad energy digestibility, *Journal of Dairy Science,* **71**, 2051-2069

Nocek, J .E. and Russell, J .B. (1988) Protein and energy as an integrated system. Relationship of ruminal protein and carbohydrate availability to microbial protein synthesis and milk production. *Journal of Dairy Science,* **71**, 2070-2107

Nolan, J. V. (1993) Nitrogen Kinetics. In *Quantitative Aspects of Ruminant Digestion and Metabolism,* pp. 123-144. Edited by J.M. Forbes and J. France. Wallingford: CAB International

O'Connor, J.D., Sniffen, C.J., Fox, D.G. and Chalupa, W. (1993) A net carbohydrate and protein system for evaluating cattle diets. IV. Predicting amino acid adequacy. *Journal of Animal Science,* **71**, 1298-1311

Oldham, J.D. (1984) Protein-energy interrelationships in dairy cows. *Journal of Dairy Science,* **67**, 1090-1114

Oldham, J.D. (1987) Efficiencies of amino acid utilisation. In *Feed Evaluation and Protein Requirement Systems for Ruminants,* pp. 171-186. Edited by R.Jarrige and G .Alderman. Luxembourg: CEC

Oldham, J.D. (1993) Evaluation of the Metabolisable Protein System. *Paper presented to the 107th Winter Meeting of the British Society of Animal Production.*

Oldham, J.D. (1994) Amino acid nutrition of dairy cows. In *Amino Acid Nutrition of Farm Animals.* Edited by J.P.F. D'Mello. Wallingford: CAB International.

Oldham, J.D. and Alderman, G. (1982) Recent advances in understanding protein-energy interrelationships in intermediary metabolism in ruminants. In *Protein and Energy Supply for High Production of Milk and Meat,* pp. 33. Oxford: Pergamon

Ørskov, E.R. and McDonald, I. (1979) The estimation of protein degradability in the rumen from incubation measurements weighted according to rate of passage. *Journal of Agricultural Science, Cambridge,* **92**, 499-503

Ørskov, E.R., Grubb, D.A. and Kay, R.N.B. (1977) Effect of post-ruminal glucose or protein supplementation on milk yield and composition in Friesian cows in early lactation and negative energy balance. *British Journal of Nutrition,* **38**, 397-405

Ørskov, Hughes-Jones and McDonald, I. (1981) Degradability of protein supplements and utilization of undegraded protein by high-producing dairy cows. In *Recent Advances in Animal Nutrition -1980,* pp. 85-98. Edited by W. Haresign. London: Butterworths

Rook, J.A.F. and Balch, C.C. (1961) The effects of intraruminal infusions of acetic, propionic and butyric acids on the yield and composition of the milk of the cow. *British Journal of Nutrition,* **15**, 361-369

Rulquin, H. and Verite, R. (1993) Amino acid nutrition of ruminants. In *Recent Advances in Animal Nutrition -1993,* pp. 55-78. Edited by P .C. Garnsworthy and D.J.A. Cole. Nottingham: Nottingham University Press

Seal, C.J. and Reynolds, C.K. (1993) Nutritional implications of gastrointestinal and liver metabolism in ruminants. *Nutrition Research Reviews,* **6**, 185-208

Schiere, J.B. and de Wit, J. (1993) Feeding standards and feeding systems. *Animal Feed Science and Technology,* **43**, 121-134

Schwab, C.G., Satter, L.D. and Clay, A.B. (1976) Response of lactating dairy cows to abomasal infusion of amino acids. *Journal of Dairy Science,* **59**, 1254-1269

Sinclair, L.A., Garnsworthy, P.C., Newbold, J.R. and Buttery, P.J. (1993) Effect of synchronizing the rate of dietary energy and nitrogen release on rumen fermentation and microbial protein synthesis in sheep. *Journal of Agricultural Science, Cambridge,* **120**, 251-264

Small, J.C. and Gordon, F.J. (1990) A comparison of the responses by lactating cows given grass silage to changes in the degradability or quantity of protein offered in the supplement. *Animal Production,* **50**, 391-398

Smith, N.E. (1988) Alteration of efficiency of milk production in dairy cows by manipulation of the diet. In *Nutrition and Lactation in the Dairy Cow,* pp.216-231. Edited by P .C.Garnsworthy. London: Butterworths

Staples, C.R., Thatcher, W.W., Garcia-Bojalil, C.M. and Lucy, M.C. (1992) Nutritional influences on reproductive function. In *Large Dairy Herd Management,* pp. 382-392. Edited by H.H. Van Horn and C.J. Wilcox. Champaign, IL.: ADSA

Strachan, P.J., Wilson, J.S. and Kelly, N.C. (1987) Response of dairy cows to compounds varying in level and profile of undegradable essential amino acids. *Animal Production,* **44,** 492-493

Sutton, J.D. (1981) Concentrate feeding and milk composition. In *Recent Advances in Animal Nutrition* -1981, pp.35-49. Edited by W. Haresign. London: Butterworths

Sutton, J.D., Bines, J.A., Morant, S.V., Napper, D.J. and Givens, D.I. (1987) *Journal of Agricultural Science, Cambridge,* **109**, 375-386

Sutton, J.D., Beever, D.E., Aston, K. and Daley, S.R. (1993) Milk N fractions in Holstein-Friesian cows as affected by amount and protein concentration of the concentrates. *Animal Production,* **56**, 429

Tamminga, S., van Vuuren, A.M., van der Koelan, C.J., Ketelaar, R.S. and von der Togt, P.L. (1990) *Netherlands Journal of Agricultural Science,* **38**, 513-526

Twigge, J.R. and van Gils, L.G.M. (1984) Practical aspects of feeding protein to dairy cows. In *Recent Advances in Animal Nutrition* -1984, pp. 201-218. Edited by W. Haresign and D.J.A. Cole. London: Butterworths

Van Saun, R.J., Idleman, S.C., and Sniffen, C.J. (1993) Effect of undegradable protein amount fed prepartum on postpartum production in first lactation Holstein cows. *Journal of Dairy Science,* **76**, 236-244

Visek, W.J. (1984) Ammonia: its effects on biological systems, metabolic hormones and reproduction. *Journal of Dairy Science,* **67**, 481-498

Waters, C.J., Kitcherside, M.A. and Webster, A.J.F. (1992) Problems associated with estimating the digestibility of undegraded dietary nitrogen from acid- detergent insoluble nitrogen. *Animal Feed Science and Technology,* **39**, 279-291

Webster, A.J.F. (1992) The Metabolisable Protein System for Ruminants. In *Recent Advances in Animal Nutrition* -1992, pp.93-110. Edited by P.C. Garnsworthy, W. Haresign and D.J.A. Cole. London: Butterworths

Whitelaw, F.G., Milne, J.S., Ørskov, E.R. and Smith, J.S. (1986) The nitrogen and energy metabolism of lactating cows given abomasal infusions of casein. *British Journal of Nutrition,* **55**, 537-556

This paper was first published in 1994

14

DEVELOPMENTS IN THE INRA FEEDING SYSTEMS FOR DAIRY COWS

R. VÉRITÉ[1], P. FAVERDIN[1] and J. AGABRIEL[2]
Institut National de la Recherche Agronomique,
[1] *Station de Recherche sur la Vache Laitière, INRA, 35590 Saint Gilles, France*
[2] *Laboratoire 'Adaptation des Herbivores au Milieu', INRA, 63122 Saint Genès-Champanelle, France*

In dairy production, optimal rationing is a most important key in controlling or improving animal performances (yield, reproduction, health, etc), milk quality, feed efficiency and N-wastage, and hence economical return. Modern feeding systems, as proposed in many countries, are useful tools for rationing. They are centred on better evaluation of nutritive values of feedstuffs and diets (mainly energy and protein) and of animal requirements or recommended allowances.

In France, the INRA feeding systems for ruminants have been elaborated from 1975 to 1977 (INRA, 1978; Vermorel, 1978; Vérité, Journet and Jarrige, 1979). They first included a net energy system (feed unit: UFL), and a metabolisable protein system (the PDI system e.g. protéines digestibles dans l'intestin). A system for predicting feed intake (the fill system) was developed slightly later (Jarrige *et al.,* 1979). They rapidly became fully functional.

They were revised ten years later (INRA, 1987; INRA, 1988; INRA, 1989), taking advantage of the information arising from research efforts as well as from their broad utilisation in practice. In addition at the same time, the above basic systems were co-ordinated in a powerful computer software package called 'INRAtion' that represents an integrated global system and allows easy rationing.

Since then several extra concepts have been developed (i.e. requirement for individual amino acids, marginal response curves) and several tools have been proposed to promote easier implementation. A new updating, based on the same scheme, is planned for the next 3-4 years. Simultaneous research projects aim at elaborating a nutrient-based model to better account for complex regulations and for differential animal responses.

As the current energy and protein systems are described in detail elsewhere (Vermorel, Coulon and Journet 1987; Vérité *et al*, 1987; INRA, 1989), only some new developments of the protein system will be presented here. The main purpose of this paper is rather to stress several other important topics that received particular attention in the INRA systems: feed intake estimation, responses to marginal input variations, integrated software as a practical tool for rationing (INRAtion).

Developments in the PDI system

The PDI system is similar to several other systems that were published later when considering the concepts and the frameworks, according to several recent comparisons; however they differ to some extent when considering available functionalities and real estimation of diets in practice (see Vérité and Peyraud, 1995 among others). With regard to the basis of the PDI system, attention should be drawn to the large experimental data set that was used for elaborating the basic relationships, the tables of feed values and the animal requirements. It should also be noted that most of the basic parameters and relationships were elaborated in a coordinated manner to prevent bias in rationing, as shown during the validation steps.

Protein degradability is basically assessed by the nylon bag method but this has some well known shortcomings: variability between laboratories, low accuracy and high cost. Therefore special attention was paid to careful standardisation, along with the use of the same reference sample in every series of measurements (Michalet-Doreau, Vérité and Chapoutot, 1987; Vérité *et al.*, 1990). Furthermore, as commercial laboratories require alternative methods, an enzymatic degradability test was developed for concentrate evaluation, standardised and then calibrated against the basic nylon bag procedure (Aufrère *et al.*, 1991). This is now implemented in French commercial laboratories. Similar work is in progress on roughages. With regard to animal requirements, much attention was paid to response curves of animal and rumen outputs to marginal N inputs (see later).

A great deal of work has been done on the concept of amino-acid profile in dairy diets. The initial interest came from a large set of INRA and foreign trials where extra supplies of lysine and methionine increased milk protein content and yield (Rulquin *et al.*, 1993). Therefore, the PDI system was expanded to include the concept of LysDI and MetDI, that evaluates the amounts of methionine and lysine digested in the small intestine (called respectively MetDI and LysDI) (Rulquin and Vérité, 1993; Rulquin *et al.*, 2001a&b). Feed values are derived from the PDI concepts with additional account of the amino-acid profiles of microbial and specific feed proteins. Recommended allowances are expressed as a percentage of PDI requirements, in accordance with the ideal protein concept. Requirements were found to be 2.5 and 7.3% PDI for MetDI and LysDI respectively. However values of 2.0 and 6.8% are considered as thresholds below which one could start considering supplementation (milk protein response vs. extra cost). This extension has been available for practical use since 1992 in advisory papers, and was included in the INRAtion software from 1995.

Predicting feed intake: the Fill Unit system

An accurate estimate of voluntary intake of roughages and/or total diet is the first and most important step when rationing because of significant variability with many factors, including rationing strategy itself. In general, direct estimates of dry matter intake rely on empirical relationships involving only a few simple characteristics of diets and animals. Such methods could work soundly in common situations, but could have important shortcomings in situations outside the range of initial data and are irrelevant to simulate the effect of different strategies (Faverdin, 1992; Faverdin, Baumont and Ingvartsen, 1995).

Several other methods are based on the widely accepted assumption that intake in ruminants is regulated through two main concomitant mechanisms involving physical and metabolic (or energy) limitations. In a first group of methods (Forbes, 1977; NRC, 1987; Mertens, 1987) both bulk and energy constraints are considered separately thus involving two independent parameters (and units) to characterise the satiating properties of the diet. For each constraint, the sum of the value of the feeds ingested cannot exceed the animal capacity; maximum intake is assessed from the first occurring limitation. In the other approach, relating to the French and Danish 'fill systems', both constraints are described with a unique parameter, the 'fill' value (FV), that accounts for all components of the satiation value of the feeds. They work like a nutritive system assuming only, with one common unit, that the diet 'fill value' equals the animal 'intake capacity'.

In the French fill system, the main basis for such a simplification relies on a relevant utilisation of the concept of substitution rate between concentrate and forage. The system works as if the satiating signals from the bulk and energy regulations interact with each other in a cumulative way, at least to some degree. Therefore the term 'satiation' would have been more appropriate than 'fill' to designate the system and its unit.

The fill system was outlined by Jarrige *et al.* (1979; 1986) and revised by Dulphy, Faverdin and Jarrige (1989). The aim was to develop a practical and additive system capable of predicting intake in cattle, sheep and goats under various circumstances. Most of the basic elements of the system were developed from several sets of feeding experiments run to determine 1) the quantity of feed that the animal is able to eat voluntarily according to its appetite in order to predict the feed intake capacity; 2) the voluntary dry matter intake (or ingestibility) of each forage when given *ad libitum* as the sole food to ruminants in order to estimate the 'fill value' of the forage' and 3) the influence of the supplementary concentrates upon the voluntary intake of forages, i.e. the substitution rate in order to calculate the 'fill value' of the concentrate. As a whole, the system appears to provide estimates of voluntary dry matter intake (VDMI) that fit reasonably well with observed data (Ostergaard, 1978) as illustrated in Figure 14.1.

BASIC PRINCIPLES

A common unit, 'the fill unit' (FU) was first defined to describe both the intake capacity (IC) of animals and the satiating properties of feedstuffs i.e. their fill value (FV). By definition, one 'fill unit' corresponds to the fill value of one kg DM of a reference forage that is an average pasture grass with specific characteristics. It works just as for the

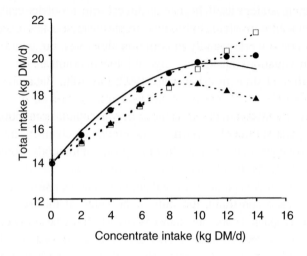

Figure 14.1 Effect of concentrate level on dry matter intake : comparison of experimental data (—) from Ostergaard (1978) with estimates from the NRC (▲···▲), the Danish Fill Unit (□···□) and the INRA Fill Unit (●···●) systems.

energy system, where the net energy content of one kg reference barley is the feed unit (UFL).

If at least one feed at least is offered *ad libitum*, the weighted sum of the fill values of all the feeds is equal to the intake capacity of the animal. Therefore on *ad libitum* feeding, calculation of diet or forage intake results from the following equation:

$$IC = \Sigma \; Q_i \; x \; FV_i \tag{1}$$

where IC is the intake capacity (FU/d), Q is feed intake levels (kg DM), FV is the feed fill value (FU/kg DM) and i refers to the different feeds in the diet.

Intake capacity is a fixed attribute of an animal in a given status whatever the diet characteristics. The fill value is a fixed attribute of a forage batch whatever the final diet and the animal characteristics. It is an inverse function of its ingestibility i.e. its VDMI when fed *ad libitum* as the sole feed to a standard animal: the higher is the ingestibility, the smaller is the fill value. The fill value (FU/kg DM) of a test forage is obtained relatively to the reference forage:

$$\text{test forage FV (FU/kg DM)} = \text{reference forage ingestibility} / \tag{2}$$
$$\text{test forage ingestibility}$$

Therefore the forages FV value accounts mainly for both physical and palatability factors.

Unlike the two others parameters, the fill value of a concentrate is not a fixed attribute for that concentrate but depends also on the current nutritional situation. This accounts for metabolic regulation mechanisms as reflected by the observed variations in the substitution rate between forage and concentrate. Adding a concentrate to forage offered *ad libitum* usually increases the total VDMI but reduces the forage VDMI. As forage FV and intake capacity are independent of concentrate intake, the FV of concentrate is a function of the substitution rate between concentrate and forages. The fill value of the concentrate (FVc) is then derived from the equation:

$$FV_c = FV_f \times SR \tag{3}$$

where FV_f is the roughage fill value and SR is the substitution rate between roughage and concentrate. In other words, one kg extra concentrate has the same 'fill' effect as the amount of forage which has disappeared, because IC is constant for a given animal situation. Contrary to the FV of forages, the FV of a concentrate reflects mainly the satiating effect through metabolic regulation i.e. mainly energy regulation.

Many experiments have shown that the substitution rate is highly variable. With different types of forages and concentrates, it has been observed that the substitution rate increases with the energy balance of the animal (Faverdin *et al.,* 1991). From these data, a model was developed to predict that substitution rate increases with the energy balance from zero up to a plateau higher than 1 according a complex function (Dulphy *et al.,* 1987). However when estimating the substitution rate, the energy balance is not known *a priori* but would arise from the resulting estimation of diet intake. Therefore the calculations should start from forage FV and energy characteristics of concentrate, forage and requirements and develop in an iterative way. The complete calculation is available within the INRAtion software.

PRACTICAL USE

All the values for animal IC and forage FV are available from tables given in reference papers (Andrieu, Demarquilly and Sauvant, 1989) or in the INRAtion software. Forage FV values could also be estimated for each batch from proximate analysis or plant characteristics such as morphological traits or age (through the estimation of VDMI by Demarquilly, Andrieu and Weiss, 1981).

The values of IC varies with animal species, physiological stage, and productive traits. In dairy cows, IC is 17 FU/d for a 600 kg cow producing 25 kg FCM and increases with milk yield (0.1 FU/kg FCM) and liveweight (0.01 FU/kg), parity (10% lower in primiparous); values are lower in early lactation (coefficients for the first 12 weeks).

The tabulated FV values for forages (Andrieu *et al*, 1989) are derived from an initial database with VDMI measurements in sheep for more than 3000 forage samples. The conversion and calculation methods for estimating FV in cattle are given by Dulphy,

Faverdin and Jarrige (1989). The FV values for forages range between 0.9 and 1.6 FU/ kg DM. They vary with many characteristics such as the initial characteristics of plants (species, physiological stage, chemical composition), the type of conservation (hay or silage), the drying method (barn-dried or field cured), the weather conditions, the harvesting method (finely chopped or flail harvested), the use of additives, and the dry matter content of the silage.

The range of FV for a given concentrate is rather large (0 to possibly more than 1) as shown in Table 14.1. Individual concentrates are not ascribed a particular FV in tables as FVc depends mainly on the energy balance of the diet (cf. above). The INRAtion software does not require FV of concentrate as an input because of automatic calculation. However the FV of a concentrate is also available from simplified tables or equations starting from forage characteristics (FV and UFL) and milk yield.

Table 14.1 VARIATION OF CONCENTRATE FILL VALUE ACCORDING TO FORAGE QUALITY AND FAT-CORRECTED MILK (FCM) YIELD FOR LACTATING DAIRY COWS FED WITH 5kg DM OF CONCENTRATES

Forage characteristics		Fill value of concentrate	
Fill value (FU)	*Energy (UFL)*	*20 kg FCM*	*35 kg FCM*
1.3	0.75	0.37	0.15
1.1	0.75	0.49	0.19
1.2	0.90	0.64	0.20
1.0	0.90	0.86	0.30

Productive responses to marginal variations in feed supply

In most modern systems, rationing starts with the desired level of animal output and works back to calculate the feed inputs required to sustain the corresponding assumed requirements (Gill, 1996). However in practice, the reverse way is of similar if not greater interest to the farmers. Most often the problem is not to elaborate an entirely new diet but rather to change some particular feed ingredient(s) in the current diet. This could arise because of problems with feedstuff availability, performance or health of animals, or economical changes (interest in deviating from the recommended allowances). Then it becomes important to know the relationships between any marginal changes in the diet and the induced changes in animal performance and efficiency.

The marginal responses could differ greatly from the theoretical ones that would be expected from average efficiency values. Productive traits usually respond according the law of diminishing return when nutritive supplies vary around requirement levels. At the moment, such input-output relationships are not easy to assess from theoretical approaches. However they could be developed from feeding trials, each comparing different input levels of a sole nutritive parameter (energy, PDI, etc).

Such response curves of intake and milk or protein yields to changes in the levels of concentrate, or energy, or metabolisable protein, or degradable protein, or specific amino acids (lysine and methionine) were obtained from relevant INRA and foreign data. Then they were either incorporated in or added as extra tools to, the basic 'energy', 'protein' and 'fill' systems. Therefore, such effects are easily simulated or anticipated with the INRAtion software.

For instance, it is generally accepted that the marginal efficiency of concentrate for milk production (extra milk/extra concentrate) decreases as concentrate allocation increases around the 'required level'. This arises from changes 1) in voluntary DM intake because of substitution, 2) in efficiency of digestive and metabolic processes and 3) in partition of available nutrients between different tissues. The INRA energy and fill systems account for such mechanisms. Firstly, the expected changes in feed intake are directly simulated by the fill system as shown in Figures 14.2 and 14.3. For a given cow, increasing concentrate allocation emphasises the negative effect on forage intake of an extra kg of concentrate and diminishes the positive effect on total DM intake. Further, when starting from a similar concentrate level, these effects are greater 1) when the yield of milk is lower (Figure 14.2) or 2) when the quality of the forage is better i.e. when forage energy concentration and ingestibility are higher as for instance, with good quality maize silage compared to medium quality grass silage (Figure 14.3). Secondly, the energy system (FU) accounts directly for a reduced digestive/metabolic efficiency when the feeding level and/or the concentrate:forage ratio are increased. These effects could account for up to 10% of the total net energy theoretically supplied (INRA, 1987). Lastly, the response curve of milk yield to changes in the real net energy availability was empirically derived from feeding trials through regression analysis (Faverdin, Hoden and Coulon, 1987). Therefore, the expected effects on animal performance (milk and protein yields and body-weight change) are directly and automatically provided, as shown in Table 14.2. In that simulation, an extra kg concentrate over requirement level would increase milk yield by only 0.5 kg FCM. The decreases in forage intake and in digestive efficiency would have accounted for approximately 45 and 10% of the net energy theoretically supplied by the extra concentrate; the remaining 45% really available would have been split between milk (2 parts) and body weight gain (1 part). If the initial situation corresponds to underfeeding, the calculated milk response is higher and the other effects are lower.

Similarly, the marginal increase in milk yield in response to a same amount of extra metabolisable protein (PDI), is lower still since the initial PDI supply, as a proportion of requirement, is higher. Data from several INRA experiments with grass and maize silage diets, each comparing several PDI levels at constant DM intake, are summarised in Figure 14.4 (Vérité, Dulphy and Journet, 1982; Vérité, unpublished). It appears that, after peak yield, the marginal responses to PDI variations is close to 0.5 kg FCM/100 g extra PDI when total input is close to requirement level. It reaches 0.9 kg FCM/100 g

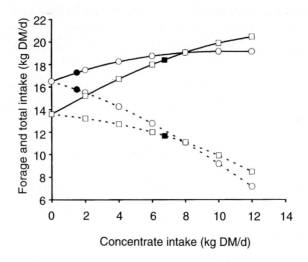

Figure 14.2 Levels of forage (---) and diet intake (—) according to the amount of concentrate supplied and the nature of forage (good quality maize silage O vs medium quality grass silage □) as simulated with INRAtion for a 25 kg FCM cow (full symbols ■, ● indicate the situations when requirements are met).

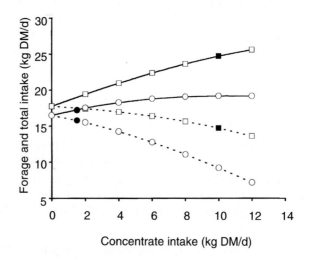

Figure 14.3 Levels of forage (---) and diet intake (—) according to the amount of concentrate supplied and milk yield level in mid lactation (25 kg O vs 40 kg □ of FCM) as simulated with INRAtion on a maize silage diet (full symbols ■, ● indicate the situations when requirements are met).

extra PDI if the initial PDI balance is negative by 200 g and only 0.2 kg FCM/100 g extra PDI if the initial PDI balance is positive by 200 g. These relationships could help in deciding if protein supply should meet requirement or deviate from it in order to optimise economical return according to the costs of energy and protein sources and to milk

Table 14.2 MARGINAL EFFECTS OF AN EXTRA KG OF CONCENTRATE AS SIMULATED BY THE INRAtion SOFTWARE FOR A 600 kg DAIRY COW PRODUCING 30 kg FCM, INITIALLY FED AT REQUIREMENT WITH 5.4 kg DM CONCENTRATE AND MAIZE SILAGE *AD LIBITUM* (15.1 kg DM)

	Marginal response	*Net energy partition (%)*
Concentrate intake	+1 kg as fed	(100)
Maize silage intake	-0.5 kg DM	50
Milk yield	+0.5 kg FCM	25
Milk protein content	+0.3 g/kg	
Body-weight change	0.05 kg/d	15
(Lower efficiency)		10

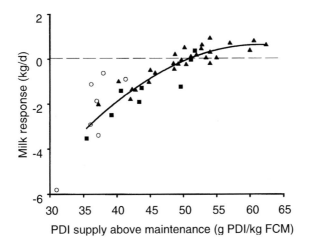

Figure 14.4 Response of milk yield to the level of PDI supply in dairy cows fed maize or grass silage diets in early (O) peak (■) or mid (▲) lactation (the regression line does not include early lactation data). Milk responses are calculated within experiments by reference to the control group fed at maintenance, i.e. 48 g PDI/kg FCM.

price. The effects are lower in early lactation because protein mobilisation could compensate to some degree. During the first 6 to 8 weeks postcalving, the cumulative negative PDI balance could reach 5 to 10 kg PDI, without significant negative effect on milk yield. Similarly, marginal response of protein content and yield to variations in lysine and methionine supply are now available (Rulquin *et al.,* 1993).

A shortage in the degradable protein supply is generally assumed to negatively affect microbial activity in the rumen and animal performance. Nitrogen recycling in the digestive tract could reduce that effect to some degree. Only few systems account for such a possibility, most often in a fixed way. However it could be modulated by other factors as shown by several INRA feeding trials, each comparing different levels of degradable protein at similar dry matter and metabolisable protein intakes (Figure 14.5). The negative effect of degradable protein shortage would depend on the animal balance for metabolisable protein. The adverse effect on milk yield of a negative 'rumen balance' (i.e. degradable protein supply as a proportion of microbial requirement) is higher when the 'animal balance' (i.e. metabolisable protein supply as a proportion of animal requirement) is lower. Further, when the 'animal balance' is positive, the rumen could afford a significant deficit in degradable protein supply. This effect is most probably related to a greater potential for nitrogen recycling because then the excess amount of amino acids is catabolised into urea. Roughly, the degradable protein supply should provide at least 100, 92 or 85% of microbial requirement if the animal balance (PDIE minus animal requirement) is respectively negative, zero or positive. Therefore, with the usual PDI parameters, the corresponding recommendation is that the PDIN/PDIE ratio in dairy diets should be at least 100, 96 or 92%.

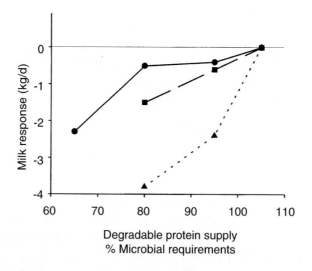

Figure 14.5 Variations of milk response to deficit in degradable protein supply according to animal balance in metabolisable protein (negative ▲⋯▲, normal ■--■ or positive ●—● balance).

The 'INRAtion' rationing software

The 'INRAtion' rationing software (INRA, 1995) has been available since 1987. It was designed as an aid to advisors and also to everyone involved in nutrition and feeding problems in cattle, sheep or goats under various physiological and productive situations. It integrates in a functional package, the intake constraint along with the nutritive constraints (energy, protein). It includes a fairly large data base on feedstuffs values (common concentrate ingredients, 600 forages from temperate areas and also 250 forages from Mediterranean, and humid or dry-tropical areas). It can also be modified by each user with his own feedstuffs analyses. Different feeding strategies can be explored, covering or deviating from requirements. Such flexibility gives a high degree of adaptation to every particular local or economical constraints. Similarly, it manages individual rationing as well as with totally mixed diets.

When starting with a given production level as a set point, it allows 'optimisation' of the diet or concentrate in terms of ingredients composition and/or amount to be supplied (possibly giving several solutions), while voluntary DM intake of forages is also predicted. The diets are directly and automatically optimised on intake, energy and protein constraints, while further optimisation on LysDI and MetDI, minerals, trace elements, vitamins can be performed when desired.

In the reverse way, when starting from a given diet, different dietary changes can be proposed and are tested for their effects on ingestion and nutritional parameters while the resulting marginal effects on production parameters are assessed from the response curves mentioned above.

Beyond its value as an aid to technical and economic problems, such software is also of good value for educational purposes, favouring the spread of common concepts and references for dairy farmers, students, advisors and feed industry. Most of the teaching, advisory or milking control services, and feed manufacturers have access to INRAtion. Furthermore, in several situations it has been included as a basic part of other software packages that were developed for broader purposes.

References

Andrieu, J., Demarquilly, C. and Sauvant, D. (1989) Tables of feeds used in France. *In Ruminant nutrition*, pp 213–303. Edited by R. Jarrige. John Libbey: London, Paris.

Aufrère, J., Graviou, D., Demarquilly, C., Vérité, R., Michalet-Doreau, B. and Chapoutot, P. (1991) Predicting in situ degradability of feed proteins in the rumen by two laboratory methods (solubility and enzymatic degradation). *Animal Feed Science and Technology*, **33**, 97–116.

Demarquilly, C., Andrieu, J. and Weiss, P. (1981) L'ingestibilité des fourrages verts et des foins et sa prévision. In *Prévision de la valeur nutritive des aliments des ruminants,* pp 155–168. Edited by C. Demarquilly. INRA Publications: Versailles.

Dulphy, J.P., Faverdin, P. and Jarrige, R. (1989) Feed Intake: the Fill Unit Systems. In *Ruminant Nutrition: recommended allowances and feed tables,* pp 61–72. Edited by R. Jarrige. INRA, John Libbey Eurotext: Paris.

Dulphy, J.P., Faverdin, P., Micol, D. and Bocquier, F. (1987) Révision du système des unités d'encombrement (UE). *Bulletin Technique du Centre de Recherches Zootechniques et Vétérinaires de Theix*, **70**, 35–48.

Faverdin, P., Baumont, R. and Ingvartsen, K.L. (1995) Control and prediction of feed intake in ruminants. In *Recent developments in the nutrition of herbivores.*

Proceeding of the IV International Symposium on the Nutrition of Herbivores, pp 95–120. Edited by M. Journet, E. Grenet, M.H. Farce, M. Theriez and C. Demarquilly. INRA Editions: Versailles.

Faverdin, P., Dulphy, J.P., Coulon, J.B., Garel, J.P., Rouel, J. and Marquis, B. (1991) Substitution of roughage by concentrates for dairy cows. *Livestock Production Science*, **27**, 137–156.

Faverdin, P. (1992) Les méthodes de prédiction des quantités ingérées. *INRA Productions Animales*, **5**, 271–282.

Faverdin, P., Hoden, A. and Coulon, J.B. (1987) Recommandations alimentaires pour les vaches laitières. *Bulletin Technique C. R. V. Z. Theix*, **70**, 133–152.

Forbes, J.M. (1977) Development of a model of voluntary food intake and energy balance in lactating cows. *Animal Production*, **24**, 203–224.

Gill, M. (1996) Modelling nutrient supply and utilization by ruminants. In *Recent developments in ruminant nutrition (3)*, pp 23–34. Edited by P.C. Garnsworthy and D.J.A. Cole. Nottingham University Press: Nottingham.

INRA (1978) *Alimentation des Ruminants*. Edited by R. Jarrige. INRA Publications: Versailles.

INRA (1987) Alimentation des Ruminants: révision des systèmes et des tables de l'INRA. *Bulletin Technique CRZV Theix, INRA*, **70**, 1–222.

INRA (1988) *Alimentation des bovins, ovins et caprins*. Edited by R. Jarrige. INRA Publications: Versailles.

INRA (1989) *Ruminant nutrition. Recommended allowances and feed tables*. Edited by R. Jarrige. John Libbey: London - Paris.

INRA (1995) *INRAtion, logiciel d'aide au rationnement des ruminants. Version 2.60*. INRA-CNERTA: Dijon.

Jarrige, R., Demarquilly, C., Dulphy, J.P., Hoden, A., Robelin, J., Beranger, C., Geay, Y., Journet, M., Malterre, C., Micol, D. and Petit, M. (1979) Le systeme des unités d'encombrement pour les bovins. *Bulletin Technique C. R. V. Z. Theix*, 38, 57–79.

Jarrige, R., Demarquilly, C., Dulphy, J.P., Hoden, A., Robelin, J., Beranger, C., Geay, Y., Journet, M., Malterre, C., Micol, D. and Petit, M. (1986) The I.N.R.A. 'fill unit system' for predicting the voluntary intake of forage-based diets in ruminants: a review. *Journal of Animal Science*, **63**, 1737–1758.

Mertens, D.R. (1987) Prediction intake and digestibility using mathematical models of ruminal function. *Journal of Animal Science*, **64**, 1548–1558.

Michalet-Doreau, B., Vérité, R. and Chapoutot, P. (1987) Méthodologie de la mesure de la dégradabilité in sacco de l'azote des aliments. *Bulletin Technique CRZV Theix, INRA*, **69**, 5–7.

NRC (1987) *Predicting feed intake of food-producing animals*. National Academic Press. Washington.

Ostergaard, V. (1978) *Strategie for concentrate feeding to attain optimum feeding level in high yielding dairy cows*. National institute of animal science. Copenhagen.

Rulquin, H. and Vérité, R. (1993) Amino acid nutrition of dairy cows: Productive effects and animal requirements. In *Recent Advances in Animal Nutrition - 1993*, pp 55–77. Edited by P.C. Garnsworthy. Nottingham University Press: Nottingham.

Rulquin, H., Pisulewski, P.M., Vérité, R. and Guinard, J. (1993) Milk production and composition as a function of postruminal lysine and methionine supply: a nutrient-response approach. *Livestock Production Science*, **37**, 69–90.

Rulquin, H., Vérité, R. and Guinard-Flament, J. (2001a) Acides animés digestibles dans l'intestin, Le système AADI et les recommandations d'apport pour la vache laitière. *INRA Prod. Anim.*, **14(4)**, 265-274.

Rulquin, H., Vérité, R. and Guinard-Flament, J. (2001b) Tables de valeurs AADI des aliments des ruminants. *INRA Prod. Anim.*, **14(4)**, supplément, 16p.

Vérité, R., Dulphy, J.P. and Journet, M. (1982) Protein supplementation of silage diets for dairy cows. In *Forage protein conservation and utilization*, pp 175–190. EEC Seminar, Dublin.

Vérité, R., Journet, M. and Jarrige, R. (1979) A new system for the protein feeding of ruminants: the PDI system. *Livestock Production Science*, **6**, 349–367.

Vérité, R., Michalet-Doreau, B., Chapoutot, P., Peyraud, J.L. and Poncet, C. (1987) Révision du système des Protéines Digestibles dans l'Intestin (PDI). *Bulletin Technique CRZV Theix, INRA*, **70**, 19–34.

Vérité, R., Michalet-Doreau, B., Vedeau, F. and Chapoutot, P. (1990) Dégradabilité en sachets des matières azotées des aliments concentrés: standardisation de la méthode et variabilités intra et interlaboratoires. *Reproduction Nutrition Développement*, **Suppl 2**, 161–162.

Vérité, R. and Peyraud, J.L. (1995) Comparison of the modern protein evaluation systems for ruminants. In *Proceedings of the 3rd International Feed Production Conference, Piacenza (Italie) - feb 1994*, pp 233–247. Edited by G. Piva. Piacenza.

Vermorel, M. (1978) Feed evaluation for ruminants. 2. The new energy systems proposed in France. *Livestock Production Science*, **5**, 347–365.

Vermorel, M., Coulon, J.B. and Journet, M. (1987) Révision du système des Unités Fourragères (UF). *Bulletin Technique CRZV Theix, INRA*, **70**, 9–18.

This paper was first published in 1997

15

THE IMPORTANCE OF RATE OF RUMINAL FERMENTATION OF ENERGY SOURCES IN DIETS FOR DAIRY COWS

D.G. CHAMBERLAIN and J-J. CHOUNG
Hannah Research Institute, Ayr, KA6 5HL, UK

Introduction

Much of the current interest in the rate of ruminal fermentation of carbohydrates stems from its relevance to the Metabolizable Protein (MP) system and related systems of protein rationing (Newbold, 1994; Beever and Cottrill, 1994). Taking a longer-term view, knowledge of the rate of fermentation of carbohydrates and the molar composition of the mixture of volatile fatty acids (VFA) produced are essential ingredients of any rationing system that attempts to predict the effects of nutrient supply on the yields of milk constituents (Newbold, 1994), but there is a more immediate interest.

Synchronizing the availability of energy and nitrogen in the rumen is seen as offering considerable potential to enhance the output of microbial protein from the rumen in certain dietary circumstances, many of which are not uncommon in practice. This idea is attractive to the feed compounder, who sees the potential to manipulate rate of fermentation by varying the sources and types of carbohydrate in formulations, thereby matching the rates at which energy and nitrogen from the basal forage and the compound become available to the microbial population.

Part of this chapter will be concerned with an examination of the extent to which microbial protein synthesis can be influenced by changes in synchrony of energy and nitrogen release in the rumen, but it is important to note that altering the rate of fermentation is likely to have a number of consequences both for the microbes and the host; some of these are listed in Figure 15.1. From the outset then, we should recognize that there are likely to be limits to our ability to manipulate rate of fermentation without incurring penalties such as reduced feed intake, changes in partition of nutrient use between the udder and other body tissues and changes in milk composition.

Synchrony of energy and nitrogen release in the rumen

The basic assumption is that a lack of synchrony between the rates at which energy

Rate of ruminal fermentation of CHO

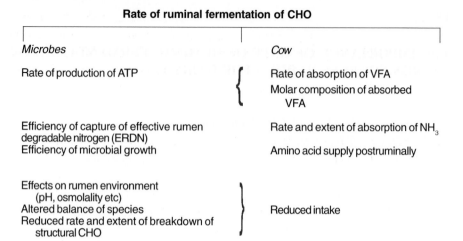

Microbes

Rate of production of ATP

Efficiency of capture of effective rumen
degradable nitrogen (ERDN)
Efficiency of microbial growth

Effects on rumen environment
(pH, osmolality etc)
Altered balance of species
Reduced rate and extent of breakdown of
structural CHO

Cow

Rate of absorption of VFA
Molar composition of absorbed
VFA

Rate and extent of absorption of NH_3

Amino acid supply postruminally

Reduced intake

Figure 15.1 Some possible elfects of rate offermentation ofCHO on rumina! microbes and the host.

and nitrogen become available to the microbes will lead to a reduced efficiency of
microbial capture of nitrogen, and ATP production from fermentation of dietary
carbohydrate being inefficiently used for microbial growth. To examine the basis of this
assumption in more detail, we may consider the extreme form of asynchrony shown
very simply in Figure 15.2.

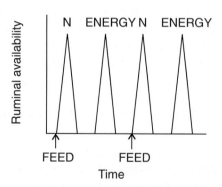

Figure 15.2 A simple diagram to show an extreme form of asynchrony between the ruminal availability
of energy and nitrogen.

A simplistic interpretation is to conclude that the peak in the availability of nitrogen (very
largely, ammonia) leads to considerable absorption of ammonia from the rumen because
there is little energy available to support microbial incorporation of ammonia (and amino
acids and peptides). Using similar reasoning, when fermentation of dietary carbohydrate
reaches its peak, the ruminal supply of available nitrogen will be markedly deficient,

leading to an 'uncoupling' of A TP production and microbial protein synthesis, such that fermentation occurs largely without the growth of microbial cells. It is clear that the soundness of this interpretation rests heavily on our knowledge of factors controlling the absorption of ammonia and the recycling of urea to the rumen, and on our knowledge of the microbial utilization of A TP generated during fermentation.

ABSORPTION OF AMMONIA AND RECYCLING OF ENDOGENOUS NIIROGEN TO THE RUMEN

It is generally assumed that the rate of absorption of un-ionized ammonia is much more rapid than that of the ammonium ion. It then follows that the rate of absorption is heavily dependent on ruminal pH: at pH values less than 7, there are only very small proportions of un-ionized ammonia present. Indeed, from an examination of the evidence available, Smith (1975) concluded that, at ruminal pH values less than 6.5, there was little evidence of appreciable absorption of ammonia from the rumen; this did not, of course, preclude absorption of ammonia from the postruminal gut, especially the omasum, following outflow of ammonia in digesta. The overall conclusion was that, under normal feeding conditions, ammonia is only slowly absorbed from the rumen, the implication being that the synchronization of ammonia and energy release in the rumen need not be anywhere near as precise as may sometimes be imagined.

Moreover, if ammonia should be in short supply during the feeding cycle, there is scope to enhance its concentration by way of recycling of urea in saliva or by entry across the ruminal epithelium. It is important to note that an increased rate of fermentation, resulting from the inclusion of readily fermentable carbohydrate in the diet, leads to an increased entry of urea into the rumen as a result of increased permeability of the ruminal epithelium (see Obara, Dellow and Nolan, 1991).

MICROBIAL UTIUZATION OF ATP GENERATED DURING FERMENTATION

Put simply, ATP generated during fermentation is used by the microbes essentially for two purposes: maintenance of cellular function and synthesis of cell constituents. However, the use of ATP for the synthesis of cell material is markedly influenced by the composition of the culture medium; cell composition can vary widely, particularly with respect to the content of storage polysaccharides (see Russell and Wallace, 1988). When the supply of fermentable carbohydrate is in relative excess of the supply of available nitrogen, rumen bacteria use the ATP produced in fermentation to synthesize storage polysaccharide, which can account for as much as 75% of cell dry matter (DM) (Stewart, Paniagua, Dinsdale, Cheng and Garrow, 1981). The energy cost of polysaccharide synthesis is only about one-third of that required for the synthesis of protein (Stouthamer, 1973) and, furthermore, the stored polysaccharide can be mobilized and the glucose metabolized to yield A TP for protein synthesis later in the feeding cycle when adequate supplies of usable nitrogen become available. Of course, this process is somewhat less efficient than the immediate use of A TP for protein synthesis, but these findings again emphasize the ability of ruminal bacteria to cope effectively with fluctuating supplies of energy and nitrogen.

We would be led to believe from the foregoing that, in general, the response of microbial protein synthesis to changes in the pattern of fermentation of carbohydrate and the release of ammonia would be small. Indeed, this view is supported by the results of experiments *in vitro,* even when the degree of mismatching between energy and nitrogen supply patterns was severe (Henning, Steyn and Meissner, 1991; Newbold and Rust, 1992), and by results of experiments *in vivo.* Changes in the frequency of intraruminal dosing with urea failed to influence the utilization of nitrogen in growing lambs (Knight and Owens, 1973; Streeter, Little, Mitchell and Scott, 1973). Again, spreading intraruminal doses of urea and starch or glucose to achieve a better matching of the rates of energy and ammonia release did not influence microbial capture of ammonia (Salter, Smith and Hewitt, 1983). Synchronizing rate of fermentation and rate of ammonia release would be expected to be beneficial only in conditions of extensive absorption of ammonia, such as might occur if ruminal pH values were high (say > 6.8) for significant periods of the feeding cycle. Whether this was the case in the experiment of Meggison, McMeniman and Armstrong (1979) which showed beneficial effects on the microbial capture of ammonia when urea was administered continuously as opposed to twice daily, is not known.

The general conclusion that a close matching of energy and nitrogen release will bring only small, if any, benefit in most practical conditions holds only if microbial growth is limited by the supplies of fermentable carbohydrate and ammonia. We must consider the possibility that other nitrogenous compounds may be limiting microbial protein synthesis, and that the supply of these other nutrients may be affected by changes in feeding strategies. Although the supply of minerals and vitamins can influence bacterial growth rates in the rumen (see Mackie and Therion, 1984), this subject will not be considered further, and attention will be focused on the role of amino acids and peptides as sources of nitrogen for microbial protein synthesis.

AMINO ACIDS AND PEPTIDES AS SOURCES OF NITROGEN FOR MICROBIAL PROTEIN

In normal circumstances, ammonia is the most abundant nitrogen compound available for microbial growth; indeed, most cellulolytic organisms have an absolute requirement for ammonia (Respell, 1984). On the other hand, starch-digesting bacteria have been shown to obtain 66% of their nitrogen from amino acids and peptides and only 34% from ammonia (Russell, Sniffen and Van Soest, 1983). The implication of findings such as these is that, although cellulolytic bacteria may need only small amounts of amino acids in ruminal fluid, provided their requirements for branched- chain amino acids are met (Bryant 1973), starch-digesting bacteria may need significant amounts of amino acids and peptides if they are to achieve their maximum growth rates, an idea developed by Russell, O'Connor, Fox, Van Soest and Sniffen, (1992).

Amino acids and peptides accumulate in ruminal fluid in the early post-feeding period, the extent of accumulation depending on the degradability of the dietary protein. Unless highly soluble proteins like casein are *fed,* the concentrations of free amino acids remain low, but concentrations of peptide can reach values in excess of 200 mg N /l just after feeding, rapidly declining to < 25 mg N/l after 2 hours (Broderick, Wallace and Ørskov, 1991).

Hence, the suggestion (Respell and Bryant, 1979) that bacterial growth may be limited by deficiencies of amino acid and peptide at times during the feeding cycle should be seen as particularly relevant when the diet is rich in starchy concentrates, and the ruminal population contains a high proportion of amylolytic bacteria. It is interesting to note that, in continuous culture studies with diets rich in starch, microbial protein output was linearly related to the intake of rumen-degradable protein up to levels in excess of 20% of DM (Hoover and Stokes, 1991).

From the above, it might be expected that, particularly with diets rich in readily fermentable carbohydrate (RFC), changes in the pattern of feeding, either of the whole diet or of protein or carbohydrate ingredients, would result in improved rates of microbial protein synthesis. To what extent such benefits have been shown to occur in practice is examined below.

EFFECTS OF CHANGES IN FEEDING PATTERN ON MICROBIAL PROTEIN SYNTHESIS

We must recognize that interpreting the results of experiments in which feeding pattern has been altered is not always straightforward, and this is especially true when the diet is rich in RFC. If the frequency of feeding of the whole diet or of the RFC component has been altered, often there are pronounced effects on ruminal pH, the molar composition of VFA etc, which may influence microbial growth in their own right. Probably, the experimental approach that offers the clearest interpretation is one in which the frequency of feeding of the protein component of the diet is altered, whilst all other components of the diet are maintained constant. We are aware of only one published study that comes close to meeting these criteria. Robinson and McQueen (1994) examined the effects on the performance of dairy cows of feeding two protein supplements either twice or five times daily. There were no effects on milk production, but no conclusions can be drawn because altering the frequency of feeding the protein supplements had no effect on the diurnal variation in ruminal concentrations of peptide. Further carefully planned experiments are needed before the question can be answered.

MISCELLANEOUS EXPERIMENTS ON SYNCHRONIZATION OF ENERGY AND NITROGEN

Experiments have been reported (McCarthy, Klusmeyer, Vicini, Clark and Nelson, 1989; Herrera-Saldana, Gomez-Alarcon, Torabi and Huber, 1990a; Sinclair, Garnsworthy, Newbold and Buttery, 1993) that claim improvements in microbial protein synthesis attributable to improved synchrony of energy and nitrogen release in the rumen. However, as pointed out by others (Henning *et al.,* 1991; Robinson and McQueen, 1994), there is a serious problem of interpretation of these results, in that changes in synchronization have been achieved by manipulation of different dietary ingredients, thereby confounding synchronization with characteristics of the feeds. This point cannot be over emphasized. Whereas it is quite permissible to put forward effects on synchrony as a possible explanation of observed differences between dietary treatments, it is not permissible to use experiments of this type to test the hypothesis that synchrony affects microbial protein synthesis.

DIETS BASED ON GRASS SILAGE

Synchronization of energy and nitrogen release has been regarded as being particularly relevant to diets based on grass silage. It has long been the view that the release of ammonia from the substantial content of non-protein nitrogen (NPN) compounds in grass silage is very rapid, and this requires a similarly rapid release of energy in the rumen to ensure the most efficient microbial capture of ammonia. The greater output of microbial protein from the rumen when sugar, as opposed to starch, supplements are given (Table 15.1) appears to derive from the faster rate of fermentation of sugars. Based on the pattern of change of ruminal pH and the concentrations of total VFA, and with the exception of lactose, the sugars were fermented more rapidly than the raw maize starch used in this experiment. Recent studies lend more support to this interpretation in that, when the starch was cooked before feeding, its effectiveness as a substrate for the production of microbial protein was increased to that of sugar (Table 15.2). Cooking maize starch had a marked effect on its rate of fermentation, as judged from its effects on ruminal pH; indeed, within the conditions of this experiment, its rate of fermentation was indistinguishable from that of the two sugars. These effects of cooking the starch are interesting also in that they lend no support to the earlier suggestion (Chamberlain, Thomas, Wilson, Newbold and MacDonald, 1985) that the inferior response to starch as opposed to sugar supplements was related to the increased numbers of protozoa that occur with starch feeding and the consequent increase in the intraruminal recycling of ammonia.

A closer examination of the increases in the output of microbial protein from the rumen in response to the addition of various carbohydrates (Table 15.3) reveals two main features. First, there are differences amongst carbohydrates, not only between

Table 15.1 EFFECTS OF VARIOUS SUGARS AND MAIZE STARCH AS SUPPLEMENTS TO A BASAL DIET OF GRASS SILAGE ON RUMINAL DIGESTION AND THE OUTPUT OF MICROBIAL PROTEIN

	Supplement					
	Silage only	*Sucrose*	*Lactose*	*Xylose*	*Starch*	*Fructose*
Ruminal pH						
Mean	6.43	6.34	6.40	6.16	6.25	6.31
Minimum	6.04	5.72	6.05	5.97	5.99	5.74
NH$_3$-N (mg/l)						
Mean	255	157	258	180	213	164
Maximum	354	240	234	240	288	233
Microbial CP*						
(g/d)	64	93	89	82	74	86

*Calculated from the urinary output of purine derivatives.
Chamberlain *et al.* (1993)

Table 15.2 EFFECTS OF MAIZE STARCH, COOKED MAIZE STARCH AND SUGAR SUPPLEMENTS TO A BASAL DIET OF GRASS SILAGE ON RUMINAL DIGESTION AND THE OUTPUT OF MICROBIAL PROTEIN

	Supplement				
	Silage only	*Starch*	*Cooked starch*	*Sucrose*	*Lactose*
Ruminal pH					
Mean	6.55	6.44	6.35	6.49	6.50
Minimum	6.43	6.39	6.07	6.24	6.24
NH$_3$-N (mg/l)					
Mean	268	233	205	217	231
Maximum	427	358	302	316	369
Protozoa					
($\times 10^5$/ml)	2.7	7.1	6.4	4.1	4.0
Microbial CP*					
(g/d)	72	79	98	86	101

*Calculated from the urinary output of purine derivatives.
Chamberlain *et al.* (1993)

starch and sugars, but also among the various sugars. Differences among the sugars may be related to the adverse effects on microbial growth of depressions of ruminal pH (Strobel and Russell, 1986) resulting from too rapid a rate of fermentation; there were

Table 15.3 SYNTHESIS OF RUMINAL MICROBIAL PROTEIN (g/kg ADDED CARBOHYDRATE) FROM CARBOHYDRATE SUPPLEMENTS TO GRASS SILAGE

Carbohydrate	g microbial N/kg added carbohydrate	Reference
Sucrose	33	Huhtanen (1987a) (cattle)
Xylose	23	
Glucose syrup	28	Rooke *et al.* (1987) (cattle)
Glucose syrup	7	
plus casein	42	
Sucrose	21	Khaili and Huhtanen (1991) (cattle)
Sucrose	23	Chamberlain, Robertson and Choung
Lactose	22	(1993) (sheep)
Xylose	15	Chamberlain, Choung and Robertson
Fructose	18	(unpublished) (sheep)
Maize starch	9	
Cooked maize starch	21	
Sucrose	25	
Barley starch	20	Chamberlain, Choung and Robertson
Cooked barley starch	28	(unpublished) (cattle)

suggestions of such effects with fructose. However, the lower response to xylose, evident in two studies, is not explicable in terms of a faster rate of fermentation, it being more slowly fermented than fructose or sucrose (Sutton, 1968), and must relate to an intrinsic difference in the microbial utilization of this sugar. The second feature that emerges from the table is that the responses to the carbohydrates are lower than the accepted maximum, especially in the studies with sheep. The suggestion is that the generally accepted low rates of microbial protein synthesis that occur with diets of silage only (Agricultural Research Council, 1984) are still evident in the incremental responses to the addition of fermentable carbohydrate. It is tempting to speculate that the rate of microbial growth is still constrained below maximum by deficiencies of other nutrients, in particular, amino acids and peptides. The very substantial response in the output of microbial protein to the continuous intraruminal infusion of casein (Rooke, Lee and Armstrong, 1987) would support this view but, on the other hand, responses to the addition of proteins to the diet have been inconsistent (Rooke, Bret, Overend and Armstrong, 1985; Dawson, Bruce, Buttery, Gill and Beever, 1988; Rooke and Armstrong, 1989; Beever, Gill, Dawson and Buttery, 1990). Obviously, further work is needed here but the inconsistent response to dietary protein supplements may reflect differences in the pattern of release of amino acids and peptides from different levels and types of protein.

Before jumping to the general conclusion that the synchronization of energy and nitrogen release can greatly affect the synthesis of microbial protein on diets containing high proportions of grass silage, it is well to consider the evidence, which boils down to: raw starch is a poorer substrate for the synthesis of microbial protein than is sugar or cooked starch. Note also that lactose and raw starch appear to have similar rates of fermentation (see later) and so a faster rate of fermentation of lactose cannot be the reason for the superiority of lactose over raw starch. It is clear that other factors are involved. Furthermore, to the extent that synchronization may be a factor to be considered, again there is no evidence that the matching of carbohydrate fermentation and ammonia release needs to be especially precise. Indeed, giving a supplement of sucrose either continuously or twice-daily resulted in a greater increase in output of microbial protein for the continuous treatment, even though a much closer matching of carbohydrate fermentation and ammonia release was obtained with the twice-daily treatment (Khalili and Huhtanen, 1989). As discussed by these workers, the twice-daily treatment may have resulted in less ATP yield per mole of sucrose fermented, since the acrylate pathway of propionate production can predominate at high rates of fermentation. There are inherent draw- backs in pursuing a very close matching of energy and nitrogen release because, even if it were necessary (and there is no evidence that it is), it can lead not only to a lower yield of ATP per mole of fermented carbohydrate with substrates such as sugars or cooked starches, but also to severe reductions of ruminal pH which have repercussions not only for microbial growth but also for the intake and digestibility of the diet.

Effects of RFC on fibre digestion and on the intake of forage

The depressions of fibre digestion, and related reductions of forage intake, that usually accompany the addition of significant amounts of RFC to the diet can be considered as made up of two components: a 'pH effect' and a 'carbohydrate effect' (Mould *et al.,* 1983). Thus we might assume that, for a given source of RFC, its 'pH effect' will be determined by its rate of fermentation and its 'carbohydrate effect' will depend on which microbial species utilize it and the interactions of these microbes with cellulolytic bacteria. It should be evident already that the 'carbohydrate effect' is not only difficult to define but is also likely to be even more difficult to measure. Again, even though the 'pH effect' might appear to lend itself more to measurement, it is important to remember that the depressions of ruminal pH resulting from the dietary inclusion of a given source of RFC will depend not only on its rate of fermentation but also on the rate of fermentation of the other components of the diet and the buffering capacity of the rumen. The picture becomes even more complex when we consider also that the 'pH effect' itself consists of at least two identifiable phases (Mould *et al.,* 1983; Hoover, 1986): one due to moderate depressions of pH, say between 6.8 and 6.2, which may relate to effects on microbial attachment to fibre; and one due to more severe depressions of pH which probably relates to severe inhibition of the growth of cellulolytic bacteria and reductions in their numbers.

It is established that replacing fibrous carbohydrate in the concentrate by starch reduces forage intake (see de Visser, 1993), but the question that concerns us here is whether different sources of RFC show different degrees of depression of forage intake. There is some evidence from experiments *in vitro* that the 'carbohydrate effect' of sugars is greater than that of starch (Simpson, 1984), which may derive from more species of cellulolytic bacteria being able to utilize soluble sugars than are able to utilize starch. Published reports of experiments *in vivo* involving direct comparisons of starch and sugars are rare, but the limited evidence would support the view that sugars have a greater intake-depressing effect than starch. Replacement of 33% of barley in an all-barley concentrate by molasses reduced silage intake by around 10% (Huhtanen, 1 987b) and a concentrate containing 38% of sucrose reduced silage intake by around 12% compared with one based on barley (Chamberlain, Martin and Robertson, 1990). However, it should be emphasized that these comparisons apply only to barley starch and sucrose, and should not be regarded as a general statement applicable to all starches and all sugars: comparisons of cooked starches and more slowly fermented sugars (e.g. lactose) might well yield a different conclusion.

There is a further, important point to make in relation to the intake-depressing effects of RFC. The results of comparisons between different sources of RFC will depend very much on the dietary conditions in which the comparisons are made. This is well illustrated in the results of Chamber-lain *et al.* (1990) referred to above (Table 15.4). Note that the reduction of silage intake induced by the high-sugar supplement was removed by the addition of a small amount offish meal to the diet. The mechanism of action of the fish meal here is not known but it might well be a simple buffering effect on ruminal pH (Choung and Chamberlain, 1993a). The message from these observations is that the intake-depressing effects of RFC should be regarded more as potential effects rather than actual: there may well be simple remedies, such as changes in compound formulation to increase buffering capacity, that could substantially lessen adverse effects of the inclusion of more rapidly fermented forms of RFC.

Table 15.4 SILAGE INTAKE (KG DM/D) OF DAIRY COWS GIVEN 5kg/d OF A BARLEY-BASED OR HIGH-SUGAR CONCENTRATE WITH OR WITHOUT FISH MEAL

	Starch				Sugar			
Fishmeal (kg/d)	0	0.5	1.0	1.5	0	0.5	1.0	1.5
Intake	8.6	8.1	8.9	8.2	7.5	8.5	8.4	8.4

Measurement of rate of fermentation

MEASUREMENT *IN VIVO*

The use of animals cannulated in the intestine can provide estimates of the extent of digestion of RFC in the rumen and in the intestines (see Theurer, 1986). However, these data are of limited use in distinguishing between different sources of RFC in terms of their rate of ruminal fermentation. Again, estimates based on the rate and extent of depression of ruminal pH or the rate of increase of VFA concentrations may provide a rough index of the rate of fermentation but, for reasons discussed earlier, such measurements are of limited accuracy, difficult to standardize and, in any case, do not lend themselves to routine use. At first sight, measurement of the rate of loss of RFC from feedstuffs held in nylon bags during incubation in the rumen (Herrera-Saldana, Huber and Poos, 1 990b; Tamminga, Van Vuuren and Van Der Koelen, 1990) is an attractive option. However, there must be serious concern over the interpretation of the data, especially with respect to the fraction that is deemed to be instantly lost from the bag (zero time loss) and hence is classed as rapidly fermented. Examination of the data presented in Table 15.5 shows that the zero-time losses certainly do not represent material that is truly soluble, and must therefore be due to the loss of particulate matter. When this undefined fraction represents at least 60% of the starch in common cereals, it is difficult to see how this technique can .provide any meaningful information on the rate of fermentation of different cereals, not to mention the effects of processing of the cereals. On a practical point, it should also be noted from Table 15.5 that the zero-time losses are not related to the method of washing the bags i.e. machine-washing versus hand-washing.

Table 15.5 SOME PUBUSHED ESTIMATES OF SOLUBILITY IN BUFFER SOLUTIONS COMPARED WITH ZERO-TIME WASHOUT VALUES FROM NYLON-BAG INCUBATIONS OF STARCH FROM SOME CEREAL GRAINS

	Solubility (%)		*Zero-time loss (%)*	
	Buffer A	*Buffer B*	*1*	*2*
Maize	4	8	28	21
Milo	2	3	33	4
Wheat	-	2	69	78
Barley	5	11	65	66
Oats	5	4	96	97

Buffers: A, acetate (Herrera-Saldana *et al.* I 990b)
              B, bicarbonate-phosphate (Herrera-Saldana, Huber and Swingle, 1986)
Nylon-bag incubations: 1, machine-washing (Tamminga *et al.* 1990a)
                               2, hand-washing (Herrera-Saidena *et al.* 1990b)

MEASUREMENT *IN VITRO*

Methods used in vitro break down essentially into two categories: those based on incubation with rumen fluid and those based on incubation with purified enzymes.

With methods based on incubation in rumen fluid, the first question is what to measure. Interest has focused mainly on the rates of production of VFA, gas or the rate of disappearance of substrate. Measuring the rate of gas production is relatively quick and easy. However, interpretation is not easy because the total production of gas derives from two sources: direct production of CO_2 and methane and indirect production of CO_2 from the action of VFA on bicarbonate in the rumen fluid and in the added buffer, and so varies with the mixture of VFA produced (Table 15.6). Hence, there is no clear relationship between the rate of fermentation and total gas production (Beuvink, 1993). On the other hand, even though the recovery of fermented sugars as VFA (and, where appropriate, lactic acid) is only around 40% (Sutton, 1968; Newbold and Rust, 1992), the rate of disappearance of sugar and the rate of appearance of fermentation acids are very highly correlated (Sutton 1968). However, most attention has been given to the fermentation of starch sources, and measurement of its disappearance from the incubation medium is easier than measuring VFA production. The results of extensive studies on the ruminal degradation of starch sources (Cone, Cline, Thiel, MarlesteirI and Van't Klooster., 1989; Cone, 1991) have shown that, although the actual values for disappearance rates vary with the diet of the donor animal, the ranking order of the starch sources is little affected (Table 15.7). Furthermore, this method has been shown to provide results that allow the effects of processing on the rate of fermentation of starch to be clearly identified (Table 15.8).

Table 15.6 DIRECT AND INDIRECT GAS PRODUCTION FROM 1 MOL OF GLUCOSE FERMENTED TO DIFFERENT END PRODUCTS

Acidic end products (mol)	Direct gas (mol)	Indirect gas (mol)	Total gas (mol)
2 Acetic acid	$2CO_2$	$2CO_2$	$4CO_2$
1 Butyric acid	$2CO_2$	$1CO_2$	$3CO_2$
2 Propionic acid	-	$2CO_2$	$2CO_2$
2 Lactic acid	-	$2CO_2$	$2CO_2$

The use of methods based on incubation with rumen fluid can pose problems for some feed compounders. Consequently, attention has been given to examining the rate of breakdown of starch using enzymes from animal and microbial sources (Cone 1991). Although, of the purified enzymes used, bacterial amylase was the most promising, its

Table 15.7 PERCENTAGE OF STARCH DEGRADED AFTER 6h INCUBATION WITH RUMEN FLUID FROM A COW FED HAY (HFC) OR HAY PLUS TWO DIFFERENT CONCENTRATES (CFC)

	HFC	*CFC (A)*	*CFC (B)*
Maize	3.5	21.6	21.6
Milocorn	5.5	23.6	25.1
Potato	6.6	25.1	36.5
Millet	6.8	25.7	31.0
Wheat	9.9	42.3	41.2
Barley	10.3	33.8	41.0
Oats	15.9	51.0	55.6
Tapioca	23.3	47.0	52.8
Paselli	55.9	60.4	58.9

Concentrates consisted mainly of tapioca and steam-flaked maize (A) and maize and milocorn (B). From Cone *et al.* (1989)

Table 15.8 THE EFFECTS OF PROCESSING ON THE PERCENTAGE OF STARCH DEGRADED AFTER INCUBATION FOR 6h WRRH RUMEN FLUID FROM A COW FED HAY (HFC) OR HAY PLUS TWO DIFFERENT CONCENTRATES

	HFC	*CFC (A)*	*CFC (B)*
Maize	3.5	21.6	21.6
Maize feed meal	11.1	36.1	36.1
Maize gluten feed	17.6	-	45.3
Steam flaked maize	14.4	34.9	42.6
Maize flake	15.8	38.5	47.7
Popped maize	31.7	49.8	52.2
Wheat	9.9	42.3	41.2
Wheat middlings	14.7	41.7	50.1
Wheat feed meal	31.3	43.5	54.9
Poppled wheat	44.0	57.8	66.4
Rice	7.8	22.4	25.3
Rice feed meal	21.8	45.3	43.4
Popped rice	50.3	57.6	56.9

Concentrates consisted mainly of tapioca and steam-flaked maize (A) and maize and milocorn (B). From Cone *et al.* (1989)

use has clear limitations when it comes to its sensitivity to some of the effects of cereal processing (Table 15.9). On the other hand, the results obtained using reconstituted freeze-dried preparations of cell-free rumen fluid agree reasonably well, in terms of the ranking order of the various maize products, with those obtained from incubations with rumen fluid (Table 15.9). Further development of this approach could provide a useful method for routine use by feed compounders.

Table 15.9 THE PERCENTAGE OF STARCH DEGRADED AFTER 6h INCUBATION IN RUMEN FLUID OR IN A CELL-FREE PREPARATION OF THE RUMEN NULD (FREEZE-DRIED AND RECONSTITUTED) OR AFTER 4h INCUBATION WITH BACTERIAL AMYLASE

	Rumen fluid	*Bacterial amylase*	*Cell-free preparation*
Maize	19.6	23.2	8.4
Maize feed meal	44.0	34.8	35.6
Maize gluten feed	37.9	52.3	41.8
Steam flaked maize	34.1	77.1	44.3
Maize flake	51.9	77.1	65.1
Popped maize	74.9	74.6	82.0

From Cone (1991)

When it comes to assigning values for the rate of fermentation of sources of RFC for rationing purposes, the best that current knowledge will allow is the construction of a provisional 'Fermentation Rate Index' derived from measurements *in vitro*. However, even this is difficult because there is insufficient information on the comparative rates of fermentation of the various starch and sugar sources. Depression of pH during incubation with rumen liquor *in vitro* was closely correlated with the production of total fermentation acids (Sutton, 1968). Under suitably controlled conditions, the rate of depression of pH might provide a useful index of the rate of fermentation. Some results from a preliminary investigation along these lines are shown in Table 15.10. The time course of changes in pH was followed over 3.5 h of incubation, during which time the depression of pH was virtually linear. Results are expressed relative to the rate of depression of pH observed for glucose as a substrate. Although the method appears promising, the provisional nature of these results must be emphasized; further more detailed experiments are needed to confirm the validity of this approach. However, it is interesting to note that the similarity in the predicted rates of fermentation of lactose and raw starch agrees with rates of depression of ruminal pH seen *in vivo* for these two substrates (Chamberlain *et al.*, 1993). This makes it difficult to argue for the superiority of lactose over raw starch, as a supplement to grass silage (Tables 15.1 and 15.2) being due to a faster rate of fermentation of lactose.

Table 15.10 THE RATE OF DEPRESSION OF PH DURING INCUBATIONS *IN VITRO* WITH RUMEN LIQUOR FOR SOME PURIFIED SUBSTRATES AND SOME FEEDS. VALUES ARE EXPRESSED RELATIVE TO THAT OF GLUCOSE (100)

Pulyitd substrates		*Feeds*	
Sucrose	100	Maize meal	49
Lactose	58	Cooked maize	78
Xylose	90	Wheat	56
Xylan	42	Cooked wheat	88
Pectin	94	Barley	54
Maize starch	52		
Cooked maize starch	80		
Barley starch	56		
Cooked barley starch	90		

Chamberlain and Choung (unpublished)

RATE OF FERMENTATION AND THE MOLAR COMPOSITION OF VFA PRODUCED

Any assessment of the rate of fermentation of energy sources should go hand in hand with a consideration of the molar composition of the mixture of VF As produced from their fermentation. This is obviously important because of effects of the molar ratio of the absorbed mixture of VFA on milk composition (see Thomas and Chamberlain, 1984), but it may be important also because of interactions between the metabolism of propionate and ammonia in the liver, that have come to light more recently. Particularly when there is a high rate of absorption of ammonia from the rumen in the early post-feeding period, propionate can reduce the capacity of the liver to detoxify the ammonia via the urea cycle, with the result that ammonia spills over into peripheral blood, leading to effects on insulin secretion, with implications for the partition of nutrients between the udder and other body tissues, and possibly also for milk composition (Choung and Chamberlain, 1995). These findings would be expected to be of relevance to the feeding of diets containing high proportions of grass silage, especially when the silage has a high concentration of crude protein. Note that these are precisely the conditions in which attempts to synchronize energy and nitrogen release in the rumen are most applicable.

Whilst there is no doubt that specific sugars are fermented to mixtures of VFA that are broadly characteristic of them as substrates (Sutton, 1968; Chamberlain *et al.*, 1993), there remains uncertainty over the extent to which such factors as the nature of the basal diet and the level of addition of the sugars to the rumen can influence the composition of the VF A mixture produced. It has been proposed (Prins, Lankhorse and Van Hoven, 1984) that the acetate: propionate ratio is controlled by the hexose flux through the cell, and that the pattern of VFA production from a given source and amount of RFC would depend on the concentration of bacteria in the rumen; the lower the number of bacteria, the higher the flux per cell. If this is true, it offers a plausible explanation of effects of the basal diet, the level of addition of RFC and the frequency of feeding of diets rich in RFC (see Sutton, 1981). Again, the hexose flux through the microbial cell would be strongly affected by the rate at which starch is degraded in the rumen, which, in turn, is dependent on the source of the starch and its treatment during processing. Hence, it is not possible, with present knowledge, to generalize about the effects of the dietary inclusion of starches or sugars on milk composition. Whilst it is known, for example, that the severity of depressions of milk fat concentration varies with the inclusion of different types of starch (see Sutton, 1981), there are no reports of systematic and sufficiently comprehensive studies of the effects of source of starch and processing treatments on milk composition; the beneficial effects that starch inclusion can have on the concentration of milk protein (Sutton, Morant, Bines, Napper and Givens, 1993) serves to emphasize the need for such studies.

Conclusions

There is no convincing evidence of a need for close synchronization of energy and nitrogen release in the rumen to ensure efficient synthesis of microbial protein. This is not to say that severe mismatching of energy and nitrogen release may not have detrimental effects on microbial protein synthesis in some dietary circumstances, notably where a rapid release of ammonia immediately after feeding is coupled with the only significant source of energy being derived from slowly fermented (usually fibrous) substrates. Such a combination would be expected to result in ruminal pH being maintained at relatively high levels, which would favour the absorption of substantial amounts of ammonia from the rumen. In such conditions, the dietary inclusion of an appropriate source of RFC would be expected to improve the efficiency of microbial capture of ammonia. However, the different effects that various types of RFC can have on microbial protein synthesis in such conditions are not explicable in terms of improved synchronization of energy and ammonia availabilities; experimental results suggest the involvement of effects of specific substrates on the activities of the microbial population, but the nature of these effects remains to be established.

Whilst it is prudent, when formulating rations, to avoid very marked mismatches in the rates of ruminal release of energy and nitrogen, there are clear potential dangers, associated with inducing wide fluctuations of ruminal pH and even ruminal acidosis, in giving too much weight to achieving close synchronization if this entails incorporating substantial amounts of certain sources of RFC. Indeed, the best approach might be to attempt to achieve the most even pattern of energy supply in the rumen (Henning, Steyn and Meissner, 1993).

To what extent the availability of amino acids and/or pep tides in the rumen can limit microbial protein synthesis remains an important question that can only be answered after further experimentation. At this stage, it is worth noting that culture studies *in vitro* indicate a clear, specific requirement of amylolytic bacteria for preformed amino acid/ peptide. Although the full implications await experimentation *in vivo,* we would do well to recognize that the nature of the energy source in the diet will influence the nutritional requirements of the microbial population in the rumen, and that the level and type of dietary protein may need to be adjusted (on the basis of considerations that go beyond the scope of the current MP system), to ensure that the requirements for maximal rates of microbial protein synthesis are met. We should remember, also, that limitations in the ruminal supply of amino acid/peptide are likely to be particularly relevant to diets containing high proportions of grass silage.

Related to the whole issue under discussion in this paper is the question: even if modest increases in the yield of microbial protein can be achieved by manipulation of compound formulation, what would be the response of milk production? Although there is no clear answer to this question at present, it is worth considering the results of recent experiments in which proteins have been infused into the abomasum in dairy cows. Note the linear increase in the yield of milk protein in response to the infusion of casein, but the very limited increase in protein yield in response to the infusion of soya protein (Figure 15.3). When we consider that microbial protein would have a lower digestibility than soya-protein isolate and, probably, a rather similar biological value, the implication of results such as these is, at the very least, to seriously question any assumption that benefits to milk production would follow, as a matter of course, from an increased ruminal output of microbial protein.

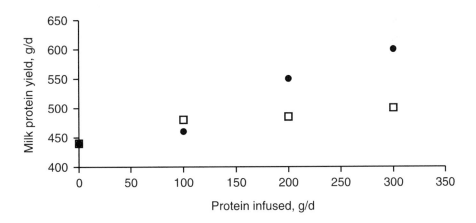

Figure 15.3 The responses in the yield of milk crude protein to the infusion of soya-protein isolate (□) or casein (●) into the abomasum in dairy cows receiving a grass silage and a cereal-based concentrate. (Choung and Chamberlain, 1993b)

Leaving aside the issue of synchronization, information on the rate and pattern of fermentation of carbohydrate sources is urgently needed if we are to uncover the mechanisms underlying the effects of diet on metabolism, and hence on milk composition, and use them to advantage in feeding the dairy cow.

Acknowledgements

We are grateful to Dr A. G. Williams for stimulating and helpful discussions.

References

Agricultural Research Council (1984) *17ze Nutrient Requirements of Ruminant Livestock* Suppl no 1 Slough: Commonwealth Agricultural Bureaux

Beever, D.E., Gill, M., Dawson, J.M. and Buttery, PJ. (1990) The effect of fish meal on the digestion of grass silage by growing cattle. *British Journal of Nutrition,* **63**, 489-502

Beever, D.E. and Cottrill, B.R. (1994) Protein systems for feeding ruminant livestock: a European assessment. *Journal of Dairy Science,* **77**, 2031-2043

Beuvink, J.M.W. (1993) Measuring and modelling in vitro gas production kinetics to evaluate ruminal fermentation of feedstuffs. Thesis, Lelystad, Netherlands: Institute for Animal Nutrition

Broderick, G.A., Wallace, RJ. and 0rskov, E.R. (1991) Control of rate and extent of protein degradation. In *Physiological Aspects of Digestion and Metabolism in Ruminants,* pp. 541-592 Edited by T. Tsuda, Y. Sasaki and R. Kawashima. London: Academic Press

Bryant, M.P. (1973) Nutritional requirements of the predominant rumen cellulolytic bacteria. *Federation Proceedings,* **32**, 1809-1813

Chamberlain, D.G., Thomas, P.C., Wilson, W.D., Newbold, CJ. and MacDonald, J.C. (1985) The effects of carbohydrate supplements on ruminal concentrations of ammonia in animals given diets of grass silage. *Journal of Agricultural Science, Cambridge,* **104**, 331-340

Chamberlain, D.G., Martin, P.A. and Robertson, S. (1990) The influence of the type of carbohydrate in the supplement on responses to protein supplementation in dairy cows receiving diets containing a high proportion of grass silage. Research Meeting No 2, British Grassland Society, Section VII, Poster 2, The British Grassland Society: Maidenhead

Chamberlain, D.G., Robertson, S. and Choung, J.-J. (1993) Sugars versus starch as supplements to grass silage: Effects on ruminal fermentation and the supply of microbial protein to the small intestine, estimated from the urinary excretion of purine derivatives, in sheep. *Journal of the Science of Food and Agriculture,* **63**, 189-194

Choung,, J.-J. and Chamberlain, D.G. (1993a) Effects of addition of lactic acid and post-ruminal supplementation with casein on the nutritional value of grass silage for milk production in dairy cows. *Grass and Forage Science,* **48**, 380-386

Choung, J.-J. and Chamberlain, D.G. (1993b) The effects of abomasal infusions of casein or soya-bean-protein isolate on the milk production of dairy cows in mid-lactation. *British Journal of Nutrition,* **69**, 103-115

Choung, J.-J. and Chamberlain, D.G. (1995) Effects of ruminal infusion of propionate on the concentrations of ammonia and insulin in peripheral blood of cows receiving an intraruminal infusion of urea. *Journal of Dairy Research,* **62**, 549-557.

Cone, J.W., Cline-Theil, W., Malestein, A. and van't Klooster, A.Th. (1989) Degradation of starch by incubation with rumen fluid. A comparison of different starch sources. *Journal of the Science of Food and Agriculture,* **49**, 173-183

Cone, J.W. (1991) Degradation of starch in feed concentrates by enzymes, rumen fluid and rumen enzymes. *Journal of the Science of Food and Agriculture,* **54**, 23-34

Dawson, J.M., Bruce, C.I., Buttery, P J., Gill, M. and Beever, D.E. (1988) Protein metabolism in the rumen of silage-fed steers: effects of fish meal supplementation. *British Journal of Nutrition,* **55**, 339-353

de Visser, H. (1993) Characterization of carbohydrates in concentrates for dairy cows. In *Recent Advances in Animal Nutrition* -1993, pp. 19-38, Edited by P.C. Garnsworthy and DJ.A. Cole. Nottingham: Nottingham University Press

Henning, P.H., Steyn, D.G. and Meissner, H.H. (1991) The effect of energy and nitrogen supply pattern on rumen bacterial growth *in vitro. Animal Production,* **53**, 165-175

Henning, P.H., Steyn, D.G. and Meissner, H.H. (1993) Effect of synchronization of energy and nitrogen supply on ruminal characteristics and microbial growth. *Journal of Animal Science,* **71**, 2516-2528

Herrera-Saldana, R., Huber, J.T. and Swingle R.S. (1986) Protein and starch solubility and degradability of several common feedstuffs. *Journal of Dairy Science,* **69** (Suppl 1), 141 (Abstr)

Herrera-Saldana, R., Gomez-Alarcon, R., Torabi, M. and Huber, J.T. (1990a) Influence of synchronizing protein and starch degradation in the rumen on nutrient utilization and microbial protein synthesis. *Journal of Dairy Science,* **73**, 142-148

Herrera-Saldana, R., Huber, J.T. and Poos, M.H. (1990 b) Dry matter, crude protein and starch degradability of five cereal grains. *Journal of Dairy Science,* **73**, 2386-2393

Hespell, R.B. (1984) Influence of ammonia assimilation pathways and survival strategy on rumen microbial growth. In *Herbivore Nutrition,* pp.346-358 Edited by F.M.C.Gilchrist and R.I. Mackie. Craighall, S. Mrica: The Science Press

Hespell, R.B. and Bryant, M.P, (1979) Efficiency of rumen microbial growth: influence of some theoretical and experimental factors on Y A TP. *Journal of Animal Science,* **49,** 1641-1647

Hoover, W.H. (1986) Chemical factors involved in ruminal fibre digestion. *Journal of Dairy Science,* **69,** 2755-2766

Hoover, W.H. and Stokes, S.R. (1991) Balancing carbohydrates and proteins for optimum rumen microbial yield. *Journal of Dairy Science,* **74,** 3630-3644

Huhtanen, P. (1987a) The effects of intraruminal infusions of sucrose and xylose on nitrogen and fibre digestion in the rumen and intestines of cattle receiving diets of grass silage and barley. *Journal of Agricultural Science in Finland,* **59,** 405-424

Huhtanen, P. (1987b) The effect of dietary inclusion of barley, unmolassed sugar beet pulp and molasses on milk production, digestibility and digesta passage in dairy cows given silage-based diet. *Journal of Agricultural Science in Finland,* **59,** 101-120

Khalili, H. and Huhtanen, P. (1991) Sucrose supplements in cattle given a grass silage-based diet. 1. Digestion of organic matter and nitrogen. *Animal Feed Science and Technology,* **33,** 247-261

Knight, W.M. and Owens, F.N. (1973) Interval urea infusion for lambs. *Journal of Animal Science,* **36,** 145-149

McCarthy, R.D., Klusmeyer, T.H., Vicini,]L., Clark,]H. and Nelson, D.R. (1989) Effects of source of protein and carbohydrate on ruminal fermentation and passage of nutrients to the small intestine of lactating cows. *Journal of Dairy Science,* **72,** 2002-2010

Mackie, R.I. and Therion,]J. (1984) Influence of mineral interactions on growth efficiency of rumen bacteria. In *Herbivore Nutrition,* pp. 455-477 Edited by F.M.C. Gilchrist and R.I. Mackie. Craighall, S. Mrica: The Science Press,

Meggison, P.A., Mcmeniman,N.P. and Armstrong, D.G. (1979) Efficiency of utilization of non-protein nitrogen in cattle. *Proceedings of the Nutrition Society,* **38,** 147A

Mould, F.L., Orskov, E.R. and Mann, S.O. (1983) Associative effects of mixed feeds. 1. Effects of type and level of supplementation and the influence of the rumen fluid pH on cellulolysis in vivo and dry matter digestion of various roughages. *Animal Feed Science and Technology,* **10,** 15-30

Newbold, J.R. (1994) Practical application of the Metabolizable Protein System. In *Recent Advancesin Animal Nutrition* 1994,pp. 231-264. Edited by P.C. Garnsworthy and DJ.A. Cole. Nottingham: Nottingham University Press

Newbold, J.R. and Rust, S.R. (1992) Effect of asynchronous nitrogen and energy supply on growth of ruminal bacteria in batch culture. *Journal of Animal Science,* **70,** 538-546

Obara, Y., Dellow, D.W. and Nolan, J.V. (1991) The influence of energy-rich supplements on nitrogen kinetics in ruminants. In *Physiological Aspects of Digestion and*

Metabolism in Ruminants, pp. 515-539. Edited by T. Tsuda, Y. Sasaki and R. Kawashima. London: Academic Press

Prins, R.A., Lankhorse, A. and van Hoven, W. (1984) Gastrointestinal fermentation in herbivores and the extent of plant cell-wall digestion. In *Herbivore Nutrition in the Sub tropics and Tropics,* pp. 408-434. Edited by F.M.C. Gilchrist and R.I. Mackie. Craighall, South Africa: The Science Press

Robinson, P .H. and McQueen, R.E. (1994) Influence of supplemental protein source and feeding frequency on rumen fermentation and performance in dairy cows. *Journal of Dairy Science,* **77**, 1340-1353

Rooke, J.A., Brett, P.A., Overend, M.A. and Armstrong, D.G. (1985) The energetic efficiency of rumen microbial protein synthesis in cattle given silage-based diets. *Animal Feed Science and Technology,* **13**, 255-267

Rooke, J.A., Lee, N.H. and Armstrong, D.G. (1987) The effects of intraruminal infusions of urea, casein, glucose syrup and a mixture of casein and glucose syrup on nitrogen digestion in the rumen of cattle receiving grass silage diets. *British Journal of Nutrition,* **57**, 89-98

Rooke, J.A. and Armstrong, D.G. (1989) The importance of the form of nitrogen on microbial protein synthesis in the rumen of cattle receiving grass silage and continuous intraruminal infusions of sucrose. *British Journal of Nutrition,* **61**, 113-121

Russell, J.B., Sniffen, CJ. and van Soest, P J. (1983) Effect of carbohydrate limitation on degradation and utilization of casein by mixed rumen bacteria. *Journal of Dairy Science,* **66**, 763-770

Russell, J.B and Wallace, RJ. (1988) Energy yielding and consuming reactions. In *The Rumen Microbial Ecosystem,* pp. 185-216 Edited by P.N, Hobson. London: Elsevier

Russell, J.B, O'Connor,j.D., Fox, D.G., van Soest, P J. and Sniffen, CJ. (1992) A net carbohydrate and protein system for evaluating cattle diets. 1. Ruminal fermentation. *Journal of Animal Science,* **70**, 3551-3561

Salter, D.N., Smith, R,H. and Hewitt, D. (1983) Factors affecting the capture of dietary nitrogen by microorganisms in the forestomachs of the young steer. Experiments with [15-N]urea. *British Journal of Nutrition,* **50**, 427-435

Simpson, M.E. (1984) Protective effect of alternative carbon sources towards cellulose during its digestion in bovine rumen fluid. *Developments in Industrial Microbiology,* **25**, 641-649

Sinclair, L.A., Garnsworthy, P.C., Newbold,J.R. and Buttery, PJ. (1993) Effect of synchronizing the rate of dietary energy and nitrogen release on rumen fermentation and microbial protein synthesis in sheep. *Journal of Agricultural Science, Cambridge,* **120**, 251-263

Smith, R.H. (1975) Nitrogen metabolism in the rumen and the composition and nutritive value of nitrogen compounds entering the duodenum. In *Digestion and*

Metabolism in the Ruminant, pp. 399-415. Edited by I. W. McDonald and A.C.I. Warner. Armidale: University of New England Publishing Unit

Stewart, C.S., Paniagua, C., Dinsdale, D., Cheng, K-J. and Garrow, S.H. (1981) Selective isolation and characteristics of Bacteroides succinogenes from the rumen of a cow. *Applied and Environmental Microbiology,* **41,** 504-510

Stouthamer, A.H. (1973) A theoretical study on the amount of ATP required for synthesis of microbial cell material. *Antonie van Leeuwenhoek,* 39,545-565

Streeter, C.L., Little, C.O., Mitchell, G.E. and Scott, R.A. (1973) Influence of rate of ruminal administration of urea on nitrogen utilization in lambs. *Journal of Animal Science,* **37,** 796-799

Strobel, HJ. and Russell, J.B. (1986) Effect of pH and energy spilling on bacterial protein synthesis by carbohydrate-limited cultures of mixed rumen bacteria. *Journal of Dairy Science,* **69,** 2941-2947

Sutton, J.D. (1968) The fermentation of soluble carbohydrates in rumen contents of cows fed diets containing a large proportion of hay. *British Journal of Nutrition,* **22,** 689-712

Sutton, J.D. (1981) Concentrate feeding and milk composition. In *Recent Advances in Animal Nutrition* -1981, pp. 35-48 Edited by W. Haresign. London: Butterworths

Sutton, J.D., Morant, S.V., Bines, J.A., Napper, DJ. and Givens, D.I. (1993) Effect of altering the starch:fibre ratio in the concentrates on hay intake and milk production by Friesian cows. *Journal of Agricultural Science, Cambridge,* **120,** 379-390

Tamminga, S., van Vuuren, A.M., van der Koelen, CJ. (1990) Ruminal behaviour of structural carbohydrates, non-structural carbohydrates and crude protein from concentrate ingredients in dairy cows. *Netherlands Journal of Agricultural Science,* **38,** 513-526

Theurer, C.B. (1986) Grain processing effects on starch utilization by ruminants. *Journal of Animal Science,* **63,** 1649-1662

Thomas, P.C. and Chamberlain, D.G. (1984) Manipulation of milk composition to meet market needs. In *Recent Advances in Animal Nutrition* - 1984, pp. 219-243 Edited by W. Haresign and DJ.A. Cole. London: Butterworths

This paper was first published in 1995

16

CARBOHYDRATE, PROTEIN AND AMINO ACID NUTRITION OF LACTATING DAIRY CATTLE

W. CHALUPA[1] and C.J. SNIFFEN[2]
[1]University of Pennsylvania, Kennett Square, Pennsylvania, USA; [2]William H. Miner Agricultural Research Institute, Chazy, New York, USA

Introduction

Rumen microbes do not provide enough protein for maximum milk production. Dietary protein must escape rumen degradation and pass to the small intestine to supply sufficient amounts of amino acids. A knowledge of amino acid requirements is important to minimize wastage of dietary protein and to optimize productivity.

Ration formulation systems described by NRC (1989), ARC (1980) and INRA (1988) require the partitioning of dietary protein into fractions degraded in the rumen (DIPIP) and resistant to rumen degradation (UIPIP). *In vivo, in situ* and *in vitro* methods are used for partitioning dietary protein into DIPIP and UIPIP.

All of these systems use different ways to estimate the organic matter fermented in the rumen. The NRC (1985) system used Total Digestible Nutrients (TDN) because that was the largest existing data base in the *USA*. This approach had problems because the high fat feeds were not accounted for and neither were the changes in the extent of digestion due to changes in rate of passage.

Tabular values in NRC (1989) are based on *in vivo* measurements with cattle fitted with cannulae in the abomasum or duodenum. Feed intake in most experiments was about 2% of body weight. However, high-producing dairy cows consume feed at 3 to 4% of body weight. Because rate of passage of feed ingredients increases with increasing feed intake, UIPIP of rations fed to lactating cows is probably greater than predicted using values in NRC (1989).

Alternatives to *in vivo* experiments are *in situ* fermentation of feeds and in *vitro* incubation with proteolytic or carbohydrate-digesting enzymes. Both methods have problems. Bacteria can enter nylon bags suspended in the rumen and contaminate the undigested residue with microbial protein. Unless undigested residues are corrected for bacterial contamination, UIPIP will be over- estimated. Like *in vivo* estimates, *in situ* methods are costly and are not readily adaptable for routine feed analyses. Enzymatic methods offer promise for routine feed analysis. However, saturation of enzyme upon substrate results in faster rates of protein degradation than occurs in the rumen. Reducing enzyme levels to limit rates of degradation can produce large analytical errors due to small variations in enzyme activity or quality. In addition, optimum time of exposure of different feed types to enzymes has not been established completely. Nevertheless, Krishnamoorthy, Sniffen, Stern and Van Soest (1983) obtained a good correlation ($R^2 =$ 0.84) between *in vivo* UIPIP and UIPIP estimated from *in vitro* incubation with protease produced by *Streptococcus griseus*. Abe (1982, 1985), Abe, Horii and Ramoeka (1979) and Abe and Nakui (1979) developed an enzymatic system to measure the digestibility of fibre and organic matter. The challenge of selecting the appropriate enzymes as well as the correct enzyme:substrate ratio is larger with the carbohydrates than with proteins.

In this report the Cornell Net Carbohydrate and Protein Model, expanded to include amino acids (Fox, Sniffen, O'Connor, Russell and Van Soest, 1990, 1992; Fox, Sniffen, O'Connor and Chalupa, 1991; Russell, O'Connor, Fox, Van Soest and Sniffen, 1992; Sniffen, O'Connor, Van Soest, Fox and Russell, 1992; O'Connor, Sniffen, Fox and Chalupa, 1993), is used to estimate feed carbohydrate and protein fractions, flows of carbohydrates, protein and amino acids to the duodenum, disappearance of carbohydrates and absorption of protein and amino acids from the small intestine, and amino acid balance of example rations.

Partition of dietary carbohydrate

The detergent system (Goering and Van Soest, 1970) is used to fractionate the carbohydrate. This approach was used because of the need to use an analytical system that was commonly used by feed-testing laboratories. The fractions are calculated as follows:

Non-fibre carbohydrate (NFC)   =   100 - (protein + fat + (NDF- NDF protein) + ash)

where NDF is neutral-detergent fibre

Sugar   =   sugar as a proportion of NFC
Starch, pectins, glucans,
volatile fatty acids (VFA)   =   NFC -sugar
Lignin

The carbohydrate fractions are as follows:
A = Sugars
B_1 = Starch, pectins, ß glucans, VFA
B_2 = Available NDF (NDF -lignin X 2.4)
C   = Unavailable fibre(lignin X 2.4)

Volatile fatty acids need to be separated from B_1. Pectins, ß glucans and other carbohydrates soluble in neutral-detergent need to be separated into as many B pools as can be determined and are found to be important in animal response. The C fraction is estimated from the work of Mertens (Sniffen *et al.,* 1992). This estimate needs to be improved. It is suggested by Abe(1982) that there are fast and slow fibre fractions and that these fractions act uniformly. There is a definite need to improve our estimates of uniform fractions of carbohydrate.

The rates of digestion of the carbohydrate fractions are based on very limited data (Sniffen *et al.,* 1992). Pool size has the greatest impact on feed digestibility. Generally, the rates of digestion of the A and B pools are orders of magnitude apart but there can be exceptions. The starch in ground shell corn and the available cell wall of a high quality grass or legume have digestion rates that are very similar. Non-fibre carbohydrates and fibre sources vary significantly in their digestion rates. These rates are affected by the source, maturity, weather, variety and processing.

Partition of dietary protein

The detergent system developed by Goering and Van Soest (1970) for analyses of carbohydrates in conjunction with extraction with borate-phosphate buffer (Fox *et al.,* 1990) offers a system to describe protein fractions (A, B1, B2, B3 and C, Figure 16.1) that, when altered in rations, will have an impact on animal responses (Sniffen, Roe, Rafferty, O'Connor, Fox and Chalupa, 1990).

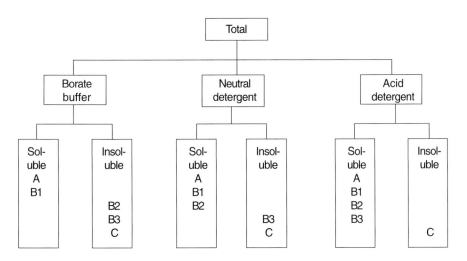

Figure 16.1 Analyses of protein fractions using borate-phosphate buffer, acid detergent and neutral detergent.

Fractions A and B1 are soluble in borate-phosphate buffer. These can be partitioned further by extraction with TCA. Fractions B2, B3 and C are insoluble in borate-phosphate buffer. Extraction with neutral detergent isolates fractions A, B1 and B2 (soluble in neutral detergent) from Fractions B3 and C (insoluble in neutral detergent). Acid detergent partitions proteins in fraction C (insoluble in acid detergent) and fractions A, B1, B2 and B3 (soluble in neutral detergent). Fraction B2 is calculated as the difference between protein insoluble in borate-phosphate buffer and that insoluble in neutral detergent. Fraction B3 is the difference between protein insoluble in neutral detergent and that insoluble in acid detergent. Proteins insoluble in acid detergent are fraction C.

Composition, rumen degradation and intestinal digestion of protein fractions are shown in Table 16.1. Fraction A contains ammonia, nitrates, amino acids and peptides; rumen degradation is instantaneous and none reaches the small intestine. Fraction Bl consists of globulins and some albumins. Because rumen degradation is 200-300 %/hour, only small amounts reach the small intestine but intestinal digestibility of Bl proteins is complete. Fraction B2 proteins contain most of the albumins and glutelins. Rumen degradation is 5-15 %/hour with intestinal digestibility of 100%. Fraction BJ proteins are prolamins, extension proteins (associated with cell walls) and heat-denatured proteins that did not undergo the Maillard reaction. They are degraded in the rumen at 0.1-1.5 %/hour; intestinal digestibility is 80%. Fraction C proteins consist of Maillard reaction proteins (heat-damaged protein) and nitrogen bound to lignin. They are not degraded in the rumen and are considered indigestible in the intestine.

Table 16.1 COMPOSITION, RUMEN DEGRADATION AND INTESTINAL DIGESTION OF PROTEIN FRACTIONS

Fraction	Rumen composition	Intestinal degradation (%/h)	Digestion (%/h)
A	NH_3, NO_3, AA peptides	Instantaneous	None reaches intestine
B_1	Globulins Some albumins	200-300	100
B_2	Most albumins Glutelins	5-15	100
B_3	Prolamins Extensin proteins Denatured proteins	0.1-1.5	80
C	Maillard products N bound to lignin	0	0

Rumen degradation of protein can be estimated from pool sizes, degradation rates of protein fractions and rates of passage of feed ingredients. Digestibility of undegraded dietary protein in the small intestine can be estimated by applying digestion rate constants (Table 16.1) to fractions B1, B2, BJ and C (Fox *et al., 1990,* Sniffen *et al., 1992).*

Protein fractions and amino acid composition of absorbed protein in feed ingredients

Protein fractions, rumen escape of protein, intestinal digestibility of undegraded dietary protein and amino acids in absorbed protein are shown in Tables 16.2 to 16.5.

Protein fractions affect both rumen undegradability and digestion of undegraded protein in the small intestine. Increasing fractions B2, BJ and C will increase undegradability but increasing Fraction C will decrease intestinal digestibility. Ensiling either forages (Table 16.2) or grains (Table 16.3) increases fraction A at the expense of fraction B2 so that undegradability is reduced. With forages, ensiling usually increases fraction C so intestinal digestibility is reduced. The effect of heat is demonstrated by comparing raw versus roasted soya beans (Table 16.4). Roasting soya beans reduces fraction A and increases fraction B2 at the expense of fraction Bl so that undegradability is increased. Because neither fraction BJ nor fraction C are affected greatly, intestinal digestibility is not changed by roasting. On the other hand, distillers grains are high in undegraded protein, but intestinal digestibility may be reduced because of the increased proportion of fraction C. In general, intestinal digestibility of un degraded protein in protein meals, whole seeds, marine and animal proteins is high (Tables 16.4 and 16.5). However, rumen undegradability of marine and animal proteins is higher because they contain higher proportions of fraction BJ.

Absorbed amino acids provided by forages are shown in Table 16.2. Legumes with crude protein contents of 200 g/kg can provide 20-40% of the crude protein required but they only provide 5-10% of absorbed essential amino acids required. This is due to low rumen escape and low intestinal digestibility of escape protein. More absorbed amino acids are provided by legumes preserved as hay rather than silage but there is little difference in absorbed amino acids provided by legumes with protein contents of 200 or 170 g/kg. This reflects changes in protein fractions. Forages, however, are important sources of highly-digestible fibre.

Absorbed amino acids provided by corn (maize) and corn products are shown in Table 16.3. Storing corn grain by ensiling reduces undegradability and supply of absorbed amino acids. Corn grain, regardless of storage method, provides less than 10% of total required absorbed essential amino acids. Because of their higher protein contents, corn gluten meal and corn distillers provide more absorbed amino acids than corn grain. In general, corn and corn products are good sources of leucine but they are low in lysine.

Absorbed amino acids provided by protein meals and whole seeds are shown in Table 16.4. Protein meals can provide 30-50% of crude protein required. Absorbed essential amino acids provided by these protein meals is 15-30% of requirements. Whole seeds are usually used because of their high net energy content due to their high fat

Table 16.2 PROTEIN FRACTIONS AND AMINO ACIDS IN FORAGES

Measurement	Legume silage early bloom	Legume hay early bloom	Legume silage mid bloom	Legume silage mid bloom	Maize silage
Protein intake (g/kg DM)	200	200	170	170	80
Protein fractions (proportion of protein intake)					
A (NPN)	0.58	0.29	0.52	0.27	0.52
B1 (true)	0	0.01	0	0.01	0
B2 (true)	0.15	0.52	0.16	0.47	0.33
B3 (true)	0.11	0.08	0.14	0.11	0.08
C (unavailable)	0.15	0.10	0.18	0.14	0.07
Undegraded	0.28	0.30	0.33	0.36	0.26
Absorbed	0.43	0.65	0.41	0.59	0.67
Absorbed protein and amino acids (g/kg)					
Protein	25	42	24	39	14
Methionine	0.30	0.52	0.29	0.47	0.12
Lysine	0.80	1.36	0.76	1.24	0.31
Arginine	0.60	1.03	0.58	0.94	0.27
Threonine	0.82	1.39	0.78	1.27	0.31
Leucine	1.59	2.70	1.51	2.46	0.92
Isoleucine	0.78	1.32	0.74	1.21	0.35
Valine	1.35	2.30	1.28	2.10	0.46
Histidine	0.16	0.27	0.15	0.24	0.15
Phenylalanine	1.04	1.77	0.99	1.61	0.42

Table 16.3 PROTEIN FRACTIONS AND AMINO ACIDS IN MAIZE PRODUCTS

Measurement	Dry grain	High-moisture grain	Gluten meal	Gluten feed	Distillers grains with solubles
Protein intake (g/kg DM)	100	100	660	260	250
Protein fractions (proportion of protein intake)					
A (NPN)	0.06	0.40	0.03	0.49	0.12
B1 (true)	0.02	0	0.01	0	0.04
B2 (true)	0.77	0.44	0.83	0.43	0.44
B3 (true)	0.10	0.11	0	0.06	0.20
C (unavailable)	0.05	0.05	0.13	0.02	0.20
Undegraded	0.59	0.34	0.65	0.34	0.65
Absorbed	0.89	0.79	0.81	0.91	0.63
Absorbed protein and amino acids (g/kg)					
Protein	55	28	357	81	104
Methionine	0.61	0.24	7.46	1.35	1.25
Lysine	0.90	0.47	4.42	1.21	2.15
Arginine	0.99	0.25	11.32	5.62	4.33
Threonine	1.53	0.82	10.45	1.38	3.25
Leucine	5.85	2.76	57.88	5.67	9.46
Isoleucine	1.47	0.70	15.49	0.72	2.90
Valine	2.05	0.69	14.99	3.22	5.46
Histidine	1.12	0.60	8.74	1.76	1.90
Phenylalanine	1.99	0.80	23.12	1.35	3.25

Table 16.4 PROTEIN FRACTIONS AND AMINO ACIDS IN PROTEIN MEALS AND WHOLE SEEDS

Measurement	Soya bean meal 48 (solvent extracted)	Cotton seed meal 44 (solvent extracted)	Soya bean (raw)	Soya bean (roasted)	Cotton seed (whole)
Protein intake (g/kg DM)	540	450	430	430	230
Protein fractions (proportion of protein intake)					
A (NPN)	0.01	0.08	0.10	0.01	0.01
B1 (true)	0.20	0.12	0.34	0.15	0.39
B2 (true)	0.77	0.70	0.51	0.72	0.52
B3 (true)	0.01	0.02	0.02	0.08	0
C (unavailable)	0.01	0.08	0.03	0.04	0.08
Undegraded	0.33	0.38	0.25	0.51	0.29
Absorbed	0.96	0.80	0.89	0.91	0.75
Absorbed protein and amino acids (g/kg)					
Protein	171	137	99	200	50
Methionine	1.56	2.80	0.92	1.75	1.08
Lysine	10.67	7.41	6.27	11.93	2.85
Arginine	15.60	17.33	9.18	17.44	6.67
Threonine	6.09	6.08	3.58	6.81	2.34
Leucine	12.53	9.79	7.37	14.01	3.77
Isoleucine	7.78	6.37	4.58	8.70	2.45
Valine	7.11	8.06	4.18	7.95	3.10
Histidine	4.52	3.52	2.66	5.06	1.36
Phenylalanine	8.23	9.67	4.84	9.20	3.72

Table 16.5 PROTEIN FRACTIONS AND AMINO ACIDS IN BREWERS GRAINS, MARINE AND ANIMAL PROTEINS

Measurement	Brewers grains (dry)	Fish meal	Meat meal	Blood meal	Feather meal
Protein intake (g/kg DM)	250	670	550	950	890
Protein fractions (proportion of protein intake)					
A (NPN)	0.03	0.05	0	0.03	0
B1 (true)	0.01	0.14	0.13	0.02	0.04
B2 (true)	0.55	0.38	0.40	0.56	0.46
B3 (true)	0.28	0.42	0.46	0.36	0.48
C (unavailable)	0.12	0.01	0.01	0.03	0.02
Undegraded	0.56	0.73	0.70	0.79	0.82
Absorbed	0.71	0.89	0.86	0.88	0.86
Absorbed protein and amino acids (g/kg)					
Protein	105	449	337	663	631
Methionine	1.32	12.76	2.83	7.10	3.09
Lysine	2.26	32.04	18.89	61.94	16.21
Arginine	2.74	32.31	27.93	33.22	46.80
Threonine	2.90	18.79	8.50	31.37	26.30
Leucine	8.90	31.51	18.42	88.86	52.42
Isoleucine	3.71	20.36	8.20	5.84	29.02
Valine	3.97	21.62	12.38	60.21	50.15
Histidine	1.55	10.34	4.86	42.77	5.93
Phenylalanine	5.05	19.46	10.22	52.12	32.86

levels. Raw soya beans provide less absorbed amino acids than soya bean meal. Roasted soya beans provide absorbed amino acids like those found in soya bean meal.

Absorbed amino acids supplied by marine and animal proteins are shown in Table 16.5. These ingredients can provide 15-30% of crude protein required and 20-40% of the total requirement for absorbed essential amino acids. Blood meal is high in absorbed lysine and leucine whereas fish meal is the best source of absorbed methionine. Meat meal and feather meal provide lower levels of absorbed methionine and lysine but these proteins may be useful in meeting requirements for other essential amino acids.

Table 16.6 contains examples of rations for high producing cows. Roasted soya beans, distillers grains, blood meal and fish meal were used as high UIPIP feeds. To avoid potential decreases in feed intake, blood and fish meals were not allowed to exceed a total of 0.8 kg/day. Nutrient constraints were 70 g/kg maximum fat, 280-300 g/kg NDF and 350-380 g/kg NFC. Rations provide sufficient peptides and ammonia so that high levels of UIPIP would not decrease microbial growth. With all rations, 40% of metabolizable protein was provided by rumen microbes and 60% by undegraded dietary protein. This was a result of the level of feed intake (24 kg/day). A high level of intake increases escape protein but decreases rumen production of bacterial protein because rumen digestion of carbohydrate is lower, due to increased rates of passage, so that less energy is available for microbial growth. Absorbed isoleucine was deficient in all rations. This may reflect the coefficient used to estimate the transfer of absorbed isoleucine to milk isoleucine (79%). However, even if a transfer coefficient of 1000;0 had been used, there would still have been a deficiency of absorbed isoleucine. Either isoleucine is the primary limiting amino acid for milk production or the model underestimates absorbed isoleucine provided by rumen microbes and/or undegraded dietary protein.

Because individual absorbed essential amino acids are required in different amounts, balances should be evaluated as percentages of requirements, rather than as absolute requirements. Deficiencies of absorbed isoleucine were discussed above. The constraint on maximum dietary fat limited distillers grains to 2.5 kg/day. Because of this, the UIPIP of the distillers ration was 0.43 and there were deficits of methionine (-17%), lysine (-17%), and valine (-10%). The UIPIP of rations containing blood and fish meal meals were 0.47-0.49. Blood meal corrects the lysine (+2%) and valine (+ 15%) deficits but methionine is still deficient (-10%). Fish meal lowers methionine (-3%), lysine (-11%) and valine (-5%) deficiencies. The best amino acid balance is with both blood and fish meals. Deficiencies of methionine and lysine are both reduced to -6%. Complete correction of amino acid balances for high levels of milk production requires the use of rumen-protected amino acids.

Protected amino acids

The primary methods developed to prevent fermentative digestion of amino acids are structural manipulation, to produce amino-acid analogues, and coating with resistant materials.

Table 16.6 EXAMPLE RATIONS TO PROVIDE ABSORBED AMINO ACIDS FOR A 650 kg COW PRODUCING 45 kg/d MILK WITH 3.2% PROTEIN AND 3.7% FAT

	Ration			
	Distillers granis	*Blood meal*	*Fish meal*	*Blood + fish meal*
Ingredients (kg DM/day)				
Maize silage	6.32	7.09	6.73	7.05
Alfalfa haylage	4.64	4.64	4.77	4.64
Maize grain	5.68	5.88	5.52	5.55
Soya bean meal	1.36	0.45	0.82	0.64
Roast soya beans	2.50	2.09	1.91	2.09
Distillers grains with solubles	2.50	1.91	2.36	2.14
Blood meal	0	0.80	0	0.30
Fish meal	0	0	0.8	0.50
Megalac	0.36	0.50	0.45	0045
Vitamins/minerals	0.45	0.45	0.45	0.45
Total	23.81	23.81	23.81	23.81
Analyses (dry matter basis)				
Protein				
Crude (%)	19.3	19.3	19.3	19.3
Undegradable (proportion)	0.43	0.49	0.47	0.48
Metabolizable (kg/day)				
Required	2.95	2.94	2.96	2.95
Supplied	2.81	3.07	2.93	2.99
Microbial	1.16	1.19	1.16	1.17
Ration	1.65	1.88	1.77	1.82
Balance	-0.14	0.13	-0.03	0.04
Net energy (Mcal/kg)	1.83	1.85	1.83	1.83
NDF (%)	28.9	28.7	29.0	29.0
NFC (%)	37.7	38.1	37.0	37.4
Fat (%)	7.0	6.9	7.0	7.0
Rumen protein balance (g/day)				
Peptides	94	42	59	52
Ammonia	167	117	140	129

Absorbed Amino Acid Requirements and Balance (g/d)

	Requirement	Balance							
Methionine	59	-10	(-17%)	-6	(-10%)	-2	(-3%)	-3	(-6%)
Lysine	192	-34	(-17%)	4	(+2%)	-22	(-11%)	-11	(-6%)
Arginine	111	60	(+54%)	65	(+59%)	66	(+59%)	67	(+60%)
Threonine	117	-1	(-1%)	17	(+14%)	6	(+5%)	10	(+9%)
Leucine	197	21	(+11%)	74	(+38%)	29	(+15%)	46	(+23%)
Isoleucine	148	-24	(-16%)	-29	(-20%)	-17	(-12%)	-21	(-14%)
Valine	155	-15	(-10%)	24	(+15%)	-7	(-5%)	4	(+3%)
Histidine	62	2	(+4%)	31	(+50%)	5	(+7%)	15	(+24%)
Phenylalanine	111	13	(+19%)	45	(+41%)	18	(+16%)	29	(+26%)

The main amino acid analogues that have been evaluated are methionine hydroxy analogue, N-(hydroxymethyl) DL-methionine calcium, and mono plus di-N-(hydroxymethyl)-L-lysine calcium. Methionine hydroxy analogue appears to be more resistant to fermentative digestion than methionine, but substantial amounts do not appear to bypass the rumen (Chalupa and Sniffen, 1991).

Amino acids have been coated with polymeric compounds, formalized protein, fat, mixtures of fat and calcium, mixtures of fat and protein, and with calcium salts of long-chain fatty acids. (Chalupa and Sniffen, 1991; Ferguson, Chalupa, Thomsen, Galligan and Cummings, 1993).

Recently, a new product (Megalac Plus®) was introduced (Church and Dwight Co. Inc., Princeton NJ). Megalac Plus® contains 3% methionine hydroxy analogue added during the manufacture of Megalac®. The calcium salts of long-chain fatty acids afford protection of the methionine hydroxy analogue. In a study on a commercial dairy (Ferguson *et al*, 1993), cows fed 0.5 kg/day Megalac Plus® versus Megalac® produced an additional 1.7 kg/day milk with modest increases in the concentration of milk protein and fat (Table 16.7). In primiparous cows, milk yield decreased (3.8 kg/day) but there was a substantial increase in the concentration of milk protein (1.2 g/kg) and a modest increase in milk fat concentration (0.8 g/kg).

Table 16.7 RESPONSES OF LACTATING COWS TO MEGALAC PLUS[1]

	Treatment	
	Megalac	*Megalac Plus*
Milk yield (kg/day)	41.4	43.0
Milk protein (g/kg)	27.9	28.3
Milk fat (g/kg)	34.2	34.7

[1] 163 multiparous cows through 168 days in milk
(Ferguson, Chalupa, Thomsen, Galligan, and Cummings, 1993)

Application

NRC (1985), ARC (1980) and INRA (1988) presented frameworks based on the biology of nitrogen metabolism in ruminants that form the basis for calculating protein requirements of lactating dairy cattle. These systems detailed protein nutrition in terms of pools and transfer coefficients between pools. Because information needed for operation of detailed models of protein nutrition was not available, initial recommendations of protein requirements were estimated from static-aggregated models. These only considered overall rumen degradation of dietary protein and synthesis of microbial protein driven only by energy available in the rumen. Although simplistic, these static-aggregated models were useful in educating dairy producers and their advisors on the dynamics of protein nutrition. Therefore, rations now fed to high-producing dairy cows usually contain by-product feed ingredients that are resistant to rumen degradation.

The Cornell net carbohydrate and protein system for evaluating cattle diets (Fox *et al*, 1990; Fox *et al.*, 1992) is a mix of empirical and mechanistic approaches that describe feed intake, rumen fermentation of protein and carbohydrate, intestinal digestion and absorption, excretion, heat production, and utilization of nutrients for maintenance, growth, lactation and pregnancy. The system can be applied at the farm level because rations are characterized according to fractions that are measured easily in most feed analyses laboratories. The system is especially valuable in estimating rumen de grad ability of dietary carbohydrates and protein and for determining whether rumen microbes are provided with proper types and amounts of nitrogenous nutrients (i.e. ammonia, peptides). The system has also been useful in providing information on amino acid requirements and identifying limiting amino acids (Fox *et al.*, 1992).

Ultimately, nutrient requirements of dairy cattle will be based on quantitative and dynamic mathematical descriptions of biochemical reactions. The efforts of Baldwin, France, Beever, Gill and Thornley (1987), Baldwin, France and Gill (1987) and Baldwin, Thornley and Beever (1987) demonstrate that biochemical data, generated from tissue level experiments *in vitro,* can be used to develop mechanistic, whole-animal models that are useful in describing utilization of nutrients and nutrient requirements.

References

Abe, A. (1982) *Japan Agricultural Research Quarterly,* **16,** 51-56

Abe, A. (1985) *Tropical Agricultural Research Series No.* 18, p. 133. Japan: Tropical Agricultural Research Center, Ministry of Agriculture, Forestry and Fisheries.

Abe, A. and Horii, S. (1979) *Journal of Japanese Grassland Science,* **25,** 70

Abe, A., Hopi, S. and Ramoeka, K. (~979) *Journal of Animal Science,* **48,** 1483

Abe, A., and Nakui, T. (1979) *Journal of Japanese Grassland Science,* **25,** 231

Agricultural Research Council (ARC;1980) *The Nutrient Requirements of Ruminant Livestock.* Slough: Commonwealth Agricultural Research Bureaux

Baldwin, R.L., France, J., Beever, D.E., Gill, M. and Thornley, J.H.M. (1987) *Journal of Dairy Research,* **54,** 133-145

Baldwin, R.L., France, J. and Gill, M. (1987) *Journal of Dairy Research,* **54,** 77-105

Baldwin, R.L., Thornley, J.H.M. and Beever, D.E. (1987) *Journal of Dairy Research,* **54,** 107-131

Chalupa, W. and Sniffen, C.J. (1991) *The Veterinary Clinics of North America- Food Animal Practice: Volume* 7, *Dairy Nutrition Management,* pp. 353-372. Philadelphia: W.B. Saundres

Ferguson, J.D., Chalupa, W., Thomsen, N., Galligan, D.T. and Cummings, K. (1993) *Journal of Dairy Science,* **76 (Supplement 1)**, 184

Fox, D.G., Sniffen, C.J., O'Connor, J.D. and Chalupa, W. (1991) Unpublished data.

Fox, D.G., Sniffen, C.J., O'Connor, J.D., Russell, J.B. and Van Soest, P.J. (1990) *The Search:Agriculture.* Ithaca: Cornell University Agricultural Experimental Station No. 34

Fox, D.G., Sniffen, C.J., O'Connor, J.D., Russell, J.B. and Van Soest, P.J. (1992) *Journal of Animal Science,* **70**, 3578-3596

Goering, H. K. and Van Soest, P.J. (1970) *Agricultural Handbook No. 379.* Washington DC: Agricultural Research Service, USDA

Institut National de la Recherche Agronomique (INRA; 1989) *Ruminant Nutrition. Recommended allowances and feed tables.* Edited by R. Jarrige. London: John Libbey Eurotext

Krishnamoorthy, U., Sniffen, C.J., Stern, M.D. and Van Soest, P.J. (1983) *British Journal of Nutrition,* **50**, 555-568

National Research Council (NRC; 1985) *Ruminant Nitrogen Usage.* Washington DC: National Research Council

National Research Council (NRC; 1989) *Nutrient Requirements of Dairy Cattle.* Washington DC: National Research Council

O'Connor, J.D., Sniffen, C.J., Fox, D.G. and Chalupa, W. (1993) *Journal of Animal Science,* **71**, 1298-1311

Russell, J.B., O'Connor, J.D., Fox, D.G., Van Soest, P.J. and Sniffen, C.J. (1992) *Journal of Animal Science,* **70**, 3551-3561

Sniffen, C.J., Roe, M.B., Rafferty, A.P., O'Connor, J.D., Fox, D.G. and Chalupa, W. (1990) *Proceedings of the University of Guelph Nutrition Conference*

Sniffen, C.J., O'Connor, J.D., Van Soest, P.J., Fox, D.G. and Russell, J.B. (1992) *Journal of Animal Science,* **70**, 3562-3577

This paper was first published in 1994

17

DEVELOPMENTS IN AMINO ACID NUTRITION OF DAIRY COWS

B. K. SLOAN
Rhône-Poulenc Animal Nutrition, 42 avenue Aristide Briand, 92164 Antony, France

What are the potential benefits to balancing dairy rations for their digestible amino acid content?

The increasing pressure in the dairy industry to produce milk more efficiently while tailoring its composition to meet the demands of different market segments has given renewed impetus to devising appropriate feed formulations and feeding strategies to meet these challenges. Optimising the amino acid balance of rations has been proposed as one approach, to enhance milk protein secretion and manipulate milk protein content. However, to be widely adopted in practice a clear definition is needed of how to balance amino acids, appropriate feed formulation constraints need to be developed and the economic benefits demonstrated.

AN ALREADY PROVEN CONCEPT IN NON RUMINANT NUTRITION

Optimising the supplies of individual amino acids has been common practice in poultry nutrition for over 30 years and in pig nutrition for the last 20 years. The principal advantage of doing this is an increase in animal performance - lean growth in broilers and growing pigs and egg production in laying hens, with an accompanying improvement in feed conversion efficiency. A similar improvement in performance may also be obtainable for ruminants by paying more attention to individual amino acid supplies, rather than trying to satisfy total amino acid supplies on a global basis. However, due to the role played by the rumen in transforming a large proportion of dietary protein into microbial protein, it has been very difficult to determine whether there is a significant performance advantage to increasing the supplies of specific individual amino acids post-ruminally for the dairy cow of high genetic merit.

In this chapter, the evidence of limitations to dairy cow performance arising from the quantity and relative proportions of individual amino acids absorbed from the small intestine of cows fed conventional rations will be reviewed. How this evidence has been transformed into a practical set of recommendations for digestible lysine and methionine concentrations in dairy rations has been outlined in Chapter 14 (Vérité *et al.*, 1997). These recommendations will be used as the basis for discussing the potential benefits of formulating rations to contain specific digestible lysine and methionine levels on various practical aspects of dairy cow performance.

DEFINITION OF THE AMINO ACID BALANCE CONCEPT FOR RUMINANTS

It should be stated from the outset, that when we talk about amino acid nutrition of ruminants, there is firstly a very important quantitative component and secondly a qualitative component that should not be neglected. Both are important in order to maximise performance and should be treated as a whole and not as alternatives. First and foremost, a ruminant needs a sufficient supply of all amino acids, essential and non essential, at the systemic level, to satisfy the large majority of amino acid demands for maintenance and production. This is normally achieved by formulating rations to satisfy the recommendations laid down in any modern protein system such as the metabolisable protein (MP) system (AFRC,1992) or the protein digested in the intestine (PDI) system described in the previous chapter. Following the principles of monogastric nutrition, a further gain in performance can be envisaged if the correct 'balance' or 'profile' of digestible amino acids is supplied. The improvement in performance in monogastrics is achieved by increasing the efficiency of total amino acid utilisation and reducing the energetic load for removing surplus amino acid nitrogen (Henry, 1993 ; Leclercq, 1996).

The qualitative component of amino acid nutrition in dairy cows will be regarded in most detail in this review. Specific reference to quantitative supplies will only be included where it is believed to be important to the understanding of certain responses observed.

Determining the limiting amino acids for milk performance

RATION PROTEIN SOURCE DETERMINES THE QUANTITY OF MILK PROTEIN SECRETED

Rulquin and Vérité (1993), from a compilation of trials where treatment differences in crude protein content and N-degradability were negligible, showed that the protein source in the diet could have a marked influence on milk protein secretion. Soya bean meal was superior to maize gluten meal and fishmeal was superior to soyabean. In fact, fishmeal-containing diets outperformed maize gluten meal rations by as much as 150 g of milk protein / cow / day. It would appear that the potential advantage of low protein degradability of maize gluten meal is compromised by its poor amino acid profile. The amino acid profile of the different protein sources would appear to have an important effect in determining the quantity of milk protein secreted.

Casein has been the mostly widely used protein source to investigate the general interest in 'improving' the quality of protein available to the dairy cow. Consistently large responses to casein infusions have been observed in terms of milk yield (1 to 4 kg per cow/day) and milk protein yield (50 to 180 g per cow/day) (Clark, 1975). There is apparently both an important quantitative as well as qualitative component to the initiation of this response. A large part of the volume response may be attributable to an increase in the total quantity of amino acids absorbed (PDI) by the dairy cow. It is also evident that the responses are very much related to the basal level of protein supply. When protein supplies are lower than requirements, a larger proportion of the additional available amino acid-N is partitioned towards milk protein synthesis relative to other productive functions compared with when requirements are already satisfied (Whitelaw, Milne, Ørskov and Smith, 1986).

However, the qualitative advantage of casein, due to its balanced amino acid profile, is also important, as demonstrated in trials comparing isonitrogenous quantities of casein and soya isolate (Choung and Chamberlain, 1993 ; Rulquin, 1986). Whereas 50 % of the extra amino acid-N from casein was found in milk protein, only 20 % was recovered as milk protein when soya isolate was infused.

NON ESSENTIAL AMINO ACIDS ARE GENERALLY NOT LIMITING

The infusion of casein has been mimicked by infusion of a solution of all its constituent individual amino acids in proportion. Improvements in milk protein secretion were essentially of the same magnitude as for casein and likewise when only the 10 so called essential amino acids were infused (Fraser, Ørskov, Whitelaw and Franklin, 1991; Schwab, Satter and Clay, 1976). This indicates that when supplies approach conventional recommendations for total amino acids (PDI or MP) there is no need for a marginal increase in non essential amino acid supplies; they are already supplied in excess and/or the animal can easily synthesize any additional requirements from other amino acids present in excess quantities.

METHIONINE AND LYSINE, THE FIRST TWO LIMITING AMINO ACIDS

Many trials have tried to identify the sequence of limiting amino acids for milk protein production by infusing individual amino acids post-ruminally. Schwab, *et al* (1976) demonstrated that methionine and lysine were likely to be the two most limiting amino acids in dairy rations for milk protein secretion. Increasing supplies of these two amino acids alone improved milk protein content by 1g/kg and milk protein secretion by 45 g/ day, which accounted for 43 % of the response to an infusion of casein.

Many experiments of a similar nature have since been carried out over a wide range of diets with the focus of the investigations being the response to increasing digestible lysine (lysDI) and methionine (metDI) supplies together. Rulquin (1992) summarized much of this work   (Table 17.1) and showed quite clearly that in the vast majority of rations, lysine and methionine must be the first two limiting amino acids. By increasing these two amino acids alone, milk protein was increased on average by 35 and 50 g/head/day in mid and early lactation cows respectively.

Table 17.1 EFFECTS OF THE STAGE OF LACTATION ON THE RESPONSES TO A POST-RUMINAL SUPPLY OF METHIONINE AND LYSINE

Stage of lactation	Early lactation	Mid lactation	SED
Week	1 to 9	10 to 29	
No. of trials	(16)	(71)	
Amino acids supplies (g/day)			
Methionine	10	8	
Lysine	24	20	
Productions			
Milk (kg/d)	+0.7	+0.1	0.9
Protein (g/d)	+56	+31	33
Fat (g/d)	+10	+1	51
Milk composition			
Protein level (g/d)	+1.2	+1.0	0.7
Fat level (g/kg)	-0.5	-0.0	1.6

Courtesy of Rulquin 1992

The relative importance of lysine limitations with respect to methionine was not so clear. Subsequent experimentation showed that for rations where maize protein was the major constituent of bypass protein supply, lysine was clearly first limiting (Rulquin, Lehenaff and Vérité, 1990; Robert, Sloan and Nozière, 1996; King, Bergen, Sniffen, Grant, Grieve, King and Ames, 1991). Protein secretion was increased by 50 to 150 g/cow/day where only lysine was increased post-ruminally. However, where maize protein made only a minor contribution and soyabean meal the major contribution to bypass protein, methionine is clearly the first limiting amino acid (Robert, Sloan and Lahaye, 1995; Rulquin and Delaby, 1994a ; Robert, Sloan and Denis, 1996; Armentano Bertics and Ducharme, 1993). In fact, supplying additional digestible lysine did not improve the milk protein response further (Sloan, 1993) on this type of diet. Where maize was the only cereal energy source and soya bean meal the principal protein source, Koch, Whitehouse, Garthwaite, Wasserstrom and Schwab (1996) showed methionine still to be clearly first limiting for milk protein synthesis, but further performance improvements could be obtained by providing extra digestible lysine.

IMPROVEMENTS IN MILK PROTEIN ARE A CONSEQUENCE OF AN INCREASE IN MILK CASEIN

The consistent increases in milk protein secretion and particularily in milk protein content observed (Rulquin, 1992) as a result of improvements in metDI and lysDI supply, are due to an increase in milk casein since the proportion of casein within milk crude protein or milk true protein is increased (Pisulewski, Rulquin, Peyraud and Vérité, 1996). Hurtaud, Rulquin and Vérité (1995) tested the cheese-making properties of milk from a range of trials where metDI and lysDI levels were increased in dairy rations and where milk protein and casein contents were improved by 1.0 to 2.0 g/kg (Rulquin, Delaby and Hurtaud, 1994). The different protein sources fed in these trials were maize gluten meal, soyabean/rapeseed meal and bloodmeal. Cheese yield was increased in line with the increase in casein content. In terms of cheese-making aptitude there was a tendency to decrease the time of firming and to enhance firmness. However, curd coagulation time increased significantly, apparently due to a decrease in the colloidal calcium/casein ratio. In practice this can be rectified by increasing the quantity of $CaCl_2$ added to milk before cheese manufacture.

Certain authors have indicated that the different milk casein fractions are improved disproportionately (Donkin, Varga, Sweeney and Muller, 1989) with increasing levels of metDI and lysDI, but this has not been observed in the majority of other trials (Hurtaud *et al.,* 1995; Colin-Schoellen, Laurent, Vignon, Robert and Sloan, 1995). Overall, balancing rations in lysDI and metDI have shown that it is possible to positively manipulate milk protein secretion through increasing milk casein synthesis. This not only provides more grams of casein to be transformed into cheese but also improves the manufacturing properties of the milk.

The first practical approach to formulating in digestible amino acids for dairy cows

The biggest breakthrough recently in practical amino acid nutrition of dairy cows was the compilation of all the relevant research work and the development of a systematic approach to estimating raw material values for digestible methionine and lysine contents and the publication of estimates for digestible lysine and methionine requirements. The methodology used has been described by Rulquin and Vérité (1993), Rulquin, Pisulewski Verite and Guinard (1993) and Chapter 14 (Vérité *et al.,* 1997).

Using this methodology, lysine and methionine requirements for the lactating dairy cow are estimated to be 7.3 % and 2.5 % of total digestible amino acid supply (PDIE) respectively. Socha and Schwab 1994, using a similar approach but based on the Cornell Net Carbohydrate and Protein system (O' Connor, Sniffen, Fox and Chalupa, 1993), estimated requirements for lysine as 16.8 % of total essential amino acids. Specific dose response studies (Robert *et al.,* 1996) have confirmed the estimation of the lysDI requirements derived by Rulquin and Vérité (1993). A precise estimate of metDI requirements has been much more difficult to establish. The marginal response to additional metDI remained positive and linear between 1.5 to 2.35 (% of PDIE) metDI where the ration provided recommended levels of lysDI (7.3 % of PDIE) (Pisulewski *et al.*, 1996; Socha, Schwab, Putnam, Whitehouse, Kierstead and Garthwaite, 1994a,b). However, Socha *et al.* (1994c) found no response to increased metDI in mid to late lactation cows. Where the lysDI level was only 6.50 % of PDIE no significant increase in milk protein secretion has been noted from additional metDI, whereas increasing simultaneously lysDI and metDI from 6.50/1.80 to a minimum of 6.80/2.15, increased milk protein secretion by 37 g/cow/day (Sloan, Robert and Lavedrine, 1994).

The estimates of 2.5 % and 7.3 % of PDIE proposed by Rulquin and Vérité (1993) would, however, appear to be very good first approximations of metDI and lysDI requirements respectively. In countries where this approach to rationing cows in terms of lysDI and metDI as a % of PDIE has been adopted, a reasonable compromise between optimising milk protein secretion and the cost of doing so, has resulted in the adoption of practical recommendations of 7.0 lysDI and 2.2 metDI (as a % of PDIE).

No major interference of other formulation constraints

A question often posed is how dependent is the response to improving digestible lysine and methionine levels on other ration formulation constraints and dietary ingredients present. The responses need to be independent, or at least predictable, in a wide range of dietary situations if lysDI/metDI formulation constraints are to be incorporated in current dairy ration formulation programmes.

RESPONSES LARGELY INDEPENDENT OF RATION ENERGY LEVEL AND SOURCE

In pigs, lysine requirements are expressed with respect to net energy (Fuller,1994); energy being needed for the process of tissue protein synthesis. Erfle and Fisher (1977) commented that an adequate energy intake also had to be provided in dairy cows to permit a response to intravenous infusions of lysine and methionine. However, where energy intakes have been varied between 90 and 110 % of conventional recommendations there has been no noticeable influence on the magnitude of the response to additional digestible methionine and lysine (Rulquin and Delaby, 1994b; Brunschwig, Augeard, Sloan and Tanan, 1995). In fact, Colin-Schoellen *et al.* (1995) observed that the improvement in milk protein secretion to extra metDI and lysDI tended to be higher (88 vs 41 g/cow/day) at low versus high energy intakes (90 vs 112 % of recommendations).

In trials where the extra energy was supplied in the form of fat (Christensen, Cameron, Clark, Drackley, Lynch and Barbano, 1994 ; Canale, Muller, McCahon, Whitsel, Varga and Lormore, 1990) the effects on milk protein content of supplying extra metDI and lysDI were significant and comparable to those obtained on a diet with no added fat. The general negative effect of added fat, independent of source, on milk protein content was counterbalanced by the positive effect of providing extra digestible lysine and methionine.

In one trial with Jersey cows, milk protein secretion was not modified when additional metDI and lysDI were supplied, independently of the presence or not of supplementary dietary fat (Karunanandaa, Goodling, Varga, Muller, McNeill, Cassidy and Lykos, 1994). Nevertheless, in very early lactation Jersey cows (Bertrand, Pardue and Jenkins, 1996) the addition of whole cottonseed depressed milk protein content by 3 g/kg. Adding supplementary metDI and lysDI inversed this decrease completely (4.6 g/kg), improving milk protein yield by 120 g/cow/day. Chow, DePeters and Baldwin (1990) confirmed that with high energy diets, whether attained by the inclusion of fat or by the feeding a high proportion of concentrate, milk protein yields were increased similarly when additional metDI and lysDI were supplied.

OVER AND ABOVE MINIMUM RECOMMENDATIONS FOR TOTAL DIGESTIBLE AMINO ACID SUPPLY (PDI) RESPONSES ARE LARGELY INDEPENDENT OF RATION PROTEIN LEVEL

The influence of the level of the protein supplied (PDI) has also been investigated. Rulquin *et al.* (1990) were able to demonstrate that dairy cows fed to meet 120 % of their recommended PDI requirements were still able to increase milk protein secretion by 150 g/cow/day with the infusion of one single amino acid, lysine. This ration was particularly imbalanced in lysine with respect to other amino acids, due to the high inclusion of maize gluten meal. When, in the same experiment, cows were fed only 100 % of their recommended PDI requirements the response to extra lysine was only 45 g/cow/day. The inclusion level of maize gluten meal was much lower, thus the relative deficit in lysDI was also lower. This was a clear indication that at the levels of protein input examined in this trial it was the relative imbalance in the profile of amino acids being absorbed by the dairy cow that was important in determining the potential response rather than the quantity of total amino acids absorbed.

Where different protein levels have been tested (100 vs 105 % of the recommendation for PDI) and the amino acid profile of protein entering the small intestine at each level was estimated to be similar, milk protein increases to a provision of extra lysDI and metDI were of the same magnitude (Sloan, Robert and Mathé, 1989; Socha *et al.* 1994; Colin-Schoellen. *et al* 1995).

FORAGE SOURCE HAS LITTLE INFLUENCE ON AMINO ACID LIMITATIONS

A major concern in Northern Europe has been that in the original database used to develop the estimates of lysDI and metDI recommendations, very few rations were based on grass silage. Would the recommendations proposed by Rulquin and Vérité (1993) be applicable for this type of diet? Earlier work where lysDI and/or metDI levels have been increased in grass-silage based diets have given very variable results (Girdler, Thomas and Chamberlain, 1988a,b; Thomas, Crocker, Fisher, Walker and Reeve, 1989; Remond, 1988). The increases in milk protein secretion were not only more variable but apparently inferior to those obtained with maize-silage based diets (Le Henaff, 1991). However, other constraints such as low dietary protein levels may have limited the capacity to respond in these trials (Girdler, 1988 a,b; Chamberlain and Thomas, 1982).

More recently, 3 trials have been carried out specifically to test the validity of the lysDI and metDI recommendations, where grass silage was the sole forage fed. In two trials, the control rations were formulated to contain approximately 7.0 lysDI and around 1.80 metDI (% of PDIE). In both trials (Robert, Sloan and Denis, 1994; Chilliard, Rouel, Ollier, Bony, Tanan and Sloan, 1995) milk protein content was improved by 1.2 g/kg which is similar to the responses (1 to 1.5 g/kg) observed with maize silage and mixed forages using similar protocols (Sloan, 1993; Brunschwig *et al*, 1995).

The control ration used in the third trial was based on grass silage and byproducts and was estimated to provide 6.70 lysDI and 1.85 metDI as a % of PDIE (Younge, Murphy, Rath and Sloan, 1995).

To test the approach of Rulquin and Vérité (1993):

1)   Only additional digestible methionine was included to achieve a ration level of at least 2.2 % metDI
2)   Additional digestible methionine and lysine were added to achieve levels of at least 7.0 % lysDI and 2.2 % metDI
3)   The ration was reformulated to achieve the 7.0 % lysDI uniquely from raw material sources, the deficit in metDI being supplied by a post-ruminal source of synthetic methionine.

As was anticipated, adding methionine alone showed virtually no increase in milk protein. Simultaneously adding digestible lysine with the additional digestible methionine permitted a significant increase in milk protein content (+ 0.8 g/kg). The largest increase was achieved by the reformulated diet (+ 1.4 g/kg).

Using the approach of Rulquin and Vérité (1993), Armentano, Bertics and Ducharme (1993) also observed similar improvements in milk protein with a lucerne-based ration, and Robert and Lavedrine (1995) with a grass-hay based ration when the predicted deficit in metDI was rectified. This tends to confirm the robustness of the sytem and the recommendations proposed by Rulquin and Vérité, (1993).

CAN OTHER AMINO ACIDS BE LIMITING ON A PRACTICAL BASIS IN DAIRY COW RATIONS

Obviously balancing dairy rations uniquely for lysine and methionine is not sufficient to achieve maximum milk performance. The comparisons of infusions of essential amino acids versus casein showed that the first two limiting amino acids could account for 40 to 50 % of the total response to casein. Thereafter other amino acids become limiting. Various amino acids have been suggested as being potentially 3rd or 4th limiting. Histidine appears to be a good candidate. Its theoretically low concentration in microbial protein would apparently suggest that mammary supplies of histidine for milk protein synthesis often look limited. In the early work of Schwab (1976) although lysine and methionine were clearly first limiting, infusion of extra histidine, in addition, tended to increase milk protein secretion through a milk volume response. Recently some Finnish work (Huhtanen, Vanhaatalo and Varvikko, 1996) indicated the potential importance of histidine as a first limiting amino acid on a grass silage, cereal/sugarbeet pulp based diet where urea was the only supplementary source of crude protein.

Another amino acid often thought to be potentially limiting on grass silage/hay based diets is leucine. In North European rations, compared with American rations which contain a large proportion of maize grain, the proportion of leucine in duodenal protein from cows fed grass-silage based rations has been shown to be up to 6 % lower (Robert, Tanan, Blanchart, Williams and Phillipeau, 1994). However although this may indicate that leucine is potentially 3rd or 4th limiting, methionine and lysine are still clearly first limiting in grass-silage based rations as indicated by the positive milk performance responses observed by Robert *et al* (1994), Chilliard *et al.* (1995), and Younge *et al.* (1995) to increasing digestible supplies of just these two amino acids.

Isoleucine has also been suggested as a potential limiting amino acid. The Cornell Net Carbohydrate and Protein system often predicts isoleucine as the first limiting amino acid. However this is probably an artefact of the low transfer coefficient (0.79) of absorbed leucine to leucine incorporated into milk protein, used in the model, compared with 0.98 and 0.88 for methionine and lysine respectively. There are no milk performance trials indicating isoleucine as a potentially limiting amino acid.

The non - essential amino acids are normally discounted as being potentially limiting for milk protein synthesis. However, Bruckental, Ascarelli, Yosif and Alumot (1991) indicated that proline could potentially increase milk yield by having a sparing effect on arginine which may contribute up to 50 % of the proline secreted in milk. Meijer, Van der Meulen and Van Vuuren (1993) proposed that glutamine could be potentially limiting, particularly in early lactation. The plasma concentration of this amino acid is extremely low compared to other amino acids at this critical period of lactation. However as yet there is no direct evidence that increasing digestible supplies of glutamine can increase any aspect of milk performance.

In practice, as we do not yet formulate to fully meet the recommendations for the two first limiting amino acids lysine and methionine, there is little point in trying to incorporate formulation constraints for the 3rd and 4th limiting amino acids based on the limited knowledge we have available today. However it is important for the future that the sequence of limitations is more clearly identified. In pigs the identification of threonine and tryptophan as 3rd and 4th limiting amino acids has given the pig nutritionist the opportunity to reduce crude protein (CP) inputs whilst maintaining performance.

The largest benefits in milk performance are achieved from balancing rations for lysDI and metDI from the beginning of lactation

BENEFITS OF CONTINUOUS APPLICATION FROM EARLY IN LACTATION

The trials used by Rulquin and Vérité (1993) to develop their recommendations virtually all used a latin square or crossover design carried out in post-peak lactation with periods sometimes as short as two weeks. Broster and Broster (1984) pointed out the dangers of directly extrapolating results of this nature into recommendations for a whole lactation. The responses to long term improvements in lysDI and metDI contents of dairy rations could as easily increase as disappear with time. The benefits could also be quite different depending on the stage of lactation at which the ration is first optimised for lysDI and metDI content. For example, Rulquin (1992) noted that in early-lactation trials, milk protein secretion responses to supplementary lysine and methionine were apparently greater than in later lactation studies (50 vs 35 g/cow/day). Schwab, Bozak, Whitehouse and Olson (1992) also noted in a repeated Latin square study, where the composition of the total mixed ration was virtually kept constant, that the response to additional lysDI and metDI was greater during the first 50 days compared with any other stage of lactation. Increases in both milk protein content (~ 2.6 vs ~ 1.3 g/kg) and milk yield (2.4 vs 0.0 kg/day) were much larger in very early lactation than any period post-peak lactation.

Brunschwig and Augeard (1994) observed that where a ration estimated to have a concentration of 6.9 lysDI and 1.75 metDI was readjusted to have 2.15 metDI (% of PDIE) from the 4th week of lactation, milk protein secretion was improved by 60 g/cow/day within a matter of days and this response was maintained at this level over the length of the trial period (until the 20th week of lactation - Figure 17.1a). This response is larger than those observed in the cross over trials summarized by Rulquin (1992). The increase in milk protein concentration (Figure 17.1b) was at first sight unexpected. An initial increase of 1 g/kg was observed at the first milk recording but by the end of the trial the difference had steadily increased to nearly 2 g/kg. This was due principally to the increased protein secretion becoming more and more concentrated in a decreasing volume of milk, post peak lactation. In addition there was an indication that milk yield was improved slightly (+ 0.5 kg/cow/day) during the first few weeks of the trial.

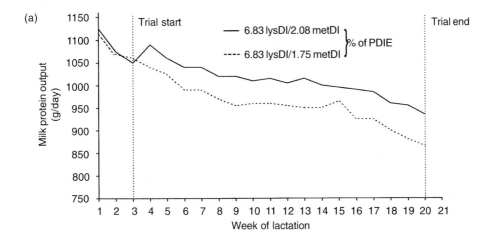

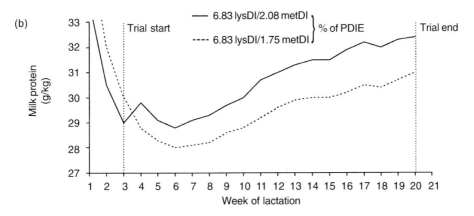

Figure 17.1 Change in milk protein output (a) and content (b) from week 4 to 20 of lactation after optimizing ration for lysDI and metDI (% of PDIE) (Brunschwig and Augeard, 1994)

In a further trial (Pabst unpublished) where ration lysDI and metDI concentrations as a % of PDIE were increased from 6.8/1.9 to 7.4/2.1, milk protein secretion was increased immediately by 75 g. This level of response was maintained until the end of the trial at the 30th week of lactation. Here the positive effect on milk protein content over time was even more pronounced than in the previous experiment; 1 g/kg at the beginning of the trial, 2.8 g/kg at the end. Polan, Cummins, Sniffen, Muscato, Vicini, Crooker, Clark, Johnson, Otterby, Guillaume, Muller, Varga, Murray, and Peirce Sandner (1991) noted an average increase of 70 g per day in milk protein secretion during days 22 to 280 of lactation when cows fed maize gluten meal as the principal dietary protein source were supplemented with extra metDI and lysDI. It appeared that the average daily increase was larger (+ 85 g) during days 22 to 112 of lactation than subsequently (+ 40 g).

However, with a similar trial design and ration, Rogers, Peirce-Sandner, Papas, Polan, Sniffen, Muscato, Staples and Clark (1989) observed an increase of over 90 g/day in milk protein secretion, which was maintained throughout the whole lactation. Thus there does seem to be an advantage to optimising lysDI/metDI levels from as early a stage of lactation as possible, not only to obtain a larger immediate effect, but also to stimulate the largest response possible over the whole lactation.

MILK VOLUME INCREASES IN EARLY LACTATION

The trials discussed previously did not start before the 4th week of lactation to provide a covariate period. It could be argued that the most stressful time of lactation has already passed. The dairy cow may, in fact, benefit even more if her amino acid nutrition is improved from Day 1 of lactation or even pre-partum.

In a recent trial involving 72 high yielding dairy cows (Socha, Schwab, Putnam, Whitehouse, Kierstead and Garthwaite, 1994d), a typical North American diet, which contained 6.50 lysDI / 1.85 meDI, was compared with a ration in which the lysDI/metDI levels were increased to 7.10 / 2.15 (as a % of PDIE) respectively from parturition until Day 105 of lactation. Milk protein yield was increased by an average of 80 g/cow/day, which, as in the trials of Brunschwig and Augeard 1994 and Pabst unpublished, was maintained consistently throughout the trial period. In the trial of Socha, *et al* (1994) the expression of the milk protein yield response was principally in terms of a milk volume response (+ 2.3 kg/day on average, + 3.5 kg/day at peak lactation) although there was some evidence by the end of the trial that the milk volume response was becoming less important and the protein content increase more important (Figures 17.2a and b).

Other trials (Rulquin, personal communication; Chilliard Ollier, Ferlay, Gruffat, Durand and Bauchart unpublished) have confirmed this large potential milk volume response where rations have been balanced for lysDI/metDI from the first week of lactation. The latter trial was also associated with a large increase in milk protein content. A further trial (partly published ; Robert, Sloan and Bourdeau, 1994) also demonstrated a large effect on milk protein yield during the first 84 days of lactation, the majority of the response being due to an increase in milk protein content (1.6 g/kg) with only a small effect on milk yield (+ 0.5 kg/day). A recently published farm study (Thiaucourt, 1996) involving 2000 cows also confirmed that balancing rations to try and achieve an objective of 7.0 lysDI / 2.2 metDI does indeed improve milk yield during the first 100 days of lactation (+ 2.2 kg/day) with the increase in milk protein content being evident (+ 1.3 g/kg) at any stage of application during the lactation.

In cows fed rations balanced for lysDI and metDI from at least the first day of lactation, milk protein secretion is increased by 60 to 100 g/cow/day. The expression of this response, which appears to remain relatively constant throughout a large part of lactation, is associated partly with a milk yield response during at least the first 100 days and an increase in milk protein content at most stages of lactation.

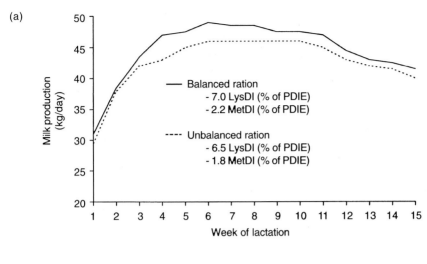

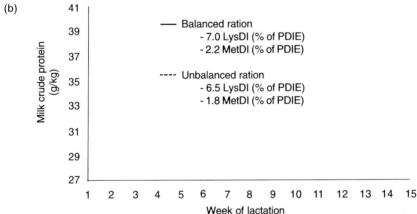

Figure 17.2 Influence of balancing rations to 7.0 lysDI and 2.2 metDI (% of PDIE) on milk yield (a) and milk protein content (b) during the first 100 days of lactation (Socha *et al.*, 1994d)

A POSITIVE INFLUENCE ON EFFICIENCY OF FEED NITROGEN AND ENERGY UTILISATION

In the trials of cross over design started post peak lactation, summarized by Rulquin (1992) the responses in daily milk protein output to supplying extra metDI and lysDI were 20 to 45 g. On average, this was achieved without a modification of feed intake. Thus the global efficiency of conversion of feed crude protein to milk protein can be estimated to be improved by the order of 0.02 to 0.05, which is not neglible. However, when the proportion of the extra metDI appearing in milk protein is calculated, it averages only 0.1. Theoretically the efficiency of utilisation for the first limiting amino acid could approach 1. However this is not realistic. Methionine is used not only for milk protein synthesis but also for maintenance functions and is implicated in other metabolic processes. Furthermore, after peak lactation a proportion of the extra metDI may be directed towards tissue protein synthesis. Realistically it cannot be expected that more than 0.6 to 0.8 of a supplementary quantity of the first limiting amino acid will be incorported into milk protein.

Similarly, in the early lactation studies (Robert, *et al* unpublished; Brunschwig and Augeard, 1994; Socha *et al.*, 1994d), improving amino acid balance had no overall effect on feed intake. However, for the same quantities of additional metDI and/or lysDI the increases in milk protein secretion were much greater (60 to 80 g/cow/day), equivalent to an improvement in effiency of feed protein use of 0.06 to 0.10. Equally the efficiency of utilisation of the supplementary quantity of the first limiting amino acid, methionine, was higher. For Brunschwig *et al.* (1995), the extra metDI was used with an efficiency of 0.2. In the trials of Pabst (unpublished) and Socha *et al.* (1994d), approximately 0.4 of the extra metDI was accounted for in extra milk protein secreted.

What is more curious is the apparent influence of balancing rations for lysDI and metDI on overall feed/energy utilisation. For 12 early-lactation trials analysed there was an improvement in apparent feed efficiency ((feed DM input/milk DM output (milk fat + milk protein)) in every case (Table 17.2). This could not be explained solely by an increase in milk protein output. In the trials where milk volume was improved, milk fat content was not reduced, thus milk fat secretion was also increased. In fact milk component yield (fat plus protein) was often increased by at least 150 g/cow/day with an increase in apparent feed efficiency of 0.04 to 0.08. Ørskov, Grubb and Kay (1975) showed that feeding fishmeal, a protein capable of providing bypass protein of a high quality, caused an increase in milk yield and milk protein secretion at the expense of mobilising more energy reserves to satisfy the increased energetic demand.

In the early lactation trials cited above there was no indication of more weight or condition score loss (where measured). This would tend to favour a hypothesis that energy yielding nutrients both of dietary origin and from body reserves are being utilised much more efficiently for milk production when rations are balanced for lysDI and metDI.

POSITIVE EFFECTS ON REPRODUCTIVE PERFORMANCE

It can be anticipated that reproductive performance of dairy cows may be influenced in various ways by balancing more correctly lysDI and metDI supplies. Any feeding practice that allows cows to return to positive energy balance sooner and/or reduce blood urea levels (Ferguson and Chalupa,1989) will create a more favourable environment for getting cows back in calf. Balancing rations in lysDI/metDI has the potential to achieve these objectives. Due to the key role that methionine plays in energy metabolism (liver function) in early lactation, cows fed diets fortified with metDI should be in a much more

Table 17.2 INFLUENCE OF RATION LYSDI/METDI CONCENTRATION ON MILK PERFORMANCE AND FEED EFFICIENCY

Reference	Trial duration (days of lactation)	Ration lysDI/metDI concentration (% PDIE)		Increase in intake (kg DM/cow/day)	Increase in milk fat plus protein yield (g/cow/day)	Apparent feed efficiency kg DM intake/kg milk DM (fat plus protein output)	
		Control	Supplemented	(Supplemented-Control)		Control	Supplemented
Robert et al, unpublished[†]	0-84	8.0/1.7	6.9/2.4	-0.1	131	7.35	6.92
Brunschwig et al 1994	21-140	6.9/1.8	6.9/2.4	0.4	149	8.67	8.29
Brunschwig et al 1995[†]	0-56	6.9/1.7	6.9/2.1	-1.1	47	7.27	6.72
Pabst unpublished[†]	21-203	6.8/1.9	7.4/2.1	0.7	187	7.86	7.50
Socha et al 1994d[†]	0-105	6.5/1.8	6.5/2.2	-1.0	-32	9.06	8.80
	0-105	6.5/1.8	7.0/2.2	0.8	158	9.06	8.85
Rulquin unpublished[†]	0-28	6.9/1.7	7.7/2.1	0.4	146	7.48	7.21
Chilliard et al unpublished[†]	5-42	6.9/1.6	6.9/2.2	0.1	291	6.48	5.87
	5-26	6.9/1.6	6.8/2.8	1.1	269	6.20	5.99
	5-26	6.9/1.6	8.2/2.6	1.7	133	6.20	6.56
Robinson et al 1995	27-305	6.2/1.9	6.8/2.2	1.0	150	10.73	10.40
	27-305	6.2/2.0	6.8/2.2	0.0	120	10.84	10.27

[†] Actual milk production values - no adjustment by covariance

favourable energy status for successful reproduction. In two recent studies Robert *et al.* (1996) found tendancies to reduce calving interval by 4 to 5 days on both maize- and grass-silage based rations where metDI levels were increased from 1.8 to 2.2 % of PDIE. In parallel field trials, Thiaucourt (1996) found the same improvement in calving interval ($P < 0.1$) in a field study involving 2000 cows that were fed a metDI-enriched concentrate.

These advantages are a logical reflection of improving energy and protein nutrition in general without necessary implicating a favourable effect of one individual amino acid on any direct aspect of reproductive function.

In the studies of Robert *et al.* (1996), the reduction in calving interval was due essentially to two factors:

1) Number of days to first insemination was reduced by 6 to 7 days
2) The number of inseminations needed per successful conception was reduced from 1.8 to 1.6

Both could be linked to the time taken for full uterine involution after calving. The proportion of cows fed the metDI-enriched diet that had completely involuted after 45 days of lactation was 0.55, compared to only 0.38 of the control animals.

Milk progesterone levels were also measured every three days during this study. Cows fed the metDI enriched diets had higher progesterone levels (16.5 vs 12.6 nmol/ litre) during the 5 to 7 days prior to the ovulation leading to a successful pregnancy. This is generally considered to be favourable to a strong ovulation and successful insemination (Folman, Rosenberg, Herz and Davidson, 1973). Subsequently after insemination higher progesterone levels are also favourable for implantation of the embryo. Robert *et al.* (1996) also observed milk progesterone levels were on average higher (4.8 vs 7.1 nmol/ litre ; $P < 0.1$) during the five days post ovulation for the metDI enriched diets.

DOES PRE-CALVING AMINO ACID NUTRITION IMPROVE SUBSEQUENT LACTATION PERFORMANCE?

During the weeks prior to calving, the dairy cow undergoes important hormonal and metabolic changes in preparation for calving and in anticipation of secreting large quantities of milk. Nutrition during this time is vital to minimising subsequent metabolic disorders and ensuring a rapid increase in intake post-calving to help satisfy the large demand for nutrients in early lactation (Grummer, 1996). Labile protein reserves can also be replenished during this time (Chilliard and Robelin, 1983) to provide a small reservoir to help meet amino acid requirements at the beginning of lactation.

As with lactation rations, it would appear that in the pre-calving ration there is first and foremost a need to ensure provision of a minimum quantity of total amino acids (PDI) which has perhaps been underestimated in the past. Moorby, Dewhurst and

Marsden (1996) have recently shown that increasing total digestible amino acid supply by approximately 100g/day during the 2 months before calving increased milk protein secretion post calving by 60 g/cow/day. There was no dietary difference post calving and intakes were similar. From where did the extra milk amino acid N secreted originate? One hypothesis is that pre-calving, the extra amino acid N fed was used in some way to constitute labile protein reserves. However, it has traditionnally been considered that the potential contribution of labile protein reserves to meet amino acid requirements is exhausted after the third or fourth week of lactation (Chilliard and Robelin, 1983). It would therefore seem likely that by some mechanism, the increased total amino acid supply pre-calving improves subsequently the efficiency of utilisation of absorbed amino acids for milk protein synthesis.

According to Rode, Fayceda, Sab, Suzuki, Julien and Sniffen (1994) attention should also be paid to the balance between rumen degradable N and bypass protein supplied in the dry cow ration. They found that feeding too high a proportion of bypass protein could in itself have potential negative effects on subsequent health and production. Both Crawley and Kilmer (1996) and Wu, Fisher and Polan (1996) showed no advantage of increasing either the proportion of crude protein in the dry cow ration or the proportion of undegradable protein in the crude protein on subsequent lactational performance.

It could be anticipated that pre-calving there would be an advantage in terms of the efficiency of utilisation of absorbed amino acid N, if the profile approached that of 'ideal protein'. Both Socha *et al.* (1994) and Rode *et al.* (1994) observed very large responses in milk protein yield, during the first hundred days of lactation, to feeding additional metDI and lysDI. Part of this response may be attributed to the additional quantities of metDI and lysDI which were also fed pre-calving.

Further evidence that not only the quantity but the balance of amino acids absorbed by the dairy cow during the dry period is important in determining lactational performance has been demonstrated by Socha *et al.* (1994), Robert *et al.* (unpublished) and Brunschwig *et al.* (1995). In these 3 trials the quantity of metDI calculated to meet the estimated deficit in the lactation ration was also fed for at least the last two weeks before parturition as part of the trial protocol. The results were not as anticipated since there was no increase in milk yield in any of the 3 trials In fact there was a decrease of 1.2 kg/day in the trial of Brunschwig *et al.* (1994), although the yield of milk components did not change. The trial of Robert *et al.* (unpublished) was carried out over two years. Overall milk component yield was increased by 140 g/cow/day. However, the results were different between the years. In year 1, a positive effect on milk volume was noted (+ 1.1kg/cow/day) whereas the effect was negative in the second year. For the trial of Socha *et al.* (1994) the addition of supplementary metDI alone was not expected to increase markedly milk performance. Although methionine was estimated to be the first limiting amino acid for the ration fed, lysDI (6.50 % of PDIE) was well below an optimum level to ensure a full response to the additional metDI. However it was surprising that there was no response at all.

The common feature of all these trials was a negative effect on feed intake (kg DM/ head/day) during early lactation (Brunschwig *et al.*, 1995,- 1.1; Robert *et al.*, unpublished, - 0.5 in the second year; Socha *et al*, -.1.0 during the first 100 days of lactation). These negative effects were evident from the first day after parturition. In fact, the problem was apparently initiated pre-calving. In all 3 trials, metDI levels pre-calving were higher than those found in lactation rations (2.4 to 3.1 as a % of PDIE) due to the feeding of a supplementary level of metDI designed for cows in lactation consuming higher quantities of PDIE. In the two trials where feed intake was measured before calving, there was no difference between treatments until 24 to 48 hours before calving. Intakes normally decrease around this time but in the case of Socha *et al.* (1994d) the decrease was spectacular for the treatment with added metDI - (Figure 17.3) and also important in the trial of Robert *et al.* (unpublished).

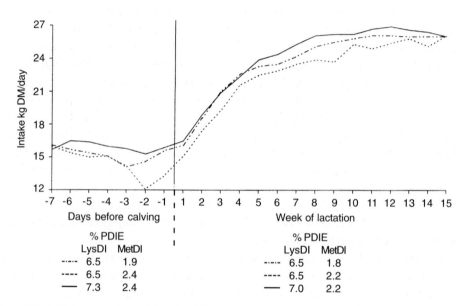

Figure 17.3 Influence of ration lysDI and metDI concentrations (% of PDIE) on dry matter intake before and after calving (Socha *et al*, 1994d; Schwab personal communication).

It would appear that it is not only the level of metDI as a proportion of total amino acids (PDIE) that is important, but also the ratio of lysDI to metDI. In the trial of Socha *et al.* (1994) the feeding of a high level of metDI in the presence of a high level of lysDI had no impact on intake in the period one to two days before calving and appeared to positively favour milk performance in the subsequent lactation. Grummer (1996) showed quite clearly that intakes post-calving, and thus lactational performance, were positively correlated with intakes immediately pre-calving. Thus it is evident that there is no interest in exceeding the normal recommendations for metDI and lysDI as a proportion of PDIE pre-calving. Despite the negative effects incurred on intake, the apparent efficiencies of utilisation of feed nitrogen and energy were still improved.

It is important to achieve a balanced profile of digestible amino acids when formulating a dry cow ration. The quantities of individual digestible amino acids necessary to balance a ration should be calculated with respect to the overall digestible protein supply, which is only approximately 0.5 of protein supply during the early lactation period.

Methionine, a key role in liver energy metabolism

The positive effects on feed utilisation cannot be explained totally by improvements in milk protein synthesis. In contrast to lysine, which is considered to have a role in protein synthesis only, methionine is known to participate in many other metabolic functions through its capacity as a methyl donor. Recently its role in liver energy metabolism has been investigated. Chilliard *et al.* (unpublished), over fed dairy cows precalving to be fat at calving and then fed an energy-deficient diet post-calving. These cows were predisposed to develop metabolic problems such as fatty liver (steatosis) and ketosis. The control diet was formulated to provide ample PDI and to meet practical requirements for lysDI (7.0 % of PDIE), but was deficient in metDI. For the test rations, additional metDI was provided to achieve a level of 2.2 % of PDIE in trial 1 and 2.8 % of PDIE in trial 2. Substantial increases in protein secretion (+ 100 g) were observed in both trials. In trial 2 this was associated with a significant reduction in plasma ketone body concentrations. Plasma ß-hydroxybutyrate and acetone concentrations were reduced by 0.33 and 0.64 respectively during week 2 of lactation, indicating fewer potential problems of energy metabolism and improved liver function. These improvements were assumed to be the result of the increased supply of metDI mediating an increase in very low density lipoproteins (VLDL), the lipoprotein complex essential for evacuating mobilised tryglycerides from the liver towards peripheral tissues, particularly the mammary gland, to provide energy nutrients for lactation.

Auboiron, Durand, Robert, Chapman and Bauchart (1995) demonstrated in calves that methionine plays a key role in assuring the synthesis of the apo protein ß complex, essential in the formation of VLDL. Likewise Durand, Chilliard and Bauchart (1992) showed in lactating cows that increasing liver supply of methionine in the presence of additional lysine resulted in the VLDL balance across the liver becoming positive rather than negative. Chilliard, Audigier, Durand, Auboiron and Bauchart (1994) observed that the supplementary metDI also decreased circulating levels of not only ß- hydroxybutyrate but also plasma triglycerides and non esterified fatty acids (NEFA) in calves. In dairy cows NEFA concentrations were also reduced in the trials of Pisulewski, Rulquin and Vérité (1996) where a ration adequate in lysDI (6.9 %) but poor in metDI was supplemented with additional amounts of metDI. Similarly, in the trial of Rulquin and Delaby (1994a), plasma NEFA were decreased from 96.2 to 74.7 and from 60.9 to 47.0 mmol/l for animals in low and normal energy status respectively, when additional metDI was added. Plasma NEFA are generally positively correlated with the level of lipid infiltration of the liver (Durand, Gruffat, Chilliard and Bauchart, 1995). Fortifying diets with metDI appears to be a positive factor towards reducing the risk of certain metabolic disorders such as steatosis and ketosis and improving the energy status of dairy cows in early lactation.

Potential to reduce nitrogen pollution

An improvement in feed nitrogen utilisation opens up the possibility of reducing urinary nitrogen excretion. This is of importance in countries where legislation is being introduced to control nitrogen usage on farms to reduce the potential negative effects of excess nitrogen on the environment. Losses through urinary excretion have been shown to increase rapidly (Wright, Moscardini, Susnel and McBride, 1996) with increasing dietary crude protein concentration, even when high bypass protein sources, with an apparently good amino acid profile, were fed. It has been shown in pigs that crude protein concentrations in rations can be reduced from 160 to 130 g/kg, without loss in performance, by judicious supplementation with synthetic amino acids. In dairy cows the same potential should exist.

At present rations for dairy cows tend to have a crude protein concentration of over 180 g/kg in the dry matter and sometimes higher. This is because it is generally recognised that there continues to be a marginal increase in milk production with increasing crude protein level (Gordon, 1980). Using the PDI, lysDI / metDI approach, reducing dietary crude protein levels to 160 g/kg DM can reduce crude protein inputs (Dinn, Fisher and Shelford, 1996) by more than 500 g/cow/day. Any marginal loss in milk yield is more than offset by the positive effect of amino acid balance on milk protein secretion (Robert, Sloan, Saby, Mathé, Dumont and Dzyzcko, 1989). However, to go further and reduce crude protein level by another 20 to 30 g/kg will be much more difficult, though not infeasible. Piva Masoero, Mancini and Fusconi (1996) fed a low crude protein diet (153 g/kg DM) to dairy cows from days 30 to 90 of lactation. With this diet, milk protein secretion was improved (+ 50 g/cow/day) when additional metDI and lysDI were included. However the increase was only 0.5 of that achieved by increasing crude protein concentration to 173 g/kg DM although the latter was at the expense of increasing milk urea N by 0.25 and reducing the efficiency of feed N utilisation. Likewise, Piepenbrink, Overton, and Clark (1996) found that supplementing a ration containing 140 g CP/ kg DM with only digestible lysine and methionine did not have any effect on milk protein secretion, whereas increasing the crude protein level to 180 g/kg DM increased it by 40 g/cow/day.

It seems likely that at low dietary crude protein concentrations more attention needs to be paid not only to lysine and methionine but to other potentially limiting amino acids. In pigs, dietary CP concentrations can be reduced from 160 to 130 g/kg DM without loss in performance, but only if, in addition to digestible lysine and methionine, the concentrations of the 3rd and 4th limiting amino acids, tryptophan and threonine, are also optimised in the ration.

Practicalities of formulating in lysDI and metDI

All raw materials can contribute to the lysDI and metDI needs of the dairy cow. It is the judicious choice of raw materials and the proportions incorporated into concentrate formulations which will be important in achieving the required overall levels of digestible lysine and methionine.

In the approach proposed by Rulquin and Vérité (1993), each raw material is assigned a lysDI and metDI value which takes into account both the microbial contribution calculated from the quantity of fermentable organic matter (FOM) digested in the rumen and the bypass contribution. All forages have relatively high lysDI values (6.8 to 7.0 % of PDIE) and above average metDI values (1.9 to 2.0 % of PDIE). This is due to the majority of the contribution to lysDI and metDI being of microbial origin. In general, rumen degradabilities of forages are high, thus the digestible amino acid contribution from bypass protein is minor. Likewise for cereals, lysDI (% of PDIE) levels tend to be slightly above average, due to their low crude protein content and high fermentable organic matter content, which again favours the microbial digestible amino acid contribution. Maize grain is an exception. Although its crude protein content is low, rumen N-degradability is very low (~ 0.40) and at least 0.2 of the FOM escapes rumen fermentation. These factors maximise the bypass digestible amino acid contribution for this raw material. With its low lysine content this results in a low value of lysDI (% of PDIE) for maize and, in general, for maize-based byproducts. Corn gluten meal has the distinction of being the raw material with the lowest lysDI concentration because of its high CP content and extremely low degradability (0.28). On the other hand, maize gluten feed has a lysDI value of 6.4 (% of PDIE) which is average. This is due to the high N-degradability (~ 0.69) of this raw material.

The raw materials that can most influence the profile of absorbed protein (PDIE) are concentrated sources of bypass protein. All protein-rich raw materials, particularly those with a low N-degradability, have the potential to modify cosiderably the amino acid profile of absorbed protein. Soya bean meal is above average in lysDI (7.0 % of PDIE). However all the other proteinaceous meals of vegetable origin tend to be low in both lysDI and metDI. Only animal protein sources have levels of either of the potential limiting amino acids superior to those required in the overall ration. Bloodmeal (now banned in the European Union) is an excellent source of lysDI, but fishmeal is the only raw material that is an excellent source of both lysDI and metDI as a % of PDIE.

In practical ration formulation it is impossible to meet both the lysDI and metDI constraints of 7.0 and 2.2 (as a % of PDIE) respectively from conventional raw materials alone; cows cannot be fed entirely on fishmeal. Unfortunately, feeding synthetic amino acids is not a potential solution. Neither DL-methionine nor the hydroxy analogue of methionine, the two commercially available forms of synthetic methionine, resist rumen degradation (Loerch and Oke 1989) and thus are not sources of bypass methionine to increase ration metDI levels. The recent availability of good quality sources of rumen protected amino acids however not only permits the lysDI and metDI constraints to be met but also gives the formulator greater choice and flexibility in the other raw materials that can be incorporated to attain these levels.

In order to formulate as accurately as possible it is important to have a reliable database of lysDI and metDI values for all the commonly used raw materials. The database issued by INRA (Rulquin Guinard Vérité and Delaby, 1993) provides the vast majority of raw material values needed. For raw materials not present in the tables, and for those recognised to be inherently variable, new lysDI and metDI values can be derived from measuring rumen N-degradability *in sacco* and from measuring the amino acid profile in the original raw materials.

The lysDI and metDI values of rumen protected amino acids cannot be measured accurately in the same way. *In sacco* degradability measurements will tend to over-estimate rumen protection to varying degrees, depending on the coating technology. Present rumen protection technologies rely on physical protection of a core of amino acids by a fat-based coating. This type of coating is more sensitive to physical pressures than chemical breakdown, thus nylon bags can create a protective environment, minimising potential losses of protection by abrasion in the rumen or by mastication. In addition, for many technologies that show excellent rumen protection, it is not evident that the amino acids can be released post-ruminally for absorption in the small intestine.

To overcome these obstacles, a specific methodology has been developed to estimate amino acid bio-availability for rumen protected amino acids. Based on the principle that what is of most importance is the bio-availability of the amino acid(s) to the host animal and not necessarily precise knowledge of the proportion resisting rumen breakdown and the proportion released and absorbed in the small intestine, a quantitative blood methodology has been developped (Rulquin, personal communication). The kinetics of appearance in the plasma of post-ruminally infused methionine is compared to the feeding of a known quantity of rumen protected product to give a quantitative estimation of bio-availability. The various rumen protection technologies tested have revealed a wide range in terms of their effectiveness (proportion of 'protected' methionine actually absorbed by the dairy cow has varied from 0 to 0.8).

It is important that manufacturers of rumen-protected amino acids provide independent measurements of amino acid bio-availability using a standardised methodology as described above. Only then can the technical and economic interest of different rumen protected amino acid technologies as sources of metDI and lysDI in dairy rations be evaluated.

Formulating for digestible amino acids can improve dairy herd performance

Paying more attention to the balance of amino acids absorbed by the dairy cows has the potential to improve milk protein yield and certain other aspects of milk performance:

1. Milk protein content can be increased immediately in cows at any stage of lactation, by 1 to 2 g/kg

2.   Milk yield can be improved by up to 2.5 kg/day in early lactation (first 100 days)
3.   Milk protein yield increases of 60 to 100 g/ day over a complete lactation are attainable
4.   Feed efficiency can be improved by 0.05.

Energy status in early lactation is improved, reducing the incidence of metabolic disturbances such as fatty liver and ketosis. Due to its specific action on the liver, digestible methionine concentrations in the ration are of particular importance at the very beginning of lactation. Furthermore, in the few trials where reproductive parameters have been studied, one of the consequences of improved nutritional status has been a shortening of the calving interval, linked to improved uterine involution and a reduction in the number of inseminations needed per conception.

To optimise these potential benefits it is essential to formulate dairy rations to contain higher levels of both lysDI and metDI than is currently practiced. The approach and recommendations proposed by Rulquin and Vérité (1993) are sufficiently robust that they can be used satisfactorally in a wide variety of dietary situations. The challenges for the future will be to refine these recommendations still further with respect to stage of lactation and milk yield potential and to determine recommendations for the dietary levels of the other essential amino acids in order to improve the efficiency of utilisation of dietary protein inputs .

References

Agricultural and Food Research Council (1992). Technical Committee on Responses to Nutrients. Report n° 9. Nutritive requirements of ruminant animals protein. *Nutrition Abstracts and Reviews*, Series B **62**, 787– 835.

Armentano, L.E. and Bertics, S.J. and Ducharme, G.A. (1993). Lactation responses to rumen-protected methionine, or methionine with lysine, in diets based on alfalfa haylage. *Journal of Dairy Science* **78,** (suppl. 1) 202.

Auboiron, S., Durand, D., Robert, J.C., Chapman, M.J. and Bauchart, D. (1995). Effects of dietary fat and L-methionine on the hepatic metabolism of very low density lipoproteins in the preruminant calf, *Bos spp. Reproduction Nutrition Development*. **35**, 167–168.

Bertrand, J.A., Pardue, F.F., and Jenkins, T.C. (1996). Effect of protected amino acids on milk production and composition of Jersey cows fed whole cottonseed. *Journal of Dairy Science* **79** (Suppl. 1), 5022.

Broster, W.H. and Broster, V. J. (1984). Reviews of the progress of dairy science and long term effects of nutrition on the performance of the dairy cow. *Journal of Dairy Research* **51**, 149–196.

Bruckental, I., Ascarelli, Y., Yosif, B. and Alumot, E. (1991). Effect of duodenal proline infusion on milk production and composition in dairy cows. *Animal Production* **53**, 299–303.

Brunschwig, P. and Augeard, P. (1994). Acide aminé protégé : effet sur la production et la composition du lait des vaches sur régime ensilage de maïs. *Journées de Recherches sur l'alimentation et la nutrition des Herbivores 16-17 mars - INRA Theix.*

Brunschwig, P., Augeard, P., Sloan, B.K., and Tanan, K., (1995). Feeding of protected methionine from 10 days pre-calving and at the beginning of lactation to dairy cows fed a maize silage based ration. *Rencontres Recherches Ruminants* **2**, 249.

Brunschwig, P., Augeard, P., Sloan, B.K., and Tanan, K. (1995). Supplementation of maize silage or mixed forage (maize and grass silage) based rations with rumen protected methionine for dairy cows. *Annales Zootechnie*, **44**, 380.

Canale, C.J., Muller, L.D., Mc Cahon, H.A., Whitsel, T.J., Varga, G.A. and Lormore, M.J. (1990). Dietary fat and ruminally protected amino acids for high producing dairy cows. *Journal of Dairy Science* **73**, 135–141.

Chamberlain, D.G. and Thomas, P.C. (1982). Effect of intravenous supplements of L-methionine on milk yield and composition in cows given silage cereal diets. *Journal of Dairy Research*, **49**, 25–28.

Chilliard, Y. and Robelin, J. (1983). Mobilisation of body proteins by early lactating dairy cows measured by slaughter and D_2O techniques. Proceedings of the fourth international symposium on protein metabolism and nutrition, Clermont-Ferrand (France). *INRA publication II (Les colloques de l'INRA, n° 16)* p 195–198.

Chilliard, Y., Audigier, C., Durand, D., Auboiron, S. and Bauchart, D. (1994). Effects of portal infusions of methionine on plasma concentrations and estimated hepatic balances of metabolites in underfed preruminant calves. *Annales Zootechnie*, **43**, 299.

Chilliard, Y., Rouel, J., Ollier, A., Bony, J., Tanan, K. and Sloan, B.K. (1995). Limitations in digestible methionine in the intestine (metDI) for milk protein secretion in dairy cows fed a ration based on grass silage. *Animal Science*, **60**, 553.

Choung, J.J. and Chamberlain D.G. (1993). The effect of abomasal infusions of casein or soya-bean-protein isolate on the milk production of dairy cows in mid lactation. *British Journal of Nutrition* **69**, 103–115.

Chow, J.M., DePeters, E. J. and Baldwin, R. L. (1990). Effect of rumen-protected methionine and lysine on casein in milk when diets high in fat or concentrate are fed. *Journal of Dairy Science* **73**, 1051–1061.

Christensen, R.A., Cameron, M.R., Clark, J.H., Drackley, J.K., Lynch, J.M. and Barbano, D.M. (1994). Effects of amount of protein and ruminally protected amino acids in the diet of dairy cows fed supplemental fat. *Journal of Dairy Science* **77**, 1618–1629.

Clark, J.H. (1975). Lactational responses to postruminal administration of proteins and amino acids. *Journal of Dairy Science* **58** , 1178–1197.

Colin - Schoellen, O., Laurent, F., Vignon, B., Robert J.C. and Sloan B.K. (1995). Interactions of ruminally protected methionine and lysine with protein source or energy level in the diet of cows. *Journal of Dairy Science* **78**, 2807–2818.

Dinn, N.E., Fisher, L.J. and Shelford, J.A. (1996). Using rumen-protected lysine and methionine to improve N efficiency in lactating dairy cows by reducing the percentage of intake N excreted in urine and feces. *Journal of Animal Science* **74**, (Suppl. 1) 11.

Donkin, S.S., Varga, G.A., Sweeney, T.F., and Muller, L.D. (1989). Rumen-protected methionine and lysine: effects on animal performance, milk protein yield, and physiological measures. *Journal of Dairy Sci*ence **72**, 1484–1491.

Durand, D., Chilliard, Y. and Bauchart, D. (1992). Effects of lysine and methionine on in vivo hepatic secretion of VLDL in the high yielding dairy cows in early lactation. *Journal of Dairy Science*, **75**, (Suppl. 1) 279.

Durand, D., Gruffat, D., Chilliard, Y. and Bauchart, D. (1995). Stéatose hépatique: mécanismes et traitements nutritionnels chez la vache laitière. *Le Point Vétérinaire* **27**, 741–748.

Erfle, J.D. and Fisher, L.J., (1977). The effects of intravenous infusion of lysine, lysine plus methionine or carnitine on plasma amino acids and milk production of dairy cows. *Canadian Journal of Animal Science* **57**, 101–109.

Ferguson, J.D. and Chalupa, W. (1989). Symposium : Interaction of Nutrition and Reproduction. Impact of protein nutrition on reproduction in dairy cows. *Journal of Dairy Sci*ence **72**, 746–766.

Folman, Y., Rosenberg, M., Herz, Z. and Davidson, M. (1973). The relationship between plasma progesterone concentration and conception in post-partum dairy cows maintained on two levels of nutrition. *Journal of Reproduction and Fert*ility, **34**, 267–278.

Fraser, D.L., Ørskov, E.R., Whitelaw, F.G. and Franklin, M.F. (1991). Limiting amino acids in dairy cows given casein as the sole source of protein. *Livestock Production Science* **28**, 235–252.

Fuller, M.F. (1994) Amino acid requirements for maintenance, body protein accretion and reproduction in pigs. *In Amino Acids in Farm Animal Nutrition* pp 155–184. Edited by J.P.F. D'Mello. CABI, Wallingford.

Girdler, C.P., Thomas, P.C. and Chamberlain, D.G. (1988a). Effect of intraabomasal infusions of amino acids or of a mixed animal protein source on milk production in the dairy cow. *Proceedings of the Nutrition Society* **47**, 50A.

Girdler, C.P., Thomas, P.C. and Chamberlain, D.G. (1988b). Effect of rumen-protected methionine and lysine on milk production from cows given grass silage diets. *Proceedings of the Nutrition Society* **47**, 82A.

Gordon, F. J. (1980). The effect of silage type on the performance of lactating cows and the response to high levels of protein in the supplement. *Animal Production* **30**, 29–37.

Grummer, R. (1996). Nutrition and physiology of the transition cow. *Proceedings of California Animal Nutrition Conference,* Fresno, 177–187.

Guillaume, B., Otterby, D.E., Stern, M.O., Linn, J.G. and Johnson, D.G. (1991). Raw or extruded soybeans and rumen-protected methionine and lysine in alfalfa based diets for dairy cows. *Journal of Dairy Science* **74**, 1912–1922.

Henry, Y., (1993). Affinement du concept de la protéine idéale pour le porc en croissance. *INRA Production Anim*ale, **6**, 199–212.

Huhtanen, P., Vanhartalo, A. and Varvikko, T. (1996). New knowledge about amino acid requirements of ruminants. *Rehuraisio Environmental Feed Symposium.*

Hurtaud, C., Rulquin, H. and Vérité, R. (1995). Effect of rumen protected methionine and lysine on milk composition and on cheese yielding capacity. *Annales Zootechnie* **44**, 382.

Karunanandaa, K., Goodling, L.E., Varga, G.A., Muller, L.O., McNeil, W.W., Cassidy, T.W. and Lykos, T. (1993). Supplementary dietary fat and ruminally protected amino acids for lactating Jersey cows. *Journal of Dairy Science* **77**, 3417–3425.

King, K.J., Bergen, W.G., Sniffen, C.J., Grant, A.L., Grieve, D.B., King, V.L. and Ames, N.K (1991). An assessment of absorbable lysine requirements in lactating cows. *Journal of Dairy Science* **74**, 2530–2539.

Koch, K.L., Whitehouse, N.L., Garthwaite, B.D., Wasserstom, V.M. and Schwab, C. G. (1996). Production responses of lactating Holstein cows to rumen-stable forms of lysine and methionine. *Journal of Dairy Science* **79**, (Suppl.1) 24.

Leclercq, B., (1996). Les rejets azotés issus de l'aviculture : importance et progrès envisageables. *INRA Production Animale* **9**, 91–101.

Le Henaff, L., (1991). Importance des acides aminés dans la nutrition des vaches laitières. Diplôme de doctorat. Thesis N° 253. *Université de Rennes,* France.

Loerch,S.C. and Oke, O. (1989). Rumen protected amino acids in ruminant nutrition. *In Absorption and Utilisation of Amino Acids.* Ed. Mendel Friedman Boca Raton, Florida Vol. III, 187–200.

Moorby, J.M., Dewhurst, R.J. and Mardsen, S. (1996). Effect of increasing digestible undegraded protein supply to dairy cows in late gestation on the yield and composition of milk during the subsequent lactation. *Animal Science* **63**, 201–213

O'Connor, J.D., Sniffen, C.J., Fox, D.G. and Chalupa, W. (1993). A net carbohydrate and protein system for evaluating cattle diets : IV Predicting amino acid adequacy. *Journal of Dairy Sci*ence **71**, 1298.

Ørskov, E.R., Grubb, D.A. and Kay, R.N.B. (1977). Effect of postruminal glucose or protein supplementation on milk yield and composition in Frisian cows in early lactation and negative energy balance. *British Journal of Nutrition* **38**, 397–405.

Piepenbrink, M.S., Overton, T.R. and Clark, J.H. (1996). Response of cows fed a low crude protein diet to ruminally protected methionine and lysine. *Journal of Dairy Science* **79**, 1638–1646.

Pisulewski, P.M., Rulquin, H., Peyraud, J.L. and Vérité, R. (1996). Lactational and systemic responses of dairy cows to post-ruminal infusions of increasing amounts of methionine. *Journal of Dairy Science* **79**, 1781–1791.

Piva, G., Masoero, F., Mancini, V. and Fusconi, G. (1996). The effect of the protected methionine and lysine suplementation on the performance of dairy cows in early lactation fed a low protein diet. *Journal of Animal Science* **74**, (Suppl.1) 278.

Polan, C.E., Cummins, K.A., Sniffen, C.J., Muscato, T.V., Vicini, J.L., Crooker, B.A., Clark, J.H., Johnson, D.G., Otterby, D.E., Guillaume, B., Muller, L.O., Varga, G.A., Murray, R.A. and Peirce-Sandner, S. (1991). Responses of dairy cows to supplement rumen-protected forms of methionine and lysine. *Journal of Dairy Science* **74**, 2997–3013.

Remond, B. (1988). Effet de l'addition de méthionine protégée à la ration des vaches laitières : influence du niveau des apports azotés. *Annales de Zootech*nie **37**, 271–284.

Robert, J.C. and Lavedrine, F. (1995). The effect of supplementation of hay plus soyabean meal diet with rumen protected methionine on the lactational performance of dairy cows in mid late lactation. *VII Symposium on protein metabolism and nutrition.* Portugal.

Robert, J.C., Sloan, B.K. and Bourdeau, S. (1994). The effect of supplementation of corn silage plus soyabean meal diets with rumen protected methionine on the lactational performance of dairy cows in early lactation. *Journal of Dairy Science* **77** (Suppl. 1), 349.

Robert, J.C., Sloan, B.K. and Denis, C. (1994). The effect of protected amino acid supplementation on the performance of dairy cows receiving grass silage plus soybean meal. *Animal Production* **58**, 437.

Robert, J.C., Sloan, B.K. and Denis, C. (1996). The effect of graded amounts of rumen protected methionine on lactational responses in dairy cows. *Journal of Dairy Science* **79** (Suppl. 1), 256.

Robert, J.C., Sloan, B.K. and Lahaye, F. (1995). Influence of increasing doses of intestinal digestible methionine (MetDI) on the performance of dairy cows in mid and late lactation. *IVth International Symposium on the Nutrition of Herbivores, Clermont-Ferrand,* France.

Robert, J.C., Sloan, B.K. and Nozière, P. (1996). Effects of graded levels of rumen protected lysine on lactational performance in dairy cows. *Journal of Dairy Science* **79**, (Suppl. 1) 257.

Robert, J.C., Sloan, B.K., Saby, B., Mathé, J., Dumont, G., Duron, M. and Dzyzcko, E., (1989). Influence of dietary nitrogen content and inclusion of rumen-protected methionine and lysine on nitrogen utilisation in the early lactation dairy cow. *Australasian Journal of Animal Science* **2**, 544–545.

Robert, J.C., Tanan, K., Blanchart, G., Williams, P. and Philippeau, C. (1994). Influence of the ration composition on the duodenal flow of amino acids in lactating dairy cows. *Procedings Society of Nutrition and Physiology* **3**, 66.

Robinson, P.H., Fredeen, A.H., Chalupa, W., Julien, W.E., Sato, H., Fujieda, T. and Suzuki, H. (1995). Ruminally protected lysine and methionine for lactating dairy cows fed a diet designed to meet requirements for microbial and post-ruminal protein. *Journal of Dairy Science* **78**, 582–594.

Rogers, J.A, Peirce-Sandner, S.B., Papas, A.M., Polan, C.E., Sniffen, C.J., Muscato, T.V., Staples, C.R. and Clark, J.H. (1989). Production responses of dairy cows fed various amounts of rumen-protected methionine and lysine. *Journal of Dairy Science* **72**, 1800–1817.

Rulquin, H. (1986). Influence de l'équilibre en acides aminés de trois protéines infusées dans l'intestin grêle sur la production laitière de la vache. *Reproduction Nutrition Développement* **26**, 347–348.

Rulquin, H. (1992). Interets et limites d'un apport de méthionine et de lysine dans l'alimentation des vaches laitières. *Production Animale* **5**, 29.

Rulquin, H. and Delaby, L. (1994a). Lactational responses of dairy cows to graded amounts of rumen-protected methionine. *Journal of Dairy Science* **77** (Suppl. 1), 345.

Rulquin, H. and Delaby, L. (1994b). Effects of energy status on lactational responses of dairy cows to rumen-protected methionine. *Journal of Dairy Science* **77** (Suppl. 1), 346.

Rulquin, H., Guinard, R., Vérité, R. and Delaby, L. (1993). Teneurs en Lysine (LysDI) et Méthionine (MetDI) digestibles des aliments pour ruminants. *Journées AFTAA Tours*.

Rulquin, H., Le Henaff, L. and Vérité, R. (1990). Effects on milk protein yield of graded levels of lysine infused into the duodenum of dairy cows fed diets with two levels of protein. *Reproduction Nutrition Development* (Suppl. 2) : 238.

Rulquin, H., Pisulewski, P.M., Vérité, R. and Guinard, J. (1993). Milk production and composition as a function of post-ruminal lysine and methionine supply : a nutrient response approach. *Livestock Production Science* **37**, 69.

Rulquin, H., and Vérité, R. (1993). Amino acid nutrition of dairy cows: Productive effects and animal requirements. In *Recent Advances in Animal Nutrition*, pp. 55–77. Edited by P.C. Garnsworthy an D.J.A. Cole. Nottingham University Press, Nottingham.

Schwab, C.G., Bozak, C.K., Whitehouse, N.L. and Olson, V.M. (1992). Amino acid limitation and flow to the duodenum at four stages of lactation. II. Extent of lysine limitation. *Journal of Dairy Science* **75**, 3503.

Schwab, C.G., Satter, L.D. and Clay, A. B. (1976). Response of lactating dairy cows to abomasal infusion of amino acids. *Journal of Dairy Science* **59**, 1254–1269.

Sloan, B. (1993). Ensilage de maïs/soja : quels acides aminés faut-il apporter pour augmenter le taux protéique chez la vache laitière ? *Journées AFTAA Tours*.

Sloan, B.K., Robert, J.C. and Lavedrine, F. (1994). The effect of protected methionine and lysine supplementation on the performance of dairy cows in mid lactation. *Journal of Dairy Science* **77** (Suppl.1), 343.

Sloan, B.K., Robert, J.C. and Mathé, J. (1989). Influence of dietary crude protein content plus or minus inclusion of rumen protected amino acids (RAA) on the early lactation performance of heifers. *Journal of Dairy Science* **72** (Suppl. 1), 506.

Socha, M.T. and Schwab, C.G. (1994). Developing dose response relationships for absorbable lysine and methionine supplies in relation to milk and milk protein production from published data using the Cornell Net Carbohydrate and Protein System. *Journal of Dairy Science* **77** (Suppl. 1), 93.

Socha, M.T., Schwab, C.G., Putnam, D.E., Whitehouse, N.L., Kierstead, N.A. and Garthwaite, B.D. (1994a). Determining methionine requirements of dairy cows during peak lactation by post-ruminally infusing incremental amounts of methionine. *Journal of Dairy Science* **77** (Suppl.1), 350.

Socha, M.T., Schwab, C.G., Putnam, D.E., Whitehouse, N.L., Kierstead, N.A. and Garthwaite, B.D. (1994b). Determining methionine requirements of dairy cows during early lactation by post-ruminally infusing incremental amounts of methionine. *Journal of Dairy Science* **77**, 246.

Socha, M.T., Schwab, C.G., Putnam, D.E., Whitehouse, N.L., Kierstead, N.A. and Garthwaite, B.D. (1994c). Determining methionine requirements of dairy cows during mid lactation by post-ruminally infusing incremental amounts of methionine. *Journal of Dairy Science* **77** (Suppl.1), 351.

Socha, M.T., Schwab, C.G., Putnam, D.E., Whitehouse, N.L., Kierstead, N.A. and Garthwaite, B.D. (1994d). Production responses of early lactation cows fed rumen-stable methionine or rumen-stable lysine plus methionine at two levels of dietary crude protein. *Journal of Dairy Science* **77** (Suppl. 1), 352.

Thiaucourt, L. (1996). L'opportunité de la méthionine protégée en production laitière. *Bulletin des GTV* 2B, 45–52.

Thomas, C., Crocker, A., Fisher, W., Walker, C. and Reeve, A. (1989). The interaction between protein level and the response to specific nutrients in high silage diets. *Animal Production* **48**, (3) 623.

Vérité, R., Faverdin, P. and Agabriel, J. (1997). Developments in the INRA feeding system for dairy cows. *In Recent Advances in Animal Nutrition*, p 153–166. Edited by P.C. Garnsworthy and J. Wiseman. Nottingham University Press, Nottingham.

Whitelaw, F.G., Milne, J.S., Ørskov, E.R. and Smith, J.S. (1986). The nitrogen and energy metabolism of lactating cows given abomasal infusions of casein. *British Journal of Nutrition* **55**, 537–556.

Wright, T.C., Moscardini, S., Susmel, P. and McBride, B.W. (1996). Effects of supplying graded levels of a fixed essential amino acid pattern on milk protein production and nitrogen utilisation in the lactating dairy cow. *Dairy Research Report*. University of Guelph - Publication N° 0396.

Younge, B.A., Murphy, J.J., Rath, M. and Sloan, B.K. (1995). The effect of protected methionine and lysine on milk production and composition on grass silage based diets. *Animal Science* **69**, 556.

This paper was first published in 1997

18

FATS IN DAIRY COW DIETS

P.C. GARNSWORTHY

University of Nottingham, Sutton Bonington Campus, Loughborough, Leics LE12 5RD

Introduction

Dairy cows have evolved an extremely efficient digestive system, principally for utilising the poor quality forages found in their natural diet. The most significant component of this system is the rumen, which is a large fermentation chamber containing billions of microorganisms. These microorganisms break down plant material to provide the energy and protein required for their growth and during this process, they produce volatile fatty acids (VFAs - principally acetate, propionate and butyrate) and ammonia as waste products. The VFAs provide the cow with the major source of energy and carbon skeletons for synthetic processes. The ammonia is converted to urea in the liver and either excreted in the urine or recycled *via* the saliva. Microbial protein is made available to the cow when the microorganisms pass out of the rumen for digestion in the small intestine.

Although moderate levels of performance can be achieved from diets containing only grass or forage, high-producing dairy cows require additional energy and protein from supplementary sources. This is particularly true in early lactation, where appetite is usually reduced to such an extent that the cow cannot eat enough to satisfy nutrient requirements for milk production. Even if body condition is controlled to minimise the reduction in appetite (Garnsworthy and Topps, 1982), diets of high energy concentration are required if cows are to achieve their potential dry matter intake (Jones and Garnsworthy, 1989). Traditional sources of supplementary energy include starchy materials such as cereals, or fibrous materials such as by-products like sugar beet pulp. High starch diets can result in rapid fermentation in the rumen and the low pH induced may inhibit forage-digesting bacteria, which are less tolerant of low pH conditions than amylolytic microorganisms. This results in lowered feed intakes and reductions in the butterfat content of milk. Fibrous supplements do not have such deleterious effects on forage digestion since they are broken down by the same cellulolytic microorganisms.

However, the relatively slow rate of digestion of these supplements limits their usefulness because of the physical effects of rumen fill on feed intake.

For diets with very high energy concentrations it is necessary to use fats. These have a gross energy content about twice that of grass and cereals; metabolisable energy is about three times as high and net energy about four times (Table 18.1). When formulating rations, fats have the advantage of creating "space" within the diet, due to their high energy content. This makes it easier, and often cheaper, to satisfy the specifications for other nutrients, such as protein, minerals and vitamins. From a compounder's point of view, fats are additionally attractive since they improve the pelleting qualities of compound feeds and reduce dust. However, dietary fats can have important effects on rumen fermentation and animal responses. These will be reviewed in the current chapter.

Table 18.1 ENERGY CONTENT OF SELECTED FEEDS FOR DAIRY COWS (MJ/KG DM)

	Gross energy	Metabolisable energy	Net energy for milk production
Grass	18.7	11.2	6.9
Grass silage	20.9	11.0	6.8
Barley grain	18.5	13.3	8.1
Fat Prills	39.0	33.0	26.4
Tallow	39.3	30.5	24.4

Sources: AFRC (1993); MAFF (1990); McDonald, Edwards, Greenhalgh and Morgan (1995); NRC (1989)

Rumen effects

The fat content of "natural" diets for ruminants is less than 50 g/kg. However, if added fat increases the total fat content of the diet to more than about 100 g/kg, digestive problems can occur.

Rumen microorganisms cannot utilise large quantities of fat. Their normal substrates are carbohydrates and proteins, although limited quantities of fatty acids can be incorporated into microorganisms during cell synthesis. More important than the quantity of fatty acids in the diet is their form, since long-chain unsaturated fatty acids have a detergent effect on bacterial cell walls. Under normal circumstances, the ester linkages of triglycerides are rapidly hydrolysed by bacterial lipases in the rumen. Once released from ester combination, unsaturated fatty acids are subsequently hydrogenated to detoxify them. The result of this is illustrated graphically in Figure 18.1. A typical diet for high-yielding dairy cows might contain twice as much unsaturated fatty acids as saturated. Analysis of rumen fluid shows that this ratio is reversed. The proportion of fatty acids in rumen bacteria that are in the unsaturated form is 0.1 and the proportion in protozoa is 0.35, although the latter may be inaccurate since it is difficult to isolate protozoa from feed particles. Because of these defence mechanisms, the current consumer demand for unsaturated fatty acids in food is difficult to satisfy in ruminant products, compared to the situation in non-ruminants, where inclusion of unsaturated fatty acids in the diet usually increases the proportion of such acids in the carcass.

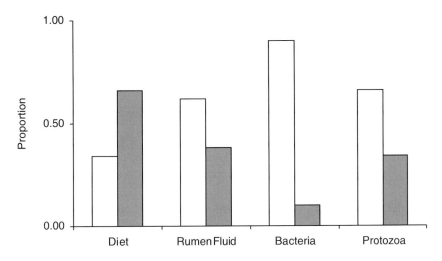

Figure 18.1 Saturation of fats in the rumen (☐ saturated, ▧ unsaturated; data from Viviani, 1970)

Fats also have a physical effect on fibre in the rumen; fibre particles become coated with fat, rendering them inaccessible for microbial attack. The magnitude of these effects depends on level, source and type of fat, dietary carbohydrate source and feed intake. A further problem is that long-chain free fatty acids can form soaps with calcium and magnesium in the rumen. This will detoxify the fatty acids, but it can also reduce the availability of the minerals.

Various products have been developed that are referred to as "protected fats". This is really a misnomer since the main requirement is to protect the rumen against detrimental effects of fat, rather than protect the fat against rumen degradation. The term "bypass fat", as used in the US, is mechanistically more accurate in this context. Protected fats offer the potential for increasing the absorption of unsaturated fatty acids from the small intestine. Rumen protection can be natural, (e.g. whole oilseeds, where the slowly digested seed coat slows the rate of fat release), chemical (e.g. encapsulation in formaldehyde-treated casein or formation of calcium soaps) or physical (e.g. selection of fatty acids with a high melting point and small particle size).

Production effects

The response by dairy cows to supplementary fat is complex and not always predictable.

Possible responses that have been reported include increased milk yields, increased or decreased milk fat content, decreased milk protein content, increased live-weight gain and decreased live-weight loss. The observed response will depend on the quantity of fat, its fatty acid profile and degree of protection, the other components of the diet and overall feeding level, the stage of lactation and genetic merit of the cow.

MILK YIELD AND LIVE WEIGHT

Milk yield responses can normally be explained by the increase in total energy intake when fats are given and the increased efficiency of utilisation of energy from fats. If rumen fermentation is disrupted, the response will not be as great as expected, since digestion of the non-fat components of the diet will be reduced. Stage of lactation and genetic merit affect both the milk yield response and the live-weight response. Cows in early lactation, and those of higher genetic merit, partition energy towards milk production at the expense of body fat reserves. Cows normally lose 0.5-1.0 kg of body weight each day for the first eight weeks of lactation and this is mostly body fat. Therefore increased energy intake at this stage of lactation could result in further increases in milk yield if the cow's genetic potential has not been reached and/or a reduction in the daily amount of body fat mobilised. In later lactation, when appetite is greater and milk yield less, partition of energy switches more towards body reserves so increased energy supply results in greater fat deposition in body reserves. Cows that have a high level of body fat reserves respond to high-fat diets by reducing fat mobilisation; cows with a low level of body reserves respond by increasing milk yield (Garnsworthy and Huggett, 1992). Cows of low genetic merit have a greater propensity for fat deposition and will partition a greater proportion of surplus energy in this direction (Holmes, 1988).

MILK FAT CONTENT

Dietary fat can affect milk fat synthesis in a variety of ways and these were summarised by Thomas and Martin (1988), as illustrated in Figure 18.2. If added dietary fats interfere with normal fibre digestion in the rumen, acetate and butyrate production will be reduced and the shortage of precursors in the mammary gland may lead to reduced *de novo* synthesis of milk fat. On the other hand, added fat may increase the quantity of fatty acids available for absorption and secretion in milk. There is also evidence that long-chain fatty acids decrease *de novo* synthesis of fatty acids in the mammary gland even when fed in the protected form so that they do not affect rumen fermentation. In most cases, when dietary fat intake is increased, the proportion of C4-16 fatty acids in milk fat will decrease and the proportion of longer-chain acids will increase. Total milk fat output will depend upon the relative magnitude of the effects on synthesis and absorption, which are affected by protection and degree of unsaturation (Thomas and Chamberlain, 1984).

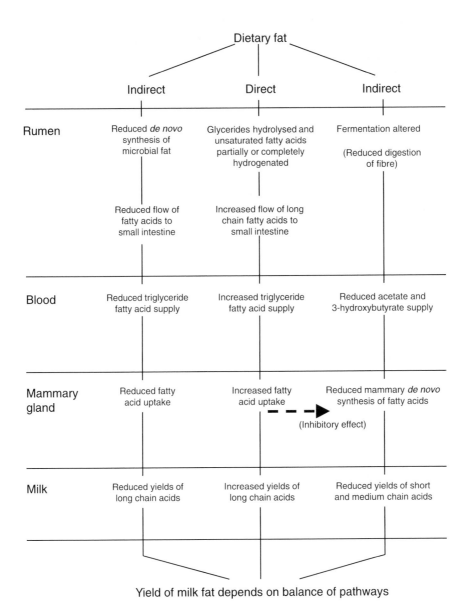

Figure 18.2 Mechanisms by which dietary fat may affect milk fat (after Thomas and Martin, 1988)

Unsaturated fatty acids can have double bonds in the *cis* or *trans* form. *Cis* fatty acids have both hydrogen atoms on the same side of the double bond; *trans* fatty acids have one hydrogen atom on each side. Naturally-occurring unsaturated fatty acids contain bonds predominantly in the *cis* form, so it is not surprising that fatty acids in the *trans* form have a much greater inhibitory effect on milk fat concentration than those in the *cis* form. *Trans* fatty acids are present in hydrogenated vegetable oils, but also arise as a result of incomplete biohydrogenation in the rumen. In addition to the general effects of unsaturated fats on fibre digestion, *trans* fatty acids also have a direct inhibitory effect on fatty acid synthesis in the mammary gland (Christie, 1981). Wonsil, Herbein and Watkins (1994) fed diets containing 330 g/kg hydrogenated tallow, menhaden oil or hydrogenated soya bean oil. The menhaden oil did not contain *trans* fatty acids, but was known to affect biohydrogenation in the rumen. The hydrogenated soya bean oil was used as a source of *trans* fatty acids. Hydrogenated tallow did not affect *trans*-oleic acid (18:1) at the duodenum or in milk and did not affect milk fat concentration. Both menhaden and soya oils significantly increased *trans*-18:1 at the duodenum and in milk. They also significantly depressed milk fat concentration (Table 18.2). This suggests that in this experiment the greatest effects of *trans* fatty acids were on milk fat synthesis, rather than fibre digestion in the rumen.

Table 18.2 EFFECT OF DIETARY CONCENTRATION AND INTAKE OF *TRANS* FATTY ACIDS ON MILK FAT CONCENTRATION

		Dietary group			
	Control	*Hydrogenated Tallow*	*Menhaden Oil*	*Hydrogenated Soya Bean Oil*	*SEM*
trans-18:1 intake (g/d)	0[a]	12[b]	0[a]	69[c]	2
trans-18:1 flow to the duodenum (g/d)	37[a]	38[a]	163[b]	152[b]	16
milk fat concentration (g/kg)	32.6[a]	31.8[a]	27.8[b]	29.5[b]	0.5
trans-18:1 in milk (g/kg fatty acids)	10[a]	18[a]	134[c]	84[b]	9

[a,b,c] means with different superscripts are significantly different (P<0.05)
Data from Wonsil, *et al.*(1994)

There is currently a great deal of interest in the manipulation of the fatty acid profile of milk fat. This results from consumer demand for unsaturated fatty acids, which are perceived to be more "healthy" than saturated fatty acids. This perception may be based on spurious evidence (Blaxter and Webster, 1992), but the demand is likely to be around for some considerable time yet and warrants attention.

It may be thought that the biohydrogenation of fatty acids in the rumen would preclude the presence of unsaturated fatty acids in the milk of cows. However, some fatty acids escape hydrogenation and some are incorporated into microbial lipids. Furthermore, some desaturation of fatty acids takes place in adipose and mammary tissue, so that typically 0.1 of the total fatty acid content of "normal" milk is unsaturated, principally in the form of oleic acid, with small proportions of linoleic. To increase this proportion, it is necessary to use protected fats, either from whole oilseeds or chemical/physical treatment.

There are numerous reports in the literature describing the effects of different fat sources on milk production, composition and fatty acid profile. Simply increasing the intake of fat can increase the proportion of unsaturated fatty acids in milk fat (e.g. Beaulieu and Palmquist, 1995), because *de novo* synthesis of short-chain fatty acids is reduced and these are all saturated. This makes it difficult to interpret the results of fatty acid profiles from studies designed to investigate a fat supplement (e.g. Garnsworthy and Huggett, 1992) or whole oilseeds (e.g. Bitman, Wood, Miller, Tyrrell, Reynolds and Baxter, 1996), where the comparison is between a low-fat control diet and a high-fat treatment diet.

Where different fat sources have been compared at equal fat intakes, convincing differences in the proportion of unsaturated fatty acids have been found. For example, Schingoethe, Brouk, Lightfield and Baer (1996) compared the effects of extruded soya beans and sunflower seeds on milk fat yield and composition. Neither oilseed increased milk fat content, compared with the low-fat control (Table 18.3), but both increased the proportion of unsaturated acids in milk fat. Interestingly, although soya beans contained nine times more linolenic acid (C18:3) than sunflower seeds, only trace amounts were found in the milk produced from either fat source, due to hydrogenation in the rumen.

Table 18.3 MAJOR FATTY ACID COMPOSITION OF MILK FROM COWS FED A LOW-FAT CONTROL DIET AND DIETS CONTAINING EXTRUDED SOYA BEANS OR SUNFLOWER SEEDS (G/KG TOTAL FATTY ACIDS).

	Diet		
	Control	*Soya bean*	*Sunflower*
C16:0[a]	295	215	208
C16:1	41	44	50
C18:0[a]	85	126	136
C18:1[a]	172	278	271
C18:2[b]	23	41	28
Total saturated[a]	716	599	612
Total unsaturated[a]	262	382	369

[a] difference between control and oilseeds P<0.01
[b] difference between control and oilseeds P<0.01 and difference between oilseeds P<0.01
Data from Schingoethe, *et al.* (1996)

Some cereals, because of their high oil content, have a depressing effect on milk fat content that is larger than might be expected simply from the normal effects of starch on rumen acetate:propionate ratios. They also affect milk fatty acid profile. In particular, naked oats (*Avena satura* var nuda) contain almost twice as much lipid as other cereals and a large proportion of this is in the form of C18:1 and C18:2. Fearon, Mayne and Marsden (1996) found that replacing barley with naked oats led to a significant decrease in milk fat content. The milk fat contained significantly higher proportions of long-chain fatty acids, particularly C18:2, which resulted in easier spreadability when the milk was subsequently made into butter. These results can be partially explained by the fact that dietary fat concentrations differed between treatments. The higher fat intake of cows given naked oats would be expected to reduce milk fat content and increase C18 proportions, as discussed above. In addition, the relatively high proportions of C18:1 and C18:2 would be expected to increase the supply of *trans*-fatty acids to the duodenum.

One of the greatest potentials for restoring consumer demand for cows' milk is to emphasise the value of the conjugated linoleic acid it contains. Conjugated linoleic acids (CLAs) are a mixture of *cis*- and *trans*- isomers of linoleic acid with alternating double and single bonds. CLAs have received much attention in the field of human health, since they exhibit anti-carcinogenic properties, reduce atherosclerosis and reduce the ratio of fat to lean in the body. The most abundant natural sources of CLAs are milk and meat from ruminant animals (Chin, Liu, Storkson, Ha and Pariza, 1992). It has been known for some time that CLAs are formed during biohydrogenation of unsaturated fatty acids by rumen microorganisms (Kepler and Tove, 1967), although recent studies have shown that approximately 80% of CLAs may be synthesised in the mammary gland by the Δ-9 desaturase enzyme (Griinari, Corl, Lacy, Chuinard, Nurmela and Bauman, 2000; Lock and Garnsworthy, 2002a). The activity of this enzyme is affected by diet composition (Bauman, Corl, Baumgad and Griinari, 2001; Lock and Garnsworthy, 2002a; 2002b) and varies between individual animals (Lock and Garnsworthy, 2002a; 2002b).

Another recent development in the context of human health has been the recommendation that intake of n3 (or omega-3) fatty acids should be increased and that the ratio of n6:n3 fatty acids should be approximately 5:1 (COMA, 1994). The best source of n3 fatty acids is marine oils. These have already been mentioned for their capacity to reduce milk fat concentration due to their propensity to increase the production of *trans*-fatty acids in the rumen (Wonsil, Herbein and Watkins, 1994). Of particular interest are the very long chain fatty acids C20:5 and C22:6, both of which are n3 fatty acids. Ashes, Siebert, Gulati, Cuthbertson and Scott (1992) found that these fatty acids were preferentially deposited in body tissue rather than in milk fat. This presents a problem when trying to increase levels of these fatty acids in milk. In the study of Wonsil, Herbein and Watkins (1994), it was found that although plasma concentrations of C20:5 and C22:6 acids were elevated after supplementation with menhaden oil, these fatty acids were not detectable in milk fat. Mansbridge and Blake (1997), found that C20:5 and C22:6 levels in milk fat were significantly increased when an unspecified fish oil was fed to dairy cows. However, the concentrations were extremely low (4 and 2 g/

kg total fatty acids respectively) and the efficiency of incorporation of these fatty acids into milk fat was very poor, with only 0.05 and 0.03 of dietary intake respectively for C20:5 and C22:6 appearing in milk fat.

As stated previously, there are many further comparisons of fat sources available in the literature. Results are quite variable, so it would be useful if the fatty acid profile of milk could be predicted from a knowledge of diet composition. Hermansen (1995) attempted to achieve this by analysing data from 35 published experiments, containing 108 treatments. None of the selected experiments used soaps or fats that were chemically protected against rumen fermentation. The best predictor of short-chain fatty acid content (<C12) was the total fatty acid content of the diet. The best predictors for C12, C14 and C16 acids were their respective concentrations in the diet. For C18:0 and C18:1, the best predictor was the total C18 content of the diet. Prediction of C18:2 and C18:3 content was poor ($r^2 = 0.29$) when a single predictor (type of fat, i.e. fats and oils *versus* oilseeds) was used, but better ($r^2 = 0.40$) when the proportion of C18:2 and C18:3 was combined with type of fat. This is not surprising since C18:2 and C18:3 would normally need a high degree of protection to avoid saturation in the rumen and subsequently appear in milk. It is unfortunate that Hermansen (1995) did not extend the analysis to include soaps and other protected fats. Such information would be very valuable when designing diets to produce milk fats tailored for specific niche markets.

MILK PROTEIN CONTENT

The majority of experiments evaluating the use of supplementary fat have found that milk protein content is reduced, although milk protein yield may be unaffected or increased. In some instances, the reduction in milk protein content may be a simple dilution effect (due to increased milk yield), but in most cases it appears to be a genuine physiological response. Wu and Huber (1994) reviewed data from 49 selected trials, involving 83 comparisons between added fat and control diets; it was observed that in most cases milk protein concentration was reduced by the addition of fat (Figure 18.3). The degree of depression seemed to be independent of fat source, although fat prills appeared to be the only fat source with positive effects on milk protein concentration. However, the six data points involving fat prills came from short-term (21 day) crossover experiments, where dry matter intake and milk yield were reduced by fat supplementation.

The control of milk protein synthesis is a complex process. Dietary protein concentration is only of relevance in deficiency situations and the response is normally determined more by the animal's glucose status. Wu and Huber (1994) discussed four possible mechanisms to explain how dietary fat depresses milk protein concentration; glucose deficiency, insulin resistence, increased energetic efficiency of milk production and somatotrophin deficiency. Of these, glucose deficiency is the strongest contender. Insulin resistence was proposed by Palmquist and Moser (1981), because elevated plasma insulin concentrations have been observed in cows given high-fat diets. However,

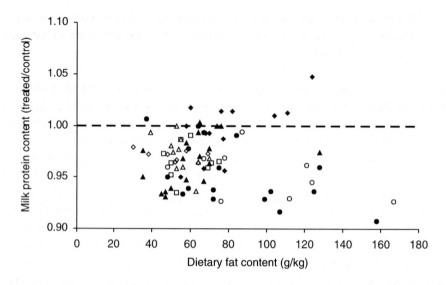

Figure 18.3 Effect of dietary fat concentration on milk protein concentration (■ animal-vegetable blend fat, ▲ calcium salts of fatty acids, ◆ prilled fat, ● protected tallow, ○ tallow, ◇ whole cottonseed, △ whole soyabean, □ yellow grease, - - - control); after Wa and Huber (1994)

Wu and Huber (1994) questioned this hypothesis since the effects of supplementary fat on plasma insulin are inconsistent and mammary tissue is not very sensitive to insulin. Increased energetic efficiency was proposed by DePeters and Cant (1992); since the direct incorporation of fatty acids into milk fat with high-fat diets would reduce acetate requirements, availability of glucose would be increased, so mammary blood flow would be decreased, thereby reducing amino acid supply. Wu and Huber (1994) found little data to support this hypothesis. Casper and Schingoethe (1989) suggested that somatotrophin production was inhibited by free fatty acids in the blood, which might reduce mammary uptake of amino acids. However, a subsequent study (Austin, Schingoethe and Casper, 1991) did not support this hypothesis.

Glucose deficiency remains the most likely explanation for the depression in milk protein concentration usually observed with dietary fat supplementation. There are several ways through which fat can affect glucose status.

- Where fat directly replaces starch in a diet, rumen propionate levels may be reduced. Propionate is the major source of glucose in ruminant metabolism.
- Microbial protein synthesis may be lower because of the reduced supply of fermentable metabolisable energy (FME). This would reduce the supply of glucogenic amino acids.
- In ruminants, fats are absorbed from the small intestine as free fatty acids. To convert these to triglycerides for transport, glycerol-3P must be synthesised from glucose present in the cells of the gut mucosae.

- Milk yield often increases after fat supplementation. This implies an increased glucose requirement for lactose synthesis, since lactose is the major osmotic component of milk.

Whether these putative effects of glucose are a direct cause of milk protein depression, or whether they act through a drain on amino acids is not clear. An attempt has been made to calculate the likely magnitude of these changes in glucose requirements, and reduced protein supply *per se*, on the protein status of a dairy cow (Figure 18.4). Some very broad assumptions have been made, but this was necessitated by lack of published data. The conversion of propionate to glucose and glucose to lactose or glycerol-3P are unlikely to be on an equi-molar basis (1.0 efficiency), since some energetic losses would occur during the synthetic processes. However, this assumption causes the magnitude of the effects to be underestimated. The assumption that all of the response to increased energy supply will be in milk production is tenuous. In practice, some shift of partitioning towards body fat reserves is usually observed. Whether this is inevitable, or simply a result of plasma protein/glucose deficiency, is not known. Evidence suggests that increasing the supply of dietary protein to cows with adequate body fat reserves shifts the partitioning of nutrients towards milk production (Garnsworthy and Jones, 1987). Whatever the exact figures are, the conclusion is the same; increasing the fat content of a diet increases glucose and protein requirements. For a cow giving 30 litres of milk per day, the 5% increase in energy supply results in an estimated 15% increase in metabolisable protein requirement. If this requirement is not met, milk protein concentration will decrease or the full potential increase in milk yield will not be realised. It is possible that in some cases the increased milk-protein yield observed with metabolisable protein supplies above theoretical requirements (Newbold, 1994) is due to correction of induced glucose deficiencies caused by high-fat diets.

In order to maintain adequate protein supplies when fats are included in a diet, the dietary protein content should be increased and consideration given to increasing the supply of fermentable carbohydrates. Even where protein supply is more than adequate, glucose status may be marginal with high-fat diets, due to insulin resistance and absorption requirements. This approach was adopted in a series of experiments conducted at Nottingham University. In the first (Garnsworthy, 1996a), the effects of replacing cereals with protected fat and/or lactose was investigated. Lactose was chosen as a source of readily-fermentable carbohydrates since it has less effect on rumen pH than sucrose and might be expected to increase microbial protein yield (Chamberlain and Choung, 1995). Replacing cereals with protected fat led to a significant increase in milk yield and a decrease in milk protein content (Table 18.4). The depression in milk protein content was partially alleviated by inclusion of lactose in the diet. In another experiment (Garnsworthy: unpublished), it was found that an increase in the supply of undegradable protein could maintain milk protein concentrations as milk yields increased in response to protected fat (Table 18.5). In a third experiment, it was found that a combination of strategies produced the best response. When cereals were replaced by a protected fat

Dietary Change

❖ Replace 0.5 kg barley with 0.5 kg calcium-salts of palm acid oil (85% fat)

Assumptions

❖ Metabolisable Energy (ME) and Metabolisable Protein (MP) are currently adequate.
❖ All the response will be in milk production, not body fat reserves.
❖ Conversions of propionate to glucose and glucose to lactose or glyercol-3P have 100% efficiency.

Direct Protein Effects

❖ ME supply increased by 10 MJ/day, sufficient for 2 litres of milk. This increase in milk yield would increase protein requirement by **90g MP**
❖ Fermentable Metabolisable Energy (FME) supply decreased by 6.1 MJ/day. This would decrease microbial protein synthesis by 67 g/day, equivalent to **43g MP**

Glucose Effects

❖ Decreased FME supply reduces propionate production in the rumen by 36 g/day, equivalent to **18 g glucose**
❖ Increased milk yield (2 l/day) contains 90 g lactose, equivalent to 90 g glucose, but it has to be assumed that this is already allowed for by the calculation of increased ME supply to avoid double accounting.
❖ 0.5 kg Ca-salts contains 1.5 M fatty acids. Conversion to triglycerides requires 0.5 M glycerol-3P, equivalent to **47 g glucose**

Indirect Protein Effects

❖ Glucose requirement has increased by 65 g/day, as shown above. If all this was supplied by glucogenic amino acids, it would be equivalent to **117 g MP**

Total increase in protein requirement = 250 g MP

Figure 18.4 Possible changes in metabolisable protein (MP) and glucose requirements when barley is replaced by fat

Table 18.4 MILK YIELD AND COMPOSITION OF COWS GIVEN PROTECTED FAT WITH OR WITHOUT LACTOSE

		Treatment group		
	Control	*Protected Fat[1]*	*Lactose[2]*	*Protected Fat[1] & Lactose[2]*
Milk yield (kg/d)	24.6	27.7	25.6	26.5
Milk fat (g/kg)	46.3	46.9	46.8	48.0
(kg/d)	1.13	1.30	1.20	1.27
Milk protein (g/kg)	32.3	30.7	32.7	31.9
(kg/d)	0.79	0.85	0.83	0.85

[1] Calcium salts of palm acid oil
[2] Whey permeate
Source: Garnsworthy (1996a)

Table 18.5 MILK YIELD AND COMPOSITION OF COWS GIVEN PROTECTED FAT WITH PROTEIN IN THE FORM OF RAPESEED MEAL, FISHMEAL OR PROTECTED RAPESEED MEAL

protein source fat source	Rapeseed Megalac[1]	Fishmeal Megalac[1]	MegaPro[2]
Milk yield (kg/d)	26.0	27.1	29.2
Milk fat (g/kg)	49.6	47.6	45.9
(kg/d)	1.29	1.29	1.34
Milk protein (g/kg)	30.0	29.9	29.1
(kg/d)	0.78	0.81	0.85

[1] Calcium salts of palm acid oil
[2] Combined product containing calcium salts of palm acid oil with rapeseed meal added during manufacture (heat-protected)
Source: Garnsworthy, unpublished

Table 18.6 MILK YIELD AND COMPOSITION OF COWS GIVEN COMBINED PROTECTED FAT AND PROTECTED RAPESEED MEAL[1] WITH OR WITHOUT LACTOSE

	Treatment Group			
	Control	Protected Fat + Protein	Lactose	Protected Fat + Protein & Lactose
Milk yield (kg/day)	21.3	23.4	22.7	27.8
Milk fat (g/kg)	42.6	41.7	42.5	41.8
Milk protein (g/kg)	33.7	33.6	33.7	33.8

[1] Calcium salts of palm acid oil combined with rapeseed during manufacture
Source: Garnsworthy (1996b)

in combination with protected rapeseed, and lactose was also added to the diet, a significant increase in milk yield was observed without any reduction in milk protein concentration (Table 18.6; Garnsworthy, 1996b).

Future possibilities

In the human food industry, dietary trends and nutritional recommendations appear somewhat volatile. It is a feature of affluent societies that consumers want plenty of choice in the foods available to them and most foods are selected for their convenience, rather than nutritional value. However, there are some instances where food fashions have been generated by nutritional considerations and certain people are willing to pay a premium for foods which more closely match their personal "ideal". Whether these nutritional considerations are justified is usually questionable, but there are often niche markets that can be profitably exploited.

One of the longer-lasting, and potentially more damaging, trends is the avoidance or reduction in consumption of animal fats. There is virtually no sound scientific evidence that animal fats harm human health more than vegetable fats. However, a generation has been advised to reduce their consumption of dairy products, with the resulting side-effect of a decrease in calcium intake. The trend towards preference for semi-skimmed or half-fat milk is probably irreversible and farmers are encouraged, through milk-pricing mechanisms, to produce milk with a low fat content. The easiest way to reduce the fat content of milk for liquid sale is to skim off some of the fat during processing. This technology has been used for centuries, but the reduction in demand for butter has reduced the economic value of milk fat. There are simple feeding techniques that can be employed to reduce the butterfat content of milk. Until the early 1980s, dairy farmers were concerned about the so-called "low fat syndrome". A simple method of reducing milk fat concentration is to feed cows on high-starch rations with little forage, which will usually have the additional benefit of maintaining high milk protein concentrations. Unfortunately, this goes against the sound economic advice (in the UK and other forage-growing countries) of producing maximum amounts of milk from home-grown forages. It also tends to increase milk yield, which could be detrimental if a volume quota is operating on milk production.

The use of dietary fat sources that increase the supply of *trans*-fatty acids to the mammary gland, such as naked oats, fish oils and hydrogenated vegetable oils may be a tempting route for farmers who want to reduce the fat content of their milk. However, these fat sources invariably increase the concentrations of *trans*-fatty acids in milk and, as it is now thought that *trans*-fatty acids increase the risk of coronary heart disease (CHD) in humans (Willett, Stampfer, Manson, Colditz, Speizer, Rosner, Sampson and Hennekens, 1993), this may seem to be a retrograde step. It is important to distinguish between *trans*-fatty acids arising from rumen biohydrogenation and those from hydrogenated vegetable oils. *Trans*-C18:1 of ruminant origin has the double bond mainly in the 11-carbon position and does not increase the incidence of CHD; hydrogenated vegetable oils have the double bond mainly in the 9-carbon position, which has been associated with increased risk of CHD (Willett, *et al.*, 1993). This may preclude the use of fats which increase *trans*-fatty acids by direct incorporation, such as hydrogenated vegetable oils, but since the position of the double bond has not been reported in studies with dairy cows, it is not possible to at this stage to draw firm conclusions.

The production of "designer" milk may be one route for adding value to milk destined for niche markets. Of particular interest are n3 fatty acids and conjugated linoleic acid. However, the poor efficiency of incorporation found with n3 acids suggests that this is not a viable option. It would be much more sensible to encourage consumers to eat fish oil directly, rather than utilise an increasingly scarce commodity by feeding it to dairy cows. The study of CLAs has yet to be actively pursued. They do offer potential for enhancing the image of milk but much more information is needed on their occurrence and the factors that affect their concentrations in milk.

References

AFRC (1993) *Energy and Protein Requirements of Ruminants* An advisory manual prepared by the AFRC Technical Committee on Responses to Nutrients. CAB International, Wallingford.

Ashes, J.R., Siebert, B.D., Gulati, S.K., Cuthbertson, A.Z. and Scott, T.W. (1992) Incorporation of n-3 fatty acids of fish oil into tissue and serum lipids of ruminants. *Lipids* **27**, 629–631

Austin, C.L., Schingoethe, D.J. and Casper, D.P. (1991)Influence of bovine somatotropin and nutrition on production and composition of milk from dairy cows. *Journal of Dairy Science* **74**:3920–3932.

Beaulieu, A.D. and Palmquist, D.L. (1995) Differential effects of high fat diets on fatty acid composition in milk of Jersey and Holstein cows. *Journal of Dairy Science* **78**, 1336–1344.

Bauman, D.E., Corl, B.A., Baumgard, L.H. and Griinari, J.M. (2001) Conjugated linoleic acid (CLA) and the dairy cow. In *Recent Advances in Animal Nutrition 2001* (eds. P.C. Garnsworthy and J. Wiseman), pp. 221-250. Nottingham University Press, Nottingham.

Bitman, J., Wood, D.L., Miller, R.H., Tyrrell, H.F., Reynolds, C.K. and Baxter, H.D. (1996) Comparison of milk and blood lipids in Jersey and Holstein cows fed total mixed rations with or without whole cottonseed. *Journal of Dairy Science* **79**,1596–1602.

Blaxter, K.L. and Webster, A.J.F. (1991) Animal production and food: real problems and paranoia. *Animal Production* **53**, 261–269.

Casper, D.P. and Schingoethe, D.J. (1989) Model to describe and alleviate milk protein depression in early lactation dairy cows fed a high fat diet. *Journal of Dairy Science* **72**,3327–3335.

Chamberlain, D.J. and Choung, J-J. (1995) The importance of rate of ruminal fermentation of energy sources in diets for dairy cows. In *Recent Advances in Animal Nutrition - 1995.* (Eds P.C. Garnsworthy and D.J.A. Cole) pp 3–27. Nottingham University Press: Nottingham.

Chin, S.F., Liu, W., Storkson, J.M., Ha, Y.L. and Pariza, M.W. (1992) Dietary sources of conjugated dienoic isomers of linoleic acid, a newly recognised class of anticarconogens. *Journal of Food Composition and Analysis* **5**, 185–197.

Christie, W.W. (1981) The effects of diet and other factors on the lipid composition of ruminant tissues and milk. In *Lipid Metabolism in Ruminant Animals* (Ed W.W. Christie) pp 193–226. Pergamon Press: Oxford.

COMA [Committee on Medical Aspects of Food Policy] (1994) Nutritional aspects of cardiovascular disease. *Report on Health and Social Subjects* No 46.

DePeters, E.J. and Cant, J.P. (1992) Nutritional factors influencing the nitrogen composition of bovine milk: a review. *Journal of Dairy Science* **75**,2043–2070.

Fearon, A.M., Mayne, C.S. and Marsden, S. (1996) The effect of inclusion of naked oats in the concentrate offered to dairy cows on milk production, milk fat composition and properties. *Journal of the Science of Food and Agriculture* **72**,273–282.

Garnsworthy, P.C. (1996a) The effects on milk yield and composition of incorporating lactose into the diet of dairy cows given protected fat. *Animal Science* **62**,1–3.

Garnsworthy, P.C. (1996b) Response by dairy cows to supplements containing protected fat and protein with and without lactose. *Proceedings of the 47ᵗʰ Annual Meeting of EAAP, Lillehammer, Norway.* **2**,166. Wageningen Pers: Wageningen.

Garnsworthy, P.C. and Huggett, C.D. (1992) The influence of fat concentration of the diet on the response by dairy cows to body condition at calving. *Animal Production* **54**,7–13.

Garnsworthy, P.C. and Jones, G.P. (1987) The influence of body condition at calving and dietary protein supply on voluntary food intake and performance in dairy cows. *Animal Production* **44**,347–353.

Garnsworthy, P.C. and Topps, J.H. (1982) The effect of body condition of dairy cows at calving on their food intake and performance when given complete diets. *Animal Production* **35**,113–119.

Griinari, J.M., Corl, B.A., Lacy, S.H., Chouinard, P.Y., Nurmela, K.V.V. and Bauman, D.E. (2000) Conjugated linoleic acid is synthesized endogenously in lactating diary cows by Δ-desaturase. *Journal of Nutrition*, 130, 2285-2291.

Hermansen, J.E. (1995) Prediction of milk fatty acid profile in dairy cows fed dietary fat differeing in fatty acid composition. *Journal of Dairy Science* **78**,872–879.

Holmes, C.W. (1988) Genetic merit and efficiency of milk production by the dairy cow. In *Nutrition and Lactation in the Dairy Cow.* (Ed P.C. Garnsworthy) pp195–215. Butterworths: London.

Jones, G.P. and Garnsworthy, P.C. (1989) The effects of dietary energy content on the response by dairy cows to body condition at calving. *Animal Production* **49**,183–191.

Kepler, C.R. and Tove, S.B. (1967) Biohydrogenation of unsaturated fatty acids. III. Purification and properties of a linoleate *cis*-12, *trans*-11 isomerase from *Butyrivibrio fibrisolvens. Journal of Biological Chemistry* **242**,5686–5692.

Lock, A.L. and Garnsworthy, P.C. (2002a) Independent effects of dietary linoleic and linolenic fatty acids on the conjugated linoleic acid content of cows' milk. *Animal Science*, **74**, 163-176.

Lock, A.L. and Garnsworthy, P.C. (2002b) Seasonal variation in milk conjugated linoleic acid and D9-desaturase activity in dairy cows. *Livestock Production Science* (in press).

MAFF (1990) *UK Tables of Nutritive Value and Chemical Composition of Feedingstuffs* Rowett Research Services, Aberdeen

Mansbridge, R.J. and Blake, J.S. (1997) The effect of feeding fish oil on the fatty acid composition of bovine milk. *Proceedings of the British Society of Animal Science,* p22, British Society of Animal Science: Edinburgh.

McDonald, P., Edwards, R.A., Greenhalgh, J.F.D. and Morgan, C.A.(1995) *Animal Nutrition* Longman, Harlow.

Newbold, J.R. (1994) Practical application of the metabolisable protein system. In *Recent Advances in Animal Nutrition - 1994.* (Eds P.C. Garnsworthy and D.J.A. Cole) pp231–264. Nottingham University Press: Nottingham.

NRC (1989) *Nutrient Requirements of Dairy Cattle* National Academy Press, Washington

Palmquist, D.L. and Moser, E.A. (1981) Dietary effects on blood insulin, glucose utilisation and milk protein content of lactating cows. *Journal of Dairy Science* **64**, 1664–1670.

Schingoethe, D.J., Brouk, M.J., Lightfield, K.D. and Baer, R.J. (1996) Lactational response of dairy cows fed unsaturated fat from extruded soybeans or sunflower seeds. *Journal of Dairy Science* **79**,1244–1249.

Thomas, P.C. and Chamberlain, D.G. (1984) Manipulation of milk composition to meet market needs. In *Recent Advances in Animal Nutrition - 1984.* (Eds W. Haresign and D.J.A. Cole) pp 219–245. Butterworths: London.

Thomas, P.C. and Martin, P.A. (1988) The influence of nutrient balance on milk yield and composition. In *Nutrition and Lactation in the Dairy Cow.* (Ed P.C. Garnsworthy) pp97–118. Butterworths: London.

Viviani, R. (1970) Metabolism of long-chain fatty acids in the rumen. *Advances in Lipid Research* **8**, 267–346.

Willett, W.C., Stampfer, M.J., Manson, J.E., Colditz, G.A., Speizer, F.E., Rosner, B.A., Sampson, L.A. and Hennekens, C.H. (1993) Intake of *trans* fatty acids and risk of coronary heart disease among women. *The Lancet* **341**, 581–585.

Wonsil, B.J., Herbein, J.H. and Watkins, B.A. (1994) Dietary and ruminally derived *trans*-18:1 fatty acids alter bovine milk lipids. *Journal of Nutrition* **124**,556–565.

Wu, Z. and Huber, J.T. (1994) Relationship between dietary fat supplementation and milk protein concentration in lactating cows: A review. *Livestock Production Science* **39**,141–155.

This paper was first published in 1997

19

MANIPULATION OF MILK FAT IN DAIRY COWS

M. DOREAU[1], Y. CHILLIARD[1], H. RULQUIN[2] and D.I. DEMEYER[3]
[1] *Institut National de la Recherche Agronomique, Unité de Recherches sur les Herbivores, Theix, 63122 Saint-Genès Champanelle, France*
[2] *Institut National de la Recherche Agronomique, Station de Recherches sur la Vache Laitière, 35590 Saint-Gilles, France*
[3] *University of Ghent, Department of Animal Production, Proefhoevestraat 10, 9090 Melle, Belgium*

Introduction

The first attempts to modify milk fat by nutritional means date from the last century. Throughout the twentieth century until the 1970s, the aim was to improve butter production by an increase in milk fat content. Numerous reviews have been devoted to the low milk fat syndrome caused by an excess of concentrates. A large change has taken place during the two past decades, with an increasing concern for milk protein, especially in countries where cheese-making is important. The aim is to increase the protein:fat ratio in milk, or at least to decrease the fat content. The present situation is motivated by the establishment of milk fat quotas, independent of milk yield quotas, or by penalties for high fat content of milk in many countries of the European Community.

The 1970s also mark the beginning of manipulation of milk fat composition. Two reasons can be evoked : 1) in developed countries milk production increased enough to ensure self-sufficiency in dairy products. For this reason interest in quality took precedence over increase in production; 2) medical research suggested a negative role of saturated fatty acids (FA) on cardiovascular diseases and the consumption of margarines was promoted at the same time. Techniques have been proposed to increase the polyunsaturated content in milk FA. More recently, other modifications of milk FA composition have been proposed, based on new research : increasing n-3 FA, decreasing *trans* FA, increasing conjugated linoleic acid (CLA) (Demeyer and Doreau, 1999). Unfortunately, as expressed by Kennelly (1996a), "the ideal milk fatty acid profile is a moving target". This is a consequence of the difficulty in establishing a scale between the different dietary factors acting positively or negatively on human health, and of accounting for the multifactorial origin of human diseases. For example, epidemiological data have shown risks of cardiovascular diseases due to *trans* FA (Willett, Stampfer, Manson, Colditz, Speizer, Rosner, Sampson and Hennekens, 1993), but other studies found no evidence of their toxicity (Wolff, 1994). In the same way, the interest in decreasing dietary saturated fats, always in effect in the United States (Havel, 1997) has been questioned in France (Apfelbaum, 1990).

Besides an effect of FA on human health, increasing attention is paid to milk organoleptic and marketing qualities. In particular, the increase in polyunsaturated FA (PUFA) in milk has negative consequences on milk quality by the development of oxidative processes and off-flavours (see Doreau and Chilliard, 1997a). The use of vitamin E to prevent oxidation, which had been found inefficient, may be positive in some cases (Focant, Mignolet, Marique, Clabots, Breyne, Dalemans and Larondelle, 1998). On another hand, different chemical constituents have been identified in the fat fraction : aldehydes, methyl ketones, esters, lactones and terpenoids (Joblin and Hudson, 1997). Although the effect of these molecules on flavour has not been clearly established, and the threshold of their concentration in milk needed to develop flavour, is unknown, attempts are made to relate their concentration in food to milk flavours. For example, it has been shown that the content of lactones may be enhanced by cereals (Urbach, 1990). In the same way, close relationships have been established between terpenoids in forages and in milk (Viallon, Verdier-Metz, Denoyer, Pradel, Coulon and Berdagué, 1999). Although fragmentary results are available in this area, it appears that in the near future a better knowledge of aromatic compounds in feeds and fat could lead to specific flavours in milk.

A new stage was reached 2-3 years ago. The BSE crisis emphasised the anxiety of the consumer over the health value of their food, and irrational behaviours appeared : blind belief in the media, especially when they predict disasters. To take into account this new behaviour, public authorities established the "precautionary principle" i.e. the quest for maximal safety, to minimize the risks of food for public health. For this reason, it is likely that the ideal milk fat composition will change in the next years, and the ideal cow's diet also.

Nevertheless, scientists must go on trying to manipulate milk fat to provide a rapid response to changes in market demand. Increased PUFA is always an objective, but human consumption of these FA can be achieved by vegetable or marine oils. At the moment, the main objective is to reduce the amount of possibly "negative" compounds in milk, such as saturated and *trans* unsaturated FA, and to increase "positive" compounds, such as CLA, which has the great advantage of being present mainly in ruminant meat and milk. It can be argued that progress in the technology of products and in *trans*genesis removes the need for developing feeding strategies to modify milk composition. The authors believe that if agricultural products are priced according to their quality, a part of the increase in value should benefit the farmer, especially if the increase in quality can be achieved by the use of "natural" diets, i.e. of vegetable origin.

Different methods of decreasing butterfat

There are two effective ways to strongly decrease butterfat : concentrate-rich diets and fish oil. Ground grass has the same effect (Clapperton, Kelly, Banks and Rook, 1980), but its use is not discussed here, due to the lack of practical use of this type of feeding. It is also possible to decrease fat in milk using sources of fat other than fish oil, or propionate-enhancing additives, but results are inconsistent.

DIETS RICH IN CEREALS

It has long been known that consumption of a large amount of concentrates decreases milk butterfat content. Many reviews have been devoted to this subject, so this section only considers the main ideas. The decrease in butterfat is generally significant (down to less than 30 g/kg) when the proportion of concentrates in the diet is more than 0.6. Milk fat content lower than 25 g/kg is almost always reached with diets containing 0.7-0.8 concentrates. However fat concentrations lower than 20 g/kg can sometimes be obtained with diets containing no more than 0.65 concentrates (Kennelly, 1996b). No threshold can be determined. Figure 19.1 illustrates the linear relationships between milk fat and proportion of concentrates in the diet on the one hand (Journet and Chilliard, 1985), and between milk fat and dietary acid detergent fibre (ADF) content on the other (Sutton, 1989). From these reviews and other more recent reviews (Grummer, 1991, Palmquist, Beaulieu and Barbano, 1993, Kennelly, 1996b, Fredeen, 1996), the main factors affecting the response of milk fat to increasing concentrates can be defined as below, provided that the proportion of concentrate is high enough to induce a significant decrease in butterfat :

1. The decrease is higher in mid-lactation than in early lactation (Jenny, Polan and Thye, 1974) because of the supply of mobilised lipids in early lactation.
2. The decrease is greater when concentrates are given 1 or 2 times a day, compared to mixed diets or concentrate distribution in multiple meals (Sutton, Hart, Broster, Elliott and Schuller, 1986).
3. The decrease is greater with cereals than with concentrates rich in fibre (Sutton, Bines, Morant, Napper and Givens, 1987) or soluble carbohydrates such as molasses, but it is similar to the decrease with sucrose (Sutton, 1989).
4. The decrease is greater when cereals are ground instead of cracked or rolled.
5. The decrease is greater when dietary starch is highly degradable (Sutton, Oldham and Hart, 1980).
6. The decrease requires the absence of a buffer in the diet (Kalscheur, Teter, Piperova and Erdman, 1997a).
7. A high individual variation is observed for the same diet (Gaynor, Waldo, Capuco, Erdman, Douglass and Teter, 1995).

Diets with a high proportion of concentrate modify milk fat composition. Short- and medium-chain fatty acids (FA), including palmitic acid, are reduced. Stearic acid is also

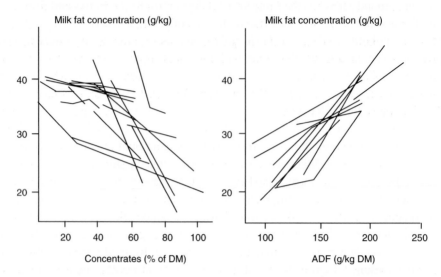

Figure 19.1 Relationship between milk fat concentration and the percentage of concentrates in the diet (Journet and Chilliard, 1985) or the ADF content of the diet (Sutton, 1989) © Journal of Dairy Science, 1989

reduced and C18:1 isomers are increased. Among them, vaccenic acid (*trans*-11 C18:1) is generally increased. In some experiments the proportion of palmitic acid did not decrease (Rémond and Journet, 1971), but output of this FA still decreased markedly.

Increasing the proportion of concentrates generally increases the energy concentration of a diet and thus milk protein content. If, in addition, milk yield increases, fat content may decrease by a dilution effect. Generally, high-concentrate diets decrease butterfat to a greater extent (often by more than 10 g/kg) than they increase protein (generally by less than 4 g/kg). Therefore, the protein:fat ratio increases.

DIETS ENRICHED WITH FISH OIL

Fish oils (and oils from marine mammals) are characterised by the presence of highly unsaturated 20- and 22-carbon FA, of which eicosapentaenoic (20:5 n-3) and docosahexaenoic (22:6 n-3) are the most important (Ackman, 1982). Among possible feeds for ruminants, only plankton and algae are also rich in these FA (Givens, Cottrill, Davies, Lee, Mansbridge and Moss, 1997).

Fish oils decrease butterfat consistently. This effect was first shown in 1894 by Sebelien, quoted by Opstvedt (1984), then largely demonstrated in the 1930s mainly with cod liver oil and recently with other oils, such as menhaden. Some experiments with specific oils, such as from salmon or shark failed to depress butterfat (review by Jarrige and Journet, 1959), but this cannot be explained by the FA composition of the oils and is perhaps due to unsuitable designs.

The minimal daily supply of fish oil needed to significantly decrease milk butterfat is low. It has been estimated as 55 g by Jarrige and Journet (1959), 75-100 g by Pike, Miller and Short (1994) and 100-150 g from results summarised by Opstvedt (1984). The decrease is frequently observed with fish meal supplements which induce rather low FA supplies (Hussein and Jordan, 1991). Most experiments with fish oil have been carried out with daily supplies of 200 to 400 g. The effect of the proportion of fish oil in the diet appears to be linear (Figure 19.2), but too few experiments have been made with two or more levels of oil inclusion for the range of linearity to be confirmed. Figure 19.2 also shows that the extent of the decrease is independent of the butterfat content of the control diet. On the other hand, the decrease could be more important when milk yield is higher : for cows producing less or more than 20 kg milk daily, it reaches 6.3 and 10.1 g/kg for a mean inclusion of 250 and 305 g fish oil, respectively. This effect has to be confirmed by direct measurements, because results with low-producing cows are generally ancient and obtained with cod liver oil, whereas results with high-producing cows have been obtained more recently with menhaden-type or mixed oils. Moreover it has been observed by Chilliard and Doreau (1997) that the decrease in butterfat is greater for primiparous than for multiparous cows. The magnitude of the decrease in butterfat may increase in diets with a high proportion of concentrates (Pike *et al.*, 1994), but this needs to be confirmed since the response was not found in the study of Nicholson and Sutton (1971).

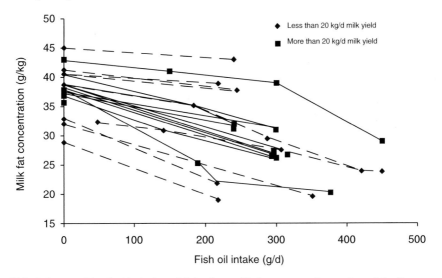

Figure 19.2 Influence of level of inclusion of fish oil on milk fat concentration: review of the literature

The decrease in butterfat has been shown to be lower when fish oil is protected by proteins (Storry, Brumby, Hall and Tuckley, 1974) or infused into the abomasum or duodenum (Pennington and Davis, 1975, Chilliard, Chardigny, Chabrot, Ollier, Sébédio and Doreau, 1999). When the added fish oil is hydrogenated, no decrease is observed

(Brumby, Storry and Sutton, 1972, Sundstøl, 1974). This shows that the decrease is related mainly to the products of biohydrogenation (which are not the same FA as those produced by industrial hydrogenation), and secondly to the naturally occurring FA.

Most of the decrease in butterfat is due to a large decrease in short- and medium-chain FA, that is not compensated for by an increase in long-chain FA. In particular, the incorporation of dietary total 20- and 22-carbon FA into milk is low, ranging from 0.15 (Brumby *et al.*, 1972) to 0.3-0.4 (Storry *et al.*, 1974, Hagemeister, Precht and Barth, 1988). With unprotected oils, the natural C20:5 and C22:6 are in very low concentrations in milk; the main 20- and 22-carbon FA are monounsaturated isomers.

Fish oil, like other lipid sources, decreases milk protein content. The feeding of fish oils with protected amino acids restores milk protein content to a similar level found in a control diet, but no interaction between fish oil and amino acid is observed (Chilliard and Doreau, 1997). On the other hand, fish oil has an adverse effect on milk taste (Lacasse, Kennelly and Ahnadi, 1998), which has to be taken into account for its use.

Algae have been recently used in dairy cow feeding. The inclusion of 910 g algae daily significantly decreased milk butterfat (Franklin, Schingoethe and Baer, 1998).

OTHER SOURCES OF FAT

Among natural or protected fats and oils of any type, except fish oil, only vegetable oils reduce milk fat, by 2.8 g/kg on average (Table 19.1). This mean value masks a high variability : Kalscheur, Teter, Piperova and Erdman (1997b) observed a decrease by 4 g/kg with soya bean oil. However, this decrease is too low to obtain low-fat milk. Feeding vegetable oils and seeds decreases the proportion and output of short- and medium-chain FA and increases the proportion and output of long-chain FA (Kennelly, 1996a).

Table 19.1 EFFECT OF LIPID SUPPLEMENTATION ON MILK FAT CONTENT ACCORDING TO THE NATURE OF DIETARY LIPIDS (REVIEWS BY CHILLIARD, 1993 AND CHILLIARD, DOREAU, GAGLIOSTRO AND ELMEDDAH, 1993)

Dietary lipids	*No of supplemented groups*	*Milk fat content (supplemented - control, g/kg)*
Animal and blended fats	22	-1.4
Protected tallow	26	+4.0**
Saturated fats	10	+0.5
Calcium salts of palm oil	29	+0.4
Vegetable oils	8	-2.8*
Oilseeds	34	-0.9*
Protected vegetable oils	26	+6.4**

* significantly different from zero, $P < 0.05$
** significantly different from zero, $P < 0.01$

Most vegetable oils and seeds (including rapeseed, soyabean, cottonseed, sunflower, safflower, maize), are rich in oleic and/or linoleic acid. Linseed oil is characterised by a high content in linolenic acid. Few experiments have been carried out with linseed oil.

According to Kennelly (1996a) linseed oil does not cause a decrease in butterfat although fat composition is modified; the decrease in short- and medium-chain FA being compensated for by an increase in long-chain FA ; moreover low amounts of *trans*-11 C18:1 are found. However, linseed oil decreased milk fat in mid-lactation but not in early lactation in a trial by Brunschwig, Kernen and Weill (1997), and increased milk fat in a trial by Nevens, Alleman and Peck (1926). A mixture of rapeseed and linseed oil decreased fat content in a trial by Focant *et al.* (1998). More information is needed on the effect of linseed oil on fat content. In rare cases, other vegetable oils provoke a strong drop in fat concentration. An example is given in Table 19.2 (Doreau and Chilliard, 1999). Curiously, the output of long-chain FA was not increased by oils or seeds. Other examples of very low fat contents have been observed by Palmquist (1984) with Ca salts of blended fat or soyabean, and Chilliard and Doreau (unpublished data) with animal fats. In the same way, a reduction of milk fat by 6 g/kg has been observed with palm oil FA (Bremmer, Ruppert, Clark and Drackley, 1998). These atypical results cannot be explained at the moment.

Table 19.2 AN ATYPICAL EFFECT OF 44 G/KG INCLUSION OF OIL AS SOYA BEAN OIL OR WHOLE SOYA BEANS ON MILK FAT (DOREAU AND CHILLIARD, 1999)

	Control	*Whole soya beans*	*Soyabean oil + soyabean meal*
Milk yield (kg/d)	21.7	21.4	20.6
Milk fat (g/kg)	35.7[a]	25.4[b]	25.5[b]
FA output (g/d)			
Total	798[a]	532[b]	528[b]
C4 to C14	212[a]	107[b]	98[b]
C16:0	207[a]	123[b]	117[b]
C18:0	90	93	81
C18:1	233	223	213
C18:2	27	30	19

Diet based on 0.6 maize silage and 0.4 concentrates.
Means on the same row with different superscripts significantly differ (P < 0.01)

FEED ADDITIVES

Ionophore antibiotics, which are propionate enhancers, are used mainly for beef cattle and very few experiments have been carried out with dairy cows. A moderate negative effect on milk fat is generally observed (reviews by Sprott, Goehring, Beverly and

Corah, 1988 and Van Amburgh, 1997 ; Cant, Fredeen, McIntyre, Gunn and Crowe, 1997). Significant decreases may occur at high ionophore supplies: more than 4 g/kg milk with 450 mg/d monensin in a trial by Van der Werf, Jonker and Oldenbroek (1998). No variation in milk protein content was observed.

Monopropylene glycol, a precursor of propionate used for the treatment or prevention of ketosis, decreases milk fat when fed in large amounts (-4 g/kg for an intake of 1.2 kg/d, Hurtaud, Vérité and Rulquin, 1991). This decrease is mainly due to a decrease in 18-carbon FA (Hurtaud, Rulquin and Vérité, 2000).

Manipulation of milk fat composition

The ideal milk fat composition would improve human health, organoleptic quality of dairy products and technological value for processing. Some of these objectives are sometimes contradictory. An increase in n-3 PUFA reduces the risk of cardiovascular diseases (Kinsella, Lokesh and Stone, 1990); PUFA increase the spreadability of butters, but also the tendency for oxidation (reviews by Palmquist *et al.*, 1993 and Doreau and Chilliard, 1997a). On the other hand, the negative effects of *trans* FA could be counterbalanced by the positive effect of CLA, which is anticarcinogenic (Kelly and Bauman, 1996), both FA being positively related (Jiang, Bjoerck, Fondén and Emanuelson, 1996). The aim of this section is to summarise methods of modifying milk fat composition, without taking a stand about the ideal composition of milk.

INCREASE IN PUFA

With natural feedstuffs the concentration of PUFA in milk fat is always low, even when high amounts of PUFA are fed, due to the high level of ruminal biohydrogenation. With diets rich in concentrates, PUFA (mainly C18:2 and C18:3), which are generally lower than 0.04 of total FA reach 0.10 of total FA (Clapperton *et al.*, 1980). Until now, the only way to increase PUFA in milk fat significantly was to use oils or oilseeds protected by encapsulation with a matrix of protected proteins. It is thus possible to obtain milk containing up to 0.35 linoleic acid with safflower oil and up to 0.22 linolenic acid with linseed oil (McDonald and Scott, 1977, Kennelly, 1996a). An increase in PUFA with 20 or 22 carbons can be achieved by the use of protected fish oils (Storry *et al.*, 1974). It must be noted that a high level of protection requires an excellent control of the process, which is not always achieved in commercial products (Ashes, Gulati, Cook, Scott and Donnelly, 1979). Other techniques for protection of oils fail to increase PUFA in significant proportions : calcium salts of PUFA (Ferlay, Chilliard and Doreau, 1992, Enjalbert, Nicot, Bayourthe, Vernay and Moncoulon, 1997) are extensively hydrogenated, fatty acyl amides from soya bean oil increase linoleic acid to a low extent, up to 6% (Jenkins, Bateman and Block, 1996). Feeding unprotected oilseeds increases PUFA in milk to a moderate extent, depending on nature of seeds : it has been observed with soya beans, especially when roasted (Tice, Eastridge and Firkins, 1994), but no effect was found in some experiments (Chouinard, Girard and Brisson, 1997a).

DECREASE IN SATURATED FA

Another objective in manipulation of milk fat is to decrease the proportion of saturated FA, i.e. to increase unsaturated FA, especially C18:1. The addition of fat to the diet generally reduces the amount of short- and medium-chain saturated FA, due to lower de novo synthesis, but does not modify the amount of saturated long-chain FA. However, substitution of palmitic acid by stearic acid is often observed (e.g. Banks, Clapperton, Kelly, Wilson and Crawford, 1980). The most efficient was to lower the ratio C16:0 : C18:0, to supply a diet with oils poor in palmitic acid, such as rapeseed or sunflower which contain less than 10% of this FA (Grummer, 1991). The reduction in de novo synthesis is thus combined with a low incorporation of exogenous C16:0. A decrease in saturated FA can also be obtained by incomplete hydrogenation of oleic acid. This has been achieved by feeding oleamide, resistant to biohydrogenation (Jenkins, 1998).

VARIATIONS IN TRANS C18:1 AND CONJUGATED C18:2 FA

Feeding oleaginous oils generally involves an increase in *trans* FA, which can be either moderate (from 3 to 6% in a trial by Banks *et al.*, 1980, from 1 to 8% in trials by Banks, Clapperton and Ferrie, 1976, and Casper, Schingoethe, Middaugh and Baer, 1988) or more pronounced (from 1 to 13% in a trial by Wonsil, Herbein and Watkins, 1994). When oleaginous seeds are fed instead of oils, the amount of *trans* FA decreases (Banks *et al.*, 1980). Calcium salts of rapeseed oil increase moderately (Enjalbert *et al.*, 1997) or do not increase (Kowalski, Pisulewski and Spanghero, 1999) *trans* C18:1. Milk fat produced from fish oil is characterised by a high content in *trans*-11 C18:1 (Wonsil *et al.*, 1994, Mansbridge and Blake, 1997, Lacasse *et al.*, 1998). The technological process of hydrogenation of fat produces *trans* FA. For this reason, feeding partially hydrogenated fats increases milk *trans* FA (Banks, Clapperton, Girdler and Steele, 1984). It has been recently shown that in this case the main isomers are *trans*-9 and *trans*-10, and that *trans*-11 represents only 15% of total *trans* C18:1 whereas *trans*-11 is the major isomer when oleaginous oils are fed (Griinari, Chouinard and Bauman, 1997a).

The CLA content of milk has been recently studied by several research groups. Various conjugated isomers of linoleic acid are present in milk, but the most important (ca. 90 - 95 %) is cis-9 *trans*-11 (Jiang *et al.*, 1996, Chilliard *et al.*, 1999). The main dietary effects on CLA content have been studied in particular by Chouinard, Corneau, Bauman, Butler, Chilliard and Drackley (1998) and reviewed by Chilliard, Ferlay, Mansbridge and Doreau (2000). It appears that the highest content of CLA in milk (more than 16 g/kg) is found with dietary supplies of fish oil (Chilliard, Ferlay and Doreau, 2001) and vegetable oils rich in linoleic (sunflower, soyabean) and linolenic (linseed) acids. Oils rich in oleic acid (peanut) are less rich in CLA; with seeds (soyabeans, cottonseeds) no increase in CLA is shown compared with control diets, at levels lower than 8 g/kg of total milk FA.

It appears that dietary factors that increase *trans* FA also increase CLA. A positive relationship has been established by Jiang *et al.* (1996). It has been shown that the majority of CLA is synthesised in the udder from *trans*-11 C18:1 by the Δ9-desaturase enzyme (Griinari, Corl, Lacy, Chouinard, Nurmela and Bauman, 2000).

Modifications of ruminal metabolism related to milk fat

The different means of modifying milk fat content or composition – increasing concentrates, supplying dietary lipids and, to a lesser extent, ionophores – induce modifications of carbohydrate fermentation and lipid metabolism in the rumen that may act on mammary lipid synthesis. All contribute to the shift of ruminal volatile FA (VFA) towards propionate and the increase in intermediate long-chain FA originating from biohydrogenation. On the other hand, concentrates and ionophores are dietary factors that reduce biohydrogenation of dietary FA.

INCREASING PROPIONATE PROPORTION

The main factors leading to an increase in propionate when concentrates are fed in large amounts are summarised on Figure 19.3. From this figure it is possible to understand

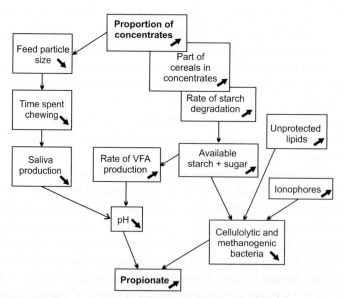

Figure 19.3 Factors modifying propionate proportion in ruminal VFA mixture

the different factors that modify the VFA pattern: amount of concentrates, amount and degradability of starch, presentation of grain and number of meals, factors modifying the ruminal pH.

Fat supplementation is also known to increase propionic acid in the VFA mixture. This is mainly a consequence of a decrease in cellulolytic and methanogenic microorganisms in the ruminal ecosystem (Prins, Van Nevel and Demeyer, 1972, Maczulak, Dehority and Palmquist, 1981). The proportion of propionate is increased more by oils than by their corresponding seeds, and more by linseed oil than by oils rich in linoleic acid (Jouany, Michalet-Doreau and Doreau, 1998). Fish oils also increase propionic acid to a large extent, although cellulolytic activity in the rumen is not depressed (Doreau and Chilliard, 1997b).

Ionophores antibiotics also enhance propionic acid production by a toxic effect on cellulolytic bacteria (Nagaraja, Newbold, Van Nevel and Demeyer, 1997). However the combination of ionophores and fat does not lead to an extra production of propionate (Zinn, 1988) whereas the addition of ionophores is less effective with a concentrate-rich diet than with a forage-rich diet (Nagajara, Newbold, Van Nevel and Demeyer, 1997).

RUMINAL BIOHYDROGENATION OF PUFA

Biohydrogenation can be defined as the sum of mechanisms related to the modification of dietary unsaturated FA, leading to saturated and intermediate unsaturated compounds. Biohydrogenation occurs only in free FA, after hydrolysis of triglycerides, phospholipids and galactolipids from the diet. The extent and the factors causing variation in biohydrogenation of 18-carbon FA have been described by Doreau and Ferlay (1994). Linolenic acid is hydrogenated to a greater extent than linoleic acid. Linoleic acid is partially taken up by bacteria (Bauchart, Legay-Carmier, Doreau and Gaillard, 1990) so that its biohydrogenation is incomplete with diets poor in linoleic acid. However, the quantity of precursors for biohydrogenation is not a major cause of variation in biohydrogenation. The disappearance of linoleic and linolenic acids in the rumen is usually reduced by high-concentrate diets, due to a low ruminal pH which limits the first step, hydrolysis of triglycerides (Van Nevel and Demeyer, 1996a). However, factors other than pH may slow down biohydrogenation with high starch intakes, suggesting that cellulolytic microorganisms are more able to hydrolyse lipids and/or to hydrogenate FA than amylolytic ones (Latham, Storry and Sharpe, 1972, Gerson, John and King, 1985). On the other hand, diurnal variations in ruminal propionic acid and in duodenal C18:1 are concomitant (Doreau, Batisse and Bauchart, 1989), suggesting a link due to microbial activity. Biohydrogenation, which has been mainly studied for 18-carbon FA, also occurs to a large extent on 20- and 22-carbon FA (Doreau and Chilliard, 1997b, Van Nevel, Fievez and Demeyer, 2000).

Biohydrogenation may be decreased by protection of lipids. The natural protection of oilseeds by their coat is of limited extent. Technological processes have thus been evaluated. The encapsulation with formaldehyde-treated proteins is the most effective (Gulati, Scott and Ashes, 1997). On the contrary, formation of Ca salts does not prevent biohydrogenation of PUFA (Ferlay *et al.*, 1992, Van Nevel and Demeyer, 1996b, Doreau, Demeyer and Van Nevel, 1997).

Antibiotics, especially ionophores, have been shown to decrease biohydrogenation (Kobayashi, Wakita and Hoshino, 1992). This is due to a limitation of lipolysis, independently of a modification of pH (Van Nevel and Demeyer, 1995).

C18:1 TRANS AND CLA

Biohydrogenation of PUFA in the rumen results in a large array of monounsaturated FA, including positional and geometric isomers (Bickerstaffe, Noakes and Annison, 1972). The most important is vaccenic acid (*trans*-11 C18:1) which is produced from hydrogenation of linoleic acid. The biochemical pathways have been described by Harfoot and Hazlewood (1997). For example, linoleic acid (cis-9, cis-12 C18:2) is rapidly isomerised to a CLA (cis-9 *trans*-11 C18:2) which is reduced to vaccenic acid (*trans*-11 C18:1) then partially to stearic acid (C18:0). Hydrogenation of linolenic acid results in the production of *trans*-11 and *trans*-15 C18:1. Although the main pathways described in the literature are simple, in practice the high number of isomers (at least 8 *trans* C18:1 according to Fellner, Sauer and Kramer, 1995) suggests that minor pathways have not yet been elucidated. Moreover, hydrogenation of *trans* C18:1 isomers to stearic acid has been shown to be high for *trans*-8, -9 and -10 and low for *trans*-11 (Kemp, Lander and Gunstone, 1984). The kinetics of production of the different intermediates of PUFA biohydrogenation suggests that the rate of conversion of vaccenic acid into stearic acid is slow (Singh and Hawke, 1979).

Compared with studies of milk composition, few experiments have been published with separation between cis and *trans* C18:1 isomers at the ruminal or duodenal level, most of them being obtained using imprecise methods. It is thus rather difficult to relate the amount of *trans* FA to characteristics of the lipid supplement. Nevertheless, it appears that the highest levels of *trans* FA are obtained with diets rich in linoleic acid or in fish oil (Wonsil *et al.*, 1994, Kalscheur *et al.*, 1997b). Compared with triglycerides, the corresponding calcium salts do not decrease the extent of *trans* FA formation (Kankare, Antila, Väätäinen, Miettinen and Setälä, 1989, Enjalbert *et al.*, 1997). Conversely, fatty acyl amides, in which linoleic acid is largely hydrogenated, do not lead to a high production of *trans* FA, for unknown reasons (Jenkins, 1995). From trials by Wonsil *et al.* (1994) and Chilliard *et al.* (1999) it appears that fish oil, although being rich in 20- and 22-carbon FA, results in large amounts of *trans*-11 C18:1. Some data are not consistent with the general trend. Steele, Noble and Moore (1971) and Børsting, Weisbjerg and Hvelplund (1992) did not observe any increase in duodenal *trans* FA when vegetable or fish oils were fed. A problem of separation between cis and *trans* isomers could have occurred in these experiments.

Increasing the proportion of concentrates in the diet is known to lead to incomplete saturation of FA, shown by increases in total C18:1. It has recently been shown that high-concentrate diets increased specifically *trans* C18:1 (Kalscheur *et al.*, 1997a). In the same way, ionophores involve incomplete biohydrogenation, with an increase in *trans* C18:1 and, only when linoleic acid is added to the medium, of CLA (Fellner, Sauer and Kramer, 1997). In addition, pasture induces high levels of *trans* FA (Rulquin, unpublished data).

The positive relationship between *trans*-11 C18:1 and CLA at the ruminal level was observed by Noble, Moore and Harfoot (1974). Recently, Jiang *et al.* (1996) deduced from this strong correlation that isomerisation and the first reduction of linoleic acid are not rate-limiting. The progressive increase in *trans* C18:1 observed when PUFA are incubated in vitro shows that the second reduction takes place at a slower rate than the first one. On the other hand, it can be observed that factors which lead to an increase in *trans* C18:1 are either factors limiting lipolysis, and thus the start of biohydrogenation (concentrates, ionophores, fish oil, etc), or high amounts of linoleic acid.

Control of milk fat secretion

The three theories described below were suggested 30 years ago and progressively enriched or invalidated as research progressed. In fact each of them does not exclude the others; a global theory remains to be proposed.

AMOUNT OF ABSORBED NUTRIENTS

The first theory elaborated to explain the decrease in butterfat is the limitation of nutrients available to mammary gland. In particular, the shift in VFA pattern towards propionate could involve a limitation to the amount of acetate and ß-hydroxybutyrate available for de novo synthesis. This explanation apparently works for all feeds which decrease butterfat : cereals, fish oil and, to a lesser extent, other sources of fat and ionophores. The potential importance of this phenomenon is stressed on Figure 19.4 which plots from available literature arterio-venous differences at the mammary level against arterial concentration (Rulquin, 1997). This figure, which confirms in particular data of Annison, Bickerstaffe and Linzell (1974), shows the constancy of the uptake rate of acetate and ß-hydroxybutyrate, even at low arterial concentrations. A limitation of de novo FA synthesis could thus arise from low arterial concentration of precursors. A positive relationship between the ruminal production of the different VFA and arterial concentration of acetate and ß-hydroxybutyrate can be established (Nozière, Martin, Rémond, Kristensen, Bernard and Doreau, 2000, Table 19.3) confirming that high-concentrate diets reduce acetate concentrations (Sutton *et al.*, 1986).

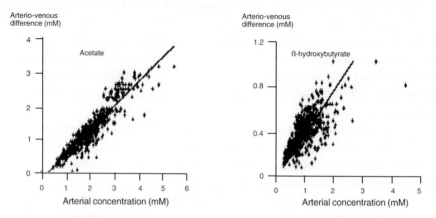

Figure 19.4 Relationship between mammary arterio-venous differences and arterial concentrations of acetate and ß-hydroxybutyrate in dairy cows: review of the literature (Rulquin, 1997)

Table 19.3 EFFECT OF RUMINAL INFUSIONS OF VFA TO SHEEP RECEIVING A HAY-BASED DIET ON ARTERIAL CONCENTRATIONS OF PRECURSORS FOR DE NOVO MILK FAT SYNTHESIS (NOZIÈRE, MARTIN, RÉMOND, KRISTENSEN, BERNARD AND DOREAU, 2000)

VFA ruminal infusion (C2:C3:C4, mmol/h)	*0:0:0*	*43:14:7*	*7:45:6*	*0:9:34*
Composition of ruminal VFA mixture (C2:C3:C4)	72:19:7	70:20:9	48:42:8	47:21:31
Acetate (m*M*)	0.59	0.81	0.59	0.53
ß-hydroxybutyrate (m*M*)	0.24	0.24	0.11	0.43
Propionate (m*M*)	0.01	0.02	0.05	0.02
Glucose (m*M*)	3.47	3.52	3.62	3.41

However, the significance of this statement is limited by the fact that, in many cases, the increases in concentrates result, in terms of VFA production, in an increase in propionate without a decrease in acetate (Annison *et al.*, 1974, review by France and Siddons, 1993). In the same way, Hurtaud, Rulquin and Vérité (1993) and Casse, Rulquin and Huntington (1994), who infused propionate in the rumen, obtained a decrease in milk fat probably related to a decrease in acetate and ß-hydroxybutyrate uptake by the udder, whereas ruminal production of acetate and butyrate was not modified. Annison *et al.* (1974) suggested that the decrease in arterial concentration of acetate with high-concentrate diets was due to a decrease in endogenous production of acetate. On the other hand, propionate may play a direct role in milk fat synthesis. Indeed by ruminal infusions of propionate Hurtaud, Rulquin and Vérité (1998a, Table 19.4) decreased milk fat, the proportion of odd-numbered FA being increased. This confirms that when propionate flow towards the mammary gland is very high, it may contribute to fat synthesis (Massart-Leën, Roets, Peeters and Verbeke, 1983).

Table 19.4 EFFECT OF PROPIONATE OR GLUCOSE INFUSIONS ON MILK FAT (HURTAUD *et al.*, 1998A)

	Control	*Propionate infusion*	*Glucose infusion*
Milk yield (kg/d)	26.7[a]	28.1[b]	26.3[a]
Milk fat (g/kg)	35.8[a]	31.5[b]	31.8[b]
FA output (g/d)			
Total	936[a]	867[b]	818[c]
C4 to C14	218[a]	196[b]	215[a]
C16:0+C16:1	287	285	286
C18:0+C18:1+C18:2	269[a]	239[b]	176[c]

Diet based on 0.6 maize silage, 0.1 hay and 0.3 concentrates.
Means on the same row with different superscripts significantly differ ($P < 0.05$)

Fat supplementation of diets results in an increase in milk long-chain FA due to incorporation of FA in milk triglycerides. These FA arise mainly from triglycerides of VLDL and chylomicrons, to a lesser extent from non-esterified FA and are generally taken up in proportion to their concentration (Gagliostro, Chilliard and Davicco, 1991, Cant, DePeters and Baldwin, 1993, Rulquin, 1997, Enjalbert, Nicot, Bayourthe and Moncoulon, 1998). It is noticeable that for low non-esterified FA concentrations their extraction rate is negative (Rulquin, 1997, Thivierge, Chouinard, Lévesque, Girard, Seoane and Brisson, 1998), due to the release of FA after partial hydrolysis by lipoprotein lipase. The possible differential uptake rate from one FA to another has not been clearly shown, results being often inconsistent because of the differences between experiments in lipid composition. For example, with diets not supplemented with lipids, vaccenic acid seems to be taken up to a greater extent than stearic acid or oleic acid (Thompson and Christie, 1991, Enjalbert *et al.*, 1998). With diets supplemented with lipids, the differences between FA become lower, limiting the consequences of the position of FA on the glycerol molecule (Enjalbert *et al.*, 1998).

ROLE OF INSULIN

The effect of increased insulin secretion was first suggested by McClymont and Vallance (1962) from the observation that intravenous infusion of glucose decreased milk fat. Insulin may act by partition of metabolites towards lipogenesis or muscle oxidation rather than towards the mammary gland. It has been recently confirmed that duodenal infusions of glucose decreased milk fat without inducing insulin resistance (Lemosquet, Rideau, Rulquin, Faverdin, Simon and Vérité, 1997, Hurtaud *et al.*, 1998a, Table 19.4). According to Hurtaud *et al.*, 1998a and Hurtaud, Rulquin and Vérité, 1998b, glucose infusions strongly decrease milk long-chain FA and slightly increase short- and medium-chain FA.

Although glucose and propionate both stimulate insulin secretion, only glucose leads to a decrease in lipid mobilisation. It seems, therefore, that the effect of insulin on milk fat is related to the nutrient balance of the animal.

The insulin hypothesis has been questioned by McGuire, Griinari, Dwyer and Bauman (1995) and Griinari, McGuire, Dwyer, Bauman and Palmquist (1997b), who did not decrease milk fat yield (but decreased milk fat percentage in the latter experiment) by raising plasma insulin level using a hyperinsulinemic – euglycemic clamp for several days. These results suggest that insulin level alone is not responsible for decreases in milk fat. On the other hand, feeding fat sometimes decreases plasma insulin level (Palmquist and Moser, 1981, Choi and Palmquist, 1996) whereas in other trials plasma insulin was not modified (review by Chilliard, 1993). Moreover, the response of milk fat to a high-concentrate diet appears independent of plasma insulin level (Gaynor *et al.*, 1995). It can be hypothesized that the increase in insulin is a consequence of the diet, when rich in concentrates and increasing propionate production, that could act on de novo FA synthesis, but that insulin may not play any role in milk fat depression independently of nutrient supply to the mammary gland.

ROLE OF LONG-CHAIN FA

The effect of long-chain FA on the decrease in de novo FA synthesis and their incorporation into triacylglycerols in the mammary gland was shown first with stearic, oleic and linoleic acid and more recently with *trans* C18:1 FA. The mode of action of FA, especially *trans* isomers, on the secretion of short- and medium-chain FA by the udder has been shown at two levels : 1) reduction of acetyl CoA carboxylase activity for de novo synthesis, suggested by Palmquist and Jenkins (1980) from the statement that butyrate secretion in milk, which does not depend on the malonyl CoA pathway, often increases when the other short- and medium-chain FA are depressed, and 2) inhibition of FA esterification (Askew, Emery and Thomas, 1971, Hansen and Knudsen, 1987).

The negative effect of *trans* FA on milk fat was suggested first by Davis and Brown (1970), then by Pennington and Davis (1975). Close negative relationships between the levels of duodenal and milk *trans* FA on the one hand, and milk fat content on the other, have then been established (Wonsil *et al.*, 1994, Griinari, Bauman and Jones, 1995). The specific role of *trans* FA has been recently proved by abomasal infusions of FA mixtures rich in cis or *trans* (250 - 300 g/d) C18:1 isomers (Gaynor, Erdman, Teter, Sampugna, Capuco, Waldo, Hamosh, 1994, Romo, Casper, Erdman and Teter, 1996) so that *trans* isomers are now considered as the main causes of milk fat depression.

In some cases, an increase in *trans* FA does not result in a milk fat depression. This has been shown with soyabeans (Chouinard *et al.*, 1997a) and calcium salts of rapeseed oil (Chouinard, Girard and Brisson, 1997b). The increase in *trans* FA, from 20 to 50-60 g/kg of total milk FA, could have been too low to decrease fat concentration, but did not avoid a decrease in short- and medium-chain FA, compensated for by an increase in long-chain FA. The absence of a decrease in milk fat, when *trans* FA was markedly increased, has been observed when partially hydrogenated fats are fed (Wonsil *et al.*, 1994, Kalscheur *et al.*, 1997b); a large supply of *trans* FA (225 g/d) was necessary to decrease milk fat in a trial by Selner and Schultz (1980).

It happens that a strong decrease in milk fat concentration corresponds to a moderate increase in *trans* FA. This has been observed by Gaynor *et al.* (1995) with concentrate-rich diets and may suggest that factors other than *trans* FA are involved in milk fat depression. The multifactorial character of milk fat depression is revealed in a trial by Griinari *et al.* (1995) who separated the effects of increasing the proportion of concentrate and the unsaturation of dietary FA in the diet. The former increases ruminal propionate:acetate ratio and plasma insulin level ; the latter raises *trans* FA in milk, but the decrease in butterfat is obtained by the combination of high concentrate and unsaturated FA in the diet. Surprising results of Focant *et al.* (1998) also question the hypothesis of the pre-eminent role of *trans* FA in milk fat depression : the inclusion of vitamin E in a diet supplemented with rapeseed and linseed oil restored milk fat to a control level without changes in FA composition, especially *trans* 18:1.

These apparent limits to the role of *trans* FA have been recently countered by Griinari *et al.* (1997a). They suggested a specific effect of *trans*-10 C18:1 instead of the well-known *trans*-11 C18:1. This hypothesis, which remains to be verified, could explain the results mentioned above. Indeed, the increase in concentrates particularly enhances *trans*-10 C18:1. On the other hand, partially hydrogenated FA in the diet contain numerous *trans* 18:1 isomers, of which *trans*-9 C18:1 is the most abundant. However, when partially hydrogenated fats are fed, the absence of a decrease in milk fat could also be related to the absence of modification of ruminal VFA pattern (Drackley and Elliott, 1993).

Apart from *trans* FA, it is likely that very long-chain FA have a specific negative action on milk fat. It has been shown that infusions of fish oil into the abomasum or duodenum decrease butterfat, although to a lesser extent than fish oil directly fed or infused into the rumen (Pennington and Davis, 1975, Léger, Sauvant, Hervieu and Ternois, 1994, Chilliard *et al.*, 1999). As neither propionic acid nor *trans* FA are increased, a direct effect of 20- and 22-carbon FA is assumed.

To a lesser extent, other sources of FA have a direct effect on milk fat. Sources of fats such as saturated fats or calcium salts from palm oil, which do not lead to the production of *trans* FA or to an increase in propionate, reduce de novo FA synthesis. By duodenal infusion of rapeseed oil, Chilliard, Gagliostro, Fléchet, Lefaivre and Sébastian (1991) reduced de novo FA synthesis, especially 10- to 16-carbon FA, suggesting that acetyl CoA carboxylase activity may decrease. Such a result was found by Drackley, Klusmeyer, Trusk and Clark (1992) with a mixture of unsaturated FA, and by Christensen, Drackley, LaCount and Clark (1994) with rapeseed, soyabean and sunflower FA. On the contrary, duodenal infusions of palmitic, stearic and oleic acid did not decrease de novo synthesis in a trial by Enjalbert *et al.* (1998).

Trans FA are not synthesised by the udder. However, a mammary synthesis of cis-9 *trans*-11 C18:2 from *trans*-11 C18-1 by the stearoyl CoA desaturase has been recently shown (Corl, Chouinard, Bauman, Dwyer, Griinari and Nurmela, 1998). This action may increase milk CLA content, but produced very little decrease in the proportion of milk *trans* FA, which is present in greater proportion than CLA in milk. By contrast, *trans*-11 C18:1 could have a negative effect on desaturation of stearic acid to oleic acid (Enjalbert *et al.*, 1998).

TOWARDS A GLOBAL THEORY

Among these mechanisms, it appears that the direct action of insulin is highly questionable. The action of *trans* FA is now sometimes considered as sufficient to explain low milk fat (Griinari *et al.*, 1997a). Although the most important decrease in milk fat appears to be due to an increase in *trans* FA, this affirmation has to be moderated by the above mentioned results obtained with infusions of propionate and glucose, and of cis FA present in lipid supplements. The comparative action of these FA could be achieved by developing techniques of abomasal or duodenal infusions of individual FA. Moreover, since factors leading to the production of *trans* FA also led to an increase in propionic acid, it is possible to find excellent positive correlations between ruminal propionate and decreases in milk fat. The specific role of *trans* FA is now evident, but the absence of a role for the limitation of precursors of *de novo* synthesis remains to be proved, for example by ruminal infusions of acetate and butyrate with high-concentrate diets.

Conclusion

Nutritional means to modify milk fat amount and composition exist. However they have to be considered together with the other consequences of their use. For example, the proportion of concentrates in dairy diets is generally determined by factors other than decreasing milk fat: economical consideratoins, risks of acidosis . . . In the same way, the use of fish oil and some other additives may adversely affect the taste of dairy products and have a negative image for the consumer. Finally, it can be considered that the decrease in milk fat content is associated with increases in *trans* FA and CLA.

Regarding composition of the fat fraction in milk, several questions have to be answered in the near future. Some of them depend on the medical profession : is the simultaneous increase in *trans* FA and CLA globally beneficial or detrimental for human health? Besides this, a large area of research remains for animal nutritionists. Knowledge of the control of ruminal lipid metabolism and of the mammary milk fat synthesis has to be increased. New techniques of protection of PUFA against ruminal microorganisms could be developed, provided they are accepted by the consumer and do not lead to problems of oxidation or off-flavours. Finally, ways to improve the organoleptic quality of milks have to be explored : maximal incorporation of specific FA in the diet, association of fats with antioxidants, development of specific flavours in milk.

References

Ackman, R.G. (1982) Fatty acid composition of fish oils. In *Nutritional Evaluation of Long-Chain Fatty Acids in Fish Oil*, pp. 25-88 Edited by S.M. Barlow and M.E. Stansby. Acad. Press, London, UK

Annison, E.F., Bickerstaffe, R. and Linzell, J.L. (1974) Glucose and fatty acid metabolism in cows producing milk of low fat content. *Journal of Agricultural Science, Cambridge*, **82**, 87-95

Apfelbaum, M. (1990) Cholestérol, c'est fou ! In *Cholestérol et Prévention Primaire*, pp. 153-157, CIDIL, Paris, France

Ashes, J.R., Gulati, S.K., Cook, L.J., Scott, T.W. and Donnelly, J.B. (1979) Assessing the biological effectiveness of protected lipid supplements for ruminants. *Journal of the American Oil Chemists' Society*, **56**, 522-527

Askew, E.W., Emery, R.S. and Thomas, J.W. (1971) Fatty acid specificity of glyceride synthesis by homogenates of bovine mammary tissue. *Lipids*, **6**, 777-782

Banks, W., Clapperton, J.L. and Ferrie, M.E. (1976) Effect of feeding fat to dairy cows receiving a fat-deficient basal diet. II. Fatty acid composition of the milk fat. *Journal of Dairy Research*, **43**, 219-227

Banks, W., Clapperton, J.L., Kelly, M.E., Wilson, A.G. and Crawford, R.J.M. (1980) The yield, fatty acid composition and physical properties of milk fat obtained by feeding soya oil to dairy cows. *Journal of the Science of Food and Agriculture*, **31**, 368-374

Banks, W. Clapperton, J.L., Girdler, A.K. and Steele, W. (1984) Effect of inclusion of different forms of dietary fatty acid on the yield and composition of cow's milk. *Journal of Dairy Research*, **51**, 387-395

Bauchart, D., Legay-Carmier, F., Doreau, M. and Gaillard, B. (1990) Lipid metabolism of liquid-associated and solid-adherent bacteria in rumen contents of dairy cows offered lipid-supplemented diets. *British Journal of Nutrition*, **63**, 563-578

Bickerstaffe, R., Noakes, D.E. and Annison, E.F. (1972) Quantitative aspects of fatty acid biohydrogenation, absorption and *trans*fer into milk fat in the lactating goat, with special reference to the cis and *trans*-isomers of octadecenoate and linoleate. *Biochemistry Journal*, **130**, 607-617

Børsting, C.F., Weisbjerg, M.R. and Hvelplund, T. (1992) Fatty acid digestibility in lactating cows fed increasing amounts of protected vegetable oil, fish oil or saturated fat. *Acta Agriculturae Scandinavica, Section A, Animal Science*, **42**, 148-156

Bremmer, D.R., Ruppert, L.D., Clark, J.H. and Drackley, J.K. (1998) Effects of chain length and unsaturation of fatty acid mixtures infused into the abomasum of lactating dairy cows. *Journal of Dairy Science*, **81**, 176-188

Brumby, P.E., Storry, J.E. and Sutton, J.D. (1972) Metabolism of cod-liver oil in relation to milk fat secretion. *Journal of Dairy Research*, **39**, 167-182

Brunschwig, P., Kernen, P. and Weill, P. (1997) Effets de l'apport d'un concentré enrichi en acides gras polyinsaturés sur les performances de vaches laitières à l'ensilage de maïs. *Rencontres Recherches Ruminants*, **4**, 361

Cant, J.P., DePeters, E.J. and Baldwin, R.L. (1993) Mammary uptake of energy metabolites in dairy cows fed fat and its relationship to milk protein depression. *Journal of Dairy Science*, **76**, 2254-2265

Cant, J.P., Fredeen, A.H., MacIntyre, T., Gunn, J. and Crowe, N. (1997) Effect of fish oil and monensin on milk composition in dairy cows. *Canadian Journal of Animal Science*, **77**, 125-131

Casper, D.P., Schingoethe, D.J., Middaugh, R.P. and Baer, R.J. (1988) Lactational responses of dairy cows to diets containing regular and high oleic acid sunflower seeds. *Journal of Dairy Science*, **71**, 1267-1274

Casse, E.A., Rulquin, H. and Huntington, G.B. (1994) Effect of mesenteric vein infusion of propionate on splanchnic metabolism in primiparous holstein cows. *Journal of Dairy Science*, **77**, 3296-3303

Chilliard, Y., Gagliostro, G., Fléchet, J., Lefaivre, J. and Sebastian, I. (1991) Duodenal rapeseed oil infusion in early and midlactation cows. 5. Milk fatty acids and adipose tissue lipogenic activities. *Journal of Dairy Science*, **74**, 1844-1854

Chilliard, Y. (1993) Dietary fat and adipose tissue metabolism in ruminants, pigs, and rodents: a review. *Journal of Dairy Science*, **76**, 3897-3931

Chilliard, Y., Doreau, M., Gagliostro, G. and Elmeddah, E. (1993) Addition de lipides protégés (encapsulés ou savons de calcium) à la ration de vaches laitières. Effets sur les performances et la composition du lait. *INRA Productions Animales*, **6**, 139-150

Chilliard, Y. and Doreau, M. (1997) Influence of supplementary fish oil and rumen-protected methionine on milk yield and composition in dairy cows. *Journal of Dairy Research*, **64**, 173-179

Chilliard, Y, Chardigny, J.M., Chabrot, J., Ollier, A., Sebedio, J.L. and Doreau, M. (1999) Effects of ruminal or postruminal fish oil supply on conjugated linoleic acid (CLA) content of cow milk fat. *Proceedings of the Nutrition Society*, **58**, 70A

Chilliard, Y., Ferlay, A., Mansbridge, R.M. and Doreau, M. (2000) Ruminant milk fat plasticity: nutritional control of saturated, polyunsatured, *trans* and conjugated fatty acids. *Annales de Zootechnie*, **49**, 181-205

Chilliard, Y., Ferlay, A. and Doreau, M. (2001) Effect of different types of forages, animal fat or marine oils in the cow's diet on milk fat secretion and composition, especially conjugated linoleic acid (CLA) and polyunsatured fatty acids. *Livestock Production Science*, **70**, 31-48

Choi, B.R. and Palmquist, D.L. (1996) High fat diets increase plasma cholecystokinin and pancreatic polypeptide, and decrease plasma insulin and feed intake in lactating cows. *Journal of Nutrition*, **126**, 2913-2919

Chouinard, P.Y., Girard, V. and Brisson, G.J. (1997a) Performance and profiles of milk fatty acids of cows fed full fat, heat-treated soybeans using various processing methods. *Journal of Dairy Science*, **80**, 334-342

Chouinard, P.Y., Girard, V. and Brisson, G.J. (1997b) Lactational response of cows to different concentrations of calcium salts of canola oil fatty acids with or without bicarbonates. *Journal of Dairy Science*, **80**, 1185-1193

Chouinard, P.Y., Corneau, L., Bauman, D.E., Butler, W.R., Chilliard, Y. and Drackley, J.K. (1998) Conjugated linoleic acid content of milk from cows fed different sources of dietary fat. *Journal of Dairy Science, **81*** (Suppl.) 1, 233

Christensen, R.A., Drackley, J.K., LaCount, D.W. and Clark, J.H. (1994) Infusion of four long-chain fatty acid mixtures into the abomasum of lactating dairy cows. *Journal of Dairy Science*, **77**, 1052-1069

Clapperton, J.L., Kelly, M.E., Banks J.M. and Rook, J.A.F. (1980) The production of milk rich in protein and low in fat, the fat having a high polyunsaturated fatty acid content. *Journal of the Science of Food and Agriculture*, **31**, 1295-1302

Corl, B.A., Chouinard, P.Y., Bauman, D.E., Dwyer, D.A., Griinari, J.M. and Nurmela, K.V. (1998) Conjugated linoleic acid in milk fat of dairy cows originates in part by endogenous synthesis from *trans*-11 octadedenoic acid. *Journal of Dairy Science, **81*** (Suppl.) 1, 233

Davis, C.L. and Brown, R.E. (1970) Low-fat milk syndrome. In *Physiology of Digestion and Metabolism in the Ruminant* pp. 545-565 Edited by A.T. Phillipson. Oriel Press, Newcastle, UK

Demeyer, D. and Doreau, M. (1999) Targets and means for altering meat and milk lipids. *Proceedings of the Nutrition Society, **58***, 593-608

Doreau, M., Batisse, V. and Bauchart, D. (1989) Appréciation de l'hydrogénation des acides gras alimentaires dans le rumen de la vache : étude méthodologique préliminaire. *Annales de Zootechnie, **38***, 139-144

Doreau, M. and Ferlay, A. (1994) Digestion and utilisation of fatty acids by ruminants. *Animal Feed Science and Technology*, **45**, 379-396

Doreau, M. and Chilliard, Y. (1997a) Digestion and metabolism of dietary fat in farm animals. *British Journal of Nutrition*, **78** (Suppl.) 1, S15-S35

Doreau, M. and Chilliard, Y. (1997b) Effects of ruminal or postruminal fish oil supplementation on intake and digestion in dairy cows. *Reproduction Nutrition Development*, **37**, 113-124

Doreau, M., Demeyer, D.I. and Van Nevel, C.J. (1997) *Trans*formations and effects of unsaturated fatty acids in the rumen. Consequences on milk fat secretion. In *Milk Composition, Production and Biotechnology* pp 73-92. Edited by R.A.S. Welch, D.J.W. Burns, S.R. Davis, A.I. Popay and C.G. Prosser. CAB International, Oxon, UK

Doreau, M. and Chilliard, Y. (1999) Un cas atypique de chute de taux butyreux du lait avec une supplementation de matières grasses végétables. *Recontres Recherches Ruminants*, **6**, 314

Drackley, J.K., Klusmeyer, T.H., Trusk, A.M. and Clark, J.H. (1992) Infusion of long-chain fatty acids varying in saturation and chain length into the abomasum of lactating dairy cows. *Journal of Dairy Science, **75***, 1517-1526

Drackley, J.K. and Elliott, J.P. (1993) Milk composition, ruminal characteristics, and nutrient utilization in dairy cows fed partially hydrogenated tallow. *Journal of Dairy Science,* **76**, 183-196

Enjalbert, F., Nicot, M.C., Bayourthe, C., Vernay, M. and Moncoulon, R. (1997) Effects of dietary calcium soaps of unsaturated fatty acids on digestion, milk composition and physical properties of butter. *Journal of Dairy Research*, **64**, 181-195

Enjalbert, F., Nicot, M.C., Bayourthe, C. and Moncoulon, R. (1998) Duodenal infusions of palmitic, stearic or oleic acids differently affect mammary gland metabolism of fatty acids in lactating dairy cows. *Journal of Nutrition*, **128**, 1525-1532

Fellner, V., Sauer, F.D. and Kramer, J.K.G. (1995) Steady-state rates of linoleic acid biohydrogenation by ruminal bacteria in continuous culture. *Journal of Dairy Science,* **78**, 1815-1823

Fellner, V., Sauer, F.D. and Kramer, J.K.G. (1997) Effect of nigericin, monensin and tetronasin on biohydrogenation in continuous flow-through ruminal fermenters. *Journal of Dairy Science*, **80**, 921-928

Ferlay, A., Chilliard, Y. and Doreau, M. (1992) Effects of calcium salts differing in fatty acid composition on duodenal and milk fatty acid profiles in dairy cows. *Journal of the Science of Food and Agriculture*, **60**, 31-37

Focant, M., Mignolet, E., Marique, M., Clabots, F., Breyne, T., Dalemans, D. and Larondelle, Y. (1998) The effect of vitamin E supplementation of cow diets containing rapeseed and linseed on the prevention of milk fat oxidation. *Journal of Dairy Science*, **81**, 1095-1101

France, J. and Siddons, R.C. (1993) Volatile fatty acid production. In *Quantitative Aspects of Ruminant Digestion and Metabolism*, pp. 107-121. Edited by M. Forbes and J. France. CAB International, Oxon, UK

Franklin, S.T., Schingoethe, D.J. and Baer, R.J. (1998) Production and feed intake of cows fed diets high in omega-3 fatty acids from unprotected and ruminally protected algae. *Journal of Dairy Science*, **81** (Suppl.) 1, 353

Fredeen, A.H. (1996) Considerations in the nutritional modification of milk composition. *Animal Feed Science and Technology*, **59**, 185-197

Gagliostro, G., Chilliard, Y. and Davicco, M.J. (1991) Duodenal rapeseed oil infusion in early and midlactation cows. 3. Plasma hormones and mammary apparent uptake of metabolites. *Journal of Dairy Science,* **74**, 1893-1903

Gaynor, P.J., Erdman, R.A., Teter, B.B., Sampugna, J., Capuco, A.V., Waldo, D.R. and Hamosh, M. (1994) Milk fat yield and composition during abomasal infusion of *cis* or *trans* octadecenoates in Holstein cows. *Journal of Dairy Science,* **77**, 157-165

Gaynor, P.J., Waldo, D.R., Capuco, A.V., Erdman, R.A., Douglass, L.W. and Teter, B.B. (1995) Milk fat depression, the glucogenic theory and *trans*-$C_{18:1}$ fatty acids. *Journal of Dairy Science*, **78**, 2008-2015

Gerson, T., John, A. and King, A.S.D. (1985) The effects of dietary starch and fibre on the *in vitro* rates of lipolysis and hydrogenation by sheep rumen digest. *Journal of Agricultural Science, Cambridge*, **105**, 27-30

Givens, D.I., Cottrill, B.R., Davies, M., Lee, P., Mansbridge R. and Moss A.R. (1997) Sources of n-3 polyunsaturated fatty acids additional to fish oil for livestock diets. *Report, MAFF project OC9514*, Ministry of Agriculture, Fisheries and Food, London, UK

Griinari, J.M., Bauman, D.E. and Jones, L.R. (1995) Low milk fat in New York Holstein herds. *Proceedings Cornell Nutrition Conference for Feed Manufacturers*, pp. 96-105, Cornell Univ., Ithaca, NY, USA

Griinari, J.M., Chouinard, P.Y. and Bauman, D.E. (1997a) *Trans* fatty acid hypothesis of milk fat depression revised. *Proceedings Cornell Nutrition Conference for Feed Manufacturers*, pp. 208-216, Cornell Univ. Ithaca, NY, USA

Griinari, J.M., McGuire, M.A., Dwyer, D.A., Bauman, D.E. and Palmquist, D.L. (1997b) Role of insulin in the regulation of milk fat synthesis in dairy cows. *Journal of Dairy Science*, **80**, 1076-1084

Griinari, J.M., Corl, B.A., Lacey, S.H., Chouinard, P.Y., Nurmela, K.V.V. and Bauman, D.E. (2000) Conjugated linoleic acid is synthesised endogenously in lactating dairy cows by $\Delta 9$-desaturase. *Journal of Nutrition*, **130**, 2285-2291

Grummer, R.R. (1991) Effect of feed on the composition of milk fat. *Journal of Dairy Science*, **74**, 3244-3257

Gulati, S.K., Scott, T.W. and Ashes, J.R. (1997) In-vitro assessment of fat supplements for ruminants. *Animal Feed Science and Technology*, **64**, 127-132

Hagemeister, H., Precht, D. and Barth, C.A. (1988) Zum *Transfer* von Omega-3-Fettsäuren in das Milchfett bei Kühen. *Milchwissenschaft*, **43**, 153-158

Hansen, H.O. and Knudsen, J. (1987) Effect of exogenous long-chain fatty acids on lipid biosynthesis in dispersed ruminant mammary gland epithelial cells: esterification of long-chain exogenous fatty acids. *Journal of Dairy Science*, **70**, 1344-1349

Harfoot, C.G. and Hazlewood, G.P. (1997) Lipid metabolism in the rumen. In: *The Rumen Microbial Ecosystem* pp. 382-426. Edited by P.N. Hobson and C.S. Stewart. Blackie Acad. Prof., London, UK

Havel, R.J. (1997) Milk fat consumption and human health: Recent NIH and other American governmental recommendations. In: *Milk Composition, Production and Biotechnology* pp 13-22. Edited by R.A.S. Welch, D.J.W. Burns, S.R. Davis, A.I. Popay and C.G. Prosser. CAB International, Oxon, UK

Hurtaud, C., Vérité, R. and Rulquin, H. (1991) Effet du niveau et de la nature des nutriments énergétiques sur la composition du lait et ses aptitudes technologiques : effet du monopropylène glycol. *Annales de Zootechnie*, **40**, 259-269

Hurtaud, C., Rulquin, H. and Vérité, R. (1993) Effect of infused volatile fatty acids and caseinate on milk composition and coagulation in dairy cows. *Journal of Dairy Science,* **76**, 3011-3020

Hurtaud, C., Rulquin, H. and Vérité, R. (1998a) Effects of level and type of energy source (volatile fatty acids or glucose) on milk yield, composition and coagulating properties in dairy cows. *Reproduction Nutrition Development*, **38**, 315-330

Hurtaud, C., Rulquin, H. and Vérité, R. (1998b) Effects of graded duodenal infusions of glucose on yield and composition of milk from dairy cows. 1. Diets based on corn silage. *Journal of Dairy Science*, **81**, 3239-3247

Hurtaud, C., Rulquin, H. and Vérité, R. (2000) Conséquences de la modification des fermentations ruminales sur la résponse des vaches laitières à des perfusions duodénales de glucose. *Recontres Recherches Ruminants*, **7**, 193

Hussein, H.S. and Jordan, R.M. (1991) Fish meal as a protein supplement in ruminant diets : a review. *Journal of Dairy Science*, **69**, 2147-2156

Jarrige, R. and Journet, M. (1959) Influence des facteurs alimentaires et climatiques sur la teneur en matières grasses du lait. *Annales de Nutrition et d'Alimentation*, **13**, A233-A277

Jenkins, T.C. (1995) Butylsoyamide protects soybean oil from ruminal biohydrogenation: effects of butylsoyamide on plasma fatty acids and nutrient digestion in sheep. *Journal of Animal Science*, **73**, 818-823

Jenkins, T.C., Bateman, H.G. and Block, S.M. (1996) Butylsoyamide increases unsaturation of fatty acids in plasma and milk of lactating dairy cows. *Journal of Dairy Science*, **79**, 585-590

Jenkins, T.C. (1998) Fatty acid composition of milk from Holstein cows fed oleamide or canola oil. *Journal of Dairy Science*, **81**, 794-800

Jenny, B.F., Polan, C.E. and Thye, F.W. (1974) Effects of high grain feeding and stage of lactation on serum insulin, glucose and milk fat percentage in lactating cows. *Journal of Nutrition*, **104**, 379-385

Jiang, J., Bjoerck, L., Fondén, R. and Emanuelson, M. (1996) Occurrence of conjugated *cis*-9, *trans*-11-octadecadienoic acid in bovine milk : effects of feed and dietary regimen. *Journal of Dairy Science*, **79**, 438-445

Joblin, K.N. and Hudson, J.A. (1997) Management of milk flavour through the manipulation of rumen microorganisms. In : *Milk Composition, Production and Biotechnology* pp. 455-463. Edited by R.A.S. Welch, D.J.W. Burns, S.R. Davis, A.I. Popay and C.G. Prosser. CAB International, Oxon, UK

Jouany, J.P., Michalet-Doreau, B. and Doreau, M. (2000) Manipulation of the rumen ecosystem to support high-performance beef cattle. *Asian-Australian Journal of Animal Science*, **13**, 96-114

Journet, M. and Chilliard, Y. (1985) Influence de l'alimentation sur la composition du lait. 1. Taux butyreux : facteurs généraux. *Bulletin Technique CRZV Theix, INRA*, **60**, 13-23

Kalscheur, K.F., Teter, B.B., Piperova, L.S. and Erdman, R.A. (1997a) Effect of dietary forage concentration and buffer addition on duodenal flow of *trans*-C18:1 fatty acids and milk fat production in dairy cows. *Journal of Dairy Science*, **80**, 2104-2114

Kalscheur, K.F., Teter, B.B., Piperova, L.S. and Erdman, R.A. (1997b) Effect of fat source on duodenal flow of *trans*-$C_{18:1}$, fatty acids and milk fat production in dairy cows. *Journal of Dairy Science*, **80**, 2115-2126

Kankare, V., Antila, V., Väätäinen, H., Miettinen, H. and Setälä, J. (1989) The effect of calcium salts of fatty acids added to the feed of dairy cows on the fatty acid composition of milk fat. *Finnish Journal of Animal Science,* **1**, 1-9

Kelly, M.L. and Bauman, D.E. (1996) Conjugated linoleic acid : a potent anticarcinogen found in milk fat. *Proceedings Cornell Nutrition Conference for Feed Manufacturers,* pp 68-74. Cornell Univ. Ithaca NY, USA

Kemp, P., Lander, D.J. and Gunstone, F.D. (1984) The hydrogenation of some *cis-* and *trans-*octadecenoic acids to stearic acid by a rumen *Fusocillus* sp. *British Journal of Nutrition,* **52**, 165-170

Kennelly, J.J. (1996a) The fatty acid composition of milk fat as influenced by feeding oilseeds. *Animal Feed Science and Technology,* **60**, 137-152

Kennelly, J.J. (1996b) Producing milk with 2.5 % fat - the biology and health implications for dairy cows. *Animal Feed Science and Technology,* **60**, 161-180

Kinsella, J., Lokesh, B. and Stone, R.A. (1990) Dietary n-3 polyunsaturated fatty acids and amelioration of cardiovascular disease : possible mechanisms. *American Journal of Clinical Nutrition,* **52**, 1-28

Kobayashi, Y., Wakita, M. and Hoshino, S. (1992) Effects of ionophore salinomycin on nitrogen and long-chain fatty acid profiles of digesta in the rumen and the duodenum of sheep. *Animal Feed Science and Technology,* **36**, 67-76

Kowalski, Z.M., Pisulewski, P.M. and Spanghero, M. (1999) Effects of calcium soaps of rapeseed fatty acids and protected methionine on milk yield and composition in dairy cows. *Journal of Dairy Research,* **66**, 475-487

Lacasse, P., Kennelly, J.J. and Ahnadi, C.E. (1998) Feeding protected and unprotected fish oil to dairy cows : II Effect on milk fat composition. *Journal of Animal Science,* **76** (Suppl.1), 231

Latham, M.J., Storry, J.E. and Sharpe, M.E. (1972) Effect of low-roughage diets on the microflora and lipid metabolism in the rumen. *Applied Microbiology,* **24**, 871-877

Léger, C., Sauvant, D., Hervieu, J. and Ternois, F. (1994) Influence of duodenal infusions of EPA and DHA on the lipidic milk secretion of the dairy goat. *Annales de Zootechnie,* **43**, 297

Lemosquet, S., Rideau, N., Rulquin, H., Faverdin, P., Simon, J. and Vérité, R. (1997) Effects of a duodenal glucose infusion on the relationship between plasma concentrations of glucose and insulin in dairy cows. *Journal of Dairy Science,* **80**, 2854-2865

Maczulak, A.E., Dehority, B.A. and Palmquist, D.L. (1981) Effect of long-chain fatty acids on growth of rumen bacteria. *Applied and Environmental Microbiology,* **42**, 856-862

Mansbridge, R.J. and Blake J.S. (1997) The effect of feeding fish oil on the fatty acid composition of bovine milk. *Proceedings of the British Society of Animal Science,* p. 22, BSAS, Penicuik, UK

Massart-Leën, A.M., Roets, E., Peeters, G. and Verbeke, R. (1983) Propionate for fatty acid synthesis by the mammary gland of the lactating goat. *Journal of Dairy Science,* **66**, 1445-1554

McClymont, G.L. and Vallance, S. (1962) Depression of blood glyderides and milk-fat synthesis by glucose infusion. *Proceedings of the Nutrition Society,* **21**, XLI-XLII

McDonald, I.W. and Scott, T.W. (1977) Foods of ruminant origin with elevated content of polyunsaturated fatty acids. *World Review of Nutrition and Dietetics,* **26**, 144

McGuire, M.A., Griinari, J.M., Dwyer, D.A. and Bauman, D.E. (1995) Role of insulin in the regulation of mammary synthesis of fat and protein. *Journal of Dairy Science,* **78**, 816-824

Nagajara, T.G., Newbold, C.J., Van Nevel, C. and Demeyer, D.I. (1997) Manipulation of ruminal fermentation. In : *The rumen microbial ecosystem,* pp. 523-632. Edited by P.N. Hobson and C.S. Stewart, Blackie Acad. Prof., London

Nevens, W.B., Alleman, M.B. and Peck, L.T. (1926) The effect of fat in the ration upon the percentage fat content of the milk. *Journal of Dairy Science,* **9**, 307-345

Nicholson, J.W.G. and Sutton, J.D. (1971) Some effects of unsaturated oils given to dairy cows with rations of different roughage content. *Journal of Dairy Research,* **38**, 363-372

Noble, R.C., Moore, J.H. and Harfoot, C.G. (1974) Observations on the pattern on biohydrogenation of esterified and unesterified linoleic acid in the rumen. *British Journal of Nutrition,* **31**, 99-108

Nozière, P., Martin, C., Rémond, D., Kristensen, N.B., Bernard, R. and Doreau, M. (2000) Effect of composition of ruminally-infused short-chain fatty acids on net fluxes of nutrients across portal-drained viscera in underfed ewes. *British Journal of Nutrition,* **83**, 521-531.

Opstvedt, J. (1984) Fish fats. In: *Fats in Animal Nutrition* pp 53-83. Edited by J. Wiseman, Butterworths, London, UK

Palmquist, D.L. and Jenkins, T.C. (1980) Fat in lactation rations for dairy: a review. *Journal of Dairy Science,* **63**, 1-14

Palmquist, D.L. and Moser, E.A. (1981) Dietary fat effects on blood insulin, glucose utilization, and milk protein content of lactating cows. *Journal of Dairy Science,* **64**, 1664-1670

Palmquist, D.L. (1984) Calcium soaps of fatty acids with varying unsaturation as fat supplements for lactating cows. *Canadian Journal of Animal Science,* **64** (Suppl.), 240-241

Palmquist, D.L., Beaulieu, A.D. and Barbano, D.M. (1993) Feed and animal factors influencing milk fat composition. *Journal of Dairy Science,* **76**, 1753-1771

Pennington, J.A. and Davis, L. (1975) Effects of intraruminal and intra-abomasal additions of cod-liver oil on milk fat production in the cow. *Journal of Dairy Science,* **58**, 49-55

Pike, I.H., Miller, E.L. and Short, K. (1994) The role of fish meal in dairy cow feeding. IFOMA *Tech. Bull.,* no 27, 26 pp., IFOMA, St Albans, UK

Prins, R.A., Van Nevel, C.J. and Demeyer, D.I. (1972) Pure culture studies of inhibitors for methanogenic bacteria. *Antonie van Leeuwenhoek,* **38**, 281-287

Rémond, B. and Journet, M. (1971) Alimentation des vaches laitières avec des rations à forte proportion d'aliments concentrés. I. Quantités ingérées et production laitière. *Annales de Zootechnie*, **20**, 165-184

Romo, G.A., Casper, D.P., Erdman, R.A. and Teter, B.B. (1996) Abomasal infusion of *cis* or *trans* fatty acid isomers and energy metabolism of lactating dairy cows. *Journal of Dairy Science*, **79**, 2005-2015

Rulquin, H. (1997) Régulation de la synthèse et de la sécrétion des constituants du lait chez les ruminants. *Rencontres Recherches Ruminants*, **4**, 327-338

Selner, D.R. and Schultz, L.H. (1980) Effects of feeding oleic acid or hydrogenated vegetable oils to lactating cows. *Journal of Dairy Science*, **63**, 1235-1241

Singh, S. and Hawke, J.C. (1979) The in vitro lipolysis and biohydrogenation of monogalactosyldiglyceride by whole rumen contents and its fractions. *Journal of the Science of Food and Agriculture*, **30**, 603-612

Sprott, L.R., Goehring, T.B., Beverly, J.R. and Corah, L.R. (1988) Effects of ionophores on cow herd production : a review. *Journal of Animal Science*, **66**, 1340-1346

Steele, W., Noble, R.C. and Moore, J.H. (1971) The effects of 2 methods of incorporating soybean oil into the diet on milk yield and composition in the cow. *Journal of Dairy Science*, **38**, 43-48

Storry, J.E., Brumby, P.E., Hall, A.J. and Tuckley, B. (1974) Effects of free and protected forms of codliver oil on milk fat secretion in the dairy Cow. *Journal of Dairy Science*, **57**, 1046-1049

Sundstøl, F. (1974) Hydrogenated marine fat as feed supplement. IV. Hydrogenated marine fat as feed supplement. *Meldinger fra Norges Landbrukshogskole*, **162**, 50 pp

Sutton, J.D., Oldham, J.D. and Hart, I.C. (1980) Products of digestion, hormones and energy utilization in milking cows given concentrates containing various proportions of barley or maize. In *Energy Metabolism*, pp. 303-306. Edited by L.E. Mount. Butterworths, London, UK

Sutton, J.D., Hart, I.C., Broster, W.H., Elliott, R.J. and Schuller, E. (1986) Feeding frequency for lactating cows : effects on rumen fermentation and blood metabolites and hormones. *British Journal of Nutrition*, **56**, 181-192

Sutton, J.D., Bines, J.A., Morant, S.V., Napper, D.J. and Givens, D.I. (1987) A comparison of starchy and fibrous concentrates for milk production, energy utilization and hay intake by Friesian cows. *Journal of Agricultural Science, Cambridge*, **109**, 375-386

Sutton, J.D. (1989) Altering milk composition by feeding. *Journal of Dairy Science*, **72**, 2801-2814

Thivierge, M.C., Chouinard, P.Y., Lévesque, J., Girard, V., Seoane, J.R. and Brisson, G.J. (1998) Effects of buffers on milk fatty acids and mammary arteriovenous differences in dairy cows fed Ca salts of fatty acids. *Journal of Dairy Science*, **81**, 2001-2010

Thompson, G.E. and Christie, W.W. (1991) Extraction of plasma triacylglycerols by the mammary gland of the lactating cow. *Journal of Dairy Research*, **58**, 251-255

Tice, E.M., Eastridge, M.L. and Firkins, J.L. (1994) Raw soybeans and roasted soybeans of different particle sizes. 2. Fatty acid utilization by lactating cows. *Journal of Dairy Science*, **77**, 166-180

Urbach, G. (1990) Effect of feed on flavor in dairy foods. *Journal of Dairy Science*, **73**, 3639-3650

Van Amburgh, M.E. (1997) Effect of ionophores on growth and lactation in cattle. *Proceedings Cornell Nutrition Conference for Feed Manufacturers* pp. 93-103, Cornell Univ., Ithaca, NY, USA

Van der Werf, J.H.J., Jonker, L.J. and Oldenbroek, J.K. (1998) Effect of monensin on milk production by Holstein and Jersey cows. *Journal of Dairy Science*, **81**, 427-433

Van Nevel, C.J. and Demeyer, D.I. (1995) Lipolysis and biohydrogenation of soybean oil in the rumen *in vitro*: inhibition by antimicrobials. *Journal of Dairy Science*, **78**, 2797-2806

Van Nevel, C.J. and Demeyer, D.I. (1996a) Influence of pH on lipolysis and biohydrogenation of soybean oil by rumen contents *in vitro*. *Reproduction Nutrition Development*, **36**, 53-63

Van Nevel, C.J. and Demeyer, D.I. (1996b) Effect of pH on biohydrogenation of polyunsaturated fatty acids and their Ca-salts by microorganisms *in vitro*. *Archives of Animal Nutrition*, **49**, 151-158

Van Nevel, C.J., Fievez, V. and Demeyer, D.I. (2000) Lipolysis and biohydrogenation of PUFA's from fish oil during in vitro incubations with rumen contents. *Proceedings of the Nutrition Society*, **59**, 193A

Viallon, C., Verdier-Metz, I., Denoyer, C., Pradel, P., Coulon, J.B. and Berdagué, J.L. (1999) Desorbed terpenes and sesquiterpenes from forages and cheeses. *Journal of Dairy Research*, **66**, 319-326

Willett, W.C., Stampfer, M.J., Manson, J.E., Colditz, G.A., Speizer, F.E., Rosner, B.A., Sampson, L.A. and Hennekens, C.H. (1993) Intake of *trans* fatty acids and risk of coronary heart disease among women. *Lancet*, **341**, 581-585

Wolff, R.L. (1994) Les isomères 18:1 *trans* dans l'alimentation des Européens. Evaluations quantitative et qualitative. *Oléagineux Corps Gras Lipides*, **1**, 209-218

Wonsil, B.J., Herbein, J.H. and Watkins, B.A. (1994) Dietary and ruminally derived *trans*-18:1 fatty acids alter bovine milk lipids. *Journal of Nutrition*, **124**, 556-565

Zinn, R.A. (1988) Comparative feeding value of supplemental fat in finishing diets for feedlot steers supplemented with and without monensin. *Journal of Animal Science*, **66**, 213-227

This paper was first published in 1999

20

UTILISATION OF RUMEN PROTECTED N-3 FATTY ACIDS BY RUMINANTS

J.R. ASHES, S.K. GULATI, S.M. KITESSA, E. FLECK AND T.W. SCOTT
CSIRO Animal Production, Locked Bag 1, Delivery Centre, Blacktown, NSW 2148, Australia

Introduction

The role of specific dietary fatty acids in the regulation of metabolic functions including membrane fluidity, prostaglandin synthesis, immunity and disease prevention, gene expression, neural and visual development is now recognised (Simopoulos, 1998). From a nutritional perspective it is considered desirable to reduce intake of total fat and saturated fatty acids, e.g. Myristic (14:0) and Palmitic (16:0) and increase the proportion of C_{18} mono and C_{18}, C_{20} and C_{22} polyunsaturated fatty acids. There is also a need to balance the proportions of n-6 and n-3 polyunsaturated fatty acids in the human diet – these are the essential fatty acids that cannot be synthesised within the tissues of most mammalian species. The average Western diet contains 10-20 times more n-6 than n-3 polyunsaturated fatty acids and this ratio is considered to be too high (Simopoulos, 1999). Recent evidence demonstrates the potential health benefit of increasing the consumption of n-3 (or omega) fatty acids particularly in individuals who are genetically linked to diseases such as diabetes, hypertension, coronary heart disease, arthritis and cancer (Leaf and Kang, 1998; Geusens *et al.*, 1995).

It is against this background that there is continuing concern about the fat content and composition of ruminant-derived foods. For example, dairy products such as milk, butter and cheese are criticised for their excessive saturated fat content including 14:0 and 16:0, which contribute to the elevation of cholesterol in the low density lipoprotein fraction of humans. Likewise ruminant meat fat also contains approximately 250-300g/ kg 16:0. The challenge is to preserve some of the unique characteristics of ruminant fat e.g. the flavouring components of butter and the reasonably high content of conjugated linoleic acid(s) (CLA), which are considered potent anti-cancer compounds (Ip, 1997), and increase the content of nutritionally desirable n-3 C_{18}, C_{20} and C_{22} fatty acids. Because of the major contribution of ruminant-derived foods to the diet of consumers throughout the world, this has stimulated research efforts with the goal of increasing their n-3 fatty acid content.

Why do n-3 fatty acids need to be protected in ruminant diets?

Grazing ruminants normally ingest significant quantities of n-3 linolenic acid (9,12,15 *cis, cis, cis,* octadecatrienoic, 18:3) as this is the principal fatty acid in the galactosyl lipids of plants (Scott and Ashes, 1993). This tri-unsaturated fatty acid is hydrogenated by rumen microbes to stearic acid (18:0) and/or C_{18} *cis* and *trans* monounsaturated isomers (Scott and Ashes, 1993). Likewise in lot-fed animals the major fatty acids in grain, e.g. linoleic acid (9,12 *cis, cis,* octadecadienoic acid, 18:2) and oleic acid (*cis* 9 octadecenoic acid, 18:1), are hydrogenated to 18:0. CLA (9 *cis, trans* 11 or 10 *trans, cis* 12 18:2) are intermediaries in the sequence of biohydrogenation and this is the principal reason for their occurrence in meat and milk, although it has been suggested that 9 *cis trans* 11 CLA can be synthesised endogenously from *trans* 11 octadecenoic acid (Chouinard *et al.*, 1999). It is also a widely accepted strategy to feed fat supplements to ruminants to increase the energy concentration of diets and overcome negative energy balance. Such fat supplements are normally composed of saturated or monounsaturated fatty acids e.g. Megalac®, because they are more rumen inert and are less toxic to rumen microbes than their polyunsaturated forms (see review by Jenkins, 1993). Despite this, it is still difficult to include fat supplements in the diet at levels greater than 30-40g/kg without causing deleterious effects on dry matter intake, rumen fermentation and animal performance (Jenkins, 1993). This is the major limitation in respect to increasing the proportion of highly unsaturated fatty acids, including C_{20} and C_{22} n-3, in the diets of ruminants.

Various studies have reported reductions in dry matter intake, milk yield, fat and protein content when C_{20} and C_{22} polyunsaturated fatty acids were fed in the diets of lactating ruminants (Cant *et al.*, 1997; Doreau and Chilliard, 1997). These effects are the result of a cascade of metabolic events that occur between the highly unsaturated fatty acid and the rumen microbial system and some of these are summarised in Table 20.1.

The amount and nature of dietary fibre appears to be a critical factor in determining the magnitude of effect that is exerted by these highly unsaturated fatty acids. Fibre sources which can bind the unsaturated fatty acid onto the surface of the feed particle would assist to reduce the cytotoxic or "detergent" like action that is occurring with the rumen microbes. Recently Keady and Mayne (1999) showed no significant effect of fish oil fatty acids on dry matter intake of grass silage made from perennial rye-grass, although there was an increase in rumen ammonia concentration, indicating a negative effect on total microbial protein synthesis. In sheep Wachira *et al.* (1998a) showed that inclusion of n-3 fatty acids, including linseed and fish oil, in the diet significantly decreased microbial protein synthesis and fibre digestion in the rumen. Microbial efficiency expressed as microbial nitrogen/kg of organic matter truly degraded in the rumen decreased from 41g to 29g and 27g as a result of including 60g linseed oil and fish oil per kg diet of sheep, respectively.

Table 20.1 METABOLIC EFFECTS OF FEEDING N-3 FISH OIL FATTY ACIDS

Site	Consequence
Rumen	Reduced dry matter intake
	Reduced cellulose digestion
	Altered VFA pattern – more propionate
	Inhibition of protein synthesis
	Inhibition of biohydrogenation – increased *trans* and hydroxy fatty acids
Blood	Reduced triacylglycerols
	Reduced cholesterol
Mammary gland	Reduced milk yield
	Reduced milk protein
	Reduced milk fat

Earlier reports suggested that the n-3 fatty acids in various sources of marine oils were not biohydrogenated by rumen micro-organisms (Ashes *et al.*, 1992; Palmquist and Kinsey, 1994); recent studies by Gulati *et al.* (1999a) and Doreau and Chilliard. (1997) have shown that significant biohydrogenation does occur at levels of fish oil inclusion equivalent to less than 2mg/ml of rumen fluid (see Figure 20.1).

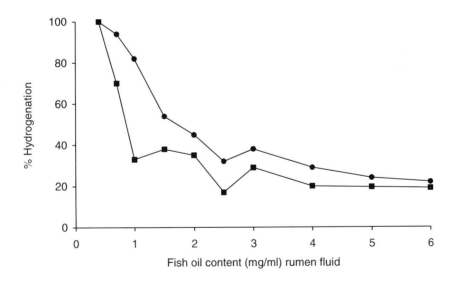

Figure 20.1 The effect of increasing levels of fish oil on the hydrogenation of 20:5 and 22:6 unsaturated fatty acids by rumen micro-organisms (● = 20:5; ■ = 22:6)

Feeding of fish oil also causes substantial changes in the pattern of ruminal biohydrogenation with the principal end-products being vaccenic acid (*trans* 11 octadecenoic acid) and 10-hydroxy stearate and not stearic acid (S. Kitessa, unpublished data) – see Figure 20.2.

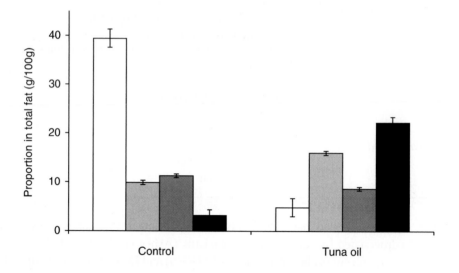

Figure 20.2   The effect of feeding tuna oil on the proportion of C_{18} fatty acids in rumen (☐ = 18:0; ☐ = 18:1 trans; ■ = 18:1 cis; ■ = hydroxy stearic acid)

The physiological significance of the increase in *trans* C_{18} fatty acids is that they cause a depression in milk fat synthesis   (Hagemeister and Voigt, 1997) and increase LDL-cholesterol when consumed by humans (Mensink and Katum, 1993). The formation of hydroxy fatty acids and their effect on microbial composition and metabolism in the rumen merits further investigation. Therefore, to reduce the deleterious effect of n-3 fatty acids, it is desirable to protect highly unsaturated fatty acid from ruminal metabolism. CSIRO researchers in Australia pioneered the development of processes to protect fat from metabolism in the rumen and in recent years have modified the technology to produce fat sources containing significant proportions of C_{18}, C_{20} and C_{22} n-3 polyunsaturated fatty acids.

Incorporation of rumen protected n-3 fatty acids into milk fat

The original research of Scott *et al.* (1970) demonstrated that rumen protected linseed oil containing linolenic acid (18:3, n-3) was readily incorporated into milk fat and levels of greater than 200g/kg were achieved. Ashes *et al.* (1997) developed a new protected fat supplement, based on a canola/soya bean oilseed blend which contained 350g fat/kg of which 0.55 was oleic (18:1, n-9), 0.28 18:2 and 0.08 18:3. Inclusion of this supplement in the diet of lactating cows produced milk fat with a very desirable fatty acid composition (see Table 20.2).

Table 20.2 FATTY ACID CONTENT OF MILK FROM COWS FED RUMEN PROTECTED RAPESEED/SOYA BEAN OIL SEEDS*

Fatty acid	Control		Canola/Soya bean	
	g/100g fat (w/w)	mg/100ml milk**	g/100 g fat (w/w)	mg/100ml milk**
Saturates				
C_{4-12}	15.1	513	12.7	432
C_{14}	10.8	367	8.0	272
C_{16}	28.0	952	18.1	615
C_{18}	12.8	435	11.1	377
Monounsaturates				
18:1 cis	21.8	741	33.0	1121
18:1 trans	2.9	99	2.5	85
Polyunsaturates				
18:2 cis n-6	1.2	41	7.8	265
18:3 cis n-3	0.7	24	2.1	71

* Protected canola soya bean oilseed supplement fed at 100g/kg DMI
** Based on a Fat content of 36g/kg.

There were substantial increases in the proportion of 18:1 n-9, 18:2 n-6 and 18:3 n-3 fatty acids and corresponding reductions in the proportions of saturated fatty acids, particularly 16:0 and 14:0. Milk products produced from this modified fat have favourable nutritional and physico-chemical properties including improved spreadability of butter and reductions in the cholesterol content of human low density lipo-proteins. For further details see Noakes *et al.* (1996); Ashes *et al.* (1997); Gulati *et al.* (1999b). Recent studies have extended these principles to prepare different forms of rumen protected fish oil containing various proportions of eicosapentaenoic (commonly referred to as EPA) (20:5) and docosahexae-noic (commonly referred to as DHA) (22:6) n-3 fatty acids. Inclusion of these rumen protected supplements in the diet of lactating cows produced milk containing 6g/kg 20:5 and 12g/kg 22:6 (Gulati, unpublished data - see Table 20.3). These changes were achieved in short-term feeding trials without depressing feed intake, or fat and protein content of milk. The proportion of 20:5 and 22:6 transferred from the diet into milk was 0.29 and 0.15 respectively; this transfer rate was lower than that achieved for 18:2 n-6 which is normally 0.40-0.45 (Ashes *et al.* 1997).

Table 20.3   FATTY ACID CONTENT OF MILK FROM COWS FED PROTECTED SOYA BEAN OILSEED/TUNA OIL*

Fatty acid	Control milk**		Protected soya bean/tuna oil***	
	g/100g fat (w/w)	mg/100ml	g/100g fat (w/w)	mg/100ml
Saturates				
$C_8 - C_{18}$	55.5	1760	50.3	1686
Monounsaturates		0		
18:1cis	25.8	818	22.0	737
18:1trans	4.5	143	5.6	188
Polyunsaturates		0		
18:2 cis n-6	2.7	86	6.6	221
18:3 cis n-3	0.9	29	1.3	44
20:5 n-3	n.d.	n.d.	0.6	20
22:6 n-3	n.d.	n.d.	1.1	37

n.d. =   Not detectable
*   Soya bean oilseed/tuna oil fed at 100g/kg DMI
**   Fat content of control milk = 34g/kg
***   Fat content of fat modified milk = 36g/kg

Preliminary organoleptic assessment of n-3 enriched cow's milk indicates no disadvantage regarding taint, flavour or oxidative stability. With respect to stability, the rumen protected n-3 fatty acid supplements were fed with 1000 IU Vitamin E per day because previous results demonstrated that the inclusion of this anti-oxidant will prevent autoxidation of milk with elevated C_{18} polyunsaturated fatty acids (Ashes *et al.*, 1997).

Previous experience with feeding rumen protected n-3 fat supplement to alter milk fat composition indicate that:

- Supplements should be as well protected as possible - e.g. *in vitro* rumen protection of >0.75 is desirable (see Gulati *et al.*,1997).
- The amount of rumen protected fish oil in the ration should be as low as possible. For example, if the recommended daily allowance for 20:5 and 22:6 n-3 fatty acids in humans is approximately 600-650mg/day then drinking 250ml of the milk described in Table 20.3 would provide 0.21 of total requirement.
- Feeding the minimal quantity of rumen protected fish oil also has the advantage of reducing or eliminating the deleterious effects on rumen fermentation, including a reduction in the formation of *trans* fatty acids. This is important because C_{18} *trans* fatty acids are potent inhibitors of milk fat synthesis in the mammary gland (Hagemeister and Voigt, 1997). Other deleterious effects including reduced dry matter intake, increased proportions of propionate, rumen ammonia and 10-hydroxy stearate would be reduced by feeding rumen protected fish oil supplements.

- Rumen protected n-3 fatty acid supplements should be fed with additional Vitamin E in the diet to prevent autoxidation of the milk fat containing increased proportions of these acids.

Incorporation of rumen protected n-3 fatty acids into meat

Lean meat derived from grass-fed ruminants contains approximately 20-80 mg of 18:3, 22-30 mg of 20:5 and 5-88 mg of 22:6 per 100 g of muscle (Wachira *et al.*, 1998b; Li *et al.*, 1998); the 20:5 and 22:6 are predominantly located in the phospholipid fraction of muscle (Ashes *et al.*, 1992). The 20:5 and 22:6 fatty acids in ruminants are normally formed by chain elongation and de-saturation from any dietary 18:3, which escapes biohydrogenation in the rumen. These steps are summarised (Spector, 1999) as follows:-

$$
\begin{array}{ccccccc}
 & \Delta\ 6\ \text{desaturase} & & & \Delta\ 5\ \text{desaturase} & & \\
18{:}3 & \rightarrow & 18{:}4 & \rightarrow & 20{:}4 & \rightarrow & 20{:}5
\end{array}
$$

$$
\begin{array}{ccccccccc}
 & & & & & & \Delta\ 6\ \text{desaturase} & & \\
18{:}3 & \rightarrow & 20{:}5 & \rightarrow & 22{:}5 & \rightarrow & 24{:}5 & \rightarrow & 24{:}6 \rightarrow 22{:}6
\end{array}
$$

As the total fat content of meat increases the proportions of n-3 fatty acids decrease because the additional fat being deposited during the growth and fattening phase is primarily triacylglycerol which contains only small quantities 20:5 or 22:6 fatty acids.

Feeding a blend of rumen protected canola and soya bean oilseeds supplement to sheep and cattle provides a practical feeding strategy to increase significantly the proportions of both C_{18} n-6 and n-3 fatty acid in meat (Ashes *et al.*, 1995; Gulati *et al.*, 1995) and an example of this is presented in Table 20.4. There is a 3 to 5 fold increase in the proportions of C_{18} polyunsaturated fatty acids and corresponding reductions in the proportion of 16:0 and 14:0. The increased polyunsaturated fatty acid content reduces the melting point of fat and assists in boning out procedures (Gulati *et al.*, 1995).

Inclusion of rumen protected fish oil supplement in the diet of lot-fed cattle and sheep increased the 20:5 content of meat from approximately 4 to 38 mg per 100g of muscle; the 22:6 content increased from a trace to 11 mg/100 g muscle (see Table 20.5). Therefore, it is feasible to significantly alter the C_{18}, C_{20} and C_{22}, n-3 fatty acid composition of ruminant meat by feeding supplements of rumen protected oil enriched with these polyunsaturated acids. More research is required to firstly, optimise the nutrient composition of diets and level of supplement to be fed to maximise the incorporation of fatty acids and secondly, to examine the organoleptic and storage properties and consumer acceptability of meat containing increased proportions of n-3 fatty acids. In studies where fish meal was included in the diet of beef cattle to increase the proportions of 20:5

Table 20.4 FATTY ACID CONTENT OF LONGISSIMUS MUSCLE FROM BEEF ANIMALS GRASS FED OR LOT FED GRAIN DIETS CONTAINING PROTECTED CANOLA/SOYA BEAN*

Fatty acid	*Grass fed*		*Protected canola/soya bean*	
	g/100g fat (w/w)	*mg/100g****	*g/100g fat (w/w)*	*mg/100g****
Saturates				
C_{14}	3.2	211	2.4	159
C_{16}	26.8	1771	21.5	1421
C_{18}	16.1	1064	14.9	985
Monounsaturates				
18:1 cis	39.9	2637	44.1	2914
18:1 trans	1.8	119	2.4	159
Polyunsaturates				
18:2 cis n-6	1.6	106	5.2	344
18:3 cis n-3	0.3	20	1.1	73

* protected canola/soya bean fed at 125g/kg DMI
** 70g fat/kg minced muscle.

Table 20.5 FATTY ACID CONTENT OF MUSCLE FROM LOT-FED CATTLE RECEIVING HIGH GRAIN DIETS SUPPLEMENTED WITH RUMEN PROTECTED MAX-EPA®*

Fatty acid	*Control*		*Protected Max-EPA*	
	g/100g fat (w/w)	*mg/100g****	*g/100g fat (w/w)*	*mg/100g****
Saturates				
C_{14}	3.2	121	4.2	159
C_{16}	22.1	834	25.5	963
C_{18}	15.3	578	17.6	665
Monounsaturates				
18:1 cis	37.1	1401	28.8	1087
18:1 trans	2.8	106	3.8	143
Polyunsaturates				
18:2 cis n-6	2.3	87	2.7	102
18:3 cis n-3	0.7	26	0.7	26
20:5 n-3	0.1	4	1.0	38
22:6 n-3	trace	<1	0.3	11

* 125g/kg DMI
** 40g fat/kg minced muscle

and 22:6 in muscle, undesirable fish aromas, flavours and after taste were present and tended to increase in amount and duration as the proportion of fish meal increased (Mandell *et al.*, 1998). Similar effects have been found in poultry and pigs where fish products have been used to increase the proportions of n-3 fatty acid (Leskanich and Noble, 1997; Leskanich *et al.*, 1997).

The future

It is clear that the fatty acid composition of ruminant-derived foods can be significantly altered by feeding rumen protected oil supplements; however, the fundamental challenge is to use this technology to produce meat and milk products with the desired n-3 and n-6 fatty acid content. Increasing their content and maintaining a ratio of n-6/n-3 of approximately 5:1 or less can be readily achieved by feeding blends of rumen protected canola/soya bean/fish oil supplements. There is also the question of the relative amounts of different n-3 fatty acids that are required – for example, if it is considered desirable to increase the proportions of 22:6 relative to 20:5, this can be readily achieved by feeding rumen protected oil supplements enriched in 22:6. The availability of a new range of n-3 and n-6 enriched meat and dairy products therefore would provide many consumers with the opportunity to balance the intake of specific dietary fats without drastically altering their eating habits. In terms of future research, the feeding of rumen protected fats allows the role of specific n-3 and n-6 fatty acids to be examined with respect to regulating gene expression, immunity, reproductive function, and manipulating body composition.

References

Ashes, J.R., Siebert, B.D., Gulati, S.K., Cuthbertson, A.Z. Scott, T.W. (1992) Incorporation of n-3 fatty acids of fish oil into tissue and serum lipids of ruminants. *Lipids* **27**, 629-631.

Ashes, J.R., Gulati, S.K. and Scott, T.W. (1995) The role of rumen-protected proteins and energy sources in the diet of ruminants. In: Ivan, M (ed.). *Animal science research and development: moving toward a new century* Ottawa, Ontario, Canada: Centre for Food and Animal Research pp.177-188.

Ashes, J.A., Gulati, S.K., Scott, T.W. (1997) Potential to alter the content and composition of milk fat through nutrition. *Journal of Dairy Science,* **80**, 2204-2212.

Cant, J. P., Freeden. A.H., MacIntyre, T., Gunn, J., Crowe, N. (1997) Effect of fish oil and monensin on milk composition in dairy cows. *Canadian Journal of Animal Science,* **77**, 125-131.

Chouinard, P.Y., Corneau, L., Barbano, D.M., Metzger., L.E. and Bauman, D.E. (1999)

Conjugated linoleic acids alter milk fatty acid composition and inhibit milk fat secretion in dairy cows. *Journal of Nutrition,* **129**, 1579-1584.

Doreau, M. and Chilliard, Y. (1997) Effects of ruminal or postruminal fish oil supplementation on intake and digestion in dairy cows. *Reproduction, Nutrition, Development,* **37**, 113-124.

Geusens, P., Wouters. C., Nigs, J., Jiang, Y., Dequeker, J. (1995) Long term effects of Omega-3 fatty acids supplementation in active rheumatoid arthritis. *Arthritic Rheumatism,* **37**, 824-829.

Gulati, S.K., Scott, T.W., Ashes, J.R., Rich, J.C. and Rich, A.C. (1995) Effects of feeding protected lipids on the chemical and physical structure of lotfed beef fat. 41st Annual International Conference of Meat Science and Technology, Texas, USA. A57.

Gulati, S.K., Ashes, J.R. and Scott, T.W. (1997) Assessing the degradation of fat supplements in ruminants. *Animal Feed Science and Technology,* **64**, 127.

Gulati, S.K., Ashes, J.R. and Scott, T.W. (1999a) Hydrogenation of eicosapentaenoic and docosahexaenoic acids and their incorporation in to milk fat. *Animal Feed Science and Technology,* **79**, 57-64.

Gulati, S.K., Ashes, J.R. and Scott, T.W. (1999b) Dietary induced changes in the physical and nutritional characteristics of butter fat. *Lipid Technology, Ed: PJ Barnes and Associates, (UK).* (January). pp10-13.

Hagemeister, H. and Voigt, J. (1997) Physiological aspects of feeding high producing dairy cows: lipid in the ration. *Archiv Fur Tierzuct,* **40**, (Supplement), 80-88.

Ip, C. (1997) Review of the effects of trans fatty acids, oleic acid, n-3 polyunsaturated fatty acids, and conjugated linoleic acid on mammary carcinogenesis in animals. *American Journal of Clinical Nutrition,* **66**, (Supplement 6), 1523s-1529s.

Jenkins, T.C. (1993) Lipid metabolism in the rumen. *Journal of Dairy Science,* **76**, 3851-3863.

Keady T.W.J. and Mayne C.S. (1999) The effects of fish oil inclusion in the diet on rumen digestion and fermentation parameters in cattle offered grass silage based diets. *Animal Feed Science and Technology,* **81**, 57-68.

Leaf, A. and Kang, J.X. (1998) w3 fatty acids and Cardiovascular Disease. *World Reviews Nutrition and Dietetics,* **83**, 24-37.

Leskanich, C.O., and Noble, R.C. (1997) Manipulation of the n-3 polyunsaturated fatty acid composition of avian eggs and meat. *World's Poultry Science Journal,* **53**, 155-183.

Leskanich, C.O., Matthews, K.R., Warkup, C.C., Noble, R.C., and Hazzeldine, M. (1997) The effect of dietary oil containing (n-3) fatty acids on the fatty acid, physiochemical and organoleptic characteristics of pig meat and fat. *Journal of Animal Science,* **75**, 673-683.

Li, D., Ng, A., Mann, N.J. and Sinclair, A.J. (1998) Contribution of meat fat to dietary arachidonic acid. *Lipids,* **33**, 437-440.

Mandell, I.B., Buchanan-Smith, J.G., Holub, B.J. (1998) Enrichment of Beef with omega 3 fatty acids. *World Review of Nutrition and Dietetics*, **83**, 144-159.

Mensink R.P. and Katum M.B. (1993) Trans monounsaturated fatty acids in nutrition and their impacts on serum lipoprotein levels in man. *Progress in Lipid Research*, **32**, 111-122.

Noakes, M., Nestel, P.J. and Clifton, P.M. (1996) Modifying the fatty acid profile through feedlot technology lowers plasma cholesterol of humans consuming the products. *American Journal of Clinical Nutrition*, **63**, 42-46.

Palmquist, D.L., and Kinsey, D.J. (1994) Lipolysis and biohydrogenation of fish oil by rumen micro-organisms. *Journal of Animal Science*, **72**, (Supplement I), 350 (Abstract).

Scott, T.W., Cook, L.J., Ferguson, K.A., McDonald, I.W., Buchanan, R.A. and Loftus Hills, G. (1970) Production of poly-unsaturated milk fat in domestic ruminants. *Australian Journal of Science*, **32**, 291-293.

Scott, T.W., and Ashes, J.R. (1993) Dietary lipids for ruminants: protection, utilisation and effect on remodelling skeletal muscle phospholipids. *Australian Journal of Agricultural Research*, **44**, 495-508.

Simopoulos, A.P. (1998) Redefining dietary reference values and food safety. *World Review of Nutrition and Dietetics*, **83**, 219-222.

Simopoulos, A.P. (1999) New Products from the Agri-Food Industry: The Return of n-3 fatty acids into the Food Supply. *Lipids*, **34** (Supplement), S297-S301.

Spector, A.A. (1999) Essentiality of fatty acids. *Lipids*, **34** (Supplement), S1-S3.

Wachira, A.N., Sinclair, L.A., Wilkinson, R.G., Hallet, K., Enser, M. and Wood, J.D. (1998a) Rumen biohydrogenation of polyunsaturated fatty acids and their effects on microbial efficiency in sheep. *Proceedings of the British Society of Animal Science*, p36.

Wachira, A.N., Sinclair, L.A., Wilkinson, R.G., Hewett, B., Enser, M. and Wood, J.D. (1998b) The effect of fat source and breed on fatty acid composition of lamb muscle. *Proceedings of the British Society of Animal Science*, p38.

This paper was first published in 2000

21

MILK ANALYSIS AS AN INDICATOR OF THE NUTRITIONAL AND DISEASE STATUS OF DAIRY COWS

B. PEHRSON
Experimental Station, Swedish University of Agricultural Sciences, P.O. Box 234, S—532 23 Skara, Sweden

Introduction

Blood profiles are commonly used in human medicine for the diagnosis of diseases and to monitor the patients' health. They are valuable because modern techniques make it possible to analyse many blood constituents simultaneously, and because in most cases there are direct and rapid routes of communication between the patients and the analytical laboratory.

Blood profiles can also be used in farm animals. The "Compton Metabolic Profile Test" was introduced by Payne, Dew, Manston and Faulks (1970) and includes a wide range of analyses. Later a "Mini Metabolic Profile Test" was introduced by Blowey (1975), in which the analyses are restricted to glucose, urea and albumin. However, it has been pointed out by, among others, Adams, Stout, Kradel, Guss, Mosel and Jung (1978) and Dirksen (1994) that blood has several practical disadvantages as a test medium.

In contrast, milk should be an ideal medium for evaluating the health and the efficiency of production of dairy cattle, because samples of milk are sent routinely to the dairy's laboratory at least once a month; there would therefore be no extra costs for sampling and transport, and farmers would be encouraged to make the best use of the information which is available so relatively cheaply. In addition, they would be able to make use of the tests carried out on the farm, either on the milk of individual cows or on the bulk milk. It is therefore not surprising that there has been an increasing interest in "Milk Profile Tests" during the last decade. The aim of this chapter is to evaluate the potential value of different constituents of milk as biological indicators of the health and productivity of dairy cows.

Somatic cell counts

Mastitis is economically the most important disease of dairy cows. The costs of treating the disease are high, but they are almost negligible in comparison with the losses due to the decreased milk yields of chronically infected cows (Taponen and Myllys, 1995). As a result great efforts are made to try to reduce the incidence of the disease, and to achieve this aim it is vital to identify any cows with chronic mastitis, so as to prevent them from spreading the infective organisms to the healthy cows in the herd.

It is well documented that chronic mastitis is characterised by an increase in the number of somatic cells in the milk. Most of them are white blood cells which have been attracted from the blood into the udder as a defence against the infection. Regular measurements of milk cell counts are therefore valuable for revealing mastitis and every effort should be made to reduce the cell count – both in samples from individual cows and in the bulk milk. Practical measures to reduce the cell count can be encouraged either by reducing the price paid for milk with a high cell count or by paying more to farmers who consistently produce milk with a low cell count. Both these methods are practised in Finland (Saloniemi, 1995), and a bonus is paid when the cell count in the bulk milk is less than 250,000/ml. In Sweden there is a price reduction for bulk milk containing more than 400,000 cells/ml, and if the cell count exceeds this value repeatedly during a period of six months the farmer is not allowed to deliver any more of the milk to the dairy. As a result farmers tend to cull cows with chronic mastitis rather than keeping them; furthermore, an important positive psychological effect is induced by the farmers' awareness of the importance of good udder health in their herds.

Fat concentration

Fat is the solid constituent of milk whose concentration is most easily affected by nutritional means, and the "low milk fat syndrome" has been studied for many years. The syndrome is not a disease but a metabolic consequence of trying to achieve a high milk yield as economically as possible. To make full use of the modern cow's genetic capacity for high milk production it is necessary to feed a ration which has a much higher energy concentration than the natural diet of a ruminant animal. Such a ration carries the risk of reducing the milk fat concentration, particularly if the ratio of forage/concentrate in the ration is low, or its concentration of acid-detergent fibre (ADF) is low, or the total dietary intake of starch is high (Sutton, 1989). The risk increases when the forage is of high nutritional quality and finely chopped, when the diet contains unsaturated fatty acids, when the concentrates are rolled or ground, or when the concentrates are fed only twice a day. The changes induced in the metabolism of the rumen by such diets tend to reduce the rumen pH, increase the production of propionic acid, reduce the ratio of acetate/propionate, and reduce the numbers of protozoa (Storry, 1970; Engvall, 1980).

However, a moderate reduction in the percentage of fat in the milk can be completely compensated by an increase in milk yield (Figure 21.1), and in these circumstances there is normally no need to change the diet. Whether a reduction in fat concentration may have a negative economic effect will depend to a great extent on the principles

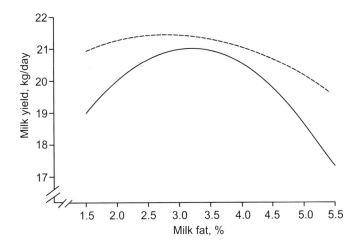

Figure 21.1 The relation between daily milk production and milk fat concentration in Swedish Red and White cows (- - -) and Swedish Friesian cows (—) during the 4th month of lactation (from Engvall, 1980)

which determine the payments for milk in a particular country; it will also depend on whether the reduced fat concentration is accompanied by a reduction in protein concentration, as has been observed in field cases by Engvall (1980), or by an increase in protein concentration, as has been observed experimentally by Emery (1978).

It is important to be aware that there may be a considerable time lag between when a diet which is liable to reduce the milk fat concentration is introduced and when the reduction occurs; Engvall (1980) found that the interval until the milk fat decreased below 2.0% varied between 34 and 65 days. However, the decrease occurred suddenly (Figure 21.2), and was accompanied by significant changes in the ruminal microbiota.

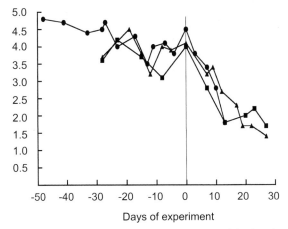

Figure 21.2 The time lag from the start of a milk fat depressing diet (2 kg long hay, 2 kg hay wafers and 10-13 kg pelletted concentrates) to the onset low milk fat syndrome in three cows (from Engvall, 1980)

Protein concentration

Changes in diet are known to have a much smaller effect on milk protein concentration than on milk fat, but nevertheless milk protein concentrations can give some indication of the efficiency of a diet. Emery (1978) concluded that increases in milk protein concentration could be achieved by feeding more energy, more crude protein and less fibre, and more recent reviews (Sutton, 1989; Spörndly, 1989) have concluded that there is a positive correlation between energy intake and milk protein concentration. Spörndly analysed the results of 53 feeding experiments and calculated that on average an increase of 1 MJ in the daily intake of metabolisable energy could be expected to increase the milk protein content by between 0.003 and 0.005 percentage points. She also concluded that the effects of the quantity of concentrates fed and of a low fibre diet were indirect effects, and that dietary fat (ether extract) had a negative effect on the protein content of milk. Furthermore, roughage in the form of hay seemed to result in higher milk protein concentrations than silage.

Severe underfeeding with protein can reduce the protein concentration of milk (Gordon, 1977), but the effects of feeding a surplus of protein appear to be variable; Emery (1978) reported a positive effect from feeding more crude protein, but Sutton (1989) considered that extra dietary protein, whether rumen-degradable or not, had no significant effect on milk protein concentration, and the results presented by Spörndly (1989) are mainly in agreement with that conclusion.

Ratio of fat/protein

Hagert (1991) and Dirksen (1994) proposed that the ratio of the concentrations of fat and protein in milk (FP ratio) could be used as an indicator of the dietary energy balance of a cow; the proposal was based on the following sequence of metabolic events:

An energy deficit during peak lactation results in the mobilisation of lipids from the body fat depots, an increase in the blood concentration of free fatty acids, and an increase in the production of fat by the udder. At the same time the energy deficit in the rumen reduces the rate of synthesis of bacterial protein; the supply of amino acids to the udder is reduced and there is a reduction in the protein concentration in the milk. They studied cows which were fed energy according to their requirement, or above or below their requirement, and found that their FP ratios provided a moderately good indication of their dietary energy balance. A FP ratio less than 1.4 indicated an optimal or positive energy balance, and a ratio above 1.4 indicated en energy deficit. During peak lactation many energy deficient cows had FP ratios above 2.1.

Lactose concentration

Severe underfeeding can result in a reduction in the lactose content of milk. There are also a few reports that a low ratio of forage/concentrate in the diet can increase milk lactose, and that high fat supplementation can cause a decrease (Sutton, 1989). However, although these changes are statistically significant, they are so small that milk lactose is of no practical value as an indicator of diseases or metabolic disturbances.

Progesterone

An optimal calving interval is vital for economic dairy production. The optimal interval may vary slightly from country to country and from farm to farm, but it should not be very far from 365 days; it is widely accepted that for every day by which the calving interval exceeds 365 days there will be a cost of approximately two pounds. It is therefore vitally important that cows are inseminated within three months of calving and at the correct time during an ovarian cycle.

By convention, each ovarian cycle (Figure 21.3) begins with an ovulation, which is defined as the release of an egg from a follicle located on the surface of one of the two ovaries. Within a few days the follicle is then transformed into a corpus luteum which secretes the hormone progesterone; during this luteal phase of the cycle high levels of progesterone are secreted into the milk where it can be detected by a suitable laboratory or on-farm test. In a normally cycling, non-pregnant cow the progesterone concentration in milk reaches a peak value about 10 days after ovulation, remains at this level for four to five days, and then decreases rapidly until 17 to 18 days after ovulation when it is barely detectable in the blood or the milk. The corpus luteum regresses, and approximately 21 days after the preceding ovulation a new follicle releases an egg to complete the ovarian cycle. The cow will be in oestrus one to two days before each ovulation.

If an egg is fertilized the corpus luteum does not regress and it continues to produce progesterone throughout the pregnancy; as a result the concentration of progesterone in the cow's milk will still be high about 19 days after it was inseminated. A progesterone concentration less than 5 ng/ml indicates the oestrus phase, a concentration more than 10 ng/ml the luteal phase, and intermediate concentrations indicate either luteolysis or the formation of a new corpus luteum (Ahlin and Larsson, 1985).

A measurement of milk progesterone concentration can therefore be used to test whether a cow is pregnant to an insemination. If the progesterone concentration is high in a milk sample taken 19 days after the cow was inseminated the cow is probably pregnant, and the pregancy would be confirmed if the concentration is still high in a sample taken five days later. However, if the concentration is low in either of the samples the cow is certainly not pregnant.

A milk progesterone measurement can also be useful at other times. For example, if the progesterone concentration is high when the cow is inseminated, the cow must have been in the luteal phase and therefore cannot become pregnant. It is also possible to predict the time of an oestrus suitable for the first insemination after calving; three samples should be taken, about one week apart, the first about 40 days after calving. In

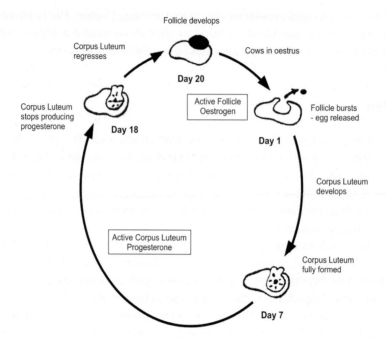

Figure 21.3 The ovarian cycle of a dairy cow

a normally cycling cow a mixture of high and low progesterone concentrations should be found, and an oestrus can be expected approximately 21 days after the day on which a low concentration was recorded.

Ketone bodies

In a high-yielding dairy cow the maximal demand for nutrients is reached within two weeks after calving, whereas the cow's voluntary food intake does not reach its maximum until several weeks later (Wiktorsson, 1971; Foster, 1988). As a result the cow is almost inevitably in negative energy balance during at least the first month of lactation. It seems to be a basic biological rule that the body reserves of an animal that has recently given birth should be regulated hormonally so that they can be mobilised to satisfy the nutritional requirements of its offspring. It is certainly no accident that in dairy cows the period of risk for ketosis coincides with the period when the cow's voluntary intake fails to balance its nutritional losses through the milk. As a result at least 98% of all cases of ketosis occur during the first eight weeks of lactation, with a peak incidence between three to five weeks after calving (Øverby, Aas Hansen, Jonsgård and Søgnen, 1974; Simensen, Halse, Gillund and Lutnaes, 1990).

The relationship between negative energy balance and ketosis was established scientifically several decades ago (e.g. Pehrson, 1966; Henkel and Borstel, 1969). However, in order to reduce the incidence of hyperketonaemia it is necessary to take into account not only the energy balance, but also the feeding regimen, as has been established by many authors, among them Gustafsson (1993), who defined some of the important dietary variables.

Besides being due to a deficiency of energy in general, ketosis in high-yielding dairy cows is related to a specific lack of glucose. The carbohydrates in the cow's diet are broken down in the rumen to volatile fatty acids, predominantly acetic and butyric acids, nether of which is glucogenic, and as a result most of the dietary carbohydrates are, from the point of view of glucogenesis, "destroyed" in the rumen. Propionic acid, which is transformed into glucose in the liver, constitutes only 15 to 20% of the volatile fatty acids produced in the rumen.

The quantity of glucose absorbed directly from the gastrointestinal tract of ruminants is negligible, and high-yielding dairy cows are therefore highly dependent on an effective system for producing glucose from other sources ("gluconeogenesis"). The main gluconeogenetic resources available are the propionic acid produced in the rumen, the glucogenic amino acids derived from the ration or mobilised from body protein, the lactate produced in the rumen and by cell metabolism, and the glycerol produced in the rumen or mobilised from body fat.

The importance of an effective level of gluconeogenesis is underlined by the fact that the level of milk production is heavily dependent on the concentration of lactose in the alveolar cells of the udder, because lactose is the major contributor to the osmotic pressure of milk; however, for the synthesis of lactose the udder cells require glucose. A cow with a high genetic capacity for milk production presumably gives its udder preference for the supply of glucose, but if there is a shortage of glucose – which is very likely during the first few weeks of lactation in an energy deficient high-yielding cow – hypoglycaemia will develop and there will be a shortage of oxaloacetate. As a result the fatty acids mobilised from the body fat cannot be used in the citric acid cycle but are transformed into ketone bodies which are secreted from the blood into the milk (Figure 21.4).

Plasma glucose concentration is thus one of the factors controlling ketogenesis and is negatively correlated with the concentration of ketone bodies (Herdt, 1988). It has been shown that cows with hypoglycaemia have a much lower pregnancy rate to the first insemination than cows with normal or high plasma glucose levels (Plym Forshell, Andersson and Pehrson, 1991; Pehrson, Plym Forshell and Carlsson, 1992; Table 21.1). At that time the risk period for ketosis has passed, but Plym Forshell *et al.* (1991) found that the cows with low fertility had been hypoglycaemic three to seven weeks after calving and were also hyperketonaemic three to five weeks after calving (Table 21.2). It should therefore be possible to evaluate the risk of a reduction in fertility by measureing either plasma glucose or milk acetone a few weeks after calving; because of the practical problems in using blood, the measurement of milk acetone is much to be preferred.

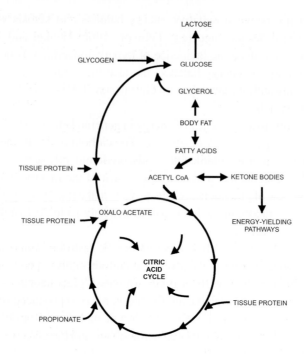

Figure 21.4 Metabolic pathways for glucose mobilization and lactose production

Table 21.1 THE NUMBERS AND PERCENTAGES OF COWS WHICH BECAME OR DID NOT BECOME PREGNANT AT THE FIRST INSEMINATION, IN RELATION TO THEIR PLASMA GLUCOSE CONCENTRATIONS (PEHRSON *et al.*, 1992).

| Plasma glucose | Pregnant | | Not pregnant | |
mmol/l	n	%	n	%
< 2.50	22	36.1	39	63.9
2.50–2.99	40	41.7	56	58.3
3.00–3.39	47	48.5	50	51.5
≥ 3.40	26	65.0	14	35.0
Significance		$p < 0.05$		

There is high correlation between the concentrations of ketone bodies in blood and acetone in milk; the abscence of significant diurnal variation even makes measurements milk acetone more suitable than measurements of blood ketone bodies (Andersson and Lundström, 1985).

Table 21.2 MEAN PLASMA GLUCOSE AND MILK ACETONE CONCENTRATIONS (MMOL/L) EARLIER IN THE LACTATION PERIOD IN COWS CLASSIFIED BY THEIR PLASMA GLUCOSE CONCENTRATION AT THE TIME OF INSEMINATION. n = NUMBER OF COWS (FROM PLYM FORSHELL *et al.*, 1991)

| | Glucose concentration at insemination | | | | | |
| | <2.50 | | 2.50–3.40 | | >3.40 | |
	n	$\bar{\times}$	n	$\bar{\times}$	n	$\bar{\times}$
Glucose week 3–4	30	2.25	218	2.73	35	2.90
Glucose week 6–7	30	2.49	217	2.74	31	2.87
Acetone week 3–4	31	0.52	214	0.21	34	0.14
Acetone week 5	18	0.91	179	0.20	28	0.17
Acetone week 6–7	34	0.21	227	0.17	31	0.16

Plym Forshell *et al.* (1991) classified the milk acetone concentrations according to the limits suggested by Andersson (1984); concentrations less than 0.41 mmol/l were considered normal, 0.41-1.00 as slightly above normal, 1.01-2.00 mmol/l as moderately above normal and more than 2.00

mmol/l as very high. Most of the cows with levels slightly above normal were not expected to show clinical signs of ketosis, whereas nearly all the cows with very high levels would have been expected to show signs which were apparent to a farmer. Gustafsson (1993) used the same FIA (flow injection analysis) technique for measuring milk acetone, but proposed that concentrations up to 0.7 mmol/l should be regarded as normal. On-farm tests based on sodium nitroprusside can give a fairly good indication of the true acetone concentration to those who have learned to interpret the colour changes with this reagent. Recently, a new test strip has been introduced by Dirksen (1994) for assessing semi-quantitatively the concentration of betahydroxybutyrate in milk. Concentrations less than 0.1 mmol/l are considered normal, and there were quite good correlations with the results of the FIA method used by Andersson (1984) for measuring milk acetone.

The relationship between hyperketonaemia – indicated by the concentration of milk acetone – and reduced fertility has been observed by several other workers. Berglund and Larsson (1983) found that there was a delay in the normalisation of the reproductive functions of hyperketonaemic cows. Andersson and Emanuelsson (1995) recorded prolonged intervals between calving and the first and last inseminations in herds with a high prevalence of hyperketonaemia, and like Refsdal (1982), they also observed an increased risk of cystic ovaries in hyperketonaemic cows. Gustafsson (1993) observed negative effects of hyperketonaemia on fertility only in cows with milk acetone concentrations above 2.0 mmol/l.

Another reason for measuring ketone bodies in milk is that, in addition to their effects on fertility, both subclinical and clinical ketosis can reduce the yield of milk. Lucey, Rowlands and Russel (1986) recorded a reduction of about 5 kg/day a few weeks before clinical signs were observed. Dohoo and Martin (1984), Andersson and Lundström (1985), and Simensen *et al* (1990) also reported reduced milk yields in subclinical cases of ketosis; the reductions were between 4–5% or 3–4 kg /day. Much larger reductions in milk yield have been recorded in cases of clinical ketosis (Andersson, 1988; Gustafsson, Andersson and Emanuelson, 1993; Figure 21.5).

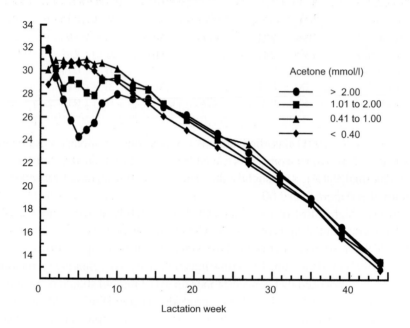

Figure 21.5 Lactation curves for daily milk yield in multiparous cows in four classes of milk acetone concentration (courtesy by Gustafsson et al., 1993)

As mentioned by Andersson (1988), measurements of ketone bodies in milk can be used either for detecting hyperketonaemia in individual animals, or for revealing suboptimal dietary regimens in herds with a high incidence of clinical and subclinical ketosis – herds which may need nutritional advice. It may also be possible to use the routine measurements of ketone bodies in the milk of dairy cows to assess the genetic contribution of the sires used for artificial insemination to the susceptibility of their daughters to ketosis.

Urea

Diets for dairy cows are calculated on the basis of tables which list the cow's requirements for different nutrients at each stage of lactation, coupled with tables which give the average nutritional composition of different feedstuffs. The calculations are based to a large extent on theoretical models of complicated biological processes, and as a result they are subject to many errors, even when the nutritional composition of each component of a diet has been analysed. It would therefore be extremely valuable if biological indicators, which would reflect the final outcome of these complicated metabolic processes, could be used to complement these theoretically calculated rations in the evaluation of the true adequacy of a diet. The appropriate indicators should preferably be simple and cheap to analyse.

Although it is not ideal, milk urea satisfies several of the criteria for a useful biological indicator. Current knowledge indicates that the concentration of urea in milk is closely related to the balance between the levels of energy and protein in the diet. Furthermore, urea is simple and cheap to analyse in the samples of bulk or individual cow's milk which are sent regularly to the dairy.

The diagram of the metabolic processes which occur in the rumen (Figure 21.6) shows that the amount of ammonia produced in the rumen is dependent on the amount of protein in the diet. This ruminal ammonia can be converted into bacterial protein, provided that there is sufficient readily fermentable energy available to the bacteria. However, any ammonia which is not used by the microbes will be absorbed from the rumen, transformed into urea in the liver, and passed into the blood; the urea in the blood will be excreted in the urine and the milk. Thus it can be predicted theoretically that the concentration of urea in milk should increase if there is a surplus of rumen-degradable protein in the diet and/or if there is a deficiency of energy in the diet, and that the concentration should decrease if there is a deficiency of protein in the diet.

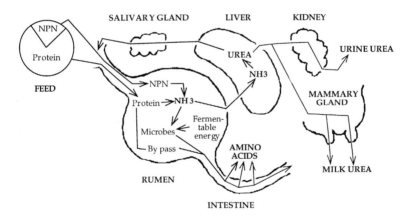

Figure 21.6 Nitrogen metabolism in ruminants. NPN = non protein nitrogen. NH$_3$ = ammonia (Carlsson, 1994)

The results of recent research seem to support the practical relevance of the theoretical model presented in Figure 21.6. Gustafsson and Palmquist (1993) observed a positive correlation between the concentration of ammonia in the ruminal fluid and the concentration of urea in blood, and several authors have reported a strong correlation between the concentrations of urea in the blood and in the milk (e.g. Oltner and Wiktorsson, 1983). It has also been shown that a surplus of crude protein in the diet gives rise to a high concentration of urea in the blood and milk (e.g. Refsdal, Baevre and Bruflot ,1985; Ferguson, Blanchard, Galligan, Hoshall and Chalupa, 1988), and Carlsson and Pehrson (1993) observed very low milk urea concentrations in samples taken from cows on farms where the rations were low in protein. Furthermore, it has been demonstrated that the concentration of urea in blood and milk is affected not only by the dietary intake of digestible crude protein, but also by the balance between the quantities of energy and protein in the diet (e.g. Oltner and Wiktorsson, 1983; Carlsson, 1994; Figure 21.7).

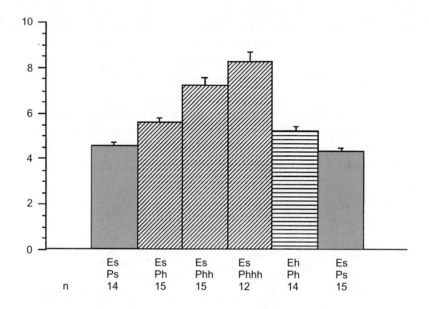

Figure 21.7 Mean milk urea concentration (mmol/l) in cows fed different amounts of metabolisable energy (ME) and digestible crude protein (DCP). EsPs = standard feeding of ME and DCP; Ph = 300 g excess DCP; Phh = 600 g excess DCP; Phhh = 900 g excess DCP; EhPh = 25 MJ excess ME and 300 g excess DCP. Bars = s.e. n = number of samples (Carlsson, 1994)

Towards the end of the 1980s a new system for the evaluation of dietary protein was introduced in the Nordic countries (Madsen, 1985). It takes into account not only the balance between the amounts of rumen-digestible protein and fermentable energy available for the synthesis of microbial protein in the rumen (PBV), but also the quantities of amino acids absorbed from the small intestine (AAT). In the light of this new system, the results of a study by Carlsson and Pehrson (1994) further illustrate the value of measurements of milk urea concentration; as expected there was a significant correlation between the milk urea concentration and PBV, but none between milk urea and AAT.

Carlsson and Pehrson (1994) concluded that when cows are fed typical Swedish rations and are milked twice a day a milk urea concentration between 4.0 and 5.5 mmol/l should indicate that their diet is balanced with respect to energy and protein. (If cows are fed other basic feedstuffs and managed in different ways then a well balanced diet might be indicated by a different range of urea concentrations, and a new "normal" range would have to be established). A similar range of normal milk urea concentrations was observed by Gustafsson and Carlsson (1993), and they also concluded that optimal fertility was achieved when the milk urea concentration was between 4.5 and 5.0 mmol/l (Figure 21.8), their results were consistent with earlier reports that the fertility of cows was reduced when their milk urea concentration was either high (e.g. Carroll, Barton, Anderson and Smith, 1988; Ferguson *et al.*, 1988; Canfield, Sniffen and Butler, 1990; Pehrson *et al.*, 1992) or low (Pehrson *et al.*, 1992; Carlsson and Pehrson, 1993).

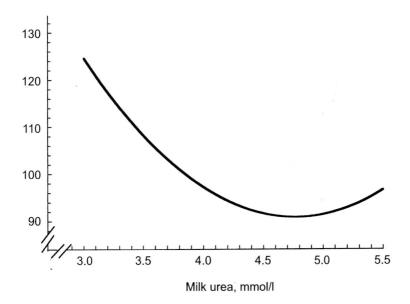

Figure 21.8 The relationship between urea concentration in milk (mmol/l) and calving to last service interval (CLI, days). (From Gustafsson and Carlsson, 1993)

Refsdal (1983) and Carlsson, Bergström and Pehrson (1995) found that the concentration of urea in bulk milk can be used as a reliable guide to the nutritional efficiency of the diet of a herd.

There is increasing interest internationally in using milk urea as a biological indicator of the efficiency of the diets fed to dairy cows. However, until more is known about the factors which affect milk urea concentration, the results must be interpreted with caution and only after taking into consideration the variations in feeding practices and management systems in different countries. It is necessary to establish the effect on milk urea of the catabolism of tissue proteins and of the amino acids absorbed from the digestive tract. It is also necessary to be aware that there is a considerable daily variation in milk urea concentration and that milk with a very high fat content may give misleading results (Carlsson and Bergström, 1994). There are also variations with the stage of lactation, particularly during the first few weeks when the milk urea concentration is lower than later in lactation (Gustafsson, 1993).

Allantoin

The synthesis of protein by the microbes in the rumen is of vital importance for the health and productivity of ruminant animals. The conventional methods for measuring the rate of synthesis of this protein require the use of animals fitted with abomasal or duodenal cannulae; these methods are not only laborious and expensive but also questionable from the point of view of the animals' welfare. During the last decade promising results have been obtained by measuring the concentrations of derivatives of purine (allantoin, uric acid, xanthine and hypoxanthine), which are the products of the breakdown of the nucleic acids DNA and RNA, as indicators of the supply of microbial protein to ruminants.

Nucleic acids are derived directly from the diet, from the rumen microbes and from endogenous catabolism. However, the bulk of the purine derivatives which are excreted is derived from the rumen microbes (Antoniewicz and Pisulewski, 1982; Giesecke, Ehrentreich, Stangassinger and Ahrens, 1994), and the other two sources contribute only a little to the total excretion. As a result the metabolic conditions are favourable for using measurements of the excretion of purine derivatives as an indicator of the rate of production of microbial protein in the rumen. Allantoin, which is the final breakdown product of nucleic acids, has been regarded as the most interesting of the purine derivatives, mainly because it appears to be the main excretory product and is excreted in the urine and the milk.

More than 90% of the allantoin excreted is excreted in the urine, and most trials have used measurements of urinary allantoin for evaluating the production of protein in the rumen. However, in spite of the fact that only 1 to 4% of total allantoin excreted appears in the milk (Giesecke *et al.*,, 1994; Gonda, 1995), several authors have preferred to use milk as the test medium.

The concentration of allantoin in milk, measured by high performance liquid chromatography, has been reported to range from about 100 to 600 μmol/l (Rosskopf and Giesecke, 1992; Giesecke *et al.* , 1994; Gonda 1995). The results have indicated that there is a non-linear relationship between milk yield and allantoin excretion, and close correlations between the dietary energy intake (Rosskopf and Giesecke, 1992) and dry matter intake (Kirchgessner and Kreuzer, 1985; Gonda, 1995) and the concentration of allantoin in milk. Giesecke *et al.* (1994) concluded that the measurement of milk allantoin appears to be a useful non-invasive method for monitoring the synthesis of rumen microbial protein; however, Gonda (1995) doubted the relevance of this conclusion because of the high correlation between the amount of allantoin excreted in milk and the milk yield.

It is evident that further research will be necessary before the value of milk allantoin as an indicator of the synthesis of microbial protein can be assessed adequately.

Vitamins and trace elements

The scientific information in this field is very restricted and further research is urgently required. However, it seems reasonable to assume that the concentration in milk of at least some of the vitamins and trace elements may be related to their nutritional balance. In the case of selenium it has been found experimentally that its concentration in milk is well correlated with the content of selenium in the diet (Aspila, 1991), and in Sweden practical experience has been in accordance with Aspila´s results. Sweden is a selenium deficient country and before 1980 the average concentration of selenium in milk supplied to consumers was about 7 µg/l; in that year it was decided to supplement all mineral additives for farm animal feedstuffs with 10 mg selenium/kg; the concentration of selenium in milk then increased to about 11 µg/l. Later the level of supplementation was increased to 30 mg/kg and the average concentration of selenium in milk is now about 15 µg/l (Pehrson, 1993).

It is expensive to analyse samples directly for selenium. However, it is much easier and cheaper to measure the activity of the selenium-containing enzyme glutathione peroxidase (GSH-Px) and this enzyme is often used instead of selenium for estimating the selenium status of blood. An ongoing project in our laboratory is aimed to evaluate the correlation between selenium concentration and GSH-Px activity also in milk.

Final conclusions

The cost of feedstuffs constitutes the largest part of the total cost of dairy production. As the demand for overall economic efficiency increases it becomes steadily more important that the efficiency of feeding a dairy herd should be maintained at an optimal level, to try to improve both the productivity and the health of the herd. This paper has shown that several of the constituents of milk which can be analysed at a reasonable cost are useful as aids to achieving this aim. The interest in the use of milk profiles is increasing, and there is good reason to believe that the information derived from the parameters so far included should become steadily more reliable. It may also be expected that new, practically useful parameters will be included in the milk profile, to the benefit of both the health of dairy herds and the profit of farmers.

References

Adams, R.S., Stout, W.L., Kradel, D.C., Guss, S.B. Jr., Mosel, B.L. & Jung, G.A. (1978) Use and limitations of profiles in assessing health or nutritional status of dairy herds. *Journal of Dairy Science*, **61**, 1671–1679

Ahlin, K.Å. and Larsson, K. (1985) Variation i mjölkprogesteron vid igångsättning av cyklicitet i äggstockarna hos mjölkkor. (Variations in milk progesterone levels at the onset of cyclicity of the ovaries in dairy cows). *Proceedings NKJ* , Mankans, Finland, pp 345–353

Andersson, L. (1984) Detection, occurrence, causes and effects of hyperketonaemia in Swedish dairy cows. *Thesis*. Swedish University of Agricultural Sciences, Skara, Sweden, 80pp

Andersson, L. (1988) Subclinical ketosis in dairy cows. In *The Veterinary Clinics of North America: Food Animal Practice*, **4**, pp 233–251. Edited by T.H. Herdt. W.B. Saunders Company, Philadelphia, PA, USA

Andersson, L. and Emanuelson, U. (1985) An epidemiological study of hyperketonaemia in Swedish dairy cows: determinants and the relation to fertility. *Preventive Veterinary Medicine*, **3**, 449–462

Andersson, L. and Lundström, K. (1985) Effect of feeding silage with high butyric acid content on ketone body formation and milk yield in postparturient dairy cows. *Zentralblatt für Veterinärmedizin A*, **32**, 15–23

Antoniewicz, A.M. and Pisulewski, P.M. (1982) Measurement of endogenous allantoin excretion in sheep urine. *Journal of Agricultural Science, Cambridge*, **98**, 221–223.

Aspila, P. (1991) Metabolism of selenite, selenomethionine and feed-incorporated selenium in lactating goats and dairy cows. *Journal of Agricultural Science in Finland*, **63**, 1–74

Berglund, B. and Larsson, K. (1983) Milk ketone–bodies and reproductive performance in post partum dairy cows. *Proceedings Fifth International Conference on Production Disease in Farm Animals*, Uppsala, Sweden, pp 153–157

Blowey, R.W. (1975) A practical application of metabolic profiles. *Veterinary Record*, **97**, 324–327

Canfield, R.W., Sniffen, C.J. and Butler, W.R. (1990) Effects of excess degradable protein on postpartum reproduction and energy balance in dairy cattle. *Journal of Dairy Science*, **73**, 2342–2349

Carlsson, J. (1994) The value of the concentration of urea in milk as an indicator of the nutritional value of diets for dairy cows, and its relationships with milk production and fertility. *Thesis*. Swedish University of Agricultural Sciences, Uppsala, Sweden

Carlsson, J. and Bergström, J. (1994) The diurnal variation of urea in cow's milk and how milk fat content, storage and preservation affects analysis by a flow injection technique. *Acta Veterinaria Scandinavica*, **35**, 67–77

Carlsson, J., Bergström, J. and Pehrson, B. (1995) Variations with breed, age, season, yield, stage of lactation and herd in the concentration of urea in bulk milk and in individual cow's milk. *Acta Veterinaria Scandinavica*, **36**, 245–254

Carlsson, J. and Pehrson, B. (1993) The relationships between seasonal variations in the concentration of urea in bulk milk and the production and fertility of dairy herds. *Journal of Veterinary Medicine A*, **40**, 205–212

Carlsson, J. and Pehrson, B. (1994) The influence of the dietary balance between energy and protein on milk urea concentration. Experimental trials assessed by two different protein evaluation systems. *Acta Veterinaria Scandinavica*, **35**, 193–205

Carroll, D.J., Barton, B.A., Anderson, G.W. and Smith, R.D. (1988) Influence of protein intake and feeding strategy on reproductive performance of dairy cows. *Journal of Dairy Science*, **71**, 3470-3481

Dirksen, G. (1994) Kontrolle von Stoffwechselstörungen bei Milchkühen an Hand von Milchparametern. (Control of metabolic disturbances in dairy cows by milk parameters). Proceedings of XVIII World Buiatrics Congress, Bologna, Italy, pp 35–45

Dohoo, I.R. and Martin, S.W. (1984) Subclinical ketosis: prevalence and associations with production and disease. *Canadian Journal of Comparative Medicine*, **48**, 1-5

Emery, R.S. (1978) Feeding for increased milk protein. *Journal of Dairy Science*, **61**, 825–828

Engvall, A. (1980) Low milk fat syndrome in Swedish dairy cows. Field and experimental studies with special reference to the rumen microbiota. *Acta Veterinaria Scandinavica*, Suppl. 72, 124pp

Ferguson, J.D., Blanchard, T., Galligan, D.T., Hoshall. D.C. and Chalupa, W. (1988) Infertility in dairy cattle fed a high percentage of protein degradable in the rumen. *Journal of the American Veterinary Medical Association*, **192**, 659–662

Foster, L.A. (1988) Clinical ketosis. In *The Veterinary Clinics of North America: Food Animal Practice*, 4, pp 253–267. Edited by T.H. Herdt. W.B. Saunders Company, Philadelphia, PA, USA

Gonda, H.L. (1995) Nutritional status of ruminants determined from excretion and concentration of metabolites in body fluids. *Thesis*. Swedish University of Agricultural Sciences, Uppsala, Sweden

Gordon, F.J. (1977) The effect of protein content on the response of lactating cows to level of concentrate feeding. *Animal Production*, **25**, 181–191

Gustafsson, A.H. (1993) Acetone and urea concentration in milk as indicators of the nutritional status and the composition of the diet of dairy cows. *Thesis*. Swedish University of Agricultural Sciences, Uppsala, Sweden, 143pp

Gustafsson, A.H., Andersson, L. and Emanuelson, U. (1993) Effect of hyperketonaemia, feeding frequency and intake of concentrate and energy on milk yield in dairy cows. *Animal Production*, **56**, 51–60

Gustafsson, A.H. and Carlsson, J. (1993) Effects of silage quality, protein evaluation systems and milk urea content on milk yield and reproduction in dairy cows. *Livestock Production Science*, **37**, 91–105

Gustafsson, A.H. and Palmquist, D.L. (1993) Diurnal variation of rurmen ammonia, serum urea, and milk urea in dairy cows at high and low yield. *Journal of Dairy Science*, **76**, 475–484

Giesecke, D., Ehrentreich, L., Stangassinger, M. and Ahrens, F. (1994) Mammary and renal excretion of purine metabolites in relation to energy intake and milk yield in dairy cows. *Journal of Dairy Science*, **77**, 2376–2381

Hagert, C. (1991) Kontinuierliche Kontrolle der Energie– und Eiweissversorgung der Milchkuh während der Hochlaktation an Hand der Konzentrationen von Azeton, Harnstoff, Eiweiss und Fett in der Milch. (Continous control of the energy and protein balance in dairy cows during peak lactation concerning acetone, urea, protein and fat in milk). *Thesis*, University of Munich, Germany

Henkel, H. and Borstel, E. v. (1969) Untersuchungen über die Abhängigkeit des Auftretens der Azetonämie vom Ernährungshaushalt hochleistender Milchkühe. (Studies on the interrelationship between the feed economy of high–yielding dairy cows and the occurrence of acetonaemia.). *Archiv für Tiernährung*, **19**, 259–272

Herdt, T.H. (1988) Fuel homeostasis in the ruminant. In *The Veterinary Clinics of North America: Food Animal Practice*, **4**, pp 213–231. Edited by T.H. Herdt, W.B. Saunders Company, Philadelphia, PA, USA

Kirchgessner, M. and Kreuzer, M. (1985) Harnstoff und Allantoin in der Milch von Kühen während und nach Verfütterung zu hoher und zu niedriges Proteinmengen. (Urea and allantoin in milk from dairy cows during and after overfeeding and underfeeding with protein). *Zeitschrift für Tierphysiologie, Tierernährung und Futtermittelkunde*, **54**, 141–151

Lucey, S., Rowlands, G.J., and Russel, A.M. (1986) Short term associations between disease and milk yield of dairy cows. *Journal of Dairy Research*, **53**, 7-15

Madsen, J. (1985) The basis for the proposed Nordic protein evaluation system for ruminants. The AAT–PBV system. *Acta Agriculturae Scandinavica*, Suppl. 25, pp 9–20

Oltner, R. and Wiktorsson, H. (1983) Urea concentrations in milk and blood as influenced by feeding varying amounts of protein and energy to dairy cows. *Livestock Production Science*, **10**, 457–467

Øverby, I., Aas Hansen, M., Jonsgård, K. and Søgnen, E. (1974) Bovine ketosis. I. Occurrence and incidence in herds affected by ketosis in eastern Norway 1967–1968. *Nordisk Veterinärmedicin*, **26**, 353–361

Payne, J.M., Dew, S.M., Manston, R. & Faulks, M. (1970) The use of a metabolic profile test in dairy herds. *Veterinary Record*, **87**, 150–158

Pehrson, B. (1966) Studies on ketosis in dairy cows. Thesis, the Royal Veterinary College, Stockholm, Sweden. *Acta Veterinaria Scandinavica*, Suppl. 15, 59pp

Pehrson, B. (1993) Selenium in nutrition with special reference to the biopotency of organic and inorganic compounds. In *Biotechnology in the Feed Industry. Proceedings of Alltech's Ninth Annual Symposium.* 71–89. Edited by T.P. Lyons. Alltech Technical Publications, Nicholasville K.Y., USA

Pehrson, B., Plym Forshell, K. and Carlsson, J. (1992) The effect of additional feeding on the fertility of high–yielding dairy cows. *Journal of Veterinary Medicine A,* **39**, 187–192

Plym Forshell, K., Andersson, L and Pehrson, B. (1991) The relationships between the fertility of dairy cows and clinical and biochemical measurements, with special reference to plasma glucose and milk acetone. *Journal of Veterinary Medicine A,* **38**, 608–616

Refsdal, A.O. (1982) Ovariecyster hos melkekyr. (Ovarial cysts in dairy cows). *Norsk Veterinär Tidsskrift,* **94**, 789–796

Refsdal, A.O. (1983) Urea in bulk milk as compared to the herd mean of urea in blood. *Acta Veterinaria Scandinavica,* **24**, 518–520

Refsdal, A.O., Baevre, L. and Bruflot, R. (1985) Urea concentration in bulk milk as an indicator of the protein supply at the herd level. *Acta Veterinaria Scandinavica,* **26**, 153–163

Rosskopf, R. and Giesecke, D. (1992) Untersuchungen an Kühen über den Einfluss der Energieaufnahme auf den Pansenstoffwechsel mittels der Allantoinausscheidung in der Milch. (Investigations in cows on the influence of energy intake on rumen metabolism by means of allantoin excretion in the milk). *Journal of Veterinary Medicine A,* **39**, 515–524

Saloniemi, H. (1995) Use of somatic cell count in udder health work. In *The Bovine Udder and Mastitis,* pp 105–110. Edited by M. Sandholm, T. Honkanen-Buzalski, L. Kaartinen and S. Pyörälä. Jyväskylä, Finland, Gummerus Kirjapaino Oy

Simensen, E., Halse, K., Gillund, P. and Lutnaes, B. (1990) Ketosis treatment and milk yield in dairy cows related to milk acetoacetate levels. *Acta Veterinaria Scandinavica,* **31**, 433–440

Spörndly, E. (1989) Effects of diet on milk composition and yield of dairy cows with special emphasis on milk protein content. *Swedish Journal of Agricultural Research,* **19**, 99–106

Storry, J.E. (1970) Reviews of the progress of dairy science. Section A. Physiology. Ruminant metabolism in relation to the synthesis and secretion of milk fat. *Journal of Dairy Research,* **37**, 139–164

Sutton, J.D. (1989) Altering milk composition by feeding. *Journal of Dairy Science,* **72**, 2801–2814

Taponen, J. and Myllys, V. (1995) The economic impact of mastitis. In *The Bovine Udder and Mastitis,* pp 261–264. Edited by M. Sandholm, T. Honkanen—Buzalski, L. Kaartinen and S. Pyörälä. Jyväskylä, Finland, Gummerus Kirjapaino Oy

Wiktorsson, H. (1971) Input/Output Relationships in Dairy Cows. The effects of different levels of nutrition, quantities of roughage and frequencies of feeding. *Thesis*, the Agricultural College, Uppsala, Sweden, 114pp

This paper was first published in 1996

22

THE USE OF BLOOD BIOCHEMISTRY FOR DETERMINING THE NUTRITIONAL STATUS OF DAIRY COWS

W.R. WARD, R.D. MURRAY, A.R. WHITE and E.M. REES
University of Liverpool, Leahurst, Neston, South Wirral, CH64 7TE, UK

Introduction

METABOLIC PROFILES

Metabolic profiles in dairy cattle were made popular by the late Jack Payne in the 1970's at the Compton Laboratory (Payne, Dew, Manston and Faulks, 1970). Despite the authors' warning that 'It must be plainly stated that the metabolic profile test is merely an aid to preventive veterinary medicine', it disappointed those who expected it to revolutionise dairy cow nutrition. The choice of metabolites may have owed more to the repertoire of the Autoanalyzer than the usefulness to the veterinarian and cattle nutritionist. The normal ranges for the metabolites were based on the standard deviations around the mean found in the herds originally tested, and believed to be normal. The early results showed interesting variations in metabolites between seasons, and during the reproductive cycle of the cow, but some of these showed no obvious relationship to subclinical problems.

Since fertility is the biggest single source of loss to dairy farmers, it is not surprising that metabolic profiles were soon investigated for their ability to detect abnormalities in the diet related to fertility. Parker and Blowey (1976) at the Central Veterinary Laboratory found that in the herds that they examined the blood measurements showed no consistent relationship either to the estimated feed intake, or to the fertility.

Early studies (Lewis, 1957) showed that blood urea concentration was closely linked to the concentration of ammonia in the portal circulation and was related to the concentration of ammonia in the rumen 4 to 6 hours earlier.

Variation in blood composition at different times of day is clearly a factor limiting the accuracy of measurement of some metabolites. Manston, Rowlands, Little and Collis (1981) showed that out of 13 metabolites betahydroxybutyrate fluctuated most, varying 2.5 fold between 0700 and 1100 hrs in lactating cows. Diurnal variation was also measured in urea, magnesium and copper, with coefficients of variation of 18 %, 7 % and 16 % respectively. Gustafsson and Palmquist (1993) found that in individual cows blood urea concentration rose from 6 to 8 or 9 mmol/l following a single daily feed. Pearson, Craig and Rowe (1992) found that bile acids varied by up to 60 mmol/l within an hour.

THE DAIRY HERD MONITORING SCHEME

The University of Edinburgh and Dalgety formed a long relationship, which lasted until the company merged. In 1991 the University of Liverpool, together with the then Amalgamated Farmers (later AF plc) set up, after a pilot study, the Dairy Herd Monitoring Scheme (DHMS). The aims of the scheme included 'To link, through the means of planned blood testing, nutrition and preventive medicine on selected dairy units. To allow a greater degree of dialogue between the AF representative and the local veterinary practice. To collate information so that it might be used by either the University of Liverpool or by Amalgamated Farmers.. .'.

From the beginning, the scheme was seen as a planned exercise. AF cattle specialists selected farmers who were willing to commit themselves to, and to pay for, a series of four sets of sampling over one year. Farmers had to select cattle at the correct stage of lactation or dry period, at the correct time relative to changes in the feed. A considerable amount of information about the herd and the individual cows tested, had to be submitted with the samples. A copy of the Input Form is shown as Figure 22.1.

One important aim of the exercise was to involve veterinarians in discussion of nutrition with farmers and nutritionists.

Blood was to be taken from 6 cows in early lactation, 5 in mid-lactation, and 6 dry cows. Three vacutainers were used, oxalate/fluoride for glucose, heparin for glutathione peroxidase and copper, and plain for other metabolites. The metabolites measured, the methods and the standard values are shown in Table 22.1. Metabolites were measured using a Specific Selective Chemistry Analyser with Supra software (Kone, Ruukintie, Finland) and kits (Randox Laboratories, Crumlin, Northern Ireland) in serum, or in whole blood for glutathione peroxidase: copper was measured in plasma, using atomic absorption spectrophotometry. Glutathione peroxidase was measured as an indicator of selenium status (Anderson, Berrett and Patterson, 1978). The concentration of glutathione peroxidase was calculated assuming a packed cell volume of 33%. External quality control (QC) was conducted by Randox Laboratories.

Other metabolites were measured on request: the most common requests have been for cobalt, when cyanocobalamin has been measured, and iodine, when thyroxine (T4) was used as the best available measure (more recently plasma inorganic iodine has been used).

Samples were almost always analysed on the day of receipt, and copies of results along with a commentary compiled by a university veterinarian (WRW or RDM) were sent to the farmer, veterinary surgeon and AF nutritionist.

DEPARTMENTS OF VETERINARY CLINICAL SCIENCE
AND VETERINARY PATHOLOGY

92L - 2242

DAIRY HERD MONITORING SCHEME
INPUT FORM

A | COW INFORMATION　　　　　CODE No. 01 - 09 - 03 - 02　　DATE 3 8 92

	Cow No.	Calving Date	Lact No.	Yield (kg)	Pred. yld (kg/lact)	App.Wt. (kg)	Cond. Sc.	Parl.Feed (kg/day)	Comments
E	719	3.7.92	2	30·0		580	2½	5·0	✱ ALL SAMPLES TAKEN
A	807	5.7.92	1	20·0		570	2½	5·0	FROM JUGULAR VEIN
R	625	15.7.92	2	35·2		600	3	5·0	
L	591	5.7.92	4	29·8		610	3½	5·0	
Y	723	1.7.92	3	27·0		580	2½	5·0	
L	650	6.7.92	3	35·2		585	3	5·0	
A	658	29.6.92	4	35·0		610	3	5·0	
C T.									
M	739	7.7.92	1	25·0		600	2½	5·0	HOME MIX
I	814	14.7.92	1	20·0		575	2	5·0	
D	690	13.7.92	3	32·0		575	3	5·0	SUGAR BEET 48%
L									MAIZE GLUTEN 24%
A	728	9.8.92	2			570	3	-	SOYA 10%
C T.	733	22.9.92	2			540	2	-	MOLASSES 12%
	702	11.8.92	2			685	3½	-	FISH 3%
	257	8.8.92	10			685	4½	-	MINS/VIT 1%
D	544	14.8.92	5			730	5	-	
R Y	489	6.8.92	5			700	4½	-	
	775	20.9.92	2			566	2½	-	

B | FEED INFORMATION

	D.M.	ME	CP	DCP	pH	'D'	NH₃N	ESTIMATED INTAKES EARLY	MID	DRY
SILAGE	20	10·6	155	103	3.7		8·0	AD LIB		-
HOME MIX								5·0		-
GRASS								AD LIB		AD LIB
DAIRYLINE 16 THROUGH PARLOUR										

C | MANAGEMENT INFORM. (tick where appropriate)　✱ PLEASE ANALYSE FOR GSH·Px
　　　　　　　　　　　　　　　　　COPPER
　　　　　　　　　　　　　　　ALL COWS　　Lead Feed

　　Self Feed　　　　　　　Easy Feed
　　Forage Box　　　　　　Flat Rate　　　　　Complete Diet
　　Group Feeding

Figure 22.1 Dairy herd monitoring scheme input form

Table 22.1 BLOOD METABOLITES MEASURED, METHODS, AND STANDARD VALUES

Metabolite	Method	Standard value
Energy		
Betahydroxybutyrate (BOHB)	Ranbut*	<0.9 mmol/l
Glucose	GOD/PAP*	>2.5 mmol/l
Protein		
Urea	Enzymatic kinetic*	3.3 to 5 mmol/l
Albumin	Bromocresol green*	30 to 40 g/l
Total protein	Biuret*	60 to 80 g/l
Globulin	Difference	30 to 40 g/l
Minerals		
Magnesium	Col'metric xylidine blue	>0.74 mmol/l
Phosphate (inorganic)	UV*	>1.8 mmol/l
(phosphate in jugular blood)		>1.6 mmol/l
Glutathione peroxidase (selenium)	Ransel*	>39 units/33% PCV
Copper	Atomic absorption	>9.4 micromol/l
(copper in serum)		>7.4 micromol/l
Liver		
Bile acids	Enzymatic colorimetric*	<60 micromol/l

*Randox Laboratories Ltd, Diamond Road, Crumlin, Co Antrim, BT29 4QY, UK

Results

OVERVIEW

A total of 145 farms registered for the scheme, in addition to those that sent single batches of samples. Most farms were in the North and Midlands of England, with 22 in Scotland (Table 22.2).

A total of 10,199 cows were tested up to September 1994. Over 1,000 cows were sampled in each lactation up to lactation 5. Cows in first lactation (heifers) accounted for 13.5% of all the cows sampled (Table 22.3). Lactation number was not recorded in 160 cases.

When lactation was divided into four stages plus the dry period, the largest group comprised the dry cows, with 2,500 cows. The smallest category consisted of the cows in late lactation (Table 22.4).

The number of cows calving in each month showed a peak in August to October, and a trough in May (Table 22.5).

Table 22.2 GEOGRAPHICAL DISTRIBUTION OF FARMS

Lancashire	31	Northumberland	6
Scotland	22	Cheshire	5
Lincolnshire	21	Hereford & Worcs	4
Yorkshire	20	Nottinghamshire	4
Cumbria	15	Cambridgeshire	1
Derbyshire	8	Humberside	1
Shropshire	6	Leicestershire	1

Table 22.3 DISTRIBUTION OF COWS BY LACATION

Lactation	Number	Percentage
1	1358	13.5
2	2072	20.6
3	1844	18.4
4	1492	14.9
5	1152	11.5
6	863	8.6
>6	1258	12.5

Table 22.4 NUMBER OF COWS AT DIFFERENT STAGES OF LACTATION

Stage	Days post-partum	Number
1. Postpartum	1 to 41	2198
2. Early	42 to 120	2217
3. Mid	121 to 199	1807
4. Late	200 to 325	1517
5. Dry	305 to calving	2460

Table 22.5 NUMBER OF COWS CALVING IN EACH MONTH

Jan	Feb	Mar	Apr	May	Jun	July	Aug	Sep	Oct	Nov	Dec
867	667	723	549	466	690	929	1067	1076	1088	945	1047

In 85 cases the month of calving was not given.

About half of all dry cows were scored above condition score 3, and only 3 % of dry cows were below condition score 2. In the group of cows calved 6 to 17 weeks, (Early group) 30% were below condition score 2.5 (Table 22.6).

Table 22.6 NUMBER AND PERCENTAGE OF COWS IN EACH BAND OF CONDITION

Category	<2.0		2 to 2.4		2.5 to 3		>3		Total
Postpartum	108	(4.9%)	401	(18.2%)	1233	(56%)	456	(20.7%)	2198
Early	195	(8.8%)	520	(23.5%)	1165	(?25%)	338	(15.2%)	2217
Mid	102	(5.6%)	329	(18.2%)	1039	(58%)	337	(18.6%)	1807
Late	74	(4.9%)	201	(13.2%)	743	(49.0%)	499	(32.9%)	1517
Dry	54	(2.2%)	76	(3.1%)	941	(38.3%)	1389	(57.0%)	2460

The daily milk yield at the time of sampling was 30 to 39 kg in over 40% of cows calved up to 6 weeks (Post-partum group) and in cows calved 6 to 17 weeks (Early group), and 20 to 29 kg in 35 to 40% of these two groups (Table 22.7).

Table 22.7 NUMBER AND PERCENTAGE OF COWS WITH DAILY MILK YIELD AT TIME OF SAMPLING IN EACH CATEGORY

Category	<19 kg		20 to 29 kg		30 to 39 kg		>40 kg		Total
P	345	(15.8%)	782	(35.9%)	901	(41.3%)	151	(6.9%)	2179
E	217	(9.9%)	861	(39.3%)	957	(43.7%)	155	(7.1%)	2190
M	495	(28.6%)	958	(55.4%)	259	(15.0%)	17	(1.0%)	1729
L	992	(68.4%)	413	(28.5%)	44	(3.0%)	0		1449

The amount of parlour compound being fed at the time of sampling ranged from under 1 to over 12 kg (Table 22.8). The mode was 6 to 6.9kg in cows calved up to 6 weeks (Post-partum) and in cows calved 6 to 17 weeks (Early); 4 to 4.9kg in cows calved 18 to 22 weeks; and 1 to 1.9kg in cows calved over 22 weeks (Late).

The percentage of cows with values outside the standard ranges varied greatly between groups of cows, and between metabolites (Table 22.9 and Figure 22.2). One third of cows in the Post-partum group and one quarter in the Early group had raised betahydroxybutyrate. One quarter of cows in the Post-partum group had low glucose. Bile acids were raised in three quarters of cows in the Post-partum, Early and Mid lactation groups, in two thirds of cows in Late lactation, but in only 38% of dry cows.

Urea was above the standard range in over half of cows in each of the groups. High globulins were seen in 15 % of cows in Mid lactation, and 22 % in dry cows and in Post-partum cows.

Table 22.8 NUMBER AND PERCENTAGE OF COWS RECEIVING PARLOUR COMPOUND OF DIFFERENT AMOUNTS AT TIME OF SAMPLING

Parlour cpd kg/day	Post partum		Early		Mid		Late		Dry	
<1	10	(0.6%)	10	(0.05%)	35	(2.2%)	64	(6.7%)	44	(90.6%)
1 to 1.9	29	(1.6%)	82	(4.2%)	169	(10.7%)	248	(26.1%)	111	(4.5%)
2 to 2.9	100	(5.5%)	134	(1.8%)	258	(16.3%)	209	(22.0%)	49	(2.0%)
3 to 3.9	136	(7.6%)	182	(9.4%)	222	(14%)	111	(11.7%)	19	(0.7%)
4 to 4.9	215	(12.0%)	225	(11.6%)	303	(19.1%)	136	(14.3%)	9	(0.4%)
5 to 5.9	231	(12.9%)	225	(11.6%)	205	(12.9%)	84	(8.9%)	0	
6 to 6.9	318	(17.7%)	320	(16.5%)	201	(12.7%)	47	(5.0%)	0	
7 to 7.9	284	(15.8%)	271	(13.9%)	86	(5.4%)	18	(1.9%)	0	
8 to 8.9	205	(11.4%)	242	(12.5%)	62	(3.9%)	22	(2.3%)	0	
9 to 9.9	130	(7.2%)	122	(6.3%)	26	(1.6%)	5	(0.5%)	0	
10 to 10.9	98	(5.5%)	71	(3.7%)	11	(0.7%)	3	(0.3%)	0	
11 to 11.9	17	(1.0%)	26	(1.3%)	2	(0.1%)	2	(0.2%)	0	
>12	21	(1.2%)	33	(1.7%)	6	(0.4%)	0		0	
Total	1794		1943		1586		949		2460	

Magnesium was below standard in 5% or less of lactating cows, and in under 9% of dry cows. Phosphate was low in around one fifth of cows in all groups.

Glutathione peroxidase was below standard in 18% of cows in the Post-partum group, 2.5% in Mid lactation and 10% in the dry cows.

BODY CONDITION AT TIME OF SAMPLING, BETAHYDROXYBUTYRATE, GLUCOSE AND BILE ACIDS

Cows were divided into those below condition score 3 at the time of sampling ('thin') and those at condition score 3 or above ('fat'). In each group of cows, mean values of beta hydroxy butyrate (BOHB), glucose and bile acids were calculated for each period of 5 days from 60 days pre-partum to 325 days post-partum having excluded extreme values (Rowlands, 1984) (Table 22.10 and Figure 22.3).

BOHB was similar in the thin and fat cows, rising steeply from calving to a peak at 25 days, and then declining through lactation. Glucose concentration declined in both groups from calving to a minimum between 6 and 20 days, then rose to a peak at 305 days in the thin group and 315 days in the fat group. Cows that were above condition score 3 had a significantly higher glucose than thinner cows between 160 and 200 days ($p < 0.01$) and after 205 days ($p < 0.05$). Bile acids rose steeply after calving to a peak at 115 days, then declined until the next calving. Bile acids were significantly higher in

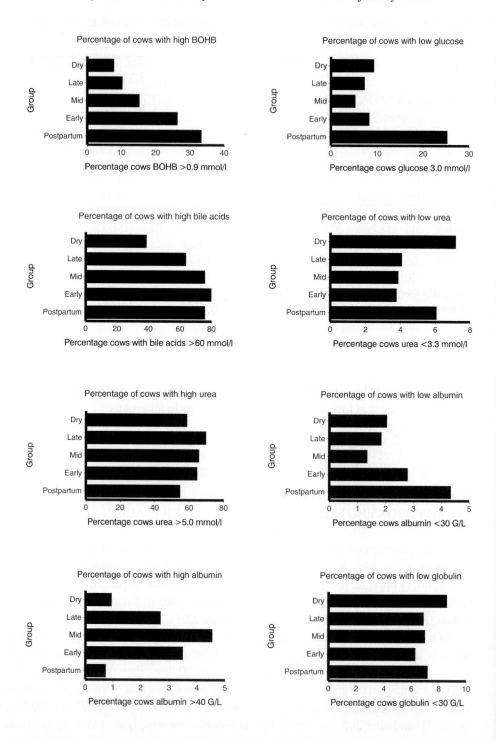

Figure 22.2　Percentage of cows with values outside the standard ranges

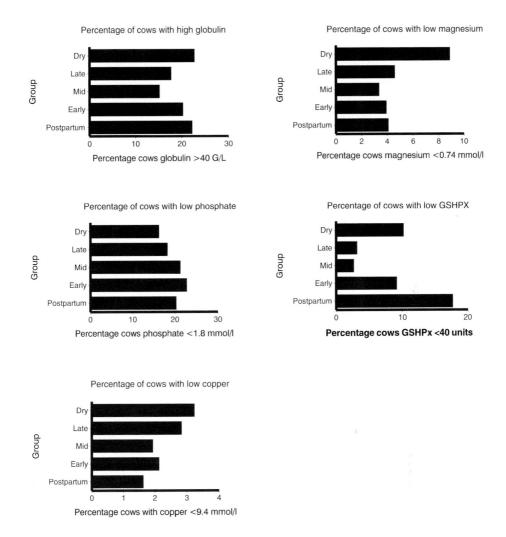

Figure 22.2 contd. Percentage of cows with values outside the standard ranges

the thin cows between 125 and 200 days post-partum (p < 0.001) and after 205 days (p < 0.01).

In the thin group, glucose concentration was negatively correlated with BOHB between 45 and 120 days post-partum (p < 0.01, r- 0.78), but positively correlated with BOHB after 205 days (p < 0.05, r 0.54), and with bile acids from 125 to 200 days (p < 0.02-0.02, r 0.42) and after 205 days (p < 0.01, r0.79). In fat cows, glucose was again negatively correlated with BOHB (p < 0.01, r -0.75), and bile acids correlated with BOHB from 125 to 200 days (p < 0.01, r 0.52).

Table 22.9 NUMBER AND PERCENTAGE OF COWS WITH VALUES OF BLOOD METABOLITES OUTSIDE STANDARD RANGES

	Post-partum	Early	Mid	Late	Dry
BOHB <0.9 mmol/l	775 34.0%	615 25.9%	280 14.8%	139 10.3%	193 7.6%
Glucose <2 mmol/l	563 24.8%	207 8.8%	96 5.1%	91 6.9%	229 9.1%
Bile acids >60 micromol/l	1697 74.7%	1853 78.5%	1406 74.5%	848 63.6%	963 38.1%
Urea <3.3 mmol/l	136 6.0%	85 3.6%	71 3.7%	54 4.0%	181 7.1%
Urea >5 mmol/l	1222 53.6%	1513 64.7%	1236 65.2%	918 67.9%	1457 57.3%
Albumin < 30 g/l	98 4.3%	64 2.7%	24 1.3%	24 1.8%	50 2.0%
Albumin >40 g/l	20 0.8%	81 3.4%	85 4.5%	37 2.7%	24 0.9%
Globulin < 30 g/l	161 7.1%	146 6.2%	128 6.8%	90 6.7%	215 8.5%
Globulin >40g/l	500 22.0%	476 20.1%	281 14.9%	237 17.6%	566 22.3%
Magnesium <0.74 mmol/l	90 4.1%	90 3.8%	63 3.3%	67 5.0%	221 8.7%
Phosphate <1.8 mmol/l	450 19.8%	526 22.3%	399 21.21%	246 18.2%	422 16.6%
GSHPx < 40 units	331 17.6%	162 8.8%	33 2.5%	28 2.8%	197 9.8%
Copper <9.4 micromol/l	25 1.6%	33 2.1%	25 1.9%	29 2.8%	79 3.2%

CONDITION SCORE, BETAHYDROXYBUTYRATE, GLUCOSE AND BILE ACIDS IN COWS SAMPLED TWICE

A total of 430 cows were found to have been tested both during the dry period and subsequently in early lactation (up to 17 weeks post-partum). A total of 73 were above condition score 3 ('fat') both when dry, and when sampled after calving: 174 were above condition score 3 when dry, but below ('thin') after calving, and 183 were below condition score 3 before and after calving. Very few cows moved from 'thin' to 'fat' after calving.

Table 22.10 BETAHYDROXYBUTYRATE, GLUCOSE AND BILE ACIDS IN COWS WITH
CONDITION SCORE AT TIME OF SAMPLING 3 OR ABOVE ('FAT') OR BELOW 3 ('THIN')

Days post partum	Thin β.hydroxybutyrate mmol/l	Fat β.hydroxybutyrate mmol/l	Thin Glucose mmol/l	Fat Glucose mmol/l	Thin Bile acids micromol/l	Fat Bile acids micromol/l
5	0.57	0.57	3.60	3.45	65.90	58.20
10	0.81	0.80	3.02	3.16	68.60	70.80
15	0.77	0.93	3.17	3.15	69.40	79.20
20	0.85	0.95	3.13	3.05	79.60	79.40
25	0.88	1.04	3.22	3.20	81.60	81.40
30	0.85	0.94	3.27	3.31	84.70	80.00
35	0.81	0.92	3.34	3.37	84.80	81.10
40	0.78	0.98	3.39	3.41	84.40	94.20
45	0.72	0.79	3.42	3.44	83.80	91.40
50	0.79	0.82	3.47	3.49	85.70	82.90
55	0.73	0.80	3.47	3.56	94.60	77.20
60	0.82	0.77	3.43	3.53	89.60	93.50
65	0.70	0.78	3.58	3.57	87.40	81.00
70	0.69	0.66	3.50	3.71	89.10	85.90
75	0.69	0.75	3.57	3.63	82.90	89.30
80	0.71	0.64	3.50	3.71	85.50	79.30
85	0.75	0.74	3.65	3.64	79.70	77.10
90	0.71	0.70	3.61	3.64	93.70	81.50
95	0.68	0.73	3.59	3.67	94.70	90.30
100	0.71	0.73	3.60	3.58	93.30	85.00
105	0.67	0.77	3.59	3.67	75.30	95.50
110	0.65	0.54	3.62	3.69	78.10	78.60
115	0.65	0.66	3.69	3.60	84.30	71.20
120	0.61	0.56	3.67	3.67	79.10	74.60
125	0.63	0.62	3.51	3.77	88.90	79.50
130	0.60	0.61	3.62	3.64	82.60	71.10
135	0.58	0.70	3.68	3.51	91.40	76.80
140	0.58	0.57	3.68	3.73	84.20	70.80
145	0.59	0.67	3.64	3.71	82.70	75.70
150	0.58	0.62	3.55	3.56	82.80	86.70
155	0.63	0.60	3.65	3.67	86.90	81.70
160	0.61	0.65	3.67	3.63	82.60	79.40
165	0.62	0.61	3.72	3.73	86.70	77.60
170	0.63	0.61	3.66	3.60	79.10	86.90
175	0.58	0.58	3.58	3.55	86.10	81.00
180	0.58	0.63	3.60	3.57	80.10	80.10
185	0.55	0.71	3.56	3.59	94.70	82.00
190	0.61	0.72	3.59	3.74	77.30	82.50
195	0.64	0.62	3.65	3.67	77.40	77.80
200	0.72	0.59	3.45	3.77	81.80	69.20
205	0.62	0.68	3.65	3.75	79.90	75.00
210	0.68	0.63	3.65	3.75	91.50	78.50
215	0.61	0.63	3.54	3.60	75.90	79.40

Table 22.10 Continued

Days post partum	Thin ß.hydroxybutyrate mmol/l	Fat ß.hydroxybutyrate mmol/l	Thin Glucose mmol/l	Fat Glucose mmol/l	Thin Bile acids micromol/l	Fat Bile acids micromol/l
220	0.62	0.60	3.73	3.84	85.40	68.50
225	0.54	0.60	3.66	3.64	84.90	67.70
230	0.55	0.52	3.70	3.77	78.50	73.40
235	0.60	0.54	3.69	3.77	77.90	81.60
240	0.61	0.62	3.55	3.78	75.60	72.80
245	0.63	0.65	3.40	3.80	80.30	71.50
250	0.50	0.49	3.57	3.59	79.60	73.00
255	0.55	0.54	3.79	3.69	77.70	69.60
260	0.47	0.59	3.68	3.62	79.10	68.10
265	0.49	0.52	3.63	3.70	74.30	65.30
270	0.56	0.61	3.67	3.71	75.60	73.30
275	0.60	0.56	3.66	3.77	70.90	63.10
280	0.66	0.57	3.47	3.70	57.10	57.40
285	0.52	0.48	3.56	3.63	67.90	65.40
290	0.49	0.53	3.32	3.60	54.40	52.20
295	0.57	0.49	3.63	3.71	75.80	59.10
300	0.47	0.53	3.36	3.73	55.10	64.00
305	0.57	0.52	3.83	3.59	87.40	68.70
310		0.43		3.60		71.60
315		0.63		3.77		76.60
320		0.44		3.76		64.00
325		0.587		3.57		56.90
-60	0.57	0.53	3.60	3.76	76.00	59.80
-55	0.59	0.54	3.61	3.67	68.10	55.50
-50	0.50	0.54	3.46	3.61	63.40	55.90
-45	0.44	0.51	3.38	3.57	62.40	54.40
-40	0.57	0.56	3.64	3.59	64.90	52.80
-35	0.53	0.53	3.29	3.58	59.00	52.10
-30	0.57	0.54	3.58	3.59	61.30	53.60
-25	0.58	0.56	3.45	3.50	60.30	53.60
-20						
-15	0.54	0.52	36.52	3.55	57.20	52.50
-10	0.57	0.55	3.40	3.48	55.30	52.30
-5	0.55	0.51	3.43	3.52	58.20	56.80
-1	0.51	0.53	3.51	3.45	51.90	59.00

For each 5-day period, mean values of ß.hydroxybutyrate, glucose and bile acids were calculated, between 1 and 16 results contributing to each mean (Figure 22.4). In cows sampled before 40 days, betahydroxybutyrate and bile acids were higher and glucose was lower ($p < 0.05$) in cows fat before calving than in those cows thin before calving.

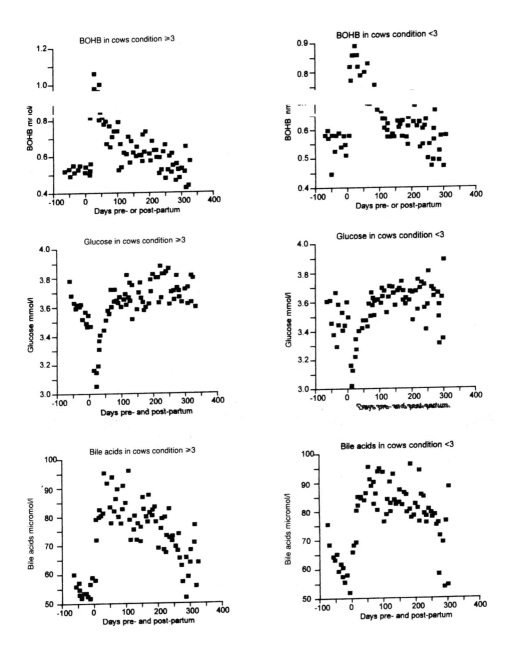

Figure 22.3 Body condition score at time of sampling, betahydroxybutyrate, glucose and bile acids

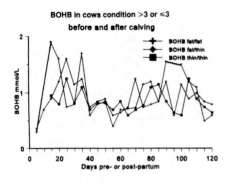

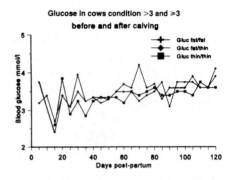

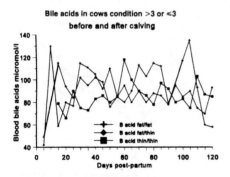

Figure 22.4 Body condition score, betahydroxybutyrate, glucose and bile acids in cows sampled twice

GLUTATHIONE PEROXIDASE AND LACTATION NUMBER

Glutathione peroxidase concentration was below standard values in over 17% of first lactation cows (heifers), whereas low values were seen in no more than 9% of mature cows (Table 22.11). During the Post-partum period in first lactation cows, 39% had low GSHPx values.

Table 22.11 NUMBER AND PERCENTAGE OF COWS IN EACH LACTATION WITH GLUTATHIONE PEROXIDASE BELOW STANDARD VALUES (40 UNITS)

Lactation	1*	2	3	4	5	6	>6
Number < 40 units	218	151	121	81	85	62	103
Total number	1254	1836	1687	1361	1042	777	1139
Percentage	17.4	8.2	7.2	6.0	8.2	8.0	9.0

*In first lactation between calving and 6 weeks post-partum, 39.1 % of cows had glutathione peroxidase below 40 units.

Discussion

Metabolites were chosen which fluctuate in a meaningful way in dairy cows. Calcium, for example was excluded because homeostatic mechanisms usually maintain the concentration within a close range except in cows with signs of clinical disease. Metabolites were also chosen where changes were likely to indicate a problem about which advice could usefully be given. Packed cell volume (PCV) for example, fluctuates in an interesting fashion during the year but the information is of limited value. Metabolites that could not withstand storage for 24 or more hours at ambient temperatures were excluded.

Bile acids were chosen to indicate liver function: Roberts, Red, Row- lands and Patterson (1981) at Compton showed the widespread existence and clinical importance of fat mobilisation syndrome, and West (1990, 1991) showed the close correlation in cattle between fatty infiltration of the liver and the concentration of bile acids in the blood.

The minerals chosen were those believed to be most frequently involved in subclinical problems, affecting productivity in British dairy cattle.

The standard ranges must be to some extent arbitrary, but are based on the best available information on the laboratory tests used, and the population of cows tested.

OVERVIEW

One aim of the DHMS was to correlate information about the herd and the cows with the blood results. The information was reasonably complete, but subsequently there was more comprehensive collection of information.

The aim of encouraging veterinarians to discuss nutrition with farmers and nutritionists was largely successful. Veterinarians were invariably involved in the collection of the blood, and received reports, which always referred to matters which the farmer was advised to discuss with the veterinarian and nutritionist. A survey was conducted to assess the perceptions of the veterinarians to the DHMS. This showed that a post-sampling meeting was invaluable.

The selection of farms was not random. It was inevitable that the distribution of farms reflected the enthusiasm of farmers and of cattle specialists and representatives. Nor would the distribution of cows sampled be random: farmers would be tempted to present the 'best cow' for sampling, in the belief that the blood sample would reveal her secret, or they might keep in a cow with a problem, thinking that the metabolic profile would explain it. Both of these practices were discouraged, but if they occurred, they would be expected to extend the range of some values.

Most of the farms were in the North and Midlands of England, with 22 from Scotland. The geographical area was limited, but the wide range of husbandry patterns and climate were representative of much of Great Britain.

The numbers of cows in each lactation and the numbers of cows calving in each month produced patterns similar to those in the area as a whole. Milk yields showed a pattern that would be common in many British herds, with 44% of those calved 6 to 18 weeks (Early lactation group) giving between 30 and 39kg a day, 40% yielding 20 to 29 kg, and 7% above 40kg.

The pattern of condition score was interesting, with 57% of dry cows above condition score 3 at the time of sampling, and only 5% below condition score 2.5. Since 23% of cows sampled up to 6 weeks after calving (Post- partum group) were below condition score 2.5, it appears that some cows were losing a considerable amount of body condition in a short time. At no stage were more than 9% of cows below condition score 2. There were clearly a lot of cows too fat in the dry period, and they would be likely to eat less after calving than leaner cows, to lose more condition and to have a lower fertility (Garnsworthy and Topps, 1982; Garnsworthy, 1988; Treacher, Reid and Roberts, 1986).

Parlour feed showed a wide range in each category of cows. For cows calved 6 to 18 weeks (Early group), the largest number were receiving 6 to 7 kg a day, while in mid lactation the greatest number were on 4 to 5 kg. Despite the trend to feed more straights, and to reduce dependence on parlour feed, over 25 % of cows in the Early group were receiving more than 8kg of parlour feed a day.

ABNORMAL VALUES

It is no surprise that BOHB was high in one third of cows up to 41 days post-partum, and in a quarter of cows between 42 and 120 days. A single individual value above the normal range is less significant than several raised values in the same group of cows, for two reasons. First, a cow may have an individual problem unrelated to the rest of the herd. Secondly, the high degree of variation found in BOHB (Manston *et al.,* 1981) must mean that a single high value may not be representative. The finding of several high values in a group, or the finding of a very high value, was however interpreted to mean that there was a significant energy deficit. The farmer was advised to discuss with the veterinarian and nutritionist possible causes, such as low palatability of silage, poor access to silage, etc.

Glucose values below 2.5 mmol/l have been regarded as below normal, but in view of the patterns seen, a cut-off point of 3.0 was adopted for this review. A quarter of cows calved less than 42 days had low glucose, similar to the findings of Rowlands, Manston, Stark, Russell, Collis and Collis (1980) whereas after that time no more than 9% did so, despite the fact that 26 % had high BOHB. Cows with high BOHB and normal glucose were commonly seen, and can be explained as cows that were mobilising fat as an energy source. It was less usual to see cows with normal BOHB and depressed glucose. Only occasionally were these thin cows, with little fat to mobilise.

Bile acids were above 60 micromol/l in a large majority of lactating cows. A maximal value of 45 micromol/l was established by West (1991). It is accepted that a high proportion of British dairy cows under current husbandry have fatty infiltration of the liver (Roberts *et at.,* 1981) and high bile acids reflected that (West, 1990, 1991). Since 57% of the dry cows in the herds studied were above body condition 3.0, these would be expected to be at risk from fat mobilisation syndrome (Garnsworthy and Topps, 1982; Roberts *et at.,* 1981). Bile acids show considerable variation in time (Pearson *et al.,* 1992) and single cows with elevated values are not regarded as significant. In many herds, however, high or very high bile acid values were seen in the majority of lactating cows.

High urea was clearly very common in these herds. While numerous studies have been published (eg. Lewis, 1957; Ropstad, Vik-Mo and Refsdal, 1989) there is room for a new study to assess urea values in cows fed according to the Metabolisable Protein system (Agriculture and Food Research Council, 1989). Further studies would be of value to assess the relationship of blood urea concentration to fertility and health, as well as to production.

Albumin is regarded as another indicator of liver function, and low values can be seen for example in liver fluke infestation. This was a rare occurrence in this population of cows. Albumin and globulin are regarded as indicators of long-term protein intake, and inadequacy was rare in these herds. High globulin can reflect various types of infection, such as chronic mastitis, when the concentration of gamma-globulin may be raised, and high globulin values were found in about one fifth of cows.

Magnesium varies little in time, and low values are regarded as significant. Very little is stored in the body. On occasion very low values were seen, and the veterinarian was then telephoned immediately so that the farmer could be warned. For dry cows, where almost 9% of cows showed low values, low magnesium is a risk factor for milk fever (Sansom, Manston and Vagg, 1983).

Low phosphate was seen in 18 to 22% of lactating cows, most of which were receiving mineralised compound, but below 17% of dry cows, presumably reflecting the higher needs of lactation. In most cases samples were taken from the tail (coccygeal) blood vessels, but when samples were taken from the jugular vein, a standard value of more than 1.6 mmol/l was adopted to allow for the lower concentration in the jugular, where some phosphate is removed by the salivary glands.

Glutathione peroxidase concentration was calculated assuming a constant packed cell volume of 33%. Our own tests agreed with Payne *et at.* (1970) that packed cell volume varies between cows and with seasons. Standard values for glutathione peroxidase differ between laboratories, and this causes confusion. Since glutathione peroxidase is incorporated into the red blood cells, the concentration reflects the amount of selenium available to the cow 4 to 6 weeks earlier. This was demonstrated in the low values seen in the dry cows, reflecting low selenium intake in late lactation, and still lower values seen in the Post-partum group, reflecting lack of mineral supplementation in many dry cows. The reports distinguished between marginally low glutathione peroxidase (20 to 40 units), and very low values (below 20 units). Selenium-responsive conditions were by no means always seen on farms where cows have marginally low values. The greater use of un- mineralised straights in place of mineralised compounds, and the more widespread feeding of maize silage in place of grass silage, might increase the prevalence of selenium-responsive problems.

Copper concentration 9.4 micromol/l and above was adopted as standard (Suttle, 1993) for plasma. When on rare occasions serum was analysed, 7.4 micromol/l was used as standard. Low copper concentration was not found to be common, but two reservations must be expressed. First, blood copper does not always directly relate to clinical problems (Suttle, 1986). Secondly, interference by molybdenum and other elements can cause clinical problems, and blood concentration of copper is not a sufficient guide.

BODY CONDITION AT TIME OF SAMPLING, BETAHYDROXYBUTYRATE, GLUCOSE AND BILE ACIDS

The fall in glucose after calving agreed with Rowlands *et al.* (1980) and the negative correlation with betahydroxybutyrate (BOHB) agreed with Mills, Beitz and Young (1986). The enormous need of the lactating mammary gland for glucose in order to produce lactose means that some energy is produced from mobilised fat, and BOHB is produced.

In general the patterns of these three metabolites were similar in the fat and thin cows. The distinction between the cows was solely the condition at the time of sampling, and it is likely that the change in condition prior to sampling is more important. Further analysis of data from the much smaller number of cows that by chance were sampled twice was therefore undertaken.

CONDITION SCORE, BETAHYDROXYBUTYRATE, GLUCOSE AND BILE ACIDS IN COWS SAMPLED TWICE

In cows sampled twice, first in the dry period and then before 40 days after calving, betahydroxybutyrate and bile acids were higher when the cows were above condition score 3 before calving than in cows that were leaner. Glucose values, and all values after 40 to 50 days appeared to show no difference. This is compatible with evidence that cows calving above condition score 3 mobilise more body tissues and are more likely to have fatty liver (Gamsworthy, 1988; Roberts *et al.,* 1981).

GLUTATHIONE PEROXIDASE AND IACTATION NUMBER

In cows (heifers) in first lactation a low glutathione peroxidase concentration was seen in 17 % of cases. An even higher proportion of first lactation cows in the Post-partum group showed low GSHPx (39%). This is a strong indication of a low selenium content in the forage fed to the heifers before their first calving, and an absence of supplementary minerals. The scheme did not set out to analyse blood from heifers before their first calving, but they could well benefit from such attention.

NORMAL VALVES OR MEAN VALVES?

Unlike Payne *et al.,* (1970) normal values were not calculated as the mean of the values found in apparently normal cows. Instead, standard values were decided upon from published data. On that basis, the mean values in some groups of cows that were tested were in many cases not normal. The results reported here suggest that a large number of British dairy cows were too fat in the dry period, lost too much condition in early lactation, and had energy deficit and fatty infiltration of the liver. An excess of urea, indicating excess rumen-degradable protein relative to fermentable energy, was very common. Low magnesium in dry cows was not uncommon, low phosphate was commonly seen, and low glutathione peroxidase was very common early in first lactation.

If mean values were taken as normal, and values more than two standard deviations from the mean as abnormal, the results of any common fault in husbandry would become accepted as normal.

FUTURE ADVANCES IN METABOLIC PROFILES

We have encouraged the use of blood samples, and a beneficial effect of that was that it necessarily involved the veterinarian. Milk samples can, however, be used for the measurement of urea, and the concentration is closely correlated with blood concentration (Oltner and Wiktorsson, 1983; Ropstad *et al.,* 1989; Gustafsson and Palmquist, 1993). Milk samples have for many years been used to measure total ketones, and the values are less variable than in urine because the concentration of urine fluctuates widely (Radostits, Blood and Gay, 1994). Other metabolites such as glucose would clearly bear no relationship to blood values. Standard ranges would need to be established for suitable metabolites. Milk has the enormous advantage that it is collected twice daily and bulk samples are regularly taken to central laboratories, and can be analysed without the expense of collection. Results can be interpreted alongside the milk protein and butterfat values, which are already routinely measured, and which are useful indicators of nutritional status. Individual samples can be collected easily by the farmer. Frequent measurement of urea could be used as a means of monitoring the balance of nitrogen and energy available to the rumen microbes.

At present, standard values are used without formal regard for the age or lactational status of the individual cow. In future, computer software could highlight values outside standard ranges depending on age, days after calving, time of year, etc.

Bile acids have been used as the best available single predictor of fatty liver (West, 1991) but it is likely that other metabolites might add to the value of the prediction. Indicators of other functions of the liver would also be of value.

Questionnaires circulated to cattle specialists and representatives, farmers and veterinarians involved in the scheme led to new developments in presentation and in substance.

Other companies have shown an interest in metabolic profiles and a different scheme has been running for several years.

Preliminary trials have been made of metabolic profiles in beef cattle and in sheep, which clearly have much in common with each other and with dairy cows. Trials have also been undertaken in pigs, where the range of useful metabolites will probably be very different: the greater variability in the diet of ruminants may mean that metabolic profiles are peculiarly valuable. Heifers have not been included in the scheme, but the evidence of low selenium in the diets of many heifers before calving suggests that extension of the scheme to heifers would be useful.

A feature of the Dairy Herd Monitoring Scheme has been to link the blood values to other information. More complete and more standardised recording of health and fertility, as in the second DAISY report (Esslemont and Spincer, 1994) could add to the value of the whole scheme.

Conclusions

The University of Liverpool Veterinary Faculty, with AF plc, showed that metabolic profiles have a place in modern dairy farming. All the parties involved benefited from a better understanding of the complex links between nutrition, health and fertility. These benefits arose to a large extent through the collection of information about the herd and the individual cows, and discussion of this information alongside the laboratory results.

Acknowledgments

Laboratory work was efficiently and meticulously performed by Malcolm Savage, Andrew Wattrett and Cynthia Dare, of the Department of Veterinary Pathology, University of Liverpool, Leahurst. Secretarial work was efficiently done by Christine Broadbent.

References

Agriculture and Food Research Council (1989) Technical Committee on Responses to Nutrients, Report No.9, Nutritive Requirements of Ruminant Animals: Protein, *Nutrition Abstracts and Reviews,* Series B, Livestock Feeds and Feeding, **62**, 787-835

Anderson, P.H., Berrett, S. and Patterson, D.S.P. (1978) Glutathione peroxidase activity in erythrocytes and muscle of cattle and sheep and its relationship to selenium. *Journal of Comparative Pathology,* **88**, 181-189

Esslemont, R.J. and Spincer, I. (1994) *DAISY Report Number* 2. Reading: University of Reading

Garnsworthy, P.C. (1988) The effect of energy reserves at calving on performance of dairy cows. In *Nutrition and lactation in the dairy cow*. Edited by P.C. Garnsworthy, pp. 157-170. London: Butterworth

Garnsworthy, P.C. and Topps, J.H. (1982) The effect of body condition of dairy cows at calving on their food intake and performance when given complete diets. *Animal Production,* **35**, 113-119

Gustafsson, A.H. and Palmquist, D.L. (1993) Diurnal variation of rumen ammonia, serum urea, and milk urea in dairy cows at high and low yields. *Journal of Dairy Science,* **76**, 475-484

Lewis, D. (1957) Blood urea concentration in relation to protein utilisation in the ruminant. *Journal of Agricultural Science,* **48**, 438-446

Manston, R., Rowlands, GJ., Little, W. and Collis, K.A., (1981) Variability in the blood composition of dairy cows in relation to time of day. *Journal of Agricultural Science,* **96**, 593-598

Mills, S.E., Beitz D.C. and Young, J.W. (1986) Characterisation of metabolic changes during a protocol for inducing lactation ketosis in dairy cows. *Journal of Dairy Science,* **69**, 352-361

Oltner, R. and Wiktorsson, H. (1983) Urea concentrations in milk and blood as influenced by feeding varying amounts of protein and energy to dairy cows. *Livestock Production Science,* **10**, 457-467

Parker, B.N.J. and Blowey, R.W. (1976) Investigations into the relationship of selected blood components to nutrition and fertility of the dairy cow under commercial farm conditions. *Veterinary Record,* **98**, 394-404

Payne, J.M., Dew, S.M., Manston, R. and Faulks, R. (1970) The use of a metabolic profile test in dairy herds. *Veterinary Record,* **87**, 150-158

Pearson, E.G., Craig, A.M. and Rowe, K. (1992) Variability of serum bile acid concentrations over time in dairy cattle, and effect of feed deprivation on the variability. *American Journal of Veterinary Research,* **53**, 1780-1783

Radostits, O.M., Blood, D.C. and Gay, C.C. (1994) *Veterinary Medicine,* 8th edition, p. 1348. London: Bailliere Tindall

Roberts, C.J., Reid, I.M., Rowlands, G.J., Patterson (1981) A fat mobilisation syndrome in dairy cows in early lactation. *Veterinary Record,* **108**, 7-9

Ropstad, E., Vik-Mo, L, and Refsdal, A. O. (1989) Levels of milk urea, plasma constituents, and rumen liquid ammonia in relation to the feeding of dairy cows during early lactation. *Acta Veterinaria Scandinavica,* **30**, 199-208

Rowlands, G.J., Manston, R., Stark A.J., Russell A.M., Collis, K.A., and Collis, S.C. (1980) Changes in albumin, globulin, glucose and cholesterol concentrations in the blood of dairy cows in late pregnancy and early lactation and relationships with subsequent fertility. *Journal of Agricultural Science,* **94**, 517-527

Rowlands, G.J. (1984) Week-to-week variation in blood composition of dairy cows and its effect on interpretation of metabolic profile tests. *British Veterinary Journal,* **140**, 550-557

Sansom, B.F., Manston, R. and Vagg, M.J. (1983). Magnesium and milk fever. *Veterinary Record,* **112**, 447-449

Suttle, N. (1986) Problems in the diagnosis and anticipation of trace element deficiencies in grazing livestock. *Veterinary Record,* **119**, 148-152

Suttle, N. (1993) Overestimation of copper deficiency. *Veterinary Record,* **133**, 123-124

Treacher, R.J., Reid, I.M. and Roberts, CJ. (1986) Effect of body condition at calving on the health and performance of dairy cows. *Animal Production,* **43**, 1-6

West H.J. (1990) Effect on liver function of acetonaemia and the fat cow syndrome in cattle. *Research in Veterinary Science,* **51**, 133-140

West H.J. (1991) Evaluation of total serum bile acid concentrations for the diagnosis of hepatobiliary disease in cattle. *Research in Veterinary Science,* **48**, 221-227

This paper was first published in 1995

23

THE INFLUENCE OF NUTRITION ON FERTILITY IN DAIRY COWS

P.C. GARNSWORTHY and R. WEBB
University of Nottingham, Division of Agriculture and Horticulture, School of Biological Sciences, Sutton Bonington Campus, Loughborough, Leics LE12 5RD, UK

Introduction

Fertility is one of the major factors influencing the profitability of dairy herds. A cow will not produce milk until after she has produced her first calf, but continued regular breeding is essential for retention of a cow in the herd. Early culling due to reproductive failure represents a waste of resources and means that the cost of rearing the animal is spread over fewer productive lactations, thereby reducing profit per litre of milk. The optimum interval between one calving and the next is normally considered to be 365 days. Interest has recently been shown in extending the length of lactation, but this should be a conscious management decision and not a result of poor reproductive performance.

The objective of this paper is to consider the influence of nutrition on fertility. Many factors influence fertility, only one of which is nutrition; it is important that putative nutritional influences are seen in the context of whole-herd management. Also, nutrition is a very broad subject area, covering not only the supply of energy and nutrients to the cow, but also the animal's requirements for total and specific nutrients. This chapter will review influences on fertility at the whole-animal level, consider the implications for nutrition, and then discuss possible mechanisms for the action of nutrition on reproductive processes.

Influences on fertility

Fertility is the reproductive performance of an individual cow or herd, measured as the number of calves produced per unit time. This presents problems for the researcher, since calving is a discrete event that only occurs once per year. Therefore, experimental designs, such as crossover or covariance designs, cannot be used and large numbers of replicates are needed. The production of a calf is a culmination of events involving follicle development, growth of a good-quality oocyte, ovulation, fertilisation, implantation and embryo survival. Failure at any stage in this sequence causes infertility, and failure might be caused by a number of animal, management and nutritional factors (Figure 23.1), many of which are inter-related.

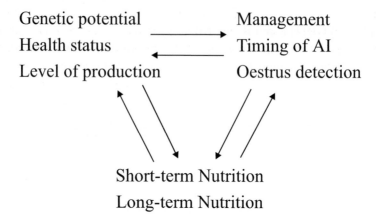

Figure 23.1 Interactions between animal, management and nutritional factors affecting fertility in dairy cows

Over the past 25 years, there have been dramatic increases in milk production in UK dairy herds, with many cows now producing over 9000 litres of milk per lactation. However, this increase in milk yield has been accompanied by a serious decline in fertility of dairy cows. Lamming, Darwash, Wathes and Ball (1998) estimated that the average conception rate to first service has declined at approximately 1% every three years.

Non-nutritional influences

Unlike other farm species, dairy cows do not exhibit strong lactational anoestrus, nor are they strongly seasonal breeders, although there is some evidence that conception rates are lower in summer (Bourchier, Garnsworthy, Hutchinson and Benson, 1987). Increased milk yields have mainly stemmed from genetic changes, with the importation of Holstein genes from North America and widespread use of bulls through artificial insemination. It is possible that single-trait selection has reduced fertility amongst dairy cows, but the move to larger herd sizes, with less attention being paid to oestrous detection, may also have contributed. Reduced fertility has been accompanied by an increased incidence of metabolic diseases and lameness.

There is no doubt that nutrition plays a key role in enabling the modern dairy cow to reach high levels of milk production. Expression of improved genetic potential has been facilitated by changes in feeding management, with increased use of complete diets fed *ad libitum*, by increased use of maize silage and better conservation of grass silage. It can probably also be claimed that our knowledge of ration formulation and the nutritive value of dietary ingredients have also improved following the publication of ARC (1980) and its successors. It could therefore be argued that the nutrition of dairy cows is better today than it was 25 years ago. However, as Agnew, Yan and Gordon. (1998) stated, the efficiency of conversion of available energy into milk energy has not increased, so high-merit animals sustain high levels of milk production partly by increased mobilisation of body reserves.

Since so many factors may have an influence on fertility, the decline in conception rates cannot be attributed solely to nutrition. It must be remembered when studying associations between two parameters, such as milk yield and conception rate, that all you can legitimately deduce is the strength of the association, not cause and effect. Both parameters may change concurrently in response to another factor. Having said that, a strong relationship shown in a survey provides a good starting point for experimental investigation.

Body reserves, food intake and milk yield

Gross measures of reproductive performance, such as conception rate to a particular service, days from calving to first oestrus and days to conception, have all been adversely associated with high milk yields, low intakes of energy and mobilisation of body reserves, which combine in the term negative energy balance. Negative energy balance is usually quoted as the main cause of poor conception rates in dairy cows.

Body reserves, milk yield and food intake are closely interrelated. If energy intake is insufficient to meets the demands of milk secretion, as it usually is in early lactation, body reserves are mobilised. If energy intake exceeds requirements, excess energy is deposited as body fat, but over the long term cows adjust their energy intake in an attempt to keep levels of body energy reserves constant (Garnsworthy, 1988). In beef cattle, calving cows in a higher body condition can improve reproductive performance (Wright, Rhind, Russel, Whyte, McBean and McMillen, 1987), but the situation is different in dairy cows. Attempts to overcome the effects of negative energy balance by increasing body condition at calving may exacerbate the problem, since there is a strong relationship between body condition at calving and the amount of condition lost in early lactation (Figure 23.2). Therefore, negative energy balance is almost inevitable in early lactation, except in cows calving with very low condition scores.

Change in body condition score is a very good indicator of energy status for a dairy cow. The University of Nottingham and ADAS conducted a survey of nearly 2000 dairy cows in high-yielding herds (average annual milk yield 7210 kg/cow); preliminary findings were reported by Bourchier *et al.* (1987). Neither condition score at calving, or at service, affected conception rate to first service, except when the condition score

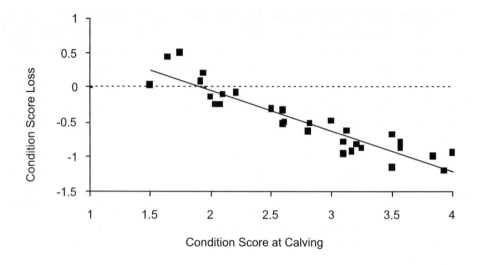

Figure 23.2   Effect of condition score at calving on loss of condition during early lactation. Each data point is a treatment mean from a published experiment (data obtained from Bourchier *et al.* (1987); Garnsworthy and Huggett (1992); Garnsworthy and Jones (1987, 1993); Garnsworthy and Topps (1982); Jones and Garnsworthy (1988, 1989); Land and Leaver (1980,1981); Treacher, Reid and Roberts (1986))

was below 1.0 (Table 23.1). Milk yield in early lactation did not significantly affect conception rate (Table 23.2), but there was a positive relationship (P<0.001) between milk yield and the length of the period from calving to first service (Days to first service = 59 + 0.0038MY, where MY is total milk yield over the first 12 weeks of lactation).

Table 23.1 EFFECCT OF CONDITION SCORE AT CALVING OR AT SERVICE ON CONCEPTION RATE TO FIRST SERVICE IN 2000 HIGH-YIELDING DAIRY COWS (BOURCHIER *et al.*, 1987).

| | *Condition Score at Calving* | | | | | |
	<1.5	*1.5*	*2*	*2.5*	*3*	*3.5+*
Conception rate	0.47	0.56	0.57	0.57	0.56	0.56

| | *Condition Score at Service* | | | | |
	<1.5	*1.5*	*2*	*2.5*	*3+*
Conception rate	0.47	0.56	0.54	0.51	0.58

Further analysis of data from this survey (Garnsworthy and Haresign, 1989) suggested that dairy cows of high genetic merit show poorest conception rates when they lose a lot of body condition between calving and service (Table 23.3). The lowest conception rates (<0.30) were found in cows that lost more than 1.5 condition-score units between calving and service but also had relatively low milk yields (<30 litres/day). This suggests

Table 23.2 EFFECCT OF MILK YIELD DURING THE FIRST TWELVE WEEKS OF LACTATION ON CONCEPTION RATE TO FIRST SERVICE IN 2000 HIGH-YIELDING DAIRY COWS (BOURCHIER *et al.*, 1987).

	Milk Yield (l/day)		
	<30	*30-36*	*>36*
Conception rate	0.47	0.56	0.56

Table 23.3 EFFECCT OF CONDITION SCORE LOSS FROM CALVING TO FIRST SERVICE ON CONCEPTION RATE TO FIRST SERVICE IN 2000 HIGH-YIELDING DAIRY COWS (BOURCHIER *et al.*, 1987).

	Condition score loss			
	>1.5	*1*	*0.5*	*<0*
Conception rate	47	56	53	63

a general upset in the metabolism of a cow that affects production and fertility concurrently, but possibly independently. Further doubt for a direct effect of energy balance on fertility stems from the fact that until the early 1980s dairy cows were managed under systems that encouraged a much greater degree of mobilisation of body reserves, yet conception rates were far higher than today.

Requirements for specific nutrients

In addition to the general effects of energy and protein balance on fertility, dairy cows have specific requirements for certain nutrients, such as vitamins and minerals. Vitamins A, D and E have been shown to have direct effects on fertility, but others, such as thiamine, niacin, vitamin B12 and choline may have act indirectly through their effects on metabolism (Bieber-Wlaschny, 1988). Many minerals can also have direct and indirect effects on fertility, often in association with vitamins (McDonald, Edwards, Greenhalgh and Morgan, 1995).

Influence of nutrition on metabolic hormones

High milk yields and/or undernutrition cause an increase in circulating concentrations of growth hormone (GH), accompanied by decreases in circulating levels of insulin and liver GH receptors. These factors reduce the production of insulin-like growth factor-I

(IGF-I) and IGF binding protein in the liver, so the net effect is that plasma concentrations of IGF-I falls, despite elevated levels of GH (Pell and Bates, 1990; Thissen, Ketelslegers and Underwood, 1994; Armstrong, Cohick, Harvey, Heimer and Campbell, 1993; Spicer, Crowe, Prendiville, Goulding and Enright, 1992). In contrast, when insulin concentration is high during overfeeding, IGF-I production increases. This is despite a decline in GH secretion and is probably due to enhanced binding of GH to its receptor, caused by insulin.

The IGF system has many components. There are two peptides, IGF-I and IGF-II, that both act on the type 1 IGF receptor (IGF-1R). The type 2 IGF receptor is thought to act as a clearance molecule for IGF-II. There is also a family of six IGF binding proteins (IGFBPs 1-6). These can either inhibit IGF activity (by reducing its bioavailability to bind to the type 1 receptor) or enhance it (by targeting IGFs to a particular tissue and acting as a local reservoir within it) (Jones and Clemmons, 1995). All of these factors may act as signals of metabolic status to the reproductive system, as discussed below. As well as being produced by the liver, these members of the IGF system are also expressed in the ovaries and the reproductive tract (Armstrong and Webb, 1997; Webb and Armstrong, 1998).

Mechanistic influences on fertility

At the mechanistic level, several reproductive stages have been identified where high milk yields, inadequate nutrition or excessive mobilisation of body reserves may have detrimental effects. These include the hypothalamus/pituitary gland, follicular growth, corpus luteum function, oocyte quality, uterine environment and embryo survival.

EFFECT OF DIET ON GONADOTROPHINS

As well as affecting metabolic hormones, diet can also influence the production of luteinising hormone (LH) by the pituitary gland, although follicle-stimulating hormone (FSH) does not seem to be affected by diet (Rhodes, Fitzpatrick, Entwistle and De'ath, 1995). Significant changes in body weight can alter the pattern of LH secretion (Gonzales-Padilla, Wiltban and Niswender, 1975; Yelich, Wettemann, Marston and Spicer, 1996). Canfield and Butler (1990) observed that baseline and mean concentration of LH and LH pulse frequency were higher in cows after the energy balance nadir compared with before the energy balance nadir. Extremes of nutrition appear to affect pituitary gonadotrophin secretion - although in most cases the pituitary gland is capable of releasing adequate amounts and patterns of gonadotrophins, the response to gonadotrophin-releasing hormone (GnRH) is reduced once a compromising body condition score is reached (Roberson, Stumpf, Wolfe, Cupp, Kojima, Werth, Kittok and Kinder, 1992). In beef cows body condition at parturition was found to be directly related to LH pulse frequency, particularly in thin cows (Bishop, Wettemann and Spicer, 1994; Wright, Rhind, Smith and Whyte, 1992).

EFFECT OF DIET ON OVARIAN FUNCTION

Follicular development in cattle is primarily controlled by the co-ordinated action of hypothalamic GnRH and pituitary gonadotrophins (Campbell, Scaramuzzi and Webb, 1995; Webb, Gong, Law and Rusbridge, 1992; Webb, Gong and Bramley, 1994; Gong and Webb, 1996). These authors have demonstrated that without pulsatile release of LH, dominant follicle development could not proceed past 7-9 mm in diameter (Gong, Campbell, Bramley, Gutierrez, Peters and Webb, 1996). When FSH concentrations were subsequently suppressed, after GnRH-agonist treatment, follicle growth stopped at 4 mm in diameter. Therefore, since follicle development depends on sustained support by gonadotrophins, nutritionally induced changes in gonadotrophin secretion will affect follicular development. Folliculogenesis in cattle is characterised by a continuous turnover of follicular waves (see Webb *et al.* 1992; Gong and Webb, 1996). Each wave of follicle development involves the simultaneous growth of a cohort of 5-7 antral follicles from the growing pool to >5 mm in diameter and then the selection of one of these follicles to grow rapidly while other cohort follicles regress. The selected follicle continues to grow to become a dominant follicle with a diameter of about 15 mm and remains at maximum size for 2-3 days before regression, followed by a new wave of follicle development. It appears that approximately 80% of cattle have three waves of follicular growth and development during each oestrous cycle and it is the dominant follicle produced during the third wave that usually ovulates. However, follicular waves have also been shown to occur during the post-partum anoestrus period (Boland, Goulding and Roche, 1991; Beam and Butler, 1997). Following ovulation and fertilisation optimum progesterone, from the newly formed corpus luteum is essential in order to provide optimal conditions in the oviduct and uterus for embryonic growth and development.

Waves of follicular development in cows are normally initiated soon after calving (Boland *et al*, 1991; Beam and Butler, 1997). During this period, the degree of negative energy balance can affect follicular development. The lower energy balance of lactating cows is accompanied by fewer follicles of >15 mm in diameter (de la Sota, Lucy, Staples and Thatcher, 1993) but higher numbers of small (3-5 mm) and medium-sized (6-9 mm) follicles (Lucy, Staples, Michel and Thatcher, 1991a, 1991b). Furthermore, when cows are fed on low energy diets, the growth rate of preovulatory follicles is slower than that of follicles from cows fed on high energy diets (Murphy, Enright, Crowe, McConnell, Spicer, Boland and Roche, 1991; Lucy, Beck, Staples, Head, de la Sota and Thatcher, 1992a).

In beef cattle, the preovulatory follicle has a smaller diameter when animals are losing weight (Murphy *et al.,* 1991; Grimard, Humblot, Ponter, Mialot, Sauvant and Thibier, 1995; Rhodes *et al.,* 1995). The reduction in follicle diameter was positively correlated with weight loss until the animals ceased ovulating (Rhodes *et al.*, 1995). In contrast, an increase in diameter of the largest follicle was seen when heifers were gaining weight (Rhodes *et al.*, 1995; Murphy *et al.*, 1991; Spicer, Enright, Murphy and Roche, 1991). These follicles were also dominant, since the number of subordinate follicles was reduced as the first ovulation postpartum approached (Gutierrez, Galina, Zarco and Rubio, 1994).

The ovarian IGF system is a key component of the regulatory system that controls folliculogenesis within the ovary (Armstrong and Webb, 1997; Webb and Armstrong, 1998). It appears that dietary energy and protein can also regulate the expression of mRNA encoding components of the ovarian IGF system. For example, diets shown previously to increase the number of small ovarian follicles in cattle (Gutierrez, Oldham, Bramley, Gong, Campbell and Webb, 1997a), decreased the expression of mRNA encoding IGFBP-2 in similar size small (<4 mm) healthy bovine follicles (Armstrong, Baxter, Sinclair, Robinson, McEvoy and Webb, unpublished observations). This is similar to the case in the development of the dominant follicle (>8 mm) in cattle, where granulosa cell IGFBP-2 mRNA expression is reduced (Armstrong, Baxter, Gutierrez, Hogg, Glazyria, Campbell, Bramley and Webb, 1998). Reduced production of IGFBP-2 probably results in upregulating the bioavailability of IGFs, leading to enhanced gonadotrophic stimulation of ovarian follicular cells (Gutierrez, Campbell and Webb, 1997b).

Factors such as GH, insulin and IGF can have a pronounced influence on ovarian follicle development in cattle (Armstrong and Webb, 1997; Webb and Armstrong, 1998). Therefore, it is likely that changes in these factors during early lactation will alter the pattern of ovarian follicle growth and development, thereby influencing reproductive function. To test this working hypothesis, possible links between metabolic changes and patterns of ovarian follicular growth and development during the early postpartum period, were studied in dairy cows on intensive and extensive systems (Gong, Logue, Crawshaw and Webb, unpublished data). No obvious differences in the pattern of ovarian follicular development between either the high and low input systems or autumn and spring calving seasons were observed. These results suggest that reproductive function need not be compromised by high milk output, providing nutritional inputs are adequate. This emphasises that it is not the absolute input or output, but the balance between input and output, which is really important.

Treatment of lactating cows with bovine somatotrophin (BST), which increases milk production and reduces energy balance, stimulated an increase in the number of follicles reaching the larger size categories and decreased the number of small (<5 mm) follicles (de la Sota *et al.*, 1993; Lucy *et al.*, 1992a). In heifers, administration of BST increased the number of small follicles (<5 mm), but did not alter the number of large follicles (>5 mm) or the dynamics of follicle turnover (Gong, Bramley and Webb, 1991; 1993). BST had no effect on circulating concentrations of FSH and LH or gonadotrophin binding to theca and granulosa cells (Gong *et al.*, 1991). The action of BST therefore appears to be via circulating insulin and IGF-I concentrations (Gong *et al.* 1993; de la Sota *et al.* 1993; Lucy, Collier, Kitchell, Dibner, Hauser and Krivi, 1993). It is likely that insulin and/

or IGF-I alter the response of follicular cells to gonadotrophins, as shown by recent *in vitro* studies culturing bovine follicular cells (Gutierrez *et al.*, 1997b) and *in vivo* dose-response studies (Gong, Baxter, Bramley and Webb, 1997). This also indicates that a change in circulating gonadotrophin concentrations is not essential.

Immunisation of prepubertal heifers against GH releasing hormone reduces the circulating concentrations of GH. The proportion of heifers developing follicles above 7 mm in diameter was only 0.22, compared with 0.77 of control heifers (Cohick, Armstrong, Withacre, Lucy, Harvey and Campbell, 1996). Recently, increased dietary intake has been associated with increased small follicle recruitment during the first follicular wave of the oestrous cycle in Holstein-Friesian heifers (Gutierrez *et al.*, 1997a). The number of small follicles returned to normal as soon as dietary treatments were terminated. The number of medium-size follicles increased in all groups, at the time when numbers of small follicles were decreasing. Taken together, these results indicate that nutrition appears to affect mainly the recruitment of small follicles.

Metabolic hormones and reproductive function were recently measured in dairy cows of High and Low genetic merit during early lactation (Gutierrez, Gong and Webb, unpublished data). Resumption of normal oestrous cycles postpartum occurred approximately 8 days later in the High-line cows, and this was associated with lower plasma insulin concentrations. A further study was designed to investigate if feeding diets to increase circulating insulin concentrations during the early postpartum period can overcome the delay in the first ovulation postpartum in animals selected for increased milk yield. Two isoenergetic diets were formulated to either stimulate or depress plasma insulin concentrations, and these were fed to cows of High or Low genetic merit. Again, the initiation of the first ovulation and the resumption of normal oestrous cycles postpartum were delayed in the cows of high genetic merit. This was associated with lower circulating insulin concentrations, but did not involve an alteration in basal plasma gonadotrophin concentrations and patterns of ovarian follicular development during the early postpartum period. Feeding the diet designed to increase circulating insulin concentrations advanced the initiation of the first ovulation postpartum so that fewer cows failed to ovulate within the first 50 days of lactation (Table 23.4; Gong, Lee, Garnsworthy and Webb, 2002).

Table 23.4 NUMBER OF ANIMALS THAT DID NOT OVULATE WITHIN 50 DAYS OF CALVING IN HIGH AND LOW GENETIC MERIT DAIRY COWS FED ON DIETS THAT INDUCED HIGH OR LOW CONCENTARTIONS OF PLASMA INSULIN (GONG, LEE, GARNSWORTHY AND WEBB; 2002).

		Diet	
		High Insulin	*Low Insulin*
Genetic merit	High	2/10	5/10
	Low	0/10	4/10

Increasing the fat content of the diet increases both the number and size of follicles present in the ovary and can also shorten the interval from parturition to first ovulation (Lucy *et al.*, 1991b; Lucy, Savio, Badinga, de la Sota and Thatcher, 1992b; Hightshoe, Cochran, Corah, Kiracofe, Harmon and Perry, 1991; Ryan, Spoon and Williams, 1992; Lammoglia, Willard, Hallford and Randel, 1997; Beam and Butler, 1997; Thomas and Williams, 1996). Raised blood cholesterol could increase precursor availability for follicular steroid synthesis. Since oestradiol-17b induces proliferation of granulosa cells this might, in turn, increase follicular progesterone (Talavera, Park and Williams, 1985; Carroll, Jerred, Grummer, Combs, Pierson and Hauser, 1990; Hawkins, Niswender, Oss, Moeller, Odde, Sawyer and Niswender, 1995; Burke, Carroll, Rowe, Thatcher and Stormshak, 1996). Another possibility is that clearance rates of progesterone from plasma may be reduced (Hawkins *et al.*, 1995). This elevation in progesterone could have a beneficial effect on fertility, as suboptimal progesterone concentrations are associated with high return rates in cows.

EFFECTS OF DIET ON OOCYTE QUALITY AND EMBRYO SURVIVAL

In sheep, it has been shown that energy intake by oocyte donors, but not dietary protein concentration, influences blastocyst production from oocytes cultured *in vitro* (McEvoy, Robinson, Aitken, Findlay and Robertson., 1997a). It has also been found that dietary energy affects blastocyst production from oocytes collected from 2-4 mm bovine follicles (McEvoy, Sinclair, Staines, Robinson, Armstrong and Webb, 1997b). This fits with the observations discussed above that nutrition affects the growth of small follicles and IGF expression.

Dietary PUFA composition may alter progesterone output via changes in the production of eicosanoids within the corpus luteum. Altering the balance of endogenous prostaglandin production within the corpus luteum could potentially alter both the production of progesterone and the overall length of the luteal phase. Maternal progesterone concentrations during the early luteal phase appear to affect development of the embryo and its ability to inhibit luteolysis through secretion of antiluteolytic trophoblast interferon (IFNL) (Mann, Lamming and Fisher, 1998).

Diets high in rumen degradable protein lead to high concentrations of rumen ammonia, which may alter uterine pH and endometrial Na and K fluxes, with reduced embryo survival. The detrimental effect of this increase in ammonia on protein synthesis in day 4 ovine embryos has been clearly shown (Robinson and McEvoy, 1996). In cattle, high ammonia levels have been associated with reduced oocyte cleavage rates (Sinclair, Kurran, Gebbie, Webb and McEvoy, 2000). Slowly degraded protein leads to lower ammonia concentrations, which may explain why fishmeal sometimes improves fertility (Armstrong, Goodall, Gordon, Rice and McGaughey, 1990). Fishmeal also supplies essential fatty acids, which may enhance embryo survival through their anti-luteolytic properties (Coelho, Ambrose, Binelli, Burke, Staples, Thatcher and Thatcher, 1997).

EMBRYO DEVELOPMENT

Maintenance of pregnancy is dependent on the embryo prolonging the lifespan of the corpus luteum by preventing luteolysis. This is achieved by secretion of IFNt by the conceptus (Roberts, Cross and Leaman, 1992) which in turn inhibits the development of oxytocin receptors (OTR) in the endometrium (Wathes and Lamming, 1995). The development of OTR is essential for pulsatile secretion of $PGF_2\mu$ to occur. Several studies in both cattle and sheep have shown that lipid infusions can alter the ability of the uterus to respond to a challenge of oxytocin in the late luteal phase in terms of $PGF_2\mu$ release and may affect cycle length (Thatcher, Staples, Danet-Desnoyers, Oldick and Schmitt, 1994; Burke *et al.*, 1996). An endometrial cyclo-oxygenase inhibitor isolated from the bovine endometrium was also identified as linoleic acid (Danet-Desnoyers, Johnson, O'Keefe and Thatcher, 1993; Thatcher, Meyer and Danet-Desnoyers, 1995) and was present at a higher concentration in pregnant compared with non-pregnant uteri. It is therefore possible that the ability of a particular cow to maintain a pregnancy by inhibiting luteolysis may be influenced by her dietary PUFA intake.

There is considerable evidence that the IGF system is important in embryo development (Wathes, Reynolds, Robinson and Stevenson, 1998). IGFs could potentially influence the embryo indirectly by altering the metabolic and secretory activity of the reproductive tract. It has been shown that many components of the IGF system are expressed in the bovine and ovine reproductive tracts (Geisert, Lee, Simmen, Zavy, Fliss, Bazer and Simmen, 1991; Stevenson, Gilmour and Wathes, 1994; Reynolds, Stevenson and Wathes, 1997; Kirby, Thatcher, Collier, Simmen and Lucy, 1996, Robinson, Mann, Lamming and Wathes, 1997). As discussed above, the main regulator of the maternal IGF system is nutrition (McGuire, Vicini, Bauman and Veenhuizen, 1992; Thissen *et al.*, 1994).

Conclusions

In conclusion, further knowledge is required before the complete relationships between milk yield, nutrition and fertility can be explained. Poor fertility is not an inevitable consequence of high genetic merit, but may be due to a combination of factors that include genetic susceptibility, management, disease, milk yield, energy balance, body reserves and specific nutritional circumstances.

The absolute requirements of an oocyte or developing embryo for energy and protein are minuscule, compared with the cow's requirements for milk production. However, nutrition can have major effects on metabolic hormones, which can cascade through the IGF system to have repercussions at the tissue or cellular level.

Because so many factors influence reproductive function in dairy cows, it is very difficult to predict whether an individual cow will be fertile under a given set of circumstances. However, it is possible to identify certain risk factors that may predispose cows to infertility (Figure 23.3). These include excesses or deficiencies of energy and

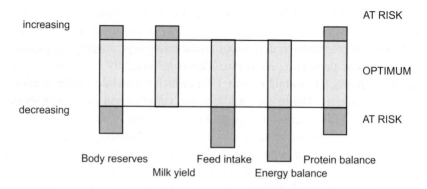

Figure 23.3 Possible risk factors causing infertility in dairy cows. For optimum fertility, all production measures should be in the central region; high or low values for these measures increase the risk of infertility

protein, severe negative energy balance and excessive weight loss. The susceptibility of a cow to these risks is influenced by her genetic merit, general health and management conditions.

References

Agricultural Research Council (1980) *The Nutrient Requirements of Ruminant Livestock*, Commonwealth Agricultural Bureaux, Slough.

Agnew, R.E., Yan, T. and Gordon, F.J. (1998) Nutrition of the high genetic merit dairy cow – energy metabolism studies. In *Recent Advances in Animal Nutrition – 1998* (eds P.C. Garnsworthy and J. Wiseman), pp 181-208, Nottingham University Press, Nottingham.

Armstrong, D. G., Baxter, G., Gutierrez, C. G., Hogg, C. O., Glazyria, A. L., Campbell, B. K., Bramley, T. A. and Webb, R. 1998. Insulin-like growth factor binding protein-2 and –4 messenger ribonucleic acid expression in bovine ovarian follicles: effects of gonadotrophins and developmental states. *Endocrinology* **139**, 2146-2154.

Armstrong, J. D., Cohick, W. S., Harvey, R. W., Heimer, E. P. and Campbell, R. M. 1993. Effect of feed restriction on serum somatotrophin, insulin-like growth factor-1 (IGF-1) and binding proteins in cyclic heifers actively immunised against growth hormone releasing factor. *Domestic Animal Endocrinology* **10**, 315-324.

Armstrong, J. D., Goodall, E. A., Gordon, F. J., Rice, D. A. and McGaughey, W. J. 1990. The effect of levels of concentrate offered and inclusion of maize gluten or fishmeal in the concentrate on reproductive performance and blood parameters of dairy cows. *Animal Production* **50**, 1-10.

Armstrong, D. G. and Webb, R. 1997. Ovarian follicular dominance: novel mechanisms and protein factors. Reviews of Reproduction **3**, 134-146.

Beam, S. W. and Butler, W. R. 1997. Energy balance and ovarian follicle development prior to the first ovulation postpartum in dairy cows receiving three levels of dietary fat. *Biology of Reproduction* **56**, 133-142.

Bieber-Wlashny, M. (1988) Vitamin requirements of the dairy cow. In *Nutrition and Lactation in the Dairy Cow* (ed P.C. Garnsworthy), pp 135-156, Butterworths, London.

Bishop, D. K., Wettemann, R. P. and Spicer, L. J. 1994. Body energy reserves influence the onset of luteal activity after early weaning of beef cows. *Journal of Animal Science.***72**, 2703-2708.

Boland, M. P., Goulding, D. and Roche, J. F. 1991. The use of ultrasound to monitor ovarian function in farm animals. *Ag. Biotechnology News Information* **2**, 841-844.

Bourchier, C. P., Garnsworthy, P. C., Hutchinson, J. M. and Benson, T. A. 1987. The relationship between milk yield, body condition and reproductive performance in high-yielding dairy cows. *Animal Production* **44**, 460 (abstract).

Burke, J. M., Carroll, D. J., Rowe, K.E., Thatcher, W.W. and Stormshak, F. 1996. Intravascular infusion of lipid into ewes stimulates production of progesterone and prostaglandin. *Biology of Reproduction* **55**, 169-175

Campbell, B.K., Scaramuzzi, R. J. and Webb, R. 1995. Control of antral follicle development and selection in sheep and cattle. *Journal of Reproduction and Fertility Supplement* **49**, 335-350.

Canfield, R. W. and Butler, W. R. 1990. Energy balance and pulsatile LH secretion in early postpartum dairy cattle. *Domestic Animal Endocrinology* **7**, 323-330.

Carroll, D. J., Jerred, M. J., Grummer, R. R., Combs, D. K., Pierson, R. A. and Hauser, E. R. 1990. Effects of fat supplementation and immature alfalfa to concentrate ratio on plasma progesterone, energy balance and reproductive traits of dairy cattle. *Journal of Dairy Science* **73**, 2855-2863.

Coelho, S., Ambrose, J. D., Binelli, M., Burke, J., Staples, C. R., Thatcher, M. J. and Thatcher, W. W. 1997. Menhaden fish meal attenuates estradiol- and oxytocin-induced uterine secretion of $PGF_2\mu$ in lactating dairy cattle. *Theriogenology* **47**, 143.

Cohick, W. S., Armstrong, J. D., Withacre, M. D., Lucy, M. C., Harvey, R. W. and Campbell, R. M. 1996. Ovarian expression of insulin-like growth factor-I (IGF-I), IGF binding proteins, and growth hormone (GH) receptor in heifers actively immunized against GH-releasing factor. *Endocrinology* **137**, 1670-1677.

Danet-Desnoyers, G., Johnson, J. W., O'Keefe, S. F. and Thatcher, W. W. 1993. Characterization of a bovine endometrial prostaglandin synthesis inhibitor (EPSI). *Biology of Reproduction* **48**, Supplement 115.

de la Sota, R. L., Lucy, M. C., Staples, C. R. and Thatcher, W. W. 1993. Effects of recombinant bovine somatotropin (Sometribove) on ovarian function in lactating and nonlactating dairy cows. *Journal of Dairy Science* **76**, 1002-1013.

Garnsworthy, P.C. (1988) The effect of energy reserves at calving on performance of dairy cows. In *Nutrition and Lactation in the Dairy Cow* (ed P.C. Garnsworthy), pp 157-170, Butterworths, London.

Garnsworthy, P. C. and Haresign, W. 1989. Fertility and nutrition. In *Dairy Cow Nutrition – The Veterinary Angles.* (Ed. A. T. Chamberlain) pp23-34. The University of Reading, Department of Agriculture.

Garnsworthy, P. C. and Huggett, C. D. 1992, The influence of the fat concentration of the diet on the response by dairy cows to body condition at calving. *Animal Production* **54**: 7-13.

Garnsworthy, P. C. and Jones, G. P. 1987. The influence of body condition at calving and dietary protein supply on voluntary food intake and performance in dairy cows. *Animal Production* **44**, 347-353.

Garnsworthy, P. C. and Jones, G. P. 1993. The effects of dietary fibre and starch concentrations on the response by dairy cows to body condition at calving. *Animal Production* **57**, 15-21.

Garnsworthy, P. C. and Topps, J. H. 1982. The effect of body condition of dairy cows at calving on their food intake and performance when given complete diets. *Animal Production* 35: 113-119.

Geisert, R. D., Lee, C., Simmen, F. A., Zavy, M. T., Fliss, A. E., Bazer, F. W. and Simmen, R. C. M. 1991. Expression of messenger RNAs encoding insulin-like growth factor-I, -II and insulin-like growth factor binding proteins-2 in bovine endometrium during the estrous cycle and early pregnancy. *Biology of Reproduction* **45**, 975-983.

Gong, J. G., Baxter, G., Bramley, T. A. and Webb, R. 1997. Enhancement of ovarian follicle development in heifers by treatment with recombinant bovine somatotrophin: a dose-response study. *Journal of Reproduction and Fertility* **110**, 91-97.

Gong, J. G., Bramley, T. A. and Webb, R. 1991. The effect of recombinant bovine somatotropin on ovarian function in heifers: Follicular populations and peripheral hormones. *Biology of Reproduction* **45**, 941-949.

Gong, J. G., Bramley, T. A. and Webb, R. 1993. The effect of recombinant bovine somatotrophin on ovarian follicular growth and development in heifers. *Journal of Reproduction and Fertility* **97**, 247-254.

Gong, J. G. and Webb, R. 1996. Control of ovarian follicle development in domestic ruminants: its manipulation to increase ovulation rate and improve reproductive performance. *Animal Breeding,* Abstract **64**, 195-204.

Gong, J. G., Campbell, B. K., Bramley, T. A., Gutierrez, C. G., Peters, A. R. and Webb, R. 1996. Suppression in the secretion of follicle-stimulating hormone and luteinizing hormone, and ovarian follicle development in heifers continuously infused with a gonadotropin-releasing hormone agonist. *Biology of Reproduction* **55**, 68-74.

Gong, J.G., Lee, W.J., Garnsworthy, P.C. and Webb, R. 2002. Effect of dietary induced increases in circulating insulin concentrations during the early postpartum period on reproductive function in dairy cows. *Reproduction* **123**, 419-427.

Gonzalez-Padilla, E., Wiltban, J. N. and Niswender, G. D. 1975. Puberty in beef heifers. 1. The interrelationship between pitiutary, hypotalamic and ovarian hormones. *Journal of Animal Science* **40**, 1091-1104.

Grimard, B., Humblot, P., Ponter, A. A., Mialot, J. P., Sauvant, D. and Thibier, M. 1995. Influence of postpartum energy restriction on energy status, plasma LH and oestradiol secretion and follicular development in suckled beef cows. *Journal of Reproduction and Fertility* **104**, 173-179.

Gutierrez, C. G., Campbell, B. K. and Webb, R. 1997b. Development of a long-term bovine granulosa cell culture system: induction and maintenance of estradiol production, response to follicle-stimulating hormone and morphological characteristics. *Biology of Reproduction* **56**, 608-616.

Gutierrez, C. G., Galina, C. S., Zarco, L. and Rubio, I. 1994. Pattern of follicular growth during prepuberal anoestrous and transition from anoestrous to oestrous cycles in *Bos indicus* heifers. *Advanced Agricultural Research* **3**, 1-11.

Gutierrez, C. G., Oldham, J., Bramley, T. A., Gong, J. G., Campbell, B. K. and Webb, R. 1997a. The recruitment of ovarian follicles is enhanced by increased dietary intake in heifers. *Journal of Animal Science* **75**, 1876-1884.

Hawkins, D. E., Niswender, K. D., Oss, G. M., Moeller, C. L., Odde, K. G., Sawyer, H. R. and Niswender, G. D. 1995. An increase in serum lipids increases luteal lipid content and alters disappearance rate of progesterone in cows. *Journal of Animal Science* **73**, 541-545.

Hightshoe, R. B., Cochran, R. C., Corah, L. R., Kiracofe, G. H., Harmon, D. L. and Perry, R.,C. 1991. Effects of calcium soaps of fatty acids on postpartum reproductive function in beef cows. *Journal of Animal Science* **69**, 4097-5004.

Holmes, C. W. 1988. Genetic merit and efficiency of milk production by the dairy cow. In *Nutrition and Lactation in the Dairy Cow*, Ed. Philip C. Garnsworthy, pp 195-215, Butterworths, London.

Jones, J. I. and Clemmons, D. R. 1995. Insulin-like growth factors and their binding proteins. *Endocrine Reviews* **16**, 3-34.

Jones, G. P. and Garnsworthy, P. C. 1988. The effects of body condition at calving and dietary protein content on dry-matter intake and performance in lactating dairy cows given diets of low energy content. *Animal Production* **47**, 321-333.

Jones, G. P. and Garnsworthy, P. C. 1989. The effects of dietary energy content on the response by dairy cows to body condition at calving, *Animal Production*, **49**, 183-191

Kirby, C. J., Thatcher, W. W., Collier, R. J., Simmen, F. A. and Lucy, M. C. 1996. Effects of growth hormone and pregnancy on expression of growth hormone receptor, insulin-like growth factor-1, and insulin-like growth factor binding protein-2 and -3 genes in bovine uterus, ovary and oviduct. *Biology of Reproduction* **55**, 996-1002.

Lamming, G.E., Darwash, A.O., Wathes, D.C. and Ball, P.J. (1998) The fertility of dairy cattle in the UK: current status and future research. *Journal of the Royal Agricultural Society of England,* **159**, 82-93.

Lammoglia, M. A., Willard, S. T., Hallford, D. M. and Randel, R. D. 1997. Effects of dietary fat on follicular development and circulating concentrations of lipids, insulin, progesterone, estradiol-17ß, 13,14-dihydro-15-keto-prostaglandin F2α and growth hormone in estrous cyclic Brahman cows. *Journal of Animal Science* **75**, 1591-1600.

Land, C. and Leaver, J.D. 1980 The effect of body condition at calving on the milk production and feed intake of dairy cows. *Animal Production,* **30**, 449 (abstract)

Land, C. and Leaver, J.D. 1980 The effect of body condition at calving on the production of Friesian cows and heifers. *Animal Production,* **32**, 362-363 (abstract)

Lucy, M. C., Beck, J., Staples, C. R., Head, H. H., de la Sota, R. L. and Thatcher, W. W. 1992a. Follicular dynamics, plasma metabolites, hormones and insulin-like growth factor (IGF-1) in lactating cows with positive or negative energy balance during the preovulatory period. *Reproduction Nutrition Development* **32**, 331-341.

Lucy, M. C., Collier, R. J., Kitchell, M. L., Dibner, J. J., Hauser, S. D. and Krivi, G. G. 1993. Immnunohistochemical and nucleic acid analysis of somatotropin receptor populations in the bovine ovary. *Biology of Reproduction* **48**, 1219-1227.

Lucy, M. C., Savio, J. D., Badinga, L., de la Sota, R. L. and Thatcher, W. W. 1992b. Factors that affect ovarian follicular dynamics in cattle. *Journal of Animal Science* **70**, 3615-3626.

Lucy, M. C., Staples, C. R., Michel, F. M. and Thatcher, W. W. 1991a. Energy Balance and size and number of ovarian follicles detected by ultrasonography in early postpartum dairy cows. *Journal of Dairy Science* **74**, 473-482.

Lucy, M. C., Staples, C. R., Michel, F. M. and Thatcher, W. W. 1991b. Effect of feeding calcium soaps to early postpartum dairy cows on plasma prostaglandin F$_2$α, luteinizing hormone, and follicular growth. *Journal of Dairy Science* **74**, 483-489.

Mann, G. E., Lamming, G. E. and Fisher, P. A. 1998. Progesterone control of embryonic interferon tan production during early pregnancy in the cow. *Journal of Reproduction and Fertility,* Abstract Series **21**, Abstract 37.

McDonald, P., Edwards, R.A., Greenhalgh, J.F.D. and Morgan, C.A. (1995) *Animal Nutrition,* 5th Edition, pp 97-127, Longman Scxientific and Technical, Harlow.

McEvoy, T. G., Robinson, J. J., Aitken, R. P., Findlay, P. A. and Robertson, I. S. 1997a. Dietary excesses of urea influence the viability and metabolism of preimplantation sheep embryos and may affect fetal growth among survivors. *Animal Reproduction Science* **47**, 71-90.

McEvoy, T. G., Sinclair, K. D., Staines, M. E., Robinson, J. J., Armstrong, D. G. and Webb, R. 1997b. *In vitro* blastocyst production in relation to energy and protein intake prior to oocyte collection. *Journal of Reproduction and Fertility,* Abstract Series **19**, Abstract **132**, page 51.

McGuire, M. A., Vicini, J. L., Bauman, D. E. and Veenhuizen, J. J. 1992. Insulin-like growth factors and binding proteins in ruminants and their nutritional regulation.

Journal of Animal Science **70**, 2901-2910.

Murphy, M. G., Enright, W. J., Crowe, M. A., McConnell, K., Spicer, L. J., Boland, M. P. and Roche, J. F. 1991. Effect of dietary intake on pattern of growth of dominant follicles during the oestrous cycle in beef heifers. *Journal of Reproduction and Fertility* **92**, 333-338.

Pell, J. M. and Bates, P. C. 1990. The nutritional regulation of growth hormone action. *Nutrition Research Reviews* **3**, 163-192.

Reynolds, T. S., Stevenson, K. R. and Wathes, D. C. 1997. Pregnancy-specific alterations in the expression of the insuli-like growth factor system during early placental development in the ewe. *Endocrinology* **138**, 886-897.

Rhodes, F. M., Fitzpatrick, L. A., Entwistle, K. W. and De'ath, G. 1995. Sequential changes in ovarian follicular dynamics in *Bos indicus* heifers before and after nutritional anoestrus. *Journal of Reproduction and Fertility* **104**, 41-49.

Roberson, M. S., Stumpf, T. T., Wolfe, M. W., Cupp, A. S., Kojima, N., Werth, L. A., Kittok, R. J. and Kinder, J. E. 1992. Circulating gonadotrophins during a period of restricted energy intake in relation to body condition in heifers. *Journal of Reproduction and Fertility* **96**, 461-469.

Roberts, R. M., Cross, J. C. and Leaman, D. W. 1992. Interferons as hormones of pregnancy. *Endocrine Reviews* **13**, 432-452.

Robinson, R. S., Mann, G. E., Lamming, G. E. and Wathes, D. C. 1997. The localization of IGF-I,-II and IGF type 1 receptor in the bovine uterus on day 16 of pregnancy. *Journal of Endocrinology* **155**, Supplement p64.

Robinson, J. J. and McEvoy, T. G. 1996. Feeding level and rumen degradable nitrogen effects on embryo survival. In "Techniques for Gamete Manipulation and Storage". ICAR Satellite Symposium, Hamilton, New Zealand.

Ryan, D. P., Spoon, R. A. and Williams, G. L. 1992. Ovarian follicle characteristics, embryo recovery and embryo viability in heifers fed high fat diets and treated with follicle stimulating hormone. *Journal of Animal Science* **70**, 3505-3513.

Sinclair, K. D., Kuran, M., Gebbie, F. E., Webb, R. and McEvoy, T. G. (2000). Nitrogen metabolism and fertility in cattle: II. Development of oocytes recovered from heifers offered diets differing in their rate of nitrogen release in the rumen. *Journal of Animal Science*, **78**, 2670-2680.

Spicer, L., Crowe, M. A., Prendiville, D. J., Goulding, D. and Enright, W. J. 1992. Systemic but not intraovarian concentrations of insulin-like growth factor-I are affected by short-term fasting. *Biology of Reproduction* **46**, 920-925.

Spicer, L. J., Enright, W. J., Murphy, M. G. and Roche, J. F. 1991. Effect of dietary intake on concentrations of insulin-like growth factor-1 in plasma and follicular fluid, and ovarian function in heifers. *Domestic Animal Endocrinology* **8**, 431-437.

Stevenson, K. R., Gilmour, R. S. and Wathes, D. C. 1994. Localization of insulin-like growth factor-I and -II messenger ribonucleic acid and type 1 IGF receptors in the ovine uterus during the estrous cycle and early pregnancy. *Endocrinology* **134**, 1655-1664.

Talavera, F., Park, C. S. and Williams, G. L. 1985. Relationships among dietary lipid intake, serum cholesterol and ovarian function in Holstein heifers. *Journal of Animal Science* **60\;** 1045.

Thatcher, W. W., Meyer, M. D. and Danet-Desnoyers, G. 1995. Maternal recognition of pregnancy. *Journal of Reproduction and Fertility (Suppl.)* **49**, 15-28.

Thatcher, W. W., Staples, C. R., Danet-Desnoyers, G., Oldick, B. and Schmitt, E. P. 1994. Embryo health and mortality in sheep and cattle. *Journal of Animal Science* **72** (suppl. 3), 16-30.

Thissen, J-P., Ketelslegers, J-M. and Underwood, L. E. 1994. Nutritional regulation of the insulin-like growth factors. *Endocrinology Reviews* **15**, 80-101.

Thomas, M. G. and Williams, G. L. 1996. Ovarian follicular characteristics, embryo recovery and embryo viability in heifers fed high-fat diets and treated with follicle-stimulating hormone. *Journal of Animal Science* **70**, 3505.

Treacher, R.J., Reid, I.M. and Roberts, C.J. 1986 Effect of body condition at calving on health and performance of dairy cows. *Animal Production,* **43**, 1-6.

Wathes, D. C. and Wooding, F. B. P. 1980. An electron microscopic study of implantation in the cow. *American Journal of Anatomy* **159**, 285-306.

Wathes, D. C. and Lamming, G. E. 1995. The oxytocin receptor, luteolysis and the maternal recognition of pregnancy. *Journal of Reproduction and Fertility Supplement* **49**, 53-67.

Wathes, D. C., Reynolds, T. S., Robinson, R. S. and Stevenson, K. R. 1998. Role of the insulin-like growth factor system in uterine function and placental development in ruminants. *Journal of Dairy Science* **81**, 1778-1789.

Webb, R. and Armstrong, D. G. 1998. Control of ovarian function; effect of local interaction and environmental influence on follicular turnover in cattle: a review. *Livestock Production Science* **53**, 95-112.

Webb, R., Gong, J. G. and Bramley, T. A. 1994. Role of growth hormone and intrafollicuar peptides in follicle development in cattle. *Theriogenology* **41**, 25-30.

Webb, R., Gong, J. G., Law, A. S. and Rusbridge, S. M. 1992. Control of ovarian function in cattle. *Journal of Reproduction and Fertility Supplement* **45**, 141-156.

Wright, I. A., Rhind, S. M., Smith, A. J. and Whyte, T. K. 1992. Effects of body condition and estradiol on luteinizing hormone secretion in post-partum beef cows. *Domestic Animal Endocrinology* **9**, 305-312.

Yelich, J. V., Wettemann, R. P., Marston, T. T. and Spicer, L.J. 1996. Luteinizing hormone, growth hormone, insulin-like growth factor-I, insulin and metabolites before puberty in heifers fed to gain at two rates. *Domestic Animal Endocrinology* **13**, 325-338.

This paper was first published in 1999

24

THE INFLUENCE OF NUTRITION ON LAMENESS IN DAIRY COWS

J.E. Offer, R.J. Berry and D.N. Logue
SAC Veterinary Science Division, Dairy Health Unit, SAC Auchincruive, KA6 5AE

Introduction

Lameness in dairy cows is widespread in all the major dairying countries and the recent Farm Animal Welfare Council report identifies lameness, reduced reproductive efficiency and mastitis as the three main causes of poor welfare in UK dairy cattle. A heightened awareness of pain in lame animals has been demonstrated (Whay, Waterman, and Webster, 1997; Whay, Waterman, Webster, and O'Brien, 1998), reinforcing the suffering that arises with the condition. Lameness is also a source of economic loss from treatment and milk loss, and through its effect on reproductive efficiency (Collick, Ward and Dobson, 1989; Sprecher, Hostetler and Kaneene 1997). It has been estimated by Logue, Offer, Chaplin, Knight, Hendry, Leach, Kempson, and Randall (1995), updating Esslemont's calculations of 1990, that lameness causes an overall loss of £100 million per year to the UK dairy industry. However it must be remembered that these estimates are based on the total losses, not the avoidable losses that may be half of this (McInerney, Howe, and Schepers, 1990). Lameness seems to be a greater problem in dairy cows than in beef suckler cows, although there are interpretative problems. There has been an apparent increase in levels of lameness in the UK over the last 20 years (Clarkson, Downham, Faull, Hughes, Manson, Merrit, Murray, Russell, Sutherst, and Ward, 1996; Esslemont and Kossaibati, 1996) that may be linked with the 15% improvement in milk production per cow per year (Dairy Facts and Figures 1980 and 1996) since a number of studies have found a negative relationship between milk production and dairy cow health and welfare (Emanuelson, 1988; Lyons, Freeman, and Kuck, 1991; Brotherstone and Hill, 1991; Hoekstra, Lugt, Werf and Ouweltjes, 1994; Gröhn, Hertl and Harman, 1994; Pryce, Veerkamp, Thompson, Hill and Simm, 1998). The widespread introduction of the Holstein to the UK, coupled with determined selection for milk production, has been recognised as a contributory factor (Veerkamp, Hill, Stott, Brotherstone and Simm 1995; Webster, 1995a). However this may only be a partial explanation, for there have been concomitant changes in general nutrition and other management factors over this period.

Thus, before discussing the role of nutrition in this multifactorial disease it is necessary to consider some of the wider issues involved in understanding one of the most intractable problems of dairy cow welfare.

Prevalence of lameness

Estimates of the level of lameness in the UK vary widely depending how the data were collected. Veterinary based surveys (Eddy and Scott, 1980; Russell, Rowlands, Shaw, and Weaver, 1982) reported lameness incidence figures of less than 10 cases per 100 cows per year, but these underestimated the problem, since figures based on farmer data (Whitaker, Smith, daRosa, and Kelly, 1983; Booth, 1989) or more intensive surveys (Prentice and Neal, 1972; Arkins 1981, Esslemont and Peeler, 1993) have shown an incidence of approximately 33 cases per 100 cows. Indeed it is likely that both the veterinary and the farmer based surveys have been underestimates as Wells, Trent, Marsh and Robinson (1993) reported farmers and herd managers only classified 40% of "lame" cows diagnosed by investigators. Thus the apparently high incidence of 55 cases per 100 cows per year reported by Clarkson, *et al.* (1996) in England is probably a more accurate reflection of the extent of the condition in the UK (Table 24.1).

Table 24.1 ESTIMATES OF THE INCIDENCE OF LAMENESS IN DAIRY COWS

		British Isles	*Rest of Europe*	*Austalia and New Zealand*
Number of publications		8	5	5
Total cows affected (estimate)		25766	3841	2070
Total cows records (estimate)		202877	13286	40598
Proportion affected	*(mean of data)*	0.13	0.29	0.05
	(mean of studies)	0.22	0.29	0.08
	(range)	0.07-0.55	0.16-0.47	0.02-0.14

The incidence in Australia and New Zealand is somewhat lower than that recorded in the UK and the rest of Europe but while this probably reflects increased grazing time it is suspected that, in some cases, there has been unwitting censorship of the data by the recording farmers.

Types of lameness

There are a variety of descriptive names for lesions associated with lameness and these have been accurately noted in some surveys but not in others. Greenough, Weaver,

Esslemont and Galindo (1997) comment that there is now a need for accuracy of recording of incidence and lesion identification. Without this, accurate epidemiological analysis and interpretation is impossible. It is recognised that for many widely based studies the categories have to be simplified. Based on present understanding of the pathogenesis of the various lesions and their risk factors, data were amalgamated into four categories; claw, interdigital, "non-foot" (upper limb, back etc.) and uncertain (Table 24.2). Using these criteria it can be seen that it is conditions of the foot that are most often observed in lameness cases and that of these claw horn lesions are the most important (Table 24.2). For this reason much lameness research has focused on understanding the development of conditions affecting the claw (Ossent, Greenough and Vermunt, 1997).

Table 24.2 FREQUENCY OF CAUSES OF LAMENESS FROM WORLD-WIDE STUDIES

	British Isles	*Rest of Europe*	*North America*	*Australia and NewZealand*
Number of publications	*6*	*6*	*1*	*5*
Number of observations	19 714	4 869	245	427
Total I/D or Digital lesions	0.20	0.27	0.09	0.18
Total Claw	0.71	0.67	0.87	0.79
White Line	*0.22*	*0.10*	*0.12*	*0.40*
Sole	*0.40*	*0.22*	*0.60*	*0.35*
Foot	*0.07*	*0.23*	*0.13*	*0.05*
Uncertain	0.04	0.07	0.01	0.01
Limb lameness	0.05	n/a	0.04	0.04

Pathogenesis

In the 1950s and 60s our understanding of claw lameness in cattle was heavily influenced by analogy with laminitis in the horse. Nilsson (1963) suggested that the appearance of haemorrhages in the sole and white line of the cow was associated with a loss of integrity of the hoof horn and that this occurred as a result of laminitis. He and later authors proposed that, although this was often insufficient to cause clinical signs (hence "subclinical laminitis"), it was nevertheless a major predisposing factor in the pathogenesis of claw lesions that caused lameness (Nilsson, 1963). This theory has been steadily refined by a series of authors (Peterse, Korver, Oldenbroek and Talmon, 1984; Bradley, Shannon and Neilson, 1989; Greenough and Vermunt, 1991; Ossent and Lischer, 1994 and 1998). Ossent and Lischer have proposed a three-stage pathogenesis to explain the sequence of sole lesion development suggesting that changes in the laminar region of the dermis lead to separation (or at least a distortion) of the dermal and epidermal layers (Stage 1). Consequently, the position of the third phalanx, the final bone of the weight-bearing column, changes relative to the softer tissues of the claw causing pressure-induced haemorrhage and necrosis in the corium of the sole so disrupting hoof horn formation (Stage 2). The predominant sign of this is the appearance of blood and cell debris within the claw horn of the sole and white line. This then leads to a loss of horn integrity and the more severe lesions of the horny capsule (Stage 3). The shape of the distal surface of the third phalanx and the angle at which it drops within the hoof capsule determines the distribution of claw lesions seen in the sole and explains the 'typical sole ulcer site' - the junction between the sole and heel caused by pressure resulting from the flexor process (the most distal point of the sunken bone) - and the development of toe ulcers from the rotation of the third phalanx. They also suggest that white line lesions are caused directly by the initial laminar damage leading to accumulation of the blood and debris in the horn. This part of the hypothesis is supported by the slightly different patterns of development between sole and white line lesions observed by Leach, Logue, Kempson, Offer, Ternent, and Randall (1997) and Offer, McNulty and Logue (1998). If disruption of the dermal-epidermal junction is severe then the change in position of the distal phalanx may be irreversible explaining how, once a cow presents with a severe claw condition such as sole ulceration, it is much more likely to present with the same condition in a subsequent lactation (Enevoldsen, Grohn and Thysen, 1991; Alban, 1995).

Aetiology

While this hypothesis fits observations of the development of claw horn lesions, especially sole and white line haemorrhages, the exact aetiology of the changes that occur in the foot that lead to the initial formation of these lesions is still unproven. Some believe that these claw horn lesions result from the physical, concussive trauma from the cow walking on hard surfaces such as concrete or rough tracks and walkways. Others favour the theory of the release of an unidentified vasoactive substance(s) that acts on the intricate blood capillary network of the corium causing vessel wall paralysis, vasodilation, venous stagnation and oedema. It is thought that this causes opening of ateriovenous anastomoses or shunts which direct the blood away from the capillary bed leading to hypoxia and further damage to capillary walls. The combination of oedema and reduced blood supply interrupts the normal oxygen and nutrient supply to the tissues underlying the basal epidermal cells. This leads to formation of poor quality horn which would be more prone to physical insult and to loss of structural integrity in the epidermal dermal junction. Once this bond is weakened the weight of the cow can cause the changes already outlined in Stage 1 of Ossent and Lischer's pathogenesis.

A third hypothesis for claw lesion aetiology has recently been proposed by Webster (1998) who suggested that hormonal changes associated with calving, particularly the increased levels of relaxin, are a major contributory factor. Since one effect of relaxin is to increase the ability of collagen and other connective tissues to deform (and so allow movement of the pelvis during birth), it is suggested that this same effect adds to the instability of the dermal-epidermal junction by allowing unusually large movement (or even breakage) in the network of collagen attachments between the distal phalanx and the basement membrane of the laminae.

In fact all of these effects may contribute to epithelial disruption since all fit our present state of knowledge. However the identity, even the existence, of such 'vasoactive substances' is still to be confirmed as is any effect of relaxin upon the collagen fibres of the foot. Because of the analogy with the horse and the observations that nutrition can influence lesion formation and lameness, most authors suggest that these "vasoactive substances" are of dietary origin: perhaps 'normal' rumen metabolites, or substances resulting from rumen dysfunction. These have included histidine or histamine (Nilsson, 1963), ammonia or other products of protein breakdown and metabolites resulting from (subclinical) rumen acidosis; D-lactate, endotoxins (Boosman, 1990; Mortensen, Hesselholt and Basse, 1986).

Nutrition and risk factors for lameness

Since rumen function or dysfunction were suspected as the main factors influencing lameness, the concentrate part of the diet was initially the subject of most research. However, these studies have not confirmed any of the theories of aetiology and pathogenesis and were reviewed by Vermunt and Greenough (1994). There have been a number of comparative experiments investigating the interrelationship between nutrition, management and lameness (Table 24.3). Most have involved a simple continuous feeding design. These studies confirmed what was until then anecdotal evidence for the effects of nutrition on lameness. They showed the importance of maintaining a stable rumen environment in limiting lameness. When high levels of protein or readily fermentable carbohydrate were fed in the concentrate, or high levels of concentrate were fed as large meals, hoof health was compromised (Table 24.3).

Table 24.3 STUDIES OF THE RELATIONSHIP BETWEEN NUTRITION AND LAMENESS

	Study	*Year*	*Effect on lameness*
Level of Concentrate:	Leaver and Webster	1983	flat rate> fed to yield
	Peterse *et al.*,	1984	high>low
	Manson and Leaver	1988a	high>low
	Kelly and Leaver	1990	rapid>slowly fermentable
	Logue, Offer and Hyslop	1994	NS
Forage:Concentrate ratio:	Livesey and Fleming	1984	high>low
	Manson and Leaver	1989	high>low
Protein:in Concentrate:	Manson and Leaver	1988b	high>low
	Offer, Roberts and Logue	1997	no sig. diff in RDP/UDP proportion

However many of these experiments had a number of deficiencies of design. A particular concern was that some lesions were the consequence of earlier disruption of the claw. Most recent studies therefore have been longitudinal observations of lesion development in first calving cows (heifers) and this approach has been generally accepted as the most suitable monitor of the extent of insult seen in the peri-parturient period and first half of first lactation (Bradley *et al.*, 1989; Chesterton Pfeiffer, Morris, and Tanner, 1989; Greenough and Vermunt, 1991; Kempson and Logue, 1993; Leach, *et al.* 1997). These studies, along with the epidemiological analysis of survey data (Clarkson *et al.*, 1996), have not to date defined the aetiology of claw horn lesions, but they have shown that such lameness is associated with a range of risk factors that includes: calving and lactation, housing in cubicles, season and higher rainfall (winter), higher yields, flat rate feeding. While various forage characteristics have been implicated (type of forage, DM, protein content) this is poorly understood and is under experimental investigation at present.

In summary these studies show that there is no single cause of lameness and that the problem is multifactorial, with many different risk factors that interact and confound the effects of other factors. The effects of calving, lactation, housing, environment and season are the major influences in lameness and lesion formation. While nutrition is a factor its effects can only be properly assessed in association with other risk factors and its relative importance is now slowly being elucidated.

NUTRITION AND CALVING

Virtually all these studies have established a clear link between the time of calving, when nutrition is changed in order to support the demands of lactation, and the formation of clinical or subclinical claw horn lesions 3 months after calving (Arkins 1981; Russell, *et al.*, 1982; Kempson and Logue, 1993). Observational studies in first calving heifers have confirmed this and shown that calving is possibly the most important risk factor for lameness associated with claw lesion formation. Figure 24.1 summarises five studies carried out at SAC and the Hannah Research Institute in which claw lesions have been measured in various groups of heifers after calving.

The majority of these lesions affected the sole/heel junction of the outer hind claw and rose to a peak at around 3 to 4 months post-calving (Figure 24.1) regardless of the environmental and management conditions. These even occurred in a small group housed on straw over winter and calved at grass in the summer (Logue, *et al.*, 1994). Analysis has shown that the pattern of lesion development after calving is similar in all claws but approximately 0.75 of all claw lesions are seen on the lateral hind claw and most of the remaining 0.25 lesions most were seen in the medial front claw. Force plate studies have shown that these two claws carry the greater proportion of the cows weight (Toussaint-Raven, 1985). Other theories for the preponderance of lesions in the lateral hind claw

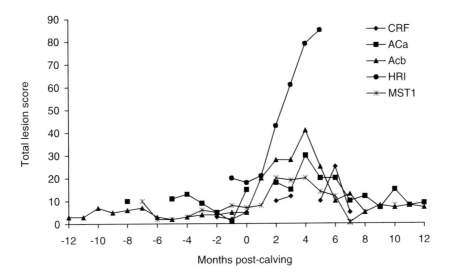

Figure 24.1 Mean total lesion score for 5 cohort studies

include the way that cows place the foot on the ground (Burgi, 1998) or the conformation of the udder in a newly calved cow forcing the cow to take a wider stance than normal and causing increased weight-bearing in the lateral claw (Webster, 1995b).

An observational study of a cohort of autumn calving cattle managed similarly either on a clover based system, receiving no artificial nitrogen, or on conventionally managed ryegrass swards showed no significant effect on the incidence of lameness. Modelling of the pooled data showed the pattern development of sole and white line lesions in the outer hind claw (Figures 24.2 and 24.3) is similar to that shown in Figure 24.1, reaching a peak at around 3 - 4 months (later in subsequent lactations) after calving and declining thereafter. Lesions were significantly worse in older animals and there was a significant interaction between time after calving and parity on lesion formation. The difference in the shape of the curves for sole and white line lesions suggests that although the aetiology may be similar, the pathogenesis may be different, as proposed by Ossent and Lischer (1998). The increased severity of lesions in older animals is supported by the increase in risk odds for lameness in older animals shown from the Liverpool Survey (Ward and French, 1997). It was suggested that the shift in timing of the peak lesion score to later in lactation was due to repeated lesion formation and animals' calving sometime after housing in later lactations instead of simultaneously as in the first lactation (Offer *et al.*, 1998). Thus already we are seeing some of the complexity of these inter-relationships.

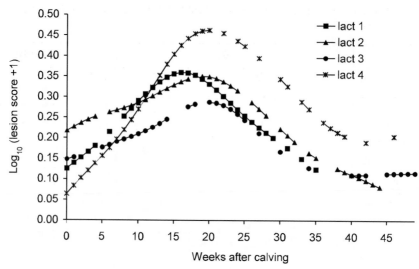

Figure 24.2   Sole lesion development in the lateral hind claws (lactations 1-4)

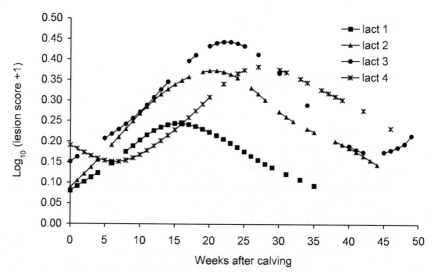

Figure 24.3   White line lesion development in the lateral hind claw (lactations 1-4)

Results from a number of more recent studies involving heifer groups have been more equivocal about the importance of nutrition than some of the earlier feeding experiments. At SAC, as part of an investigation into Metabolic Stress (Logue, Berry, Offer, Chaplin, Crawshaw, Leach, Ball and Bax, 1999) the two Acrehead herds (each of 70 cows, housed in adjacent halves of the same shed and milked by the same person, through the same milking parlour) were fed considerably different concentrate inputs (Table 24.4).

Table 24.4 DIETS OF ANIMALS IN ON LOW INPUT (LI) AND HIGH OUTPUT (HO) MANAGEMENT SYSTEMS

Composition (kg FW)	1994/5		1995/6		1996/7	
	LI	*HO*	*LI*	*HO*	*LI*	*HO*
Silage	40	40	26	35	32	36
Grainbeet	10	15	7.5	10	4	8
Barley straw	-	-	3	-	-	-
Maize gluten	4.2	-	-	-	-	-
Wholecrop barley	-	-	-	-	7.5	6.5
Fodder beet	-	-	-	-	17.5	20
Fishmeal	0.7	-	-	-	-	-
Blended concentrate	-	4	-	-	-	-
Parlour concentrate	1	2	1.5	3	2	3
Fresh weight mix	55.9	61	38	48	63	73.5
Mix ration						
kg DM	19.5	21.2	12.9	16.7	15.9	21
ME (MJ/kg DM)	12.0	11.3	10.5	11.7	11.7	11.8
CP (g/kgDM)	171	184	139	160	131	135
OIL (g/kgDM)	53	51	47	53	40	43
NDF (g/kgDM)	442	402	540	476	365	404
Starch and Sugar (g/kgDM)	94	81	85	92	221	207
Ash (g/kgDM)	82	102	77	84	99	80

Figure 24.4 summarises the claw lesion scores for first lactation heifer groups during the last 2 months pre-calving and first 6 months post-calving of either a low input herd (LI, yielding 5,000kg/cow/year) or high output herd (HO, yielding 8,500kg/cow/year) during the years 1994-97. In summary, while there were significant differences between the 3 years and between the two herds in 96/97, the general picture is one of little major difference between herds despite quite dramatic differences in concentrate input (0.5 vs. 2.0 tonnes/cow/year). It is suggested that the increased lesion scores for both herds in 96/97 relate to the higher levels of starch/sugar and lower NDF in the ration compared with previous years. Interestingly, claw lesions in those receiving only 0.5 tonnes/cow/year concentrate were significantly worse than for those receiving 2.0 tonnes/cow/year in that year. Two factors may have influenced this: firstly, LI started with a higher lesion score at calving; secondly, the metabolic challenge for LI was greater than for HO and they were consequently less able to withstand the additional challenges of calving and the higher starch/sugar rations. Put simply, this is the cumulative results of the interaction of several risk factors for lesion formation (calving, nutrition and metabolic challenge).

These data seem to follow a somewhat similar pattern to that described by Bergsten (1995), Bergsten and Frank (1996) and Olsson, Bergsten and Wiktorsson (1998) in

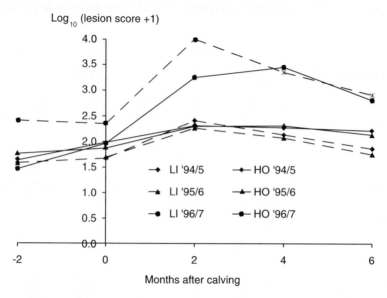

Figure 24.4　Total lesion score in first lactation heifers on low input (LI) or high output (HO) management systems 1994-1997

Sweden. They were unable to show any significant effect of concentrate level on lameness or lesion formation. Conversely, the CVL/ADAS/RCVS group at Bridgets have reported a highly significant effect of concentrate input upon heifer claw lesion score development (Livesey, Harrington, Johnston, May and Metcalf, 1998). However in their 2×2 factorial experiment comparing the effects on lameness of high with low levels of concentrate and straw yards with cubicles, they found much greater differences due to housing type than to level of concentrate; where cubicles gave a higher lesion score than a straw yard. Thus the results from these more recent studies involving heifer groups have been more equivocal about the importance of nutrition than some of the earlier feeding experiments.

A further aspect of the effects of nutrition on lameness is supplementation with mineral and vitamins. Recently there has been an upsurge of interest in the effects of biotin supplementation on dairy cow lameness. In a very well controlled experiment Midla, Hoblet, Weiss and Moeschberger (1998a and b) monitored claw lesion development using heifer groups supplemented or not with biotin. Although no significant difference in overall lesion score was found between treatments (Midla *et al.,* 1998a) there was significantly less white line separation in supplemented animals (Midla *et al.,* 1998b). There is also some tentative evidence that biotin can increase the rate at which claw lesions heal (Koller, Lischer, Geyer, Ossent, Schulze and Auer, 1998) and supplementation with organic forms of zinc may improve the tensile strength of hoof horn and thus increase the resistance of the hoof capsule to physical trauma (Stern and Guyer, 1998).

Generally these additives may have some positive qualities but their value to the farm depends on their cost.

NUTRITION AND HOUSING

When the clinical cases of lameness in all cows (not just first lactation animals) on the 'Metabolic Stress' project were analysed, the results were not as would be expected from the data on lesion score in heifers. Overall HO had a higher incidence of clinical lameness (p<0.05) despite there being no difference in lesion scores for first lactation heifers (Table 24.5). In 1995-96 a major contributor to this difference was an outbreak of foul in the foot in HO during the autumn. Although both herds were affected, HO was much more severely affected than LI and this was considered as the major contributor to the poorer mobility of cows in HO. Over the three years there was a higher incidence of lameness caused both by digital and interdigital dermatitis and by claw lesions in HO.

Table 24.5 NUMBER OF LESIONS/YEAR IDENTIFIED AT CLINICAL EXAMINATIONS FOR LAMENESS

	Low input	*High output*
(Inter) digital dermatitis	18	36
Claw Horn Lesion	27	38
Other	1	2
Total	46	76

We believe that, thanks to the use of both extended grazing in the late autumn and daylight grazing in the spring and early autumn, the lower time spent indoors (25% less) by the LI herd and also the more broken nature of this housing, reduced the challenge to the feet and the prevalence of both digital and interdigital and claw horn lesions in this group. In addition there may have been a cumulative effect of the management and feeding regimes on cow hoof health since lesions are known to be more severe and are also repeated in later lactations. While we also believe that the environmental challenge was a principle component in the greater development of claw horn lesions in the older cattle we cannot rule out an indirect nutritional interaction.

Nutrition can indirectly affect lameness by influencing the quantity and characteristics of the slurry and underfoot conditions within the housing. There is now ample evidence that by far the most important risk factor for these digital and interdigital lesions is a dirty environment (Rodriguez-Lainz, Hird, Carpenter and Read, 1996). Furthermore it is known that slurry greatly increases the permeability of the intertubular horn of the sole and the heel (Kempson, Langridge and Logue 1998), leaving the horn of the sole and particularly the heel vulnerable to microbial invasion and physical trauma. Heel erosion is ubiquitous amongst housed cattle and although not a primary cause of lameness, can, if severe, change the conformation and biomechanics of the foot in such a way as to make lesion formation more likely. Figure 24.5 shows how heel erosion in autumn calving dairy cattle housed on concrete develops over the winter months and is at a peak by April/May when the animals are turned out for spring grazing again. Once out at grass and away from the influence of slurry and concrete the heels begin to recover until the next housing in autumn.

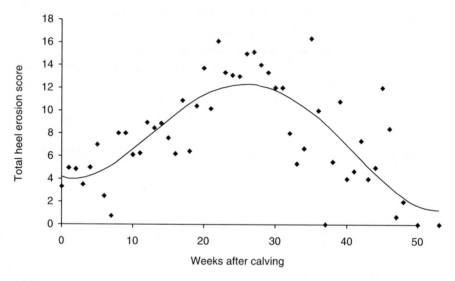

Figure 24.5 Heel erosion score in autumn calving cattle housed from mid October to late April in a concrete based cubicle house

There is often a net hoof wear in autumn calved cattle, and hooves become steeper over the winter housing period, but no direct relationship with diet has been established. Measurements of hoof hardness, which is notoriously difficult to measure, have shown little if any effect of nutrition. The *in vitro* measurement of claw horn epithelial cell proliferation and keratinization from small groups of mid-lactation cattle has shown that the initiation of a silage based diet and introduction to housing (cubicles and concrete) causes a cumulative reduction in DNA synthesis by the laminar epithelium (MacCallum, Knight, Wilde, Kim, and Logue, 1996). This fall in the rate of epidermal growth may reduce the ability of the claw horn to withstand damage and again demonstrates the multifactorial nature of lameness.

A further aspect of nutrition which may influence lameness and lesion formation is the quality of the diet and the way that this interacts with cow behaviour. On the Metabolic Stress project animals in LI were fed a diet with a large proportion of forage. As a result the animals had to spend a greater proportion of their time feeding and sacrificed time lying down in cubicles (as shown in Figure 24.6). Lack of adequate

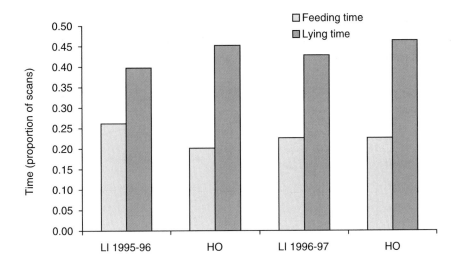

Figure 24.6 Summary time budget for low input (LI) and high output (HO) cohorts in Metabolic Stress study (1995-1997)

cubicle comfort and a consequent reduction of lying time have been considered by some as the major aetiological factors influencing severe claw lesions. (Colam-Ainsworth, Lunn, Thomas and Eddy 1989; Singh, Ward, Lautenbach, Hughes and Murray,1993 Singh, Ward and Murray, 1993). However, since in this study there was a substantial difference in lying time in 1995/6, but no obvious difference in the effect on claw lesion development in the first calving heifer groups over their first housed period, it is clear that the matter is not that simple! (Berry, Logue, Waran, Appleby and Offer, 1997). The even more extreme heifer cohort studies of Leonard, O'Connell and O'Farrell (1994 and 1995) confirm this view point. Without more detailed investigations it is only possible to speculate about the various inter-relationships which might explain this further.

NUTRITION AND SEASON

Season has a big influence on lameness and lesion formation closely related to many of the other management factors, nutrition and housing that are changed because of the season and outdoor environmental conditions. Season has other effects, largely outwith management control, such as rainfall, humidity and day length. Whilst rainfall has been shown by epidemiological evidence to influence lameness (Russell, *et al.*, 1982), the direct effect of day length is currently under investigation. It has been shown that the interaction with season and calving can have a major influence on lesion formation.

Animals from the Metabolic Stress project mentioned earlier were split into autumn-calving and spring-calving groups for analysis (i.e. calving before and after Christmas respectively). Autumn-calving animals had significantly higher total lesion scores than spring-calvers at 2, 4, and 6 months post calving (p<0.01) (Figure 24.7)

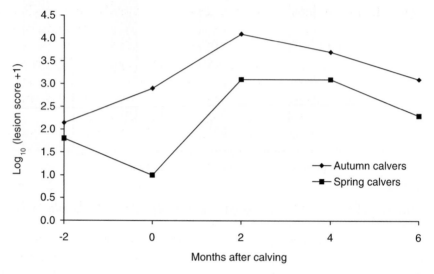

Figure 24.7 Effect of season of calving on total lesion score (1996-1997)

Overall, autumn-calving cows had a higher incidence of lameness than spring calving animals (p<0.05). Cows calving in the autumn, at or close to housing for the winter, experience two known risk factors (both housing and calving) together and lesion scores rise higher than they otherwise would. This effect is exacerbated by the reduction in laminar epithelium DNA synthesis rates during winter (MacCallum, Knight, Wilde and Hendry, 1998). This suggests that cows calving in spring are able to recover from the initial challenge of housing before they calve and consequently lesion scores tend not to increase to the levels seen in autumn-calving animals. Additionally, autumn-calving animals are at increased risk of infectious causes of lameness whilst at peak milk production, whereas spring-calving animals have the added advantage of being out at grass for at least half of their lactation when lesions may be expected to be at their worst.

Summary

The general nutrition of dairy cows has improved over the last 20 years as our understanding of the problems facing the high yielding cow increases. Improvements in ration formulation and feeding practice has allowed dairy cows to meet the metabolic demands of calving and lactation despite being asked to work harder as profit margins are squeezed. We have shown in our studies of metabolic stress that cows can meet the demands of either low input or high output systems (towards the extremes of dairy cow management in Scotland) but that high levels of production may be detrimental to hoof health because of the increased environmental challenge rather than the level of feeding *per se* (provided that nutrition is well formulated). The increased interest in welfare and lameness in particular has meant that we are getting better at monitoring lameness. We believe that measurement of lameness must be standardised in order to assess this apparent increase more fully. However if, as epidemiology suggests, there is an increase in the prevalence and incidence of lameness, it seems that nutrition is not as important as a risk factor as was once thought and that other, in some cases related, factors already discussed such as quality and length of housing may be responsible.

We are still far from understanding the full intricacies of this problem but several matters have been clarified. We now know that calving, housing and season are the primary risk factors for lameness and claw lesion formation. When animals are well managed, fed balanced rations and the rumen is functioning optimally, nutrition is can vary quite widely without adversely affecting their feet provided that the environmental challenge is also limited. However when the animal is exposed to known nutritional risks (rapid change in diet, large meals of rapidly fermentable carbohydrate, high levels of protein) and at the same time is experiencing other risk factors, (calving, housing on concrete) then hoof health can be compromised. Ideally the number of risk factors faced by a dairy cow at any particular time should be minimised. This is especially important in the dairy heifer; the lower the baseline lesion score prior to calving the better for hoof health. All the evidence is that this should be obtained by steady growth rates and training the animals to the various management regimes they are likely to encounter in later life. Care is also needed with the introduction of newly calved cows, especially first calving heifers, into a cubicle house. Good cubicle comfort and adequate access to forage is essential. Care of the young cow will mean fewer lesions in older ones!

Acknowledgement

We gratefully acknowledge help and advice from SAC, Edinburgh University and BioSS colleagues. One of us (RB) was in receipt of a MAFF studentship and SAC receives funding from SOAEFD.

References

Alban, L. (1995) Lameness in Danish dairy cows- frequency and possible risk factors. *Preventative Veterinary Medicine* **22,** 213-225.

Anon. (1996) Dairy facts and figures 1996. A National Dairy Council Publication, London.

Anon. (1997) Report on the welfare of dairy cattle. FAWC, Tolworth, Surrey (MAFF publication PB3426).

Anon. (1980) United Kingdom dairy facts and figures 1980. The Federation of United Kingdom Milk Marketing Boards, Milk Marketing Board of England and Wales, Surrey.

Arkins, S. (1981). Lameness in dairy cows. *Irish Veterinary Journal* **35,** 135 - 140 and 163-170.

Bergsten, C. and Frank, B. (1996) Sole haemorrhages in tied primiparous cows as an indicator of periparturient laminitis: effects of diet, flooring and season. *Acta Veterinaria Scandinavia* **37,** 383- 394.

Bergsten, C. (1995) Management and nutritional effects on foot health in dairy cows. *Proceedings of the 46th Annual Meeting of the European Association of Animal Production* 1995, Prague, 4 - 7th Sept Abstr. p82

Berry R.J., Logue, D.N., Waran, N.K., Appleby, M.C. and Offer, J.E. (1997) Effect of high and low production regimes on the behaviour of dairy cows. *Proceedings of the 51st Scientific meeting of the Association of Veterinary Research Workers* Abst. 1B20 p 20

Boosman, R. (1990) Bovine laminitis: Histopathologic and arteriographic aspects, and its relation to endotoxaemia. Proefschrift, Utrecht, 1990

Booth, J.M. (1989) Lameness and mastitis losses. *Veterinary Record* **125,** 161

Bradley, H.K., Shannon, D. and Neilson, D.R. (1989) Subclinical laminitits in dairy heifers. *Veterinary Record,* **125,** 177 - 179

Brotherstone, S. and Hill, W. G. (1991) Dairy herd life in relation to linear type traits and production 1. Phenotypic and genetic analyses in pedigree type classified herds. *Animal Production* **53,** 279-287

Burgi (1998) Determine maintenance hoof trimming by observing movement *Proceedings of the Xth International Symposium on Lameness in Ruminants, Lucerne, Switzerland.* (Eds. Lischer, Ch. J. and Ossent, P.) 20 - 22

Chesterton, R.N., Pfeiffer, D.U., Morris, R.S. and Tanner, C.M. (1989) Environmental and behavioural factors affecting the prevalence of foot lameness in NewZealand Dairy Herds - a case control study. *New Zealand Veterinary Journal,* **37,** 135 - 142

Clarkson, M. J., Downham, D. Y., Faull, W. B., Hughes, J. W., Manson, F. J., Merrit, J. B., Murray, R. D., Russell, W. B., Sutherst, J. and Ward, W. R. (1996) Incidence and prevalence of lameness in dairy cattle. *Veterinary Record* **138,** 563-567

Colam-Ainsworth, P., Lunn, G. A., Thomas, R. C. and Eddy, R. G. (1989) Behaviour of cows in cubicles and its possible relationship with laminitis in replacement dairy heifers. *Veterinary Record* **125,** 573-575

Collick, D. W., Ward, W. R. and Dobson, H. (1989) Association between types of lameness and fertility. *Veterinary Record* **125,** 103-106.

Eddy, R.G. and Scott, C.P. (1980) Some observations on the incidence of lameness in dairy cattle in Somerset *Veterinary Record* **106**, 140-144.

Emanuelson, U. (1988) Recording of production diseases in cattle and possibilities for genetic improvements: a review. *Livestock Production Science* **76**, 89-106

Enevoldsen, C., Grohn, Y. T. and Thysen, I. (1991) Sole ulcers in dairy cattle: associations with season, cow characteristics, disease and production. *Journal of Dairy Science* **74**, 1284-1298

Esslemont, R.J. and Peeler, E.J. (1993) The scope for raising margins in dairy herds by improving fertility and health. *British Veterinary Journal* **149**, 537-547.

Greenough, P. R. and Vermunt, J. J. (1991) Evaluation of subclinical laminitis in a dairy herd and observations on associated nutritional and management factors. *Veterinary Record* **128**, 11-17

Greenough, P. R., Weaver A. D., Esslemont R. J. and Galindo F. A. (1997) Basic concepts of bovine lameness. In: *Lameness in cattle* (3rd edition). (Eds., Greenough, P. R. and Weaver, A. D.) London. p3-13

Gröhn Y. T., Hertl J. A. and Harman J. L. (1994) Effect of early lactation milk yield on reproductive disorders in dairy cows. *American Journal of Veterinary Research* **55**, 1521-1528

Hoekstra, J., Lugt, A. W. van der, Werf, J. H. J. ven der and Ouweltjes, W. (1994) Genetic and phenotypic parameters for milk production and fertility traits in upgraded dairy cattle. *Livestock Production Science* **12**, 225-232

Kelly, E.F. and Leaver, J.D. (1990) Lameness in dairy cattle and the type of concentrate given. *Animal Production*, **51**, 221 - 227

Kempson, S.A., Langridge, A. and Logue, D.N. (1998) Laminitis versus papillaryitis. *Proceedings of the 10th International Symposium on Lameness in Ruminants.* Sept 7 - 10, 1998 Lucerne, Switzerland pp 153 - 154

Kempson, S.A. and Logue, D.N. (1993) Ultrastructural observations of hoof horn from dairy cows: changes in the white line during the first lactation. *Veterinary Record*, **132**, 524 - 527

Koller, U., Lischer, C.J., Geyer, H., Ossent, P., Schulze, J. and Auer J.A.(1998) The effect of biotin in the treatment of uncomplicated sole ulcers in cattle. A controlled study. *Proceedings of the Xth International Symposium on Lameness in Ruminants, Lucerne, Switzerland.* (Eds. Lischer, Ch. J. and Ossent, P.) 230 - 232

Leach, K. A., Logue, D. N., Kempson, S. A., Offer, J. E., Ternent, H. E. and Randall, J. M. (1997) Claw horn lesions in dairy cattle: development of sole and white line haemorrhages during the first lactation. *The Veterinary Journal* **154**, 215-225

Leaver, J.D and Webster, D.M (1983) Assessment of lameness in dairy cattle on different systems of concentrate feeding. In *SAC Crichton Royal Annual Report (1983)* pp 27 - 29

Leonard F. C., O'Connell J. and O'Farrell K. (1994) Effect of different housing conditions on behaviour and foot lesions in Friesian heifers. *Veterinary Record* **134**, 490-494

Leonard F. C., O'Connell J. and O'Farrell K. (1995) Effect of overcrowding on claw health in first-calved Friesian heifers. *British Veterinary Journal* **152**, 459-472

Livesey, C. T. and Fleming, F. L. (1984) Nutritional influences on laminitis, sole ulcer and bruised sole in Friesian cows. *Veterinary Record* **114**, 510-512

Livesey, C. T., Harrington, T., Johnston, A. M., May, S. A. and Metcalf, J. A. (1998) The effect of diet and housing on the development of sole haemorrhages, white line haemorrhages and heel erosions in Holstein heifers. *Animal Science* **67**, 9-16

Logue, D.N., Offer, J.E., Leach, K.A. Kempson, S.A. and Randall. J.M. (1994) Lesions of the hoof in first-calving dairy heifers. *Proceedings of the 8th International Symposium on Disorders of the Ruminant Digit*, Banff, Canada, Ed. Greenough P.R. 272

Logue, D.N., Berry, R.J., Offer, J.E., Chaplin. S.J., Crawshaw, W.M., Leach, K.A., Ball, P.J.H. and Bax, J. (1999) Consequences of 'metabolic load' for lameness and disease. *Proceedings of the International Symposium on Metabolic Stress in Dairy Cows* 28 - 30 Oct 1998, British Society of Animal Science, Edinburgh

Logue, D.N., Offer, J.E. and Hyslop, J.J. (1994) Relationship of diet, hoof type and locomotion score with lesions of the sole and white line. *Animal Production*, **59**, 173 - 181

Logue, D.N., Offer, J.E., Chaplin, S.J., Knight, C.H., Hendry, K.A.K., Leach, K.A., Kempson, S.A. and Randall, J.M. (1995) Lameness in dairy cattle. *Proceedings of the 46th Annual Meeting of the European Association of Animal Production* 1995, Prague, 4 - 7th Sept Abstr. p218

Lyons, D. T., Freeman, A. E., and Kuck, A. L. (1991) Genetics of health traits. *Journal of Dairy Science* **74**, 1092-1100

MacCallum, A.J., Knight, C.H., Wilde, C.J., Kim, J.S. and Logue, D.N. (1996) Environmental and nutritional influences on bovine laminitis. *Hannah Research Institute Report* (1996) Abst

MacCallum, A.J., Knight, C.H., Wilde, C.J. and Hendry, K.A.K. (1998) Cell proliferation and keratinization in bovine hoof during the development of the cow and during lameness challenge. *Proceedings of the Xth International Symposium on Lameness in Ruminants, Lucerne, Switzerland.* (Eds. Lischer, Ch. J. and Ossent, P.) p 236 - 238

Manson, F. J. and Leaver, J. D. (1988a.)The influence of concentrate amount on locomotion and clinical lameness in dairy cattle. *Animal Production* **47,** 185-190

Manson, F. J. and Leaver, J. D. (1988b) The influence of dietary protein intake and of hoof trimming on lameness in dairy cattle. *Animal Production* **47**, 191-199

Manson, F. J. and Leaver, J. D. (1989) The effect of concentrate:silage ratio and of hoof trimming on lameness in dairy cattle. *Animal Production* **49,** 15-22

McInerney, J.P., Howe, K.S. and Schepers, J.P. (1990) A framework for the economic analysis of disease in farm livestock. *Report of a research project (ref CSA 873) funded by MAFF*. The University of Exeter, Agricultural Economics Unit. 87pp

Midla, L.T., Hoblet, K.H., Weiss, W.P. and Moeschberger, M.L. (1998a) Supplemental dietary biotin for prevention of lesions associated with aseptic subclinical laminitis (*pododermatitis aseptica diffusa*) in primiparous cows. *American Journal of Veterinary Research*, **59**, 733 - 737

Midla, L.T., Hoblet, K.H., Weiss, W.P. and Moeschberger, M.L. (1998b) Biotin feeding trial to prevent lesions associated with pododermatitis aseptica diffusa in lactating cattle). *Proceedings of the Xth International Symposium on Lameness in Ruminants, Lucerne, Switzerland*. (Eds. Lischer, Ch. J. and Ossent, P.) p 225 - 226

Mortensen, K., Hesselholt, M and Basse, A. (1986) Pathogenesis of bovine laminitis (*pododermatitis aseptica diffusa*). Experimental models. *Proceedings of the 14th World Congress on Diseases in Cattle*, Dublin, Ireland, 1025 - 1030

Nilsson, S.A. (1963) Clinical, morphological and experimental studies of laminitis in cattle. *Acta Veterinaria Scandinavica*, **4**, Suppl 1, 1 - 276

Offer, J. E., McNulty, D. And Logue, D. N. (1998) Modelling lesion development in a cohort of Holstein-Friesian cows (lactations 1 to 4). *Proceedings of the Xth International Symposium on Lameness in Ruminants, Lucerne, Switzerland.* (Eds. Lischer, Ch. J. and Ossent, P.) p 159-160

Offer, J.E., Logue, D.N. and Roberts, D.J. (1997) The effect of protein source on lameness and solear lesion formation in dairy cattle. *Animal Science*, **65**, 143 - 149

Olsson, G., Bergsten, C. and Wiktorsson, H. (1998) The influence of diet before and after calving on the food intake, production and health of primiparous cows, with special reference to sole haemorrhages. *Animal Science*, **66**, 77 - 86

Ossent, P., Greenough P.R. and Vermunt J.J. Laminitis (1997) In *Lameness in cattle* (3rd edition). (Eds., Greenough, P. R. and Weaver, A. D.) London. 277 - 292

Ossent, P. and Lischer, C. J. (1994) Theories on the pathogenesis of bovine laminitis. *Proceedings of the 8th International Symposium on disorders of the Ruminant Digit*, Banff, Canada. 207-209.

Ossent, P. and Lischer, C.J. (1998) Bovine laminitis: the lesions and their pathogenesis. *In Practice* **20**, 415 - 427

Peterse, D. J., Korver, S., Oldenbroek, J. K. and Talmon, F. P. (1984) Relationship between levels of concentrate feeding and the incidence of sole ulcers in dairy cattle. *Veterinary Record* **115**, 629-630.

Prentice, D.E. and Neal, P.A. (1972) Some observations on the incidence of lameness in dairy cattle in West Cheshire *Veterinary Record* **91**, 1 - 7

Pryce, J. E. Veerkamp, R. F. Thompson, R. Hill W.G. and Simm, G. (1998) Genetic parameters of common health disorders and measures of fertility in Holstein Friesian dairy cattle. *Animal Science* **65**, 353-360.

Rodriguez-Lainz, A. J., Hird, D. W., Carpenter, T. E. and Read, D. H. (1996) Case control of papillomatous digital dermatitis in Southern California dairy farms. *Preventive Veterinary Medicine* **28**, 117-131.

Russell, A. M., Rowlands, G. J., Shaw, S. R. and Weaver, A. D. (1982) Survey of lameness in British dairy cattle. *Veterinary Record* **111**, 155-160.

Singh, S. S., Ward, W. R., Lautenbach, K., Hughes, J. W. and Murray, R. D. (1993a) Behaviour of first lactation and adult dairy cows while housed and at pasture and its relationship with sole lesions. *Veterinary Record* **133**, 469-474.

Singh, S. S., Ward, W. R. and Murray, R. D. (1993b) Aetiology and pathogenesis of sole lesions causing lameness in cattle: a review. *Veterinary Bulletin* **63**, 303-315.

Sprecher, D. J., Hostetler, D. E. and Kaneene, J. B. (1997) A lameness scoring system that uses posture and gait to predict dairy cattle reproductive performance. *Theriogenology* **47**, 1179 -1187

Stern, A., Guyer, H., Morel, I. and Kessler, J. (1998) Effect of organic zinc on horn quality in beef cattle *Proceedings of the Xth International Symposium on Lameness in Ruminants, Lucerne, Switzerland.* (Eds. Lischer, Ch. J. and Ossent, P.) 233 - 235

Toussaint-Raven, E. (1985) *Cattle footcare and claw trimming.* Farming Press, Ipswich.

Veerkamp, R. F., Hill, W.G., Stott A. W., Brotherstone S. and Simm, G. (1995) Selection for longevity and yield in dairy cows using transmitting abilities for type and yield. *Animal Science* **61**, 189-198.

Vermunt, J.J. and Greenough, P.R. (1994) Predisposing factors of laminitis in cattle. *British Veterinary Journal,* **150**, 151 - 164

Ward, W.R. and French N.P. (1997) Foot lameness in cattle. *Proceedings of the 51st Scientific meeting of the Association of Veterinary Research Workers* Abst. 1B17 p 19

Webster, A.J.F. (1998) *Report on the biology of lameness workshop.* Funded by SOAEFD and MDC, SAC Report (*In press*)

Webster, A. J. F. (1995a) Welfare strategies in future selection and management strategies. In *Breeding and feeding the high genetic merit dairy cow. Occasional publication No 19 British Society of Animal science 1995* (Eds T J L Lawrence, Gordon FJ and Carson A.) p 87- 93

Webster A.J.F. (1995b) Animal Welfare - a cool eye towards Eden. Blackwell Science, Oxford

Wells, S. J., Trent, A. M., Marsh, W. E. and Robinson, R. A. (1993) Prevalence and severity of lameness in lactating dairy cows in a sample of Minnesota and Wisconsin herds. *Journal of the American Veterinary Medical Association* **202**, 78-82.

Whay, H.R., Waterman, A. E., Webster, A. J. F. and O'Brien, J. K. (1998) The influence of lesion type on the duration of hyperalgesia associated with hindlimb lameness in dairy cattle. *The Veterinary Journal* **156**, 23-29.

Whay, H.R., Waterman, A. E. and Webster, A. J. F. (1997) Associations between locomotion, claw lesions and nociceptive threshold in dairy heifers during the peri-partum period. *Veterinary Journal* **154**, 155-161.

Whitaker, D. A., Smith, E. J. daRosa, G. L., and Kelly, J. M. (1993) Some effects of nutrition and management on the fertility of dairy cattle. *Veterinary Record* **133**, 61-64.

This paper was first published in 1999

25

FEEDING AND MANAGING HIGH-YIELDING DAIRY COWS — THE AMERICAN EXPERIENCE

CARL E. COPPOCK

Coppock Nutritional Services, Laredo, Texas 78045, USA

Introduction

It was but a few years ago that average annual milk yields of 10,000 kg/cow were achieved only by the best managed herds; today yields of 13,500 kg and more are becoming widespread. New individual milk production records seem to be set nearly every year. Just recently, a new world milk record was set in Wisconsin with 28,804 kg of milk produced in 365 days by a cow milked twice daily. Walton (1983) predicted that by the year 2000, top individual milk production records would approach 32,000 kg per cow per year, and the best herd averages would approach 16,000 kg per cow per year. Although in 1983 this prediction seemed unduly optimistic, it now seems like a near certainty. Although the Holstein breed dominates the dairy cow population in the U.S. (94% of the cows), the Jersey breed is making strong progress. Recently it was noted (Halladay, 1996) that one Jersey herd with the 5th highest production in the U.S., averaged 8,550 kg milk, 420 kg fat and 325 kg of protein per year, considerably higher than the U.S. average for Holsteins (7,530 kg).

For at least a decade, the genetic progress in Holsteins for milk has been about 118 kg per year or 1180 kg for the 10-year interval. In Jerseys, the genetic change for milk was estimated to be 76 kg annually from 1960 to 1987, but 137 kg from 1983 to 1987 (Nizamani and Berger, 1996). An important advantage of the pervasive genetic merit for high milk yields is that dairy cows are highly responsive to good environment in the broad sense of that word. In more markets, price incentives for low somatic cells encourage better control of udder infections; more precise engineering of milking systems and environmental management systems have reduced these constraints. Development of repartitioning agents especially bovine somatotropin (BST) now focus attention on the constraints associated with nutrition and feeding management which often now limit higher but economic yields of milk. The objectives for this chapter are to describe several key features of nutrition and management in high-yielding U.S. dairy herds and suggest several areas for improved efficiency.

Dairy management practices

The U.S. is fortunate to now have a National Animal Health Monitoring System which includes a major emphasis on dairy cows. In May, (Anonymous, 1996), Part I: Reference of 1996 Dairy Management Practices, was published and this document contains a large array of data concerning the management and conditions of U.S. dairying. Twenty states participated, representing 83.1% of the U.S. milking cows. The data were obtained from 2,542 dairy producers who were surveyed with an on-farm questionnaire to provide a representative sample. A few of the results are shown in Table 25.1 and others will be referred to in subsequent sections.

Table 25.1 EXAMPLES OF U.S. DAIRY INFORMATION AND MANAGEMENT PRACTICES[a]

	Percent Operations	*Percent Dairy Cows*
Record-Keeping System		
Hand written (as ledger)	80.7	73.3
Dairy Herd Improve. (DHIA)	43.4	54.6
Computer at the location	15.1	36.9
Computer — off location	9.9	13.2
Other system	6.0	5.1
Any system	100.0	100.0
Identification Type		
Ear Tags (all types)	81.2	87.3
Collars	22.3	16.3
Photograph or sketch	17.4	10.3
Branding (all methods)	4.9	12.3
Implanted electronic ID	0.3	0.2
Tattoo (other than brucellosis)	6.5	7.8
Other	10.1	6.4
None	8.8	2.5

[a]Part I: Reference of 1996 Dairy Management Practices (NAHMS) Anonymous (1996)

Feed sources

Although corn (maize), sorghum, barley and oats continue to be dominant feed grains for cattle and soya bean meal and cottonseed meal are important plant protein supplements, many alternative feeds, sometimes called by-products, and more recently and correctly called co-products are used in cattle feeds in the U.S. A regional bulletin (Bath *et al.*, 1980) listed 357 tabular entries with 49 feedstuffs discussed individually. Many are well known, including molasses, brewers' grains, hominy feed, wheat bran and maize distillers' grains. Others are less well known including almond hulls, apple pomace, buckwheat middlings, caproco, peanut skins, cow peas, vetch seeds and many more. Most are available only in specific regions, for example California, and some only during certain seasons. Probably no more than 10 to 15 are consistently available in most of the U.S. Two national alternative feeds symposia have been held (1991 and 1995) to address the issues of these feedstuffs in the rations of dairy and beef cattle.

Grasser *et al.* (1995) surveyed an array of industry representatives to evaluate the importance of 9 major by-products used in livestock feeding in California in 1992. These are listed in Table 25.2 with their individual tonnage and market value at that time. California is now the No. 1 milk producing state in the U.S. and these 9 by-products accounted for more than 2.5 million tonnes and about 27% of all concentrates used in California that year. Whole cottonseed was the most important by-product studied and it accounted for 31% of the total tonnage. It provided about 66% of the total crude protein (CP) and 53% of the total net energy for lactation (NE$_l$) of the 9 by-products. Moreover, cottonseed constitutes about 62% of the total cotton crop yield (lint plus seed). It has become such a respected and sought after feed that now nearly 78% of the California cottonseed crop is fed to cattle, with 20% crushed for oil and the remainder is used for planting seed. Although it is grown across the southern U.S., it is valued so highly that it is shipped into all of the major dairy states on the northern tier. Brewers' grains are used exclusively (100%) for cattle feed. It was determined that these 9 by-products could have provided the CP or NE$_l$ for more than 31% of the milk produced in California during 1992.

Table 25.2 NINE IMPORTANT BY-PRODUCTS USED IN CALIFORNIA IN 1992[a]

By-product	Total as fed tons (1000)	Percentage of total Concentrate (%)	Market Price ($/ton)	Total Value $ (1000)
Almond hulls	498	5.19	66	32,881
Beet pulp	267	2.78	132	35,191
Brewers' grains (wet)	409	4.26	35	14,318
Citrus pulp, (17% DM)	336	3.50	13	4,372
Citrus pulp, (30% DM)	91	0.95	35	3,182
Maize gluten feed, (wet)	15	0.15	57	829
Maize gluten meal, (dry)	16	0.17	358	5,853
Whole cottonseed	814	8.48	154	125,356
Rice bran	127	1.33	77	9,802
Total	2,573	26.81		231,786

[a] Grasser *et al.*, (1995)

A nationwide survey of feedstuffs fed to lactating dairy cattle was recently completed by Mowrey and Spain (1996). Dairy nutritionists from 28 states responded and the results were grouped into 5 regions, midwest (MW), northeast (NE), northwest (NW), southeast (SE), and southwest (SW). The predominant concentrate energy feed was corn followed by barley, sorghum, oats and wheat. The primary protein supplements were soyabean meal, cottonseed meal, soyabean seed, and canola (rapeseed) meal. The predominant by-products were whole cottonseed, soya bean hulls, wheat milling by-products and field maize milling by-products. Alfalfa (hay plus silage) was the principal forage fed, followed by maize forage (silage) and grass forage (hay plus silage) and 15 other forages. Probably the majority of U.S. dairy producers believe that to achieve top production, some alfalfa hay or silage must be part of the forage programme. A recent article (Merrill, 1996) described a forage program without either alfalfa or corn silage in which production averaged 10,900 kg per year. A combination of grasses (primarily stored) provided the forage for this herd.

As part of a symposium which addressed management for herds to produce 13,620 kg of milk per cow per year, Jordan and Fourdraine (1993) sent survey forms to 128 producers who had been identified as high milk producing herds, and from 61 surveys returned, found that maize silage was the dominant forage fed followed by legume hay, legume silage, and grass hay. The average producer supplemented these forages with 6.7 different feed additives (sodium bicarbonate, yeast, tallow, niacin, minerals, etc) and 3.5 different alternative feeds (cottonseed, distillers grains, blood meal, fishmeal, etc). As part of the same symposium, Chase (1993) reviewed some of the practices and applications of using the NRC (1989) recommendations for high-yielding cows. In general, the nutrient guidelines were in relatively close agreement with the rations fed in herds with high production.

Several examples of rations fed to high-producing herds in Wisconsin are shown in Table 25.3 (Gunderson, 1992). A wide array of feedstuffs is apparent, in concert with the high dry matter intake (DMI) necessary to support such intense lactation.

Feed management systems

Forty years ago pasture was a dominant forage for most dairy herds in the U.S., followed by hay and silage. Nearly all dairies fed concentrates in the barn at the time of milking so that eating occurred during milking. In the late 1950s and early 1960s it was discovered that many lactating dairy cows would respond to additional concentrates above the feeding standards used then. As herd sizes increased during the 1960s there was an increased emphasis on labour efficiency and a corresponding increase in the construction of milking parlours. But as production increased there was also greater mechanization in the parlour which further reduced the time cows spent there to be milked. Even when additional time was provided and precision equipment was operated carefully, there was no way to ensure that the appetite of the cow would induce her to consume the required

Table 25.3 SOME RATIONS OF HIGH-YIELDING HERDS IN WISCONSIN WITH PRODUCTION >11,350 KG/COW PER YEAR[a]

Ingredient	Dairy					
	A	B	C	D	E	F
Hay						1.6
Haylage	9.9	10.0	8.5	11.3	5.5	7.9
Maize silage		1.9	3.5		5.5	
High-moisture shelled maize		6.5	7.2		6.0	9.4
High-moisture ear maize	7.5			7.0		
High-moisture barley					2.9	
Distillers' grains		0.4	0.1			0.5
Wet brewers' grains			2.6			
Maize gluten meal	0.5	0.3	0.3	0.3	0.2	
Liquid molasses		0.1				
Soya beans (roasted)	3.5	0.3	2.2	0.9	2.4	0.5
Soya beans (raw)				1.3		
Soya bean meal	0.4	1.3	1.0		1.0	
Soya bean meal (expeller)		0.6				0.5
Fish meal	0.4				0.5	
Whole cottonseed		2.1		2.1		3.4
Meat & bone meal	0.5			1.0	0.3	
Blood meal	0.2	0.1		0.2		0.4
Tallow	0.5	0.5		0.3		
Urea (46%)	0.09		0.06		0.16	
Sodium bicarbonate			0.16		0.23	
Dicalcium phosphate	0.25	0.10	0.39	0.12	0.25	0.25
Limestone		0.11	0.09	0.02	0.16	0.17
White salt	0.11	0.04	0.11	0.08	0.11	0.11
Magnesium oxide	0.05	0.03		0.04	0.04	0.05
Zinc methionine	0.005		0.005		0.005	
Micromins/Vits	0.04	0.02	0.04	0.02	0.04	0.06
Yeast			0.11		0.11	

[a]Gunderson, 1992; High group rations, kg dry matter per day.

concentrate. Most parlour concentrate feeding then became free choice feeding for two 10-minute intervals per day. And the resulting "slug feeding" of highly soluble protein and carbohydrate must have been highly disruptive to a ruminal fermentation system which functions best as a steady state system.

The resolution of the parlour concentrate feeding dilemma has taken several forms: 1) feed some concentrate outside the parlour separate from or blended with forage; 2) use computer controlled concentrate feeders (CCCF); 3) feed all of the concentrate outside the parlour either through the computer feeders or blended with forage as a totally mixed ration (TMR). The TMR system of feeding has been reviewed by Coppock *et al.* (1981); and Spain (1995). A TMR is identified as a quantitative blend of all dietary ingredients, mixed thoroughly enough to prevent separation and sorting, formulated to specific nutrient concentrations and offered *ad libitum.* The national survey (Anonymous, 1996) showed that although among all operations only 35.6% fed a TMR, but among the operations with 200 or more cows, 83.5% fed a TMR. Muller (1992) notes that both research and farmer experiences have shown that from 450 to 900 kg or more increases in milk production per cow per year, when herds were switched to a well formulated TMR.

The CCCF was developed to resolve the dilemma of parlour concentrate feeding and under some conditions it has been quite successful. Its greatest application is in smaller herds and where pasture is a dominant forage programme. The feeders may restrict the cow's rate of eating and the proportion of the 24-hr allotment which a cow can receive at any one meal. Some allow 25% of the day's allowance to be eaten during each 6-hr quadrant of the day. But the CCCF deals only with the concentrate portion of the ration; forage(s) must be dealt with by another system. The problem of feeding concentrates separately from forage is that some cows seem to prefer concentrates to forage and other cows vice versa, and it is difficult to ensure that a cow will eat her needed forage if she is given a large allotment of concentrates which is increasingly necessary as higher production becomes the norm. Moreover, a few cows never learn to use the feeders and social dominance may cause disturbances around the feeders. The feeders are relatively expensive and require routine maintenance and frequent resetting as cows' requirements change.

There are at least three cogent reasons for feeding different TMR rations within the milking herd: 1) The cows can be fed rations which are formulated so that their *ad libitum* consumption will result in more closely meeting the cows' nutrient requirements than some average formulation; 2) Feed costs can usually be reduced by feeding rations of lower nutrient concentration to the lower producing cows; 3) There will be less transfer of certain nutrients (e. g., nitrogen, phosphorus and sodium) to the manure by using formulations tailored to requirements, primarily milk production.

Ideally cows would calve in close calendar proximity so that they could remain in the same group for their entire lactation and the diet composition could be adjusted gradually as lactation advanced. This is most feasible for first lactation cows whose pregnancies were synchronized when they were heifers and who reside in large herds. But most cows will need to change groups as they advance in lactation in order to prevent overcondition and to reduce feed costs. Albright (1983) recommends that farmers should "Move small groups of cows. . . Not only is there social pressure on the cow in her new group, but she may have different amounts of feed, a new milker and a different milking time. Try to keep group size stable and no larger that 100 cows".

Frequency of milking

The Dairy Records Processing Laboratory in North Carolina (Butcher, 1996) reported that 757 herds out of a total of 11,557 herds (6.5%) milked their cows 3 times per day (3X). However, the 3X herds averaged 334 cows compared to an all-herds average of 113 cows. Therefore, 19.4% of the cows whose records are processed by that centre are milked 3X. It is not known whether this number is representative of the whole U.S., but because many larger herds are in the southwest and west, it is probably a low estimate.

DePeters *et al.* (1985) used 38 multiparous cows and 15 primiparous cows (Holsteins) in full lactation studies to compare the effects of twice-daily milking (2X) with three times daily milking (3X) on production, and reproductive performance. The older cows milked 3X produced 15% more milk during the complete lactation and the young cows produced 6% more milk during their first lactation. In both groups, neither dry matter nor energy intakes were affected by milking frequency, but neither group gained as much weight during the lactation as their herdmates milked 2X. Reproductive performance of the cows was not affected. These authors emphasized that herds milked 3X successfully will need careful nutrition and reproductive management.

From a study of 28 California herds (average size, 537), Gisi *et al.* (1986) compared the response of these herds to 2X milking for 3 to 17 months, and after a switch to 3X milking for 36 months. In California during 1984, 11% of the herds and 15% of the cows were being milked 3X. In this study, milk production of all herds increased by 12% above that when they were milked 2X. First lactation cows increased their production by 14%, but the range in response among herds was -2 to +32%. It was further noticed that most of the increased response occurred during the first 3 months that the herds were milked 3X. It was emphasized that if increased response to 3X milking is to be sustained over a long term, better nutrition, especially improved forage and perhaps increased feeding frequency, may be essential. It is not known how soon after a 3X milking regimen appetite will increase. The increase in feed energy which is necessary to support a 15% increase in milk production is shown in Table 25.4. For 27 kg of milk, about 10% more energy is required of the same ration. There is no reason to assume an increased metabolic efficiency, so the increased milk production must be supported with greater dietary nutrient intake.

A study from Michigan (Speicher *et al.*, 1994) shows that the effects of BST and 3X milking are largely additive, although primiparous cows responded more to the combination of BST and 3X milking than did the multiparous cows. If both of these factors are imposed simultaneously, dairy producers should be prepared for the large increase in appetite which will eventually occur.

Table 25.4 EFFECT OF A 15% INCREASE IN MILK YIELD ON FEED REQUIRED TO MAINTAIN BODY ENERGY STATUS

	Initial yield		*15% increase*
		(kg/day)	
	30.0		34.5
		NE_l *(MJ/day)*	
Net energy required for[a]:			
Maintenance[b]	40.58		40.58
Growth (+10%)	4.06		4.06
Milk	86.61		99.58
Total NE_l required	131.25		144.22
Difference		12.97	
Percentage increase in feed required[c]		9.88	

[a] From NRC (1989).
[b] Calculated for 600 kg second lactation, nonpregnant cow, giving milk of 35 g/kg fat.
[c] Assumes no change in digestive or metabolic efficiency and a diet of uniform composition.

Bovine Somatotrophin (BST)

BST has been used commercially in the U.S. for nearly 3 years. The national survey (Anonymous, 1996) showed that of all operations only 9.4% used BST, but in herds of 100-199 cows, 18.5% used this product, and in herds with >200 cows, 31.9% had used BST. So resistance to use was greatest in the small herds of <100 cows. And the percentage of cows that are receiving BST is considerably larger than 10%. Use of BST causes an increase in milk yield within 2-4 days of its first use, although maximal response usually takes from 4 to 6 weeks of sustained use. One survey showed that dairymen were getting an average increase of 4.8 kg of milk per cow per day from BST use. At today's relatively high milk prices, this additional milk is worth about $1.68. With a product cost of about $0.40 per cow per day, and increased feed required of about 2 kg ($0.35) and extra labor of $0.10, the return is highly favorable. Studies with the respiration chambers at USDA-Beltsville, MD (Tyrrell *et al.*, 1988), showed that neither digestive nor metabolic efficiency was changed when BST was used. Therefore, the increased milk which occurs with BST use must be paid for with increased feed. Additional milk of 4.8 kg will require about 2 kg more of feed DM of a well balanced TMR. There is no free lunch with the use of this product. One feature of a cow's appetite, is that there is a lag of 4 to 6 weeks after the first BST injection, before the appetite increases for the additional feed. During this lag period, the nutrients to pay for the additional milk must come from body stores, feed, or a combination of the two. Feed nutrients must be available when the appetite increases so that cows have the chance to replenish nutrient reserves as lactation advances. As with 3X milking, some dairy producers have felt that the sharp response to the initial use of BST has not been sustained, but it is likely in these cases, that the dietary nutrients were not available to sustain the increased milk yields which occurred.

So cows respond to BST in 3 ways; a) they produce more milk; b) after a lag period they eat more feed; and c) when they eat more feed, they produce more heat. Therefore, use of BST affects 2 primary management systems: a) nutritional management, and b) environmental management.

Cornell workers (Van Amburgh *et al.*, 1996) have suggested that because of the increased persistency of cows treated with BST, it may be economically desirable and feasible to deliberately extend the calving interval to as much as 18 months. These workers used nine herds to address this subject with some cows assigned to treatments which allowed extended calving intervals and some cows were never rebred, but all treatment cows received BST beginning at 63 days postpartum. In a preliminary report of this study, it was found that as lactation advanced, milk yield response to BST increased, so that an important difference in persistency occurred. Profitability was greater by nearly $0.75 per cow per day for cows that had an 18-month calving interval vs. those with a 13.2-month interval. This increase in profitability occurred because of greater persistency, fewer postpartum metabolic problems and less culling with fewer replacements required. If the results of this study are confirmed and if they receive wide acceptance, major changes in the management of dairy cows will occur.

Implications of continued emphasis on high yield for cow health, reproduction and longevity

Grohn, Eicker and Hertl (1995) examined the relationship between previous 305-day milk yield and disease in 8070 Holstein cows of second and later parity from within 25 herds in New York State. It was felt that because many disorders occur early in lactation, it was better to use the previous 305-day mature equivalent production. Cows that calved between June 1990 and November 1993 were used in this analysis. A separate statistical model was used to study the occurrence of each of 7 disorders including: retained placenta, metritis, ovarian cysts, milk fever, ketosis, abomasal displacement, and mastitis. Table 25.5 shows the incidence risk as a percentage and the median day of occurrence postpartum. Only mastitis showed an increased incidence with increasing milk yield. However, it was cautioned that this did not necessarily mean a cause and effect relationship. It was explained that often cows with mastitis and low production are culled, whereas higher producing cows with mastitis may be kept in the herd as treatment is applied. Therefore, the continued presence of higher yielding cows with mastitis in the herd may cause an apparent relationship even if none is present.

Although studies reported prior to 1975 showed little relationship of higher milk yields to reproductive performance, later work has accumulated a considerable volume of

Table 25.5 LACTATIONAL INCIDENCE RISKS AND THE MEDIAN DAYS TO THE POSTPARTUM OCCURRENCE OF DISORDERS IN HOLSTEIN COWS[a]

Disorder	Lactational incidence risk (%)	Median post partum day of occurrence (day)
Retained placenta	7.4	1
Metritis	7.6	11
Ovarian cyst	9.1	97
Milk fever	1.6	1
Ketosis	4.6	8
Displaced Abomasum	6.3	11
Mastitis	9.7	59

[a] Grohn *et al.*, (1995); 8070 cows in New York State

research to show that some antagonistic relationship exists between high milk production and reproduction (Nebel and McGilliard, 1993). As these workers have noted, recent studies have described a detrimental effect of high yields particularly through a delay in ovarian activity and by a lower conception rate. But it was emphasized that managerial actions can have a major effect which greatly minimize the effect of the high milk production. In this context, adverse effects of an extended negative energy balance (NEB) can be minimized by formulation strategems such as use of supplemental fat to reduce the interval and degree of NEB. No doubt some of this antagonism is expressed as dairy producers try to achieve the dogma of an ideal calving interval (CI) of 12 to 13.5 months. As noted above, if through the use of BST and/or other management tools, persistency can be maintained at a higher level and a CI of 13 months is no longer sought, then this antagonism may diminish greatly or even disappear.

There is much interest and concern for the nutrition and management of the transition cow, defined as the peripartum period from about 21 days prepartum to 15 to 30 days postpartum. Some work suggests that using low potassium diets and/or adjusting the cation/anion relationship to near zero or slightly negative during the 2 to 3 week prepartum, will result in less subclinical as well as clinical hypocalcemia and less depression in feed intake at parturition which will result in reducing the magnitude of NEB in the early postpartum. If this strategem is successful, it will probably diminish the degree of antagonism between high yields and reproductive performance.

Heat stress and high yields

For those of us who live in the sub-tropics or tropics, another dimension to higher milk yields is that the greater the feed intake, the greater the metabolic heat production. As Dennis Armstrong says, "a cow is a little furnace". And the greater the feed intake, the hotter the furnace. In summer the modern dairy cow does not belong in the sun, so shades, sprinklers and fans are all important for the alleviation of heat stress. But the primary reason for a decline in milk yield in hot weather is a voluntary reduction by the cow in feed intake. From a nutritional perspective, Chandler (1994) states that some feed ingredients have a lower heat increment (the heat associated with the metabolism of nutrients) than others. These include the fats especially, and in general, the lower fibre ingredients. But apart from nutrition, it is clear that if dairy producers in the warmer regions of the world are to keep up with the pace of increasingly higher production, then technologies which reduce heat stress will become increasingly mandatory.

Problems of formulation

The Cornell Net Carbohydrate and Protein System (CNCPS) is our most advanced system of feed formulation, but it too is undergoing a nearly constant revision (Barry *et al.*, 1994). It uses both carbohydrate and protein fractions that are partitioned according to their ease and speed of degradation in the rumen. However, nearly all formulation programs require definitions of degradable intake protein (DIP) and undegradable intake protein (UDP). The National Research Council (NRC) for dairy cattle (1989) recommends 35% UIP and 60% DIP for a cow producing 40 kg of milk per day. Recently, Huber and Santos (1996) summarized the responses of a number of research studies from the literature which compared diets in which soya bean meal protein was replaced with a less degradable protein such as blood meal, brewers grains, feather meal, fish meal and blends of these. From 97 comparisons which involved lactation trials published from 1985 to 1994, it was found that milk yield increased in only 19% of the comparisons, there was no significant change in 73% and there was a significant decline in 9% of the trials. And if better protein nutrition was the goal in these studies, it was not reflected in the milk protein percentage because there was no change or even decreases in most of the trials. This comparison shows that much more care and refinement is needed in the successful application of the UIP/DIP system. Because microbial protein produced in the rumen has the best amino acid profile for milk synthesis, much more effort should be directed to those conditions which maximize the growth of ruminal microbes. In addition, the UIP protein needs an amino acid profile which complements the ruminal microbes. In the above comparison, fish meal substituted for soyabean meal resulted in greater milk yields in 46% of the trials. A major problem for feed formulators is that there is no well accepted method for the determination of DIP/UIP. Therefore, too often we are faced with using best estimates based on book values or from laboratory methods which are at best, compromises.

To provide optimal substrate for ruminal microbes in formulation, an expression for non-fibre carbohydrates (NFC) is needed. Again, lack of rapid, inexpensive laboratory procedures presents a serious obstacle. As Hoover and Miller (1996) note, the determination of NFC, also called nonstructural carbohydrate (NSC) by the difference method (easier method used frequently by feed testing laboratories compared to the enzymatic method which is more tedious), shows large differences for some feedstuffs. The objective is to measure or designate the sugars and starches, the rapidly digestible carbohydrates, but until more data become available from the enzymatic method, or another more rapid determination becomes available, progress is seriously hampered.

Another formulation quandary relates to the appropriate energy expression to use at the production intakes of lactating cows. The problem arises because there is a substantial disagreement between two authorities, the NRC (1989) for dairy cattle and Van Soest, Rymph and Fox (1992), especially for certain co-products. The disagreement arises over the amount of the depression in digestibility which occurs as intakes go from maintenance to 3 or 4 times maintenance. This depression occurs as cows eat more feed which results in a faster rate of passage through the digestive tract and a hence a lower digestibility for the feed. But how much less? The NRC assumes 8% less for all feeds at an intake of 3 times the intake equal to that required for maintenance. Van Soest *et al.* (1992) say that each feed ingredient differs, based on its own special characteristics. In Table 25.6 a comparison of the 2 systems is shown for several co-products. Some large differences are obvious. So what is a dairy producer or a ration formulator to do in light of this controversey? For the time being NRC (1989) is recommended, but it must be remembered that the energy values attached to some of the co-products may not truly reflect their real energy values, especially under some conditions. When a substitution is made to include a certain commodity, do high producers at their peak maintain their production well or even increase, or do they decline? Although this is very subjective, it may be the best indication we have that an appropriate energy value has been used for that co-product.

Conclusions

An old saying seems as true today as it was 50 years ago: "cows are better bred than fed". Geneticists have done an incredible job with their science; but this is good news to nutritionists and those in the feed business. Now when ration changes are made which are true improvements, cows usually respond with greater milk yields.

The food industry generates a large array of by-products which ruminants can use productively to produce milk and meat. This is not to suggest that there are a lot of free lunches out there, because in a free market feed ingredients tend to be sold at a price which reflects their true nutritive value as buyers see them. Yet the availability of these products extends the feed supply and in some cases make special contributions to the diet.

About the time that dairy producers began to expand their herds, and mixer wagons with electronic load cells became available, the TMR system of feeding evolved and

Table 25.6 COMPARISON OF NET ENERGY FOR LACTATION BY VAN SOEST *et al.* (1992) AND NRC FOR DAIRY CATTLE (1989)

Feed	Discount[a] (%)	(NE_l) 3M [a] — (MJ/kg DM) —	NRC [b]
Molasses-Cane	0.0	6.19	6.86
Bakery Waste	2.0	9.00	8.62
Alfalfa Hay	3.2	6.57	6.30
Whole Cottonseed	4.0	9.20	9.33
Soya bean Meal (44%)	5.1	7.45	8.17
Rice Bran	6.6	6.49	6.69
Wheat middlings	7.0	7.95	6.57
Brewers Grains (wet)	10.7	5.61	6.28
Maize Distillers (wet)	14.0	6.90	8.33
Maize Hominy	15.0	6.74	8.41
Pineapple Bran	18.0	4.35	6.49
Soya Hulls	18.0	5.40	7.41

[a] Van Soest *et al.* (1992);
[b] NRC (1989), discounted by 8% for 3M (see text for details).

now is used widely. At first it was used before its inherent advantages were recognized, but today a large majority of enthusiastic users attest to its value. In larger herds, cows are housed in groups for managerial reasons, so that different formulations of TMRs can be used without special housing.

A number of dairymen have tried 3X milking but have returned to 2X milking. The primary reason seems to be that the initial increase in milk seen did not seem to persist, or cows were required to stand on concrete for an extended period and feet and leg problems developed. But an increase in milk yield must be paid for at some point with additional feed nutrients, and the opportunity for cows to eat that extra feed may not have been there in some cases.

The approval of BST for commercial use in the U.S. was accompanied by some controversey, despite years of research done in quadruplicate. Most of the controversey has disappeared or at least it has quietened down. The consistency of response of cows to this product and its successful use by some of the best herds has not yet caused its widespread adoption, despite a clear economic payback. This will probably come with time.

Despite a rather general impression that high yields are accompanied by increased incidence of metabolic problems, except for mastitis, this does seem to occur. There is some antagonism between reproductive competence and high yields, but most dairy producers seem willing to accept this downside. If current research comparing 13.5

month calving intervals with 18 months in conjunction with BST use is supported by additional work, even the lower reproductive performance may diminish or disappear.

Hot weather is a major constraint during summer in many parts of the U.S. If herd owners in the more humid and hotter areas of the world are to keep pace with their colleagues in more temperate regions, major expenditures must be made on technologies for heat stress abatement.

Feed formulators could be much more precise in the construction of diets if more precise values could be used for DIP/UIP, NSC, and net energy. Today, much uncertainty exists for some of the numbers which we use for these nutrient expressions. The bottom line is that much excess supplementation results and considerable money is wasted. Despite these uncertainties, production continues upwards with no limit in sight.

References

Albright, J.L. (1983) Putting together the facility, the worker and the cow. *Proceedings 2nd National Dairy Housing Conference*, 15–22.

Anonymous (1996) *Part I. Reference of 1996 Dairy Management Practices*. National Animal Health Monitoring System.APHIS-VS, U. S. Dept. Agriculture.

Barry, M.C., Fox, D.G., Tylutki, T.P., Pell, A.N., O'Connor,J.D., Sniffen, C.J. and Chalupa, W. (1994) *A manual for using the Cornell Net Carbohydrate and Protein System for evaluating cattle diets*. Revised for CNCPS Release 3, Sept. 1, Cornell University 14853–4801.

Bath, D.L., Dunbar, J.R., King, J.M., Berry, S.L., Leonard, R.O. and Olbrich, S.E. (1980) Byproducts and unusual feedstuffs in livestock rations. *W. Regional Ext. Publ.* 39.

Butcher, K.R. (1996) Personal Communication.

Chandler, P. (1994) Is heat increment of feeds an asset or liability to milk production? *Feedstuffs*, **66**, No. 15 12–17.

Chase, L.E. (1993) Developing nutrition programs for high producing dairy herds. *Journal of Dairy Science*, **76**, 3287–3293.

Coppock, C.E., Bath, D.L. and Harris, Jr., B. (1981) From feeding to feeding systems. *Journal of Dairy Science*, **64**, 1230–1249.

DePeters, E.J., Smith N.E. and Acedo-Rico, J. (1985) Three or two times daily milking of older cows and first lactation cows for entire lactation. *Journal of Dairy Science*, **68**, 123–132.

Gisi, D.D., DePeters, E.J. and Pelissier, C.L. (1986) Three times daily milking of cows in California dairy herds. *Journal of Dairy Science*, **69**, 863–868.

Grasser, L.A., Fadel, J.G., Garnett, I. and DePeters, E.J. (1995) Quantity and economic importance of nine selected by-products used in California dairy rations. *Journal of Dairy Science*, **78**, 962–971.

Grohn, Y.T., Eicker, S.W. and Hertl, J.A. (1995) The association between previous 305-day milk yield and disease in New York State dairy cows. *Journal of Dairy Science*, **78**, 1693–1702.

Gunderson, S. (1992) How six top Wisconsin herds are fed. *Hoard's Dairyman*, **137**, 686–687.

Halladay, D. (1996) Small wonders. *The Western Dairyman*, **77**, (No.9) 8–12.

Hoover, W.H. and Miller, T.K. (1996) Feeding for maximum rumen function. *Proceedings of Mid-South Ruminant Nutrition Conference*, 33–46. Texas Animal Nutrition Council, Dallas, TX

Huber, J.T. and Santos, F.P. (1996) The role of bypass protein in diets for high producing cows. *Proceedings of Southwest Nutrition and Management Conference*, 55–65. U. Arizona.

Jordan, E.R. and Fourdraine, R.H. (1993) Characterization of the management practices of the top milk producing herds in the country. *Journal of Dairy Science*, **76**, 3247–3256.

Merrill, L.S. (1996) 24,000 pounds of milk...no corn silage, no alfalfa. *Hoard's Dairyman*, **141**, 436.

Mowery, A. and Spain, J.N. (1996) Results of a nationwide survey of feedstuffs fed to lactating dairy cattle. *Journal of Dairy Science*, **79**, (Suppl. 1) 202. (Abstr.)

Muller, L.D. (1992) Feeding management strategies. In *Large Dairy Herd Management - 1992*, pp 326–335. Edited by H.H. Van Horn and C. J. Wilcox. Management Services, ADSA, Champaign, IL.

National Research Council (1989) *Nutrient Requirements of Dairy Cattle. 6th Revised Edition, National Academy of Science*, Washington, DC.

Nebel, R.L. and McGilliard, M.L. (1993). Interactions of high milk yield and reproductive performance in dairy cows. *Journal of Dairy Science*, **76**, 3257–3268.

Nizamani, A.H. and Berger, P.J. (1996) Estimates of genetic trend for yield traits of the registered Jersey population. *Journal of Dairy Science*, **79**, 487–494.

Spain, J.N. (1995) Management strategies for TMR feeding systems. *Proceedings 2nd Western Large Herd Management Conference*, 161–168. Las Vegas, NV.

Speicher, J.A., Tucker, H.A., Ashley, R.W., Stanisiewski, E. P., Boucher, J.R. and Sniffen, C.J. (1994) Production responses of cows to recombinantly derived bovine somatotrophin and to frequency of milking. *Journal of Dairy Science*, **77**, 2509–2517.

Tyrrell, H.F., Brown, A.C.G., Reynolds, P.J., Haaland, G.C., Peel, C.J. and Steinhour, W.D. (1988) Effect of Somatotropin on metabolism of lactating cows:energy and nitrogen utilization as determined by respiration calorimetry. *Journal of Nutrition*, **118**, 1024–1030.

Van Amburgh, M.E., Galton, D.M., Bauman, D.E. and Everett, R.W. (1997) Management and economics of extended calving intervals with use of BST. *Livestock Production Science,* **50**, 15-29.

Van Soest, P.J., Rymph, M.B. and Fox, D. (1992) Discounts for net energy and protein - fifth revision. *Proceedings Cornell Nutrition Conference* 40–68. Ithaca, NY.
Walton, R.E. (1983) A glimpse at dairying in the year 2000. *Dairy Science Handbook*, **15**, 511.

This paper was first published in 1997

26

NUTRITION OF THE HIGH GENETIC MERIT DAIRY COW — PRACTICAL CONSIDERATIONS

C. P. FERRIS[1], D. C. PATTERSON[1,2,3] and C. S. MAYNE[1,2,3]
[1] *Agricultural Research Institute of Northern Ireland, Hillsborough, Co Down*
[2] *The Department of Agriculture for Northern Ireland*
[3] *The Queen's University of Belfast*

Introduction

The rapid increase in genetic merit of the dairy herd in the United Kingdom (UK) and Ireland has been described by Agnew, Yan and Gordon (1998). In addition, these workers have reported that, although the efficiency with which metabolisable energy (ME) is converted to milk energy increases with increasing genetic potential, genotype has no effect on the partial efficiency of ME use for lactation (k_1). Thus the higher milk yields of high-merit animals are a consequence of their greater ability to partition ME intake to milk output rather than tissue gain, coupled with their higher intakes (Ferris, Gordon, Patterson, Mayne and Kilpatrick, 1999). While this change in partitioning results in higher milk yields in the short term through the depletion of body tissue, a much longer term approach must be adopted when considering the nutrition of the dairy cow.

In North America, the source of many of the high genetic merit bloodlines currently being used in the UK and where yields of 13500 kg are becoming widespread (Coppock, 1997), alfalfa hay/silage and maize silage are the two most common forages offered (Mowery and Spain, 1996). In addition, relatively high inputs of supplementary concentrates are used. Consequently dry matter (DM) intakes greater than proportionally 0.04 of body weight are common for the cows in many high-producing herds in the United States (US) (Chase, 1993). In contrast, in northern and western areas of the UK, grass-silage based systems, coupled with relatively low concentrate inputs, are common. Since nutrient intakes associated with these systems are considerably less than those achieved in the US, the development of strategies through which nutrient intakes can be economically increased would appear to be a major requisite in feeding the high-merit cow. While increased nutrient intakes can be achieved through increasing the nutrient concentration of the diet and/or increasing total dry matter intake, it is important to note that milk production systems developed in these areas have evolved to suit local climatic conditions and the cost-price relationships between the various inputs and outputs.

Thus questions arise as to whether high-merit animals can be successfully managed on these conventional systems to ensure that improvements in genetic merit ultimately result in increased profit, and if so, how? This paper will examine some of the practical implications of feeding high-merit dairy cows during the winter period in systems based on grass silage and supplementary concentrates. Grazing considerations for these animals were examined previously by McGilloway and Mayne (1996).

Forage quality for cows of high genetic merit

Grass silage remains the principal form of conserved forage offered to dairy cattle during the winter period in the UK. However, low voluntary food intake is a particular problem with grass-silage based diets as it is generally accepted that the intake potential of herbage is reduced as a result of the ensilage process (Mayne and Cushnahan, 1995). Consequently, there is considerable interest at present in opportunities to increase dry matter intake, either through increasing the digestibility of the crop, wilting prior to ensiling or modification of the fermentation process.

FIELD WILTING

Field wilting of herbage prior to ensiling is now widely adopted in silage making systems throughout Europe, primarily as a means of reducing effluent production during ensilage. A number of previous reviews have shown that whilst pre-wilting has generally increased intake of the resulting silage, on average it has marginally reduced animal performance (Rohr and Thomas, 1984). This reduction in animal performance reflects nutrient loss and proteolysis during wilting, particularly with the prolonged field-wilting periods that are often required to achieve DM concentrations of 250-300 g/kg under the prevailing climatic conditions of northern and western regions of Europe.

Recent research has examined opportunities to enhance the rates of crop drying in the field, using either conventional techniques such as conditioning and tedding (Bosma, 1991; Patterson, 1993) or forage-mat making techniques involving maceration and pressing of herbage during cutting (Savoie, Burgess, Knight and McGeechan, 1994; Frost, Poots, Knight, Gordon and Long, 1995). Whilst forage matting has given small improvements in rates of grass drying during wilting, no effects on the chemical composition of silage or DM intake and digestibility by sheep have been observed (Frost *et al.*, 1995).

Yan, Patterson and Gordon (1996) examined the effect of rapid wilting using conventional procedures on food intake and performance of dairy cows over a total of 8 silage harvests. Pre-wilted material was conditioned at mowing, spread immediately, and tedded during the wilting period, with a mean field-wilting period of 39 hours. On average, wilting increased silage DM intake and fat plus protein yield by proportionately

0.2 and 0.05 respectively (Table 26.1). These results suggest that improvements in food intake and animal performance can be achieved with rapid-wilting systems. However, an examination of the data for individual harvests within this experiment indicates a wide range in response; for example, increases in food intake ranged proportionally from 0.10 to 0.35 and changes in fat plus protein yield ranged from -0.01 to +0.18. Thus, while the intake and performance benefits associated with wilting may be considerable, they are not always found, so it is necessary to examine the factors determining the outcome of the wilting process. To this end, the data from the eight harvests presented in Table 26.1, together with data from a further 46 comparisons of wilted and unwilted silages undertaken at Hillsborough, were examined (D. Wright, Personal communication). This analysis showed that the intake response from wilting is primarily related to the extent and rate of water loss from the crop during the wilting process, together with the fermentation quality of the unwilted silage. Therefore, a system of grass analysis should be developed that enables the magnitude of the response from wilting to be predicted, based on the chemical composition of the standing grass crop, the prevailing climatic conditions and the method of crop management in the field.

Table 26.1 EFFECT OF RAPID WILTING OVER 8 HARVESTS ON SILAGE COMPOSITION AND DAIRY COW PERFORMANCE (YAN *et al.*, 1996)

	Unwilted	*Wilted*	*s.e.*
Silage composition			
Dry matter (g/kg)	176	316	2.5
pH	4.14	3.92	0.065
NH_3-N (g/kg total N)	130	74	8.9
Animal performance			
Silage intake (kg DM/d)	10.6	12.7	0.13
Milk yield (kg/d)	21.8	22.4	0.16
Fat + protein yield (kg/d)	1.68	1.77	0.017

DIGESTIBILITY AND FERMENTATION

In addition to DM concentration, the other key factors influencing food intake, and hence animal performance with grass-silage based diets, are digestibility of herbage at harvest and the effects of ensiling on the nitrogen and carbohydrate fractions of the resulting material. The effect of silage digestibility on animal performance was reviewed by Gordon (1989) who concluded that a 10 g/kg decrease in digestible organic matter concentration in silage DM (D-value) resulted in reductions in silage intake and milk yield of 0.16 and 0.37 kg/day respectively. Unfortunately, the production of silage with high digestibility necessitates early and frequent harvesting of grass during the growing season, thereby increasing the cost per unit forage DM relative to low-digestibility silage.

Alternatively, intake can be increased by harvesting grass less frequently and minimising changes in the nitrogen and carbohydrate fractions during ensilage, for example, by the use of high levels of formic acid.   Doherty and Mayne (1996) demonstrated a 0.17 proportionate improvement in intake with a restricted relative to an extensively fermented grass silage. Dawson, Steen and Ferris (1998) examined interactions between grass maturity at harvest, fermentation characteristics and effects of concentrate supplementation on silage DM intake of growing steers. Results for the unsupplemented silages offered in this study indicate that a silage digestible energy (DE) intake of 90 MJ/day could be achieved either by early harvesting (D-value 694) with no additive, or by later harvesting (D-value 640) and applying high levels of organic acids (8.5 litres/tonne of fresh grass) prior to ensiling (Figure 26.1).   These results highlight the range of options that are available to the farmer to achieve a given level of forage DE intake. However, the implications of providing supplementary concentrates to these silages have yet to be clarified.

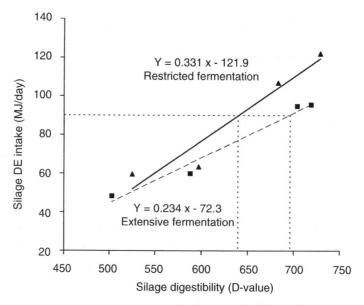

Figure 26.1 Effect of silage digestibility and fermentation pattern on silage digesible energy intake (derived from Dawson *et al.*, 1998)

PREDICTING INTAKE OF FORAGES

A number of studies (Wilkins, Fenlon, Cook and Wilson, 1978; Rook and Gill, 1990) have attempted to produce multi-factor relationships to predict the intake of silage when offered to sheep or cattle. However, the accuracy of these predictive relationships was limited by the fact that they were based on historical data across a range of experiments and consequently confounded a large number of animal and food factors. More recent studies (Offer, Thomas and Dewhurst, 1995; Steen, Gordon, Mayne, Poots, Kilpatrick,

Unsworth, Barnes, Porter and Pippard, 1995) attempted to overcome these confounding effects by feeding large numbers of silages to sheep or cattle within a common feeding management and statistical design. Steen *et al.* (1995), in a study involving 136 grass silages offered to growing cattle, observed that voluntary feed intake was either unrelated, or poorly related, to factors previously considered to have a major effect on intake, for example, pH, buffering capacity, total acidity and lactic and volatile fatty acid concentrations. Factors of moderate importance included DM and ammonia nitrogen concentrations. The key factors influencing intake were the protein and fibre fractions within the silage and, in particular, their relative rates and extent of digestion within the animal. However, the most important finding in this study was the fact that near infrared reflectance spectroscopy (NIRS) on both dried and fresh samples provided a very accurate prediction of silage intake as the sole feed (Park, Gordon, Agnew, Barnes and Steen, 1997).

Concentrate supplements in the diets of high-merit cows

Although generally more expensive than conserved forages, concentrates increase the nutrient concentration of the diet, promote total dry matter intake, and consequently increase nutrient intake and milk output. Their role in dairying systems can be viewed either as a means of allowing the nutritional requirements of the cow to be met, or of controlling nutrition to the point that maximises economic returns. While the former may appear to be an ideal biological concept, reality dictates that the dairy farmer keeps cows with a view to making profit. Consequently, in this paper supplementation will be examined in terms of its ability to improve the profitability of a dairying enterprise. Within this concept the optimum or 'break even' level of supplementation is defined as the point where the value of the extra milk produced, plus savings in forage costs achieved from an additional increment of concentrate feed, is equivalent to the cost of the additional supplement offered. This approach depends on defining the relationships between supplement feed level and silage intake, together with the associated milk output responses. Using this information, breakeven levels of supplementation can be calculated for any feed cost-milk price scenario.

GENOTYPE X SUPPLEMENT LEVEL INTERACTIONS

Supplement-input, milk-output relationships, such as those defined for spring and autumn calving cows by Gordon (1980 and 1984), have been used previously to determine optimum levels of supplementation for dairy cows. In addition, it has been argued that the input-output relationships for groups of high- and low-yielding animals within a herd are parallel, differing only in intercept (Gordon 1984: Mayne and Gordon, 1995). This concept has been the basis of the flat-rate feeding approach to the feeding of concentrates to cows within a herd. However, the animals involved in these comparisons would be considered as low to medium genetic merit today, while animals within trials were genetically quite similar. The rapid increase in the genetic merit of dairy cows in recent years has prompted a re-examination of these input-output relationships. For example, Ferris *et al.*, (1999) compared the responses of high-and medium-merit cows (PTA$_{95}$ fat + protein = 43.3 and 1.0 kg respectively) offered grass-silage based diets containing a range of supplement proportions in the overall diet (0.37, 0.48, 0.59 and 0.70 total DM). Individual response relationships for each genotype indicated a proportionally 0.48 greater fat plus protein yield response with the high- compared with the medium-merit animals (Figure 26.2). These effects are supported by work undertaken at the Langhill Dairy Cattle Research Centre in Scotland, in which 'Control' and 'Selection' line animals (Pedigree index (PI) for fat plus protein = 4.3 and 18.8 kg respectively) have been compared on 'low' and 'high' concentrate regimens (Veerkamp, Simm and Oldham, 1994). When these authors regressed milk production against PI for fat plus protein yield, significantly different regression coefficients for the high- and low-concentrate diets were obtained. This provides additional evidence to support a genotype x nutrition interaction, indicating that the milk yield response to additional feed, increases with genetic merit.

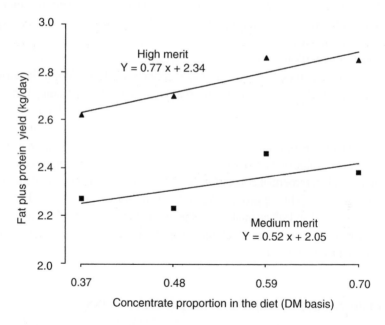

Figure 26.2 Fat plus protein yield responses of high and medium merit cows to increasing the concentrate proportion in the diet (derived from Ferris *et al.*, 1999)

Whilst the previous two sets of data have been obtained under controlled experimental conditions, there is also on-farm evidence that the response to level of concentrate feeding in a herd is influenced by the genetic merit of the individual cow (Cromie, 1999).

This is provided by a study currently in progress at Hillsborough in conjunction with University College Dublin. In this study, concentrate input levels for each herd and milk production and genetic index data for individual animals were obtained from 702 farms throughout Northern Ireland and the Republic of Ireland for the four-year period from 1992—1995. These records were subdivided into herds with high feed inputs, defined as the top quartile of herds in terms of average concentrate input/cow/year, and low feed inputs, defined as the bottom quartile of herds in terms of concentrate input. The mean concentrate inputs were 1.50 and 0.49 t/cow/year for the high and low feed input herds respectively and this provided 21,220 and 11,549 cow records for each of the respective groups.

Within each of these groups Best Linear Unbiased Prediction (BLUP) breeding values were calculated for all sires. Twenty-three sires that had daughters common to both high- and low-input herds had proofs of greater than 60% reliability in both systems and also had official Interbull proofs in the US. Within each of the two herd environments (high- and low-concentrate inputs) the calculated BLUP breeding values were regressed against the Interbull proofs from the US. These relationships were described by the following equations:

High-input	$Y_1 = 0.57x + 198$	$R^2\ 0.65$	Equation 26.1
Low-input	$Y_2 = 0.26x + 113$	$R^2\ 0.54$	Equation 26.2

where Y_1 and Y_2 are the proofs (kg milk) calculated in the high- and low-input systems respectively and x (kg milk) is the Interbull proof in US (Figure 26.3).

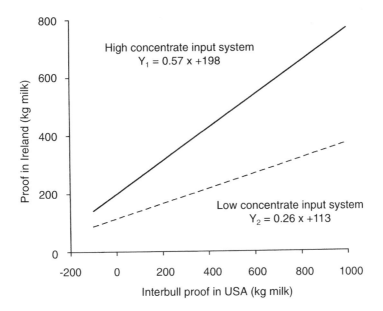

Figure 26.3 Influence of herd concentrate input on BLUP performance of sires (Cromie, 1999)

There are two relevant aspects to these relationships. Firstly the product-moment correlations between proofs in high- and low-input herds with official Interbull proofs in the US were 0.81 and 0.74 respectively. These correlations suggest that for both levels of herd concentrate input there was little evidence of a genotype x environment interaction arising from re-ranking between the countries. However there was a considerable scaling effect, both between the two countries and between the two systems (high *vs* low inputs) within Ireland. The b-values for high- and low-input herds within the US were 0.57 and 0.26 respectively.

The relationships in Equations 26.1 and 26.2 can be used to explore one of the key elements of this review - the effect of genetic merit on the response to additional concentrate input within a practical context. For any given genetic merit (Interbull US) the difference in the response in bull proofs is given by the following equation:

$$Y_1 - Y_2 \quad = \quad 0.57x + 198 - (0.26x + 113)$$
$$= \quad 0.31x + 85 \qquad\qquad \text{Equation 26.3}$$

where x = Interbull proof and $Y_1 - Y_2$ is the response to additional concentrate input.

The relationship in Equation 26.3 demonstrates that at farm level the response in milk yield between the two herd concentrate inputs increases linearly with genetic merit. However, these data are based on breeding values and therefore the enhanced performance of an individual dairy cow will be double those shown in this relationship, i.e. the response in milk output, over the total lactation, between the two concentrate inputs, will be 0.62 kg milk per kg increase in PTA for milk. Assuming a lactation length of 305 days this represents a mean response due to concentrate level (0.49 *vs* 1.50 t) of 0.20 kg milk/day per increase of 100 kg in PTA for milk. The results from this large-scale analysis of herd data therefore strongly support the results established from controlled studies (Veerkamp *et al.*, 1994; Ferris *et al.*, 1999).

It is also of interest to note that the b-value obtained for high-input herds in Ireland (0.57, Equation 26.1) is similar to the value currently applied in the UK formula for converting US bull proofs to UK PTA equivalents (ADC, 1997). This is not surprising given that the average level of concentrate input/cow/year for recorded herds in the UK is similar to that used in the high-input herds in this study (Genus, 1996)

The studies outlined above strongly support the view that there is an interaction between genotype and concentrate feed level, with much greater responses in yield to increased concentrate feeding with animals of high genetic merit. A theoretical representation of these concepts is presented in Figure 26.4. Differences in milk output responses between genotypes must be attributed either to differences in intake and/or differences in nutrient partitioning, based on the *a priori* assumption that cow genotype has no effect on the partial efficiency of ME utilisation for lactation (Agnew *et al.*, 1998).

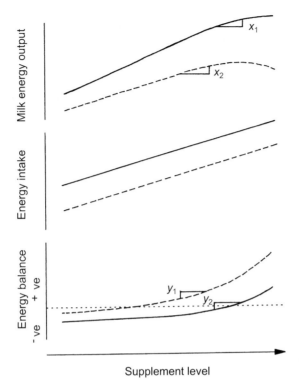

Figure 26.4 Theoretical representation of genotype x supplement level interactions for animals of high (——) and medium (- - -) genetic merit

Figure 26.4 indicates that high-merit cows produce more milk than medium-merit animals at low levels of supplementation, a consequence of more extensive tissue mobilisation and higher feed intakes. The latter is likely to reflect higher rumen capacity and greater intake drive in high-merit animals, a function of their larger body size and higher milk output respectively. It is assumed that body size is positively correlated with genetic merit. Body size effects on intake, through associated effects on rumen capacity, are likely to be most pronounced with bulky diets containing a high proportion of forage. As level of supplementation increases, it could be argued that rumen capacity is likely to become less important in determining intake with control moving towards physiological feedback mechanisms which could be driven by milk yield. However the exact nature of these effects of diet quality on the intake of cows of differing genetic merit is unclear. Ferris *et al.* (1999) observed that the feed intakes by high- and medium-merit cows tended to converge at high levels of supplementation, while Veerkamp *et al.* (1994) recorded the opposite effect when PI (fat plus protein) was plotted against intake for high and low input systems. In the light of these conflicting results, intakes of both genotypes are assumed to be parallel at all levels of supplementation in Figure 26.4.

The relationships shown in Figure 26.4 indicate that at low levels of supplementation high-merit cows experience a greater degree of negative energy balance than medium-merit cows. However, as the proportion of supplement in the diet increases, medium-merit animals exhibit a higher rate of partitioning of nutrients to body-tissue reserves and a lower milk energy output than animals of high genetic merit. Although it is unclear which of these two parameters, milk yield or tissue deposition, is the driving force behind this effect, the outcome remains the same. The milk output response of medium-merit animals begins to exhibit a marked decline (x_2) at a lower level of supplementation than for the high-merit animals (x_1). The reduced milk output responses with both genotypes will be mirrored by a more rapid increase in tissue deposition (y_1 and y_2 for the medium- and high-merit cows respectively). In the scenario postulated in Figure 26.4, differences between genotypes in milk output responses are therefore driven largely by differences in the rate of change of nutrient partitioning between milk and body tissue.

RESPONSE TO SUPPLEMENTATION

The practical implications of a genotype x nutrition interaction are that higher inputs of supplement can be economically justified with animals of higher genetic potential. Determining the optimum level of supplementation for high-merit animals requires a knowledge of supplement-input, milk-output relationships for these animals. While input-output data for high genetic merit cows given grass-silage based diets are limited, a response curve has been developed by combining the data from two trials undertaken at Hillsborough (Ferris *et al.*, 1999; Ferris *et al.*, 2001) (Figure 26.5). In addition, data from two previous trials (Gordon, 1984; Mayne, 1989) involving animals of much lower genetic potential have also been combined to produce a similar response curve for low-merit animals. Experimental effects have been removed by parallel curve analysis. The relationships obtained are described by the following equations:

High genetic merit	$MY = 37.77 - (11.97(0.9065^x))$	Equation 26.4
Low genetic merit	$MY = 25.76 - (12.56(0.7684^x))$	Equation 26.5

in which MY = milk yield (kg/day) and x = concentrate dry matter intake (kg/day).

Although derived from a range of experiments, these response curves demonstrate the markedly differing response to concentrates for animals of high and low genetic merit. In addition, using differential equations derived from the response equations it is possible to quantify the effect of genetic merit on the responses to additional increments of concentrates. These data (Table 26.2) confirm the more rapid decrease in marginal milk yield responses with animals of low, compared with animals of high genetic merit. Using these differential equations, and assuming that a milk-yield response of 0.5 kg milk per kg additional supplement (DM basis) offered is required to 'break even' on an

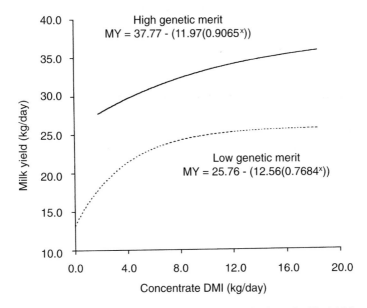

Figure 26.5 Diminishing response relationship between concentrate intake and milk yield for animals of high and low genetic merit (derived from Gordon, 1984; Mayne, 1989; Ferris *et al.*, 1999; Ferris *et al.*, 2001)

Table 26.2 DIRECT RESPONSES IN MILK YIELD TO INCREMENTAL CHANGES IN SUPPLEMENTATION (KG DM/DAY) FOR ANIMALS OF HIGH AND LOW GENETIC MERIT (DERIVED FROM EQUATIONS 26.4 AND 26.5)

Basal level of supplementation (kg DM/day)	*Direct response (kg milk/day) per kg additional supplement DM*	
	High genetic merit	*Low genetic merit*
4	0.79	1.15
6	0.65	0.68
8	0.54	0.40
10	0.44	0.24
12	0.36	0.14
14	0.30	0.08
16	0.24	0.05

economic basis, the optimum inputs of supplement for animals of high and low genetic potential would be 8.7 and 7.2 kg DM/day respectively.

In addition, data presented in Table 26.2 indicate that as the level of supplementation increases the milk yield responses to additional concentrates are small relative to the increased quantity of ME that the concentrates should contribute to the overall diet. While this is likely to be due in part to an increased partitioning of additional nutrients to tissue gain, it is worth noting that the increase in total ME intake (MEI) with additional concentrate ME offered may be relatively small. The latter can be attributed to the fact that the increase in total MEI follows a diminishing response curve as ME from concentrates is increased. For example, when total MEI (MJ/kg DM) was regressed against concentrate DMI (kg/day) for the 4 experiments included in Figure 26.5 (Gordon, 1984; Mayne, 1989; Ferris *et al.*, 1999; and Ferris *et al.*, 2001), experimental effects having been removed by parallel curve analysis, the following relationship was obtained:

$$MEI = 272.7 - (160.9 \ (0.850^x)) \hspace{2cm} \text{Equation 26.6}$$

in which MEI = intake of metabolisable energy (MJ/day) and x = concentrate DMI (kg/day).

The differential of this relationship also provides the incremental response in ME intake to increases in the concentrate DMI throughout the entire range of concentrate feeding levels. This is described by the following equation:

$$d \ MEI/d \ \text{concentrate DMI} = -160.5 \ (\ln \ (0.851)) \ x \ (0.851^x) \hspace{1cm} \text{Equation 26.7}$$

Using this relationship, it is seen that the marginal increase in MEI to 1 kg additional concentrate DM decreases from 13.6 to 2.0 MJ/day when the basal level of concentrate input increases from 4 to 16 kg DM/day (Figure 26.6). This major decline in response is likely to be a function of the increased substitution rate of grass silage by concentrates with increasing levels of supplementation, although at higher levels of supplementation the metabolisability of the diet offered may also be reduced through effects on rumen function. These relationships clearly highlight the fact that offering increasing levels of supplementation has limitations in terms of achieving ever greater ME intakes.

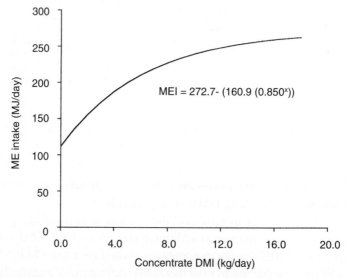

Figure 26.6 Metabolisable energy intake response to concentrate supplementation (derived from Gordon, 1984; Mayne, 1989; Ferris *et al.*, 1999; Ferris *et al.*, 2001)

With the evidence presented in this paper indicating the existence of a genotype x supplement level interaction, the whole question of flat-rate systems of feeding concentrates must be reconsidered. Leaver (1986) compared different systems of concentrate allocation (flat rate vs feed to yield) and concluded that provided forage was offered *ad libitum*, similar total milk outputs were achieved when a constant level of concentrates was offered using either system. However this review did not consider the high genetic merit animals that are available today. As discussed earlier, the concept of flat rate feeding is based on the premise that low- and high-yielding animals within a herd exhibit similar marginal responses in milk yield per unit of additional feed offered, thus allowing a single optimum level of supplementation to be used for all animals. This approach may no longer hold true in herds with a wide range of genetic merit, due to differing optimum levels of supplementation between animals. This statement must however be considered in light of the relatively small differences in optimum levels of supplementation identified between animals of very different genetic potentials, together with the management implications associated with the adoption of more complex regimens of concentrate allocation.

FORAGE QUALITY X SUPPLEMENT LEVEL INTERACTIONS

While the implications of improved forage quality and increased levels of supplementation have already been discussed separately, interactions between the two must also be considered. Results from studies involving animals of low/medium genetic potential are somewhat conflicting, with Steen and Gordon (1980), Castle, Retter and Watson (1980) and Phipps, Weller and Bines (1987) observing no interaction between silage quality and response to supplement level, and other workers (Moisey and Leaver, 1984; and Aston, Thomas, Daley, Sutton and Dhanoa, 1994) finding an increased response in milk yield to increasing concentrate level with medium- compared with high-quality silages. However, the majority of these studies tended to focus on concentrate levels below 10 kg per day (fresh basis). In a recent study, Ferris *et al.* (2001) offered lactating cows of high genetic merit (PTA_{95} fat + protein 40.0 kg) silages of high (D value 747) and medium (D value 661) quality. The former was supplemented with concentrates at proportional inclusion rates of 0.10, 0.30, 0.50 and 0.70, and the latter at 0.32, 0.48, 0.64 and 0.80 total DM. The milk output responses are described by the following equations:

High-quality silage	$MY = 34.15 - (11.94 (0.0101^x))$	Equation 26.8
Medium-quality silage	$MY = 34.22 - (28.46 (0.0101^x))$	Equation 26.9

where MY = milk yield (kg/day) and x = concentrate proportion in the diet (DM basis).

The milk output responses plotted in Figure 26.7 indicate that at low levels of concentrate inclusion the benefit in milk yield associated with offering the high-quality silage is considerable, but this benefit is greatly reduced as the concentrate proportion in

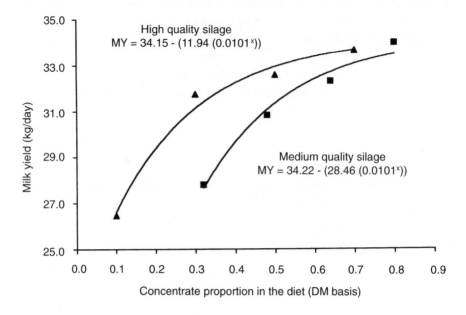

Figure 26.7 Milk yield responses to increasing proportion of concentrate in the diet with silages of two different qualities (Ferris *et al.*, 2001)

the diet increases. The direct effects of silage type on milk output can be derived from the study by Ferris *et al.* (2001) by regressing milk output against concentrate dry matter intake. In this analysis milk yield has been expressed on a standard milk basis (40 g/kg fat, 32 g/kg protein), thus overcoming differences between silages in terms of milk composition:

High-quality silage	$SMY = -0.084x^2 + 1.91x + 26.3$	Equation 26.10
Medium-quality silage	$SMY = -0.081x^2 + 2.11x + 22.2$	Equation 26.11

where SMY = yield of standard milk (40 g/kg fat, 32 g/kg protein) and x = concentrate DMI (kg/day)

The effect of silage quality on the output of standard milk, as derived from 26.10 and 26.11, has been presented in Table 26.3 for a range of concentrate levels. The higher milk output associated with the high-quality silage is a function of its higher intake together with its higher nutritive value. However, as the concentrate level is increased from 4 to 16 kg DM/day, the benefit in milk yield associated with offering the high-quality silage declines from 3.25 kg to 0.21 kg milk/day. While part of this effect may be attributed to the reduction in the quantity of silage in the diets (proportional reduction of 0.47 and 0.43 for the high- and medium-quality silages respectively), the proportional decline in milk

Table 26.3 RESPONSE IN YIELD OF STANDARD MILK (40 G/KG FAT, 32 G/KG PROTEIN) FROM IMPROVING SILAGE QUALITY AT A RANGE OF LEVELS OF CONCENTRATE SUPPLEMENTATION (DERIVED FROM FERRIS *et al.*, 2001)

Supplement DMI (kg/day)	Additional milk produced from high-quality silage
4	3.25
6	2.80
8	2.33
10	1.83
12	1.31
14	0.77
16	0.21

yield response to the higher quality silage was 0.94. This supports the view that other factors were involved. For example, at high levels of MEI there is a much greater partitioning of nutrients to body tissue gain rather than milk yield (Agnew *et al.*, 1998). From a practical point of view, these results suggest that for milk producers operating systems with low inputs of supplements, producing a high-quality silage remains of paramount importance. However, when supplements are offered in excess of 0.5 of total dry matter intake, the quality of silage offered becomes less critical. In fact, the economics associated with offering a high-quality silage with high concentrate inputs must be questioned. For example, at a concentrate input of 16 kg DM/day, intakes of the high- and medium-quality silages were 8.0 and 6.5 kg DM/day respectively, while the benefit in milk yield associated with the high-quality silage was only 0.21 kg milk/day. A full economic appraisal of these alternative scenarios can be undertaken when the effects of concentrate DMI on silage DMI and milk yield are fully quantified. The relationships derived for milk yield are presented above (Equations 26.10 and 26.11), while linear relationships for silage DMI are given below:

High-quality silage	$DMI = -0.603x + 17.66$	Equation 26.12
Medium-quality silage	$DMI = -0.409x + 13.06$	Equation 26.13

where DMI = silage DMI (kg/day) and x = concentrate DMI (kg/day)

Using these equations, 'break-even' levels of supplementation have been calculated for a number of milk price/supplement cost scenarios (Table 26.4). In these calculations the high- and medium-quality silages have been costed at £100 and £75 per tonne DM respectively. The data presented in Table 26.4 indicate that optimum levels of supplement input are influenced by fluctuations in supplement cost and milk price. In addition, for any given costing scenario in this analysis, silage quality has relatively little impact on

Table 26.4   BREAK-EVEN LEVELS OF SUPPLEMENTATION (KG CONCENTRATE DM/
DAY) FOR HIGH- AND MEDIUM-QUALITY SILAGES FOR A RANGE OF MILK PRICE-
SUPPLEMENT COST SCENARIOS (DERIVED FROM FERRIS *et al.*, 2001)

	High-quality silage	*Medium-quality silage*
Milk @ 24 p/l, supplement @ £184/t DM	8.4	9.1
Milk @ 24 p/l, supplement @ £137/t DM	9.5	10.3
Milk @ 18 p/l, supplement @ £184/t DM	7.3	7.8
Milk @ 18 p/l, supplement @ £137/t DM	8.9	9.4

the break-even levels of supplementation. The decision on whether to produce milk
from high- or medium-quality silage will be influenced by many factors. For example, at
the break-even levels of supplementation within any of the scenarios presented in Table
26.4, a higher milk output will be produced with the high-quality silage, thus necessitating
fewer animals to achieve a given output of milk. In addition, the silage costs used in
these calculations include an opportunity cost of £247/ha for the land used. However
this figure will be influenced by many local factors, including land availability and the
profitability of alternative enterprises that could be conducted on a farm. The use of a
lower opportunity cost for land would reduce the costs involved in producing milk from
a high-quality silage to a greater extent than for a medium-quality silage. Taking a
longer-term perspective, while milk price and supplement costs are likely to fluctuate
depending on a large range of factors, the trend in silage production costs seems likely to
continue upwards. If this trend continues, the long-term feasibility of high-quality silage
systems may be questionable.

   Furthermore, marginal milk yield responses may not be the only factor influencing
optimum levels of supplement input. For example, offering supplements at feed levels
above the break-even level may be justified should additional benefits be identified, such
as improved longevity, health or fertility.

RESIDUAL RESPONSES TO SUPPLEMENTATION

The preceding discussion has been primarily concerned with the direct response to
changes in feed input, ie responses during the period over which the feed input changes
have been in place. In addition to the direct responses to concentrate feeding during the
winter period, it has been recognised for a long time that additional nutrients fed at one
stage in the lactation may result in more milk being produced later in the lactation, or
indeed during subsequent lactations (Broster, 1972). These residual responses may have
considerable implications for the economics of supplement feeding. Gordon (1980),
reviewing the findings of a number of studies undertaken with animals which would now
be considered of low genetic potential, noted that the largest residual effects were

recorded when levels of nutrition during the post-calving period were low. Ferris, Gordon, Patterson and Mayne (1997) measured the effects of winter concentrate allowance on performance of high-merit cows after turnout to pasture and observed a positive residual response in milk yield during one study but no effect in another. Indeed, in the former study the magnitude of the residual response was approximately half of the direct response to concentrate feeding. Such a residual response would have a major effect on the economic break-even point. The later mobilisation of tissue reserves deposited at higher levels of supplementation, or the replenishment of reserves lost following periods of underfeeding, together with residual effects on udder secretory tissue, seem likely explanations for residual milk yield effects. However current understanding of factors affecting residual responses, or indeed of the likely magnitude of any residual response, is insufficient to enable this to be accurately considered when planning feed levels to be used in winter.

RESPONSE TO SYSTEM OF FEEDING CONCENTRATE SUPPLEMENTS

In traditional indoor feeding systems in the UK, the concentrate supplement is offered separately from the silage, as two in-parlour meals per day. However, the alternative practice of intimately mixing the concentrate supplement with the forage component of the diet to form a homogeneous blend, termed a complete diet or TMR, is becoming increasingly popular. Benefits claimed for complete-diet feeding are often attributed to improved synchronisation of the supply of dietary fermentable energy and nitrogen in the rumen, and minimising fluctuations in rumen fermentation patterns. The former has been reported to increase the efficiency of microbial synthesis in the rumen (Sinclair, Garnsworthy, Newbold and Buttery, 1993). In addition, the use of complete-diet equipment provides opportunities to use a range of alternative feeds.

Mixing the concentrate and forage components prior to feeding, in comparison with feeding the forage and concentrate separately, has been widely investigated during the last two decades. A summary of the results from 14 such studies, with a similar intake of concentrate on both systems, is presented in Table 26.5. Over these studies the mean responses in DM intake and milk yield to complete diet feeding were positive, with proportional increases of 0.09 and 0.03 respectively. While there is evidence within some of these studies that improvements in DM intake with complete diet feeding were more likely to be obtained at higher concentrate proportions (Phipps, Bines, Fulford and Weller, 1984; Istasse, Reid, Tait and Ørskov, 1986), this was not universal, with no increase being obtained in the studies of Villavicencio, Ruscoff, Girouard and Waters (1968) and Holter, Urban, Haynes and Davies (1977). In addition, positive intake responses have been obtained in some studies which used a low proportion of concentrates in the diet (Dulphy, Rouel, Bony and Andrieu, 1994; Agnew, Mayne and Doherty, 1996). However, when the responses in milk yield are examined a clearer picture unfolds, with improvements in milk yield generally being obtained when the proportion of concentrates

Table 26.5 COMPARISONS OF THE EFFECTS OF COMPLETE DIET (CD) AND SEPARATE FEEDING OF THE FORAGE AND CONCENTRATE (SF) ON DRY MATTER (DM) INTAKE AND MILK YIELD

Forage type and concentrate proportion of DM	Days†	DM intake (kg DM per day)		Milk yield (kg/day)		Milk fat (g/kg)		Milk protein (g/kg)		References
		CD	SF	CD	SF	CD	SF	CD	SF	
Pineapple bran, 0.50	42	13.6	13.6	14.8	14.3	39.6	40.7	34.6	35.4	Stanley and Morita (1967)
Alfalfa hay, 0.70	50	20.4	19.8	28.5	27.2	27.7	29.1	31.5	34.5	Villavicencio et al. (1968)
Wilted grass silage, 0.56	14	16.6	16.1	25.0	24.5	42.2	42.7			Wiktorsson and Bengtsson (1973)
Grass/maize silage, 0.61	43	15.3	15.0	24.1	22.8	36.5	38.0	31.5	31.4	Holter et al (1977)
Maize/lucerne silage, 0.60	21	16.5	14.3	22.2	22.1	39.2	31.6	33.5	32.1	Phipps et al (1984)
Grass silage, 0.50	21	16.4	16.1	23.6	24.2	40.7	40.1	32.8	32.4	
Maize/lucerne silage, 0.50	120	21.5	20.0	28.3	28.5	35.7	35.5	33.2	33.6	Nocek, Steele and Braund (1986)
Hay, 0.40	2	17.0	15.4	24.3	23.3	38.7	38.2			Istasse et al (1986)
Hay, 0.65	2	18.6	14.9	28.2	24.3	34.4	36.6			
NH₃-treated straw, 0.60	2	15.5	14.6	25.3	24.0	37.5	38.3			
Grass silage, 0.28	na	16.3	12.9	28.5	27.4	39.4	40.6	31.5	31.2	Dulphy et al (1994)
Grass silage, 0.29	na	13.0	11.6	21.9	22.6	35.1	37.5	27.6	32.3	
Grass silage, 0.33	11	13.9	12.9	20.0	19.8	39.1	37.8	27.3	27.6	Agnew, Mayne and Doherty (1996)
Grass silage, 0.43	12	15.8	15.7	22.7	22.8	39.4	39.2	31.1	30.7	
Mean	28	16.5	15.2	24.1	23.4	37.5	37.6	31.5	32.1	

†Number of days after calving at start of experiment (na - not available)

was 0.6 or higher (Villavicencio *et al.,* 1968; Holter *et al.,* 1977; Istasse *et al.,* 1986), the exception being the first experiment by Phipps *et al.* (1984).

It should be noted that in most of the studies involving a concentrate proportion in the diet of >0.6, and where a milk yield benefit was recorded with complete diet feeding, forages other than grass silage were offered. This is particularly relevant in view of the importance of grass silage in the UK, and the trend to offer ever increasing levels of supplementation to animals of high genetic merit. Furthermore, at these high levels of supplementation traditional in-parlour concentrate feeding systems, in which the daily allowance is normally consumed in two or three brief time periods, have their limitations. However, modern computerised out-of-parlour systems for concentrate feeding allow the concentrates to be offered in a large number of small meals throughout each 24 hour period. Consequently, it is possible that the benefits claimed for complete diet feeding in terms of synchrony of supply of fermentable energy and nitrogen to the microbial population in the rumen, could equally be achieved with a computerised concentrate feeding system.

A series of three experiments, involving animals which were mainly of high genetic merit, has been undertaken to compare two methods of offering concentrate supplements, i.e. either fed separately from the silage using a computerised out-of-parlour feeding system or within a complete diet (Gordon, Patterson, Yan, Porter, Mayne and Unsworth, 1995; Yan, Patterson and Gordon, 1998). The mean proportion of concentrates in the total diet across the three experiments was 0.61, and in all studies the forage offered was good quality grass silage. The weighted overall mean responses across the three experiments are summarised in Table 26.6. In contrast to the majority of studies reviewed in Table 26.5, data presented in Table 26.6 indicates that complete diet feeding decreased total DM intake by 0.03 proportionally. This difference may be due to the concentrate being offered throughout the day in the studies in Table 26.6, thus minimising the disturbance to rumen digestion, compared with twice-daily feeding, as used in most studies presented in Table 26.5. However in the present series of studies milk yield was increased by 1.9 kg/day (0.06 proportionally) through offering the concentrate as a complete diet rather than by an out-of-parlour feeding system, while fat plus protein yield was increased by only 0.02 proportionally. The latter reflects the reduced concentration of milk fat with the complete diet system, which is in agreement with the results of a number of studies presented in Table 26.5 (Villavicenio *et al.,* 1968; Holter *et al.,* 1977; Istasse *et al.,* 1986). This reduction in milk fat may be due to a reduced concentration of fat precursors in the rumen. For example, when the two methods of concentrate feeding were simulated with rumen-fistulated steers with a concentrate proportion of 0.61 total DM, the ratio of lipogenic/non-lipogenic rumen fatty acids (Sutton, 1981) were 3.11 and 3.56 for complete diet and separate feeding respectively (Yan *et al.,* 1998), in agreement with the findings of Agnew *et al.* (1996).

The increase in milk yield associated with complete diet feeding in the present series of studies occurred despite a reduction in total DM intakes, and cannot be explained by treatment effects on the digestibility of dietary energy (Gordon *et al.,* 1995; Yan *et al.,* 1998). In addition, one of these studies (Gordon *et al.,* 1995) involved placing a number

Table 26.6 RESPONSES TO COMPLETE-DIET FEEDING VERSUS COMPUTERISED OUT-OF-PARLOUR FEEDING OF THE CONCENTRATE SUPPLEMENT - WEIGHTED OVERALL MEAN RESPONSES ACROSS THREE EXPERIMENTS (GORDON *et al.*, 1995 ; YAN *et al.*, 1998)

	Silage intake (kg DM/day)	Concentrate intake (kg DM/day)	Total intake (kg DM/day)	Milk yield (kg/day)	Fat (g/kg)	Protein (g/kg)	Yield of fat plus protein (kg/day)
Weighted mean	7.5	11.5	19.0	32.7	39.8	33.9	2.40
Response to complete diet	-0.9	0.3	-0.6	1.9	-1.7	-0.1	0.05
Proportional response	-0.11	0.03	-0.03	0.06	-0.04	0.01	0.02

of animals in respiration chambers, with the results indicating that the partial efficiency of ME use for lactation (k_l) was the same (0.58) for both the complete diet treatment and the out-of-parlour feeding treatment. Nevertheless, when the ratio of milk energy output/ME intake was calculated for the three studies (assuming methane energy to be 0.08 of gross energy intake and estimating milk energy output after Tyrell and Reid (1965) in the experiments by Yan *et al.* (1998)), the mean values indicate a higher energetic efficiency with complete diet feeding of concentrates (0.46) compared to out-of-parlour feeding of concentrates (0.43). However, this type of calculation ignores the potential effects of treatments on body-tissue reserves. It must also be remembered that these benefits were obtained at high concentrate levels (mean of 11.5 kg DM/day), which is above any of the break-even levels of supplementation calculated for a range of milk price/concentrate cost/silage quality scenarios (Table 26.4). At a concentrate proportion in the diet of less than 0.6 total DM, lower performance responses to complete diet feeding would be expected.

Conclusions

The current trend towards increasing genetic merit of the UK dairy herd must be matched by improvements in animal nutrition. However, any improved nutritional regimen must not nullify the potential economic advantages associated with the higher overall efficiencies of ME conversion to milk production of high-merit animals. The efficient production and utilization of grass silage is therefore likely to remain a central part of feeding strategies for high genetic merit dairy cows in northern and western areas of the UK for the foreseeable future. Options for increasing nutrient intakes from grass silage include harvesting earlier to produce a crop of higher digestibility, adoption of field techniques to enable rapid wilting to be achieved, and restriction of the fermentation process. However, there are increased costs involved with each of these options and it is important that clear decisions, based on sound economics, are made in relation to the best way forward at an individual farm level.

The role of concentrate feedstuffs as supplements to grass silage for animals of high genetic merit is likely to increase, although it is essential that this takes place within a scenario of improved profitability. The greater responses in milk yield to increments of additional concentrates identified for animals of high compared with low genetic merit, suggests a higher economic break-even level of supplementation for animals as genetic merit increases. However, even with high-merit animals, offering concentrates at levels beyond the economic break-even level makes little economic sense, especially as there is no evidence that animal longevity, health or fertility are positively correlated to concentrate feed level. In addition, although residual responses during the grazing period may influence the break-even level of supplementation, both the occurrence and magnitude of these responses are difficult to predict, and therefore cannot be readily incorporated into prediction models for calculating optimum levels of concentrate input. It must also be noted that offering increased levels of supplementation is not necessarily a means of achieving ever increasing ME intakes, as the response in ME intake to supplementation decreases markedly at high concentrate feed levels. This effect accounts in part for the decreasing marginal response in milk yield to concentrate supplementation that occurs as level of supplementation increases. Similarly, improving silage quality at the same time as increasing the level of supplementation also has its limitations, since the benefit in milk yield from feeding a high-quality silage decreases with increasing levels of supplementation. Small improvements in animal performance and efficiency have been identified when concentrates were offered in the form of a complete diet rather than through an out-of-parlour feeding system. However these benefits have only been obtained when concentrate feeding levels were above the break-even levels of supplementation identified for a wide range of milk price/concentrate cost scenarios.

References

Animal Data Centre (ADC) (1997). UK Statistics for genetic evaluation (Dairy). August 1997

Agnew, K.L., Mayne, C.S. and Doherty, J.G. (1996). An examination of the effects of method and level of concentrate feeding on milk production in dairy cows offered a grass silage-based diet. *Animal Science* **63,** 21-31.

Agnew, R.E., Yan, T. and Gordon, F.J. (1998). Nutrition of the high genetic merit dairy cow - energy metabolism studies. In: *Recent Advances in Animal Nutrition* (Eds. P.C. Garnsworthy and J. Wiseman), pp. 181-208, Nottingham University Press : Nottingham.

Aston, K., Thomas, C., Daley, S.R., Sutton, J.D. and Dhanoa, M.S. (1994). Milk production from grass silage diets : effects of silage characteristics and the amount of supplementary concentrate. *Animal Production*, **59,** 31-41.

Bosma, A.H. (1991). Efficient field treatment for silage and hay. In: G. Pahlow and H. Honig (eds.), *Landbauforschung Volkenrode, Sonderheft 123 Forage Conservation Towards 2000*, pp. 71-85.

Broster, W.H. (1972). Effect on milk yield of the cow of the level of feeding during lactation. *Dairy Science Abstracts*, **34,** 265-288.

Castle, M.E., Retter, W.C. and Watson, J.N. (1980). Silage and milk production : a comparison between three grass silages of different digestibilities. *Grass and Forage Science*, **35,** 219-225.

Chase, L.E. (1993). Developing nutrition programmes for high producing dairy herds. *Journal of Dairy Science*, **76,** 3287-3293.

Coppock, C.E. (1997). Feeding and managing high-yielding dairy cows - the American experience. In: *Recent Advances in Animal Nutrition - 1997* (Eds. P.C.

Garnsworthy and J. Wiseman), pp. 135-151, Nottingham University Press : Nottingham.

Cromie, A.R. (1999). *Genotype by environmental interactions for milk production traits in Holstein Friesian dairy cattle in Ireland.* PhD Thesis. Queens University, Belfast.

Dawson, L.E.R., Steen, R.W.J. and Ferris, C.P. (1998). The effect of stage of grass maturity at harvesting and restricting fermentation on the intake of grass silage by beef cattle. In: *Proceedings of the British Society of Animal Science, Winter Meeting, 1998. Scarborough,* Page 43.

Doherty, J.G. and Mayne, C.S. (1996). The effect of concentrate type and supplementary lactic acid or soya oil on milk production characteristics in dairy cows offered grass silages of contrasting fermentation type. *Animal Science*, **62,** 187-198.

Dulphy, J.P., Rouel, J., Bony, J. and Andrieu, J.P. (1994). Feeding value of complete diets based on grass silage for dairy cows. *Annales de Zootechnie* **43,** 113-123.

Ferris, C.P., Gordon, F.J., Patterson, D.C. and Mayne, C.S. (1997). The effects of winter concentrate feed level on the post-turnout performance of high merit cows. In: *Proceedings of the Irish Grassland and Animal Production Association, 23rd Annual Research Meeting, Dublin.*

Ferris, C.P., Gordon, F.J., Patterson, D.C., Mayne, C.S. and Kilpatrick, D.J. (1999). The influence of dairy cow genetic merit on the direct and residual responses to level of concentrate supplementation. *Journal of Agricultural Science, Cambridge*, **132**, 467-481.

Ferris, C.P., Gordon, F.J., Patterson, D.C., Kilpatrick, D.J., Mayne, C.S. and McCoy, M. (2001). The response of dairy cows of high genetic merit to increasing proportion of concentrate in the diet with a high and medium feed value silage. *Journal of Agricutlural Science, Cambridge*, **136**, 319-329.

Frost, J.P., Poots, R., Knight, A.C., Gordon, F.J. and Long, F.N.J. (1995). Effects of forage matting on rate of grass drying, rate of silage fermentation, silage intake and digestibility of silage by sheep. *Grass and Forage Science*, **50,** 21-30.

Genus (1996). Genus milk minder Annual Report, 1995-1996.

Gordon, F.J. (1980). Feed input - milk output relationships in the spring-calving dairy cow. In: *Recent Advances in Animal Nutrition - 1980* (Ed. W. Haresign), pp. 15-32, London : Butterworths.

Gordon, F.J. (1984). The effect of level of concentrate supplementation given with grass silage during the winter on total lactation performance of autumn-calving dairy cows. *Journal of Agricultural Science, Cambridge*, **102,** 163-179.

Gordon, F.J. (1989). The principles of making and storing high quality, high intake silage. In: C.S. Mayne (Ed.). *Silage for Milk Production. Occasional Symposium of the British Grassland Society No. 23*, pp. 3-19.

Gordon, F.J., Patterson, D.C., Yan, T., Porter, M.G., Mayne, C.S. and Unsworth, E.F. (1995). The influence of genetic index for milk production on the response to complete diet feeding and the utilisation of energy and nitrogen. *Animal Science* **61,** 199-210.

Holter, J.B., Urban, W.E., Haynes, H.H. and Davies, H.A. (1977). Utilisation of diet components fed blended or separately to lactating cows. *Journal of Dairy Science* **60,** 1288-1293.

Istasse, I., Reid G.W., Tait, C.A.G. and Ørskov, E.R. (1986). Concentrates for dairy cows: effects of feeding method, proportion in diet and type. *Animal Feed Science and Technology* **15,** 167-182.

Leaver, J.D. (1986). Systems of concentrate distribution. In: *Principles and practice of feeding dairy cows*. Eds. W.H. Broster, R.H. Phipps and C.L. Johnston, pp. 113-131, *Technical Bulletin 8, NIRD Reading*.

Mayne, C.S. (1989). Effect of protein content of the supplement on the response to level of supplementation for diary cows with *ad libitum* access to grass silage. Proceedings of the British Society of Animal Production Winter Meeting 1989. Paper 24.

Mayne, C.S. and Cushnahan, A. (1995). The effects of ensilage on animal performance from the grass crop. *68th Annual Report of the Agricultural Research Institute of Northern Ireland*, pp. 30-41.

Mayne, C.S. and Gordon, F.J. (1995). Implications of genotype x nutrition interactions for efficiency of milk production systems. In: *Breeding and Feeding the High Genetic Merit Dairy Cow* (Eds. T.L.J. Lawrence, F.J. Gordon and A. Carson), pp. 67-77. *Occasional Publication No. 19, British Society of Animal Production, 1995.*

McGilloway, D.A. and Mayne, C.S. (1996). The importance of grass availability for the high genetic merit dairy cow. In: *Recent Advances in Animal Nutrition* (Eds. P.C. Garnsworthy, J. Wiseman and W. Haresign), pp. 135-169, Nottingham University Press : Nottingham.

Moisey, F.R. and Leaver, J.D. (1984). A study of two cutting strategies for the production of grass silage for dairy cows. *Research and Development in Agriculture*, **1,** 47-52.

Mowery, A. and Spain, J.N. (1996). Results of a nationwide survey of feedstuffs fed to lactating dairy cattle. *Journal of Dairy Science*, **79,** (Suppl.1) 202 (Abstract).

Nocek, J.E., Steele R.L. and Braund, D.G. 1986. Performance of dairy cows fed forage and grain separately versus a total mixed ration. *Journal of Dairy Science,* **69,** 2140-2147.

Offer, N.W., Thomas, C. and Dewhurst, R.J. (1995). Validation of advisory models for the prediction of voluntary intake of grass silage by lambs and dairy cows. *Proceedings of the British Society of Animal Science Winter Meeting 1995,* pp. 22.

Park, R.S., Gordon, F.J., Agnew, R.E., Barnes, R.J. and Steen, R.W.J. (1997). The use of near infrared reflectance spectroscopy on dried samples to predict biological parameters of grass silage. *Animal Feed Science and Technology*, **68,** 235-246.

Patterson, D.C. (1993). The effects of grass and swath treatment factors on the rate of drying of silage grass, pp. 52-53, *Proceedings of the 10th International Silage Research Conference, Dublin.*

Phipps, R.H., Bines, J.A., Fulford, R.J. and Weller, R.F. (1984). Complete diets for dairy cows; a comparison between complete diets and separate ingredients. *Journal of Agricultural Science, Cambridge,* **103,** 171-180.

Phipps, R.H., Weller, R.F. and Bines, J.A. (1987). The influence of forage quality and concentrate level on dry matter intake and milk production of British Friesian heifers. *Grass and Forage Science,* **42,** 49-58.

Rohr, K. and Thomas, C. (1984). In Eurowilt: Efficiency of silage systems - a comparison between unwilted and wilted systems. *Landbauforschung Volkenrode, Sonderheft,* 69, pp. 64-70.

Rook, A.J. and Gill, M. (1990). Prediction of the voluntary intake of grass silages by beef cattle. 1. Linear regression analysis. *Animal Production,* **50,** 425-438.

Savoie, P., Burgess, L.R., Knight, A.C. and McGeechan, M.B. (1994). Drying and physical characteristics of matted ryegrass. *Grass and Forage Science,* **49,** 257-263.

Sinclair, L.A., Garnsworthy, P.C., Newbold, J.R. and Buttery, P.J. (1993). Effects of synchronising the rate of dietary energy and nitrogen on rumen fermentation and microbial protein synthesis in sheep. *Journal of Agricultural Science, Cambridge,* **120,** 251-263.

Stanley, R.W. and Morita, K. (1967). Effects of frequency and method of feeding on performance of lactating dairy cattle. *Journal of Dairy Science,* **50,** 585-586.

Steen, R.W.J. and Gordon, F.J. (1980). The effect of type of silage and level of concentrate supplementation offered during early lactation on total lactation performance of January/February calving cows. *Animal Production,* **30,** 341-354.

Steen, R.W.J., Gordon, F.J., Mayne, C.S., Poots, R.E., Kilpatrick, D.J., Unsworth, E.F., Barnes, R.J., Porter, M.G. and Pippard, C.J. (1995). Prediction of the intake of grass silage by cattle, pp. 67-89. In: P.C. Garnsworthy and D.J.A. Cole (eds.). *Recent Advances in Animal Nutrition 1995,* Butterworths, London.

Sutton, J.D. (1981). Concentrate feeding and milk composition. In *Recent Advances in Animal Nutrition* (ed. Haresign, W.), pp. 35-48. Butterworths, London.

Tyrell, H.F. and Reid, J.T. (1965). Prediction of the energy value of cow's milk. *Journal of Dairy Science,* **48,** 1215-1223.

Veerkamp, R.F., Simm, G. and Oldham, J.D. (1994). Effects of interaction between genotype and feeding system on milk production, feed intake, efficiency and body tissue mobilization in dairy cows. *Livestock Production Science,* **39,** 229-241.

Villavicencio, E., Ruscoff, L.L., Girouard, R.E. and Waters, W.H. (1968). Comparison of complete feed rations to a conventional ration for lactating cows. *Journal of Dairy Science,* **51,** 1633-1638.

Wiktorsson, H. and Bengtsson, A. (1973). Feeding dairy cattle during the first part of lactation. 2. Comparison of *ad lib.* feeding of wilted hay silage and concentrate blended or separate. *Swedish Journal of Agricultural Research,* **3,** 161-166.

Wilkins, R.J., Fenlon, J.S., Cook, J.E. and Wilson, R.F. (1978). A further analysis of relationships between silage composition and voluntary intake by sheep. *Proceedings 5th Silage Conference, Ayr,* pp. 34-35.

Yan, T., Patterson, D.C. and Gordon, F.J. (1996). The effects of bacterial inoculation of unwilted and wilted grass silages on digestibility by sheep and intake and performance by dairy cows. *Proceedings British Society of Animal Science Winter Meeting 1996,* p. 66.

Yan, T., Patterson, D.C. and Gordon, F.J. (1998). The effect of two methods of feeding the concentrate supplement to dairy cows of high genetic merit. *Animal Science,* **67,** 395-403.

This paper was first published in 1998

27

HEIFER REARING FOR OPTIMUM LIFETIME PRODUCTION

C.S. PARK

Laboratory of Growth and Lactation, North Dakota State University, Fargo, USA

Introduction

The success of feeding and management programmes for replacement heifers must not only be measured in terms of efficiency of body growth but, more importantly, must be assessed by the milk-yield potential of the heifer. Milk-yield capacity in turn is largely influenced by the degree of mammary development (Knight and Wilde, 1993; Park and Jacobson,1993). Nutritional status is critical to mammary development, especially during hormone-sensitive developmental stages, including from before puberty through early lactation (Swanson and Poffenbarger, 1979; Park and Jacobson, 1993). To develop an effective nutrition regimen for developing heifers, it is necessary to have a better understanding of how the nutritional conditions during various physiological stages modulate mammary development and subsequent lactation potential. In an effort to understand the role of nutritionally-directed mammary development and lactation, stair-step compensatory nutrition regimens have been studied for dairy (Park *et al.,* 1987, 1989; Ford, 1997; Ford and Park, 2001) and beef (Park *et al.,* 1998) heifers, gilts (Crenshaw *et al.,* 1989) and laboratory animal species (Park *et al.,* 1988,1994; Kim *et al.,* 1998; Moon and Park, 1999).

Mammary gland development

MAMMOGENESIS DURING HORMONE-SENSITIVE STAGES

Mammary growth is a major determinant of milk-yield potential and persistency of lactation (Park and Jacobson, 1993; Forsyth, 1996). Growth of the mammary gland (mammogenesis) takes place during various reproductive epochs beginning prenatally and lasting through early lactation. Mammary growth and development from puberty until the end of pregnancy are mostly under the influence of hormonal control (Jacobson, 1961). From birth to puberty, mammary tissue undergoes relatively little development; mammary growth rate is consistent with body growth rate (isometric growth) until the onset of ovarian activity preceding puberty and increase in mammary size is mainly due to an increase in connective tissue and fat.

Beginning just before the first oestrous cycle (puberty), mammary parenchyma (secretory alveolar tissues) begins to grow at a faster rate than whole-body growth. Rapid allometric mammary growth continues for several oestrous cycles and then returns to an isometric pattern until conception. During each recurring oestrous cycle, the mammary gland is stimulated by oestrogen from the ovary and prolactin and somatotropin from the anterior pituitary gland. In species that experience long oestrous cycles with a functional luteal phase (cattle, goat, pig, horse, and human), progesterone is produced by the corpus luteum and is available to synergise with oestrogen, prolactin, and somatotropin to stimulate growth and differentiation of mammary ducts into a lobulo-alveolar system. At this stage of development, the parenchyma usually contains 10 to 20% epithelial cells, 40 to 50% connective tissue, and 30 to 40% fat cells (Sejrsen *et al.*, 1982). In comparison, lactating parenchyma consists of 40 to 50% epithelial cells (ducts and alveoli), about 40% connective tissue, 15 to 20% lumen, and almost no fat cells (Harrison *et al.*, 1983).

Allometric growth begins again at conception and continues, in most species, after parturition for variable periods of time. The majority of mammary growth occurs during pregnancy (Knight and Peaker,1982) and the rate of growth remains exponential throughout gestation. During this phase, the mammary gland consists of ductular and secretory alveolar epithelial cells embraced in a heterogenous matrix of cells (stroma) which include myoepithelia, adipocytes, and fibroblasts. As mammary ducts elongate further and development reaches its peak, parenchymal tissues gradually replace stroma, resulting in an extensive development of the lobulo-alveolar system. Accelerated mammary growth during pregnancy is probably due to increased and synchronous secretion of oestrogen and progesterone, with coincidental secretion of prolactin and perhaps somatotropin. Placental lactogen secretion also stimulates substantial mammary growth (Topper and Freeman, 1980).

The mammary gland continues to develop in early lactation, although the extent of growth varies from less than 10% in ruminants to as much as 50% in rats. In first-calf dairy heifers, the degree of mammary parenchyma tissue development around parturition is a major determinant of milk-yield capacity during the first and succeeding lactation cycles (Swanson and Poffenbarger, 1979; Park and Jacobson, 1993). Estimates of the correlation between milk yield and mammary alveolar epithelial cell numbers range between 0.50 and 0.85. Conversely, increased proportions of fibroblasts and adipocytes in the mammary gland are associated with reduced milk yield in cows (Park and Jacobson, 1993).

INFLUENCE OF NUTRITION ON MAMMOGENESIS

Nutritional status plays an important role in mammary development, differentiation, and subsequent lactation. Changes in feeding level (mainly energy concentration) can alter the secretion of hormones such as somatotropin and corticoids and greatly affect mammary growth and differentiation during hormone-dependent stages of development (from peripuberty to late gestation) as growth shifts from isometric to allometric (Forsyth, 1996). Careful control of energy allowances during peripuberty and gestation can significantly enhance mammary growth and succeeding lactation potential of heifers.

In growing dairy heifers, restricting energy intake delays the normal rate of development of the mammary gland. However, a delay in mammary development, controlled by dietary energy, does not impair subsequent development and differentiation of parenchymal tissue during pre-lactational mammogenesis, provided energy requirements are met (Park *et al.*, 1988,1989,1994,1998; Peri *et al.*, 1993; Kim *et al.*, 1998). Restricting the energy intake of growing animals brings about physiological adaptation whereby energy flow is redirected to energy-conserving activities, mainly maintenance and repair functions (Weindruch and Walford, 1988). Energy restriction also reduces certain energy-wasteful metabolic systems (e.g. re-esterification), which may not be metabolically essential for growth and maintenance (Newsholme, 1980).

Re-alimentation following energy restriction induces compensatory growth, which is characterised by accelerated metabolism, reduced maintenance requirement by depression of the basic metabolic rate, an activated endocrine status, and altered tissue composition of mammary gland (Wilson and Osbourn,1960; Blum *et al.*, 1985; Park *et al.*,1987). If compensatory growth is induced during the peripubertal period, the greater induction of hormones stimulates ovarian function, encouraging earler conception (Shetty,1990). Furthermore, a cascade of up-regulated genes involved in cell proliferation intensify fuller parenchymal tissue growth and development in the mammary gland, especially during gestation; mammary epithelial cell numbers increase and fat deposition decreases (Park *et al.*, 1988, 1989, 1998). In particular, the nutritional status of dairy heifers during the two to three months before parturition is important to maximise proliferation of secretory alveolar cells (Park and Jacobson, 1993).

Nutritionally-directed compensatory growth and development

BACKGROUND

The proper use of a time-dependent and closely-controlled nutrition regimen during hormone-sensitive growth phases prior to first calving can significantly affect animal growth, mammogenesis, and performance in subsequent lactations. The stair-step compensatory nutrition (SSCN) regimen is a rearing scheme with a unique combination of alternating dietary energy-restriction and re-alimentation (re-feeding) phases. Various SSCN models have been examined for developing dairy and beef heifers, gilts, steers, and rats.

The basic concept of the SSCN regimen is to exploit the nature of both dietary energy restriction and the compensatory growth phenomenon in concert with one or more hormone-dependent phases of mammary development. The consequence of this interaction is to bring about maximum growth of mammary parenchyma tissue and to permanently enhance milk synthesis and secretion and persistency of lactation for the first and subsequent lactations (Figure 27.1).

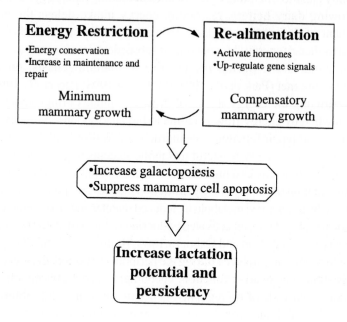

Figure 27.1 The stair-step compensatory nutrition regimen for the enhancement of mammary development and subsequent lactation.

The SSCN regimen has been studied, together with its effect on 1) efficiency of body growth; 2) mammary development and differentiation; 3) lactation potential during the first and succeeding lactation cycles; 4) apoptosis of mammary cells and persistency of lactation. In addition, considerable effort is being directed towards the adaptation of this nutritional programme to large or commercial livestock operations.

The stair-step compensatory nutrition regimen

Figure 27.2 illustrates a 3-2-4-2-5-2-month stair-step nutrition model for dairy heifers. Holstein heifer calves, weighing an average of 160 kg (approximately 6 months of age), were assigned to one of two dietary treatments: control and the SSCN regimen. Throughout the study, the control heifers were offered *ad libitum* access to a diet meeting the energy and nutrient requirements recommended by the National Research

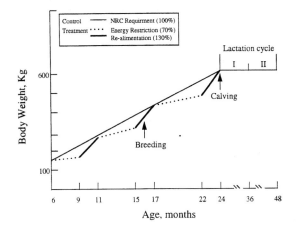

Figure 27.2 A stair-step compensatory nutrition regimen for dairy heifers. The control group is offered ad *libitum* access to a diet meeting the nutrient requirements recommended by NRC (1989). Treatment heifers are subjected to a stair-step feeding regimen according to an alternating 3-2-4-2-5-2-month schedule beginning with the energy restriction diet (0.7 of NRC ME requirements) followed by the re-alimentation diet (1.3 of NRC ME requirements). Animals are mated during the second re-alimentation period to calve at 24 months of age.

Council (NRC, 1989) and adjusted for an age at first calving of 24 months and a live-weight gain of 0.78 kg/day. During the first stair-step, which lasted for three months and encompassed the prepubertal period, the SSCN heifers were fed on a diet that was formulated to reduce the intake of metabolisable energy by 30%. Protein supply was maintained at levels recommended by NRC (1989) by increasing the crude protein from 120 to 170 g/kg dry matter. Following three months of energy restriction, the animals received a re-alimentation diet (1.3 times the metabolisable energy recommended by NRC, 1989). Compensatory growth occurred during this re-alimentation period which was also associated with an allometric phase of mammary development. The second step (puberty and breeding) consisted of energy restriction for four months (11 to 15 months of age) followed by re-alimentation for two months (15 to 17 months of age). In the third and final step, heifers were subjected to energy restriction for five months (17 to 22 months of age) followed by re-alimentation for two months. The stair-step heifers received an average of 0.9 of the energy allowance (average from all stair-step periods) given to the control group. Both low-energy and re-alimentation diets were formulated to provide intakes of protein, vitamins, and minerals equal to the control diet except energy intake which was varied. (Table 27.1). Heifers were mated during the second re-alimentation period (16 months of age) to calve at approximately 24 months of age.

Table 27.1 NUTRIENT CONTENT OF EXPERIMENTAL DIETS FOR DAIRY HEIFERS

Treatment variable	Protein (g/kg)	Metabolisable Energy (MJ/kg)	Energy intake
Control	120	9.83	1.0 x NRC[a]
Stair-step			
Energy restriction	170	9.83	0.7 x NRC
Re-alimentation	120	12.76	1.3 x NRC

[a] National Research Council (1989)

Heifer growth potential

Measurements of growth in dairy heifers subjected to a SSCN regimen are summarised in Table 27.2. Heifers raised on the SSCN regimen displayed characteristic compensatory responses. Stair-step heifers gained more body weight and consumed less feed than heifers fed conventionally. While live-weight gains were depressed during the period of energy restriction, heifers showed good recovery during the re-alimentation phase, resulting in significant improvements overall in feed, energy and protein conversion ratios. Beef heifers responded similarly on a 2-3-2-month stair-step rearing scheme (Table 27.3).

Table 27.2 PRODUCTION MEASUREMENTS OF DAIRY HEIFERS AVERAGED BY GROUP

	Control	Stair-step
Live weight (W, kg)		
Initial	281	278
Final	553	575
Live-weight gain (LWG, kg/day)	0.68	0.98*
Dry matter intake (DMI, kg/day)	9.3	7.5
DMI (g/kg $W^{0.75}$/day)	110.2	87.1*
Overall conversion efficiency		
Feed (g LWG/kg DMI)	73	130*
Energy (g LWG/MJ intake)	7.8	13.8*
Protein (g LWG/kg intake)	542	965*

Source: Park *et al.* (1987)

*Mean values (n=20) are significantly different from those of the control group (P<0.05)

Table 27.3 LEAST SQUARE MEANS FOR GROWTH MEASUREMENTS OF BEEF HEIFERS DURING VARIOUS PHASES OF THE STAIR-STEP COMPENSATORY NUTRITION REGIMEN[a]

Nutritional status	Control			Stair-step			SE[b]	P[b]
	ad libitum	ad libitum	ad libitum	High energy	Restricted energy	High energy		
Month of diet regimen	2	3	2	2	3	2		
Live-weight gain (kg/day)	0.75	0.50	0.32	1.00	0.14	0.68	0.12	0.042
Dry matter intake (kg/day)	7.7	9.6	10.0	8.3	7.2	9.8	0.20	0.126
Growth efficiency (g LWG/kg DMI)	97	52	32	120	20	70	11	0.001

Source: Park et al. (1998)

[a] Beef heifer calves, averaging 8 months of age, were assigned to either a control or stair-step regimen. Control diet met National Research Council (1989) standards for growing beef heifer calves. Stair-step regimen consisted of two diets: high energy diet (30% above the energy provided by the control diet) and restricted energy diet (30% below the energy provided by the control diet)

[b] SE = standard error of the mean, where n=4; P = significance level of F-test for equality of three nutrition phases from two study groups

Nutritional status and feed intake markedly influence growth hormone secretion. Feed restriction may cause changes in the secretion of growth hormone-releasing and growth hormone-inhibiting factors from the hypothalamus, resulting in an increase in the level of growth hormone (Gregory *et al.*, 1991). As shown in Table 27.4, serum growth hormone in dairy heifers was increased during the energy-restriction phase but decreased during the compensatory phase compared with that of the control group. Low energy intake increases growth hormone concentrations in beef heifers (Houseknecht *et al.*,1988). There is a negative relationship between growth hormone and deposition of adipose tissue (Peel *et al.*,1981). Increases in growth hormone concentrations during restricted feeding are probably the result of attempts by the animal to mobilise energy reserves from adipose tissue and thereby offset the effects of a negative energy balance (Bauman *et al.,* 1982).

Table 27.4 SERUM INSULIN AND GROWTH HORMONE CONCENTRATIONS OF DAIRY HEIFERS

Study group	Nutritional phase (months)	Months of age	Hormone	
			Growth hormone (ng/ml)	Insulin (μIU/ml)
Control	ad libitum	15	2.9	22.7
	ad libitum	18	3.4	25.1
Stair-step	Restricted	15	4.7 *	10.6 *
	Re-alimented	18	3.0	38.3 *

Source: Ford (1997)
*Mean values (n=5) are significantly different from the control values (P<0.05)

In contrast to growth hormone, the concentrations of insulin in blood are positively correlated with feed or energy intake (Bassett, 1974). Serum insulin concentrations in stair-step heifers were lower during feed restriction but were higher during refeeding, compared with controls, indicating a dual role of insulin as both lipogenic and antilipolytic in cattle (Table 27.4). Steers (both dairy and beef) reared on a stair-step regimen have a substantial reduction (10 to 15%) in fat deposition in the *biceps femoris* muscle (Ford *et al.,* 1996; Maddock *et al.,* 1996).

In summary, a controlled stair-step compensatory nutrition model can certainly enhance the growth potential of heifers. During the energy-restriction phase, the rate of growth lags behind the body weight of traditionally-fed animals. During the energy re-alimentation phase following energy restriction, animals consume energy far in excess of that needed for maintenance thereby redirecting the energy flow to the metabolic process of growth. Thus, these animals exhibit an accelerated rate of growth that exceeds the normal growth curve.

Mammary tissue development and gene expression

TISSUE COMPOSITION

The extent of mammary hyperplasia and hypertrophy induced by a compensatory nutrition regimen is clearly reflected in the higher nucleic acid and protein content of the tissue (Park *et al.*, 1988,1989,1998). Table 27.5 shows the composition of mammary tissue obtained from dairy heifers in late gestation. Mammary tissue from the stair-step group had 1.3 times the DNA and 2.05 times the RNA of mammary tissue from control animals. The mammary tissue from the stair-step group also had higher protein concentrations and higher ratios of RNA/DNA and protein/DNA. Mammary tissues from beef heifers in early lactation (30 days) raised on the SSCN regimen had 1.15 times the DNA and 1.30 times the RNA concentrations of those from the control group (Park *et al.*, 1998). Mammary tissues from these SSCN heifers also had higher protein contents and ratios of protein/DNA compared with those on the control regimen.

Table 27.5 CHEMICAL COMPOSITION OF MAMMARY TISSUE FROM DAIRY HEIFERS IN LATE GESTATION

Composition[a]	*Control*	*Stair-step*	*SE*[b]	*P*[b]
DNA (mg/g)	4.3	5.6	0.5	0.047
RNA (mg/g)	14.5	29.7	2.3	0.001
Protein (mg/g)	217.1	308.4	31.6	0.016
RNA/DNA	3.2	5.3	0.4	0.029
Protein/DNA	49.2	55.0	2.5	0.088
Lipid (mg/g)	730.7	628.3	36.4	0.067

Source: Park *et al.* (1989)
[a] mg/g denotes dry matter tissue
[b] SE = standard error of the mean, where n=4; P = significance of F-test for equality of two study groups

In growing animals the lipolytic and antilipid synthetic effects of growth hormone minimise fat deposition and promote oxidation of fat. Data from these studies (Park *et al.*, 1988, 1989, 1994, 1998), as well as others (Choi *et al.*, 1997), have consistently shown that mammary tissue from animals that have been reared on a compensatory-growth regimen contained more parenchyma and less fat than their counterparts (Table 27.5). This decrease in lipid level is likely due to an increased lipolytic activity associated with elevated growth hormone (Park *et al.*, 1989).

MILK PROTEIN GENE EXPRESSION

The caseins are major proteins of milk and are secreted only by differentiated mammary tissues. Induction and expression of milk protein genes are controlled by complex multi-hormonal and enzymatic stimulations of transcriptional events, RNA processing, nucleocytoplasmic transport efficiency, stability of mRNA, and the rate of translation (Guyette *et al.*, 1979). The concentrations of β-casein mRNA were 2 to 5-fold higher in mammary tissues from heifers reared on a compensatory nutrition regimen than in those of conventionally-reared heifers (Ford, 1997; Park *et al.*, 1998l; Ford and Park, 2001). The α, β, and γ-casein and whey acidic protein mRNA were also 2 to 4-fold higher in lactating mammary tissues from rats reared on the SSCN regimen (Park *et al.*, 1988). Increased expression of the major milk protein genes indicates increased mammary differentiation and functional activity in these mammary tissues; SSCN heifers had 1.05 times the total protein and 1.15 times the casein in milk than the control heifers (Park *et al.*, 1998).

In addition to gene expression *in vivo*, acini (alveoli) isolated and cultured from mammary tissues of early lactating heifers on the SSCN regimen had proportionally 0.45 higher α_{S1} casein and 0.52 higher β-casein mRNA than those from the control group (Park *et al.*, 1989). Acini from the stair-step group also had a 0.14 increase in uptake of amino acids and a 0.21 increase in secretion of milk protein (Table 27.6). The increase in milk protein secretion, with a concurrent elevation in casein mRNA in mammary alveolar epithelial cells, provides evidence that the SSCN regimen modulates the expression of milk protein genes at both the transcriptional and translational levels.

Table 27.6 MILK PROTEIN mRNA, AMINO ACID UPTAKE, AND MILK PROTEIN SECRETION IN BOVINE MAMMARY ACINI CULTURE

	Control	*Stair-step*	*SE*[a]	*P*[a]
Cytoplasmic mRNA (specific activity)				
α_{S1}-casein	17.5	25.4	2.2	0.042
β-casein	31.7	48.2	3.4	0.027
Secreted protein (dpm/mg x 10^{-2})	21.3	25.8	3.0	0.039
Amino acid uptake (nmol/mg protein)	30.6	34.8	2.5	0.052

Source: Park *et al.* (1989)
[a] SE = standard error of the mean, where n=4; P = significance level of F-test for equality of two study groups during early lactating stage

Lactation potential

MILK YIELD

Table 27.7 provides a summary of the results of a study on stair-step nutrition of dairy heifers. Twenty heifers were utilised in each of two studies. The lactation records represent an average of eight cows per study group. The average of four lactations are reported for Study 1 and three lactations for Study 2. Lactation performance is significantly enhanced in cows reared on a stair-step scheme versus those fed according to the standard linear growth curve of NRC (1989). Stair-step heifers produce 1.1 times the milk of conventionally-reared control animals; this increase represents approximately 900 kg milk over 250 days whilst achieving post-calving body weights close to control heifers (Park et al., 1989). Peri et al. (1993) demonstrated an 0.18 increase in milk yield in first-lactation dairy heifers using a similar dietary regimen. Milk yield of beef heifers raised on the SSCN regimen was proportionally 0.06 greater than that of heifers on the control regimen (Park et al., 1998). Also, calves suckled by heifers on the SSCN regimen were approximately 5.5 kg heavier at weaning than calves from heifers on the control regimen. Even greater increases in milk production (measured as litter weight) have been found in pigs and rats, 0.27 and 0.14, respectively (Crenshaw et al., 1989; Park et al., 1988). It must be noted that this increase in milk yield from the compensatory-growth animals is derived from multiple-lactation records of heifers and rats that had previously undergone the SSCN regimen. Therefore, the enhancement of lactation potential by compensatory growth persists in succeeding lactation cycles (Park et al., 1989; Moon and Par, 1999; Ford and Park, 2001).

Table 27.7 MILK YIELD AND COMPOSITION OF MILK FROM DAIRY COWS

Study no.	No. lactation records	Response	Control	Stair-step	SE[a]	P[a]
1	4	Milk (kg)	7,913	8,715	244	0.001
		Fat (g/kg)	36.2	34.5	1.0	0.034
		Protein (g/kg)	31.1	31.9	0.4	0.242
2	3	Milk (kg)	8,533	9,251	268	0.001
		Fat (g/kg)	33.7	32.6	0.8	0.542
		Protein (g/kg)	32.7	33.0	0.7	0.356

Source: Park et al. (1989)

[a] SE = standard error of the mean. Each value represents the mean of 4 lactation records (average 7.6 cows/record) and 3 records (8.3 cows/record), for Studies 1 and 2, respectively; P = significance level of F-test for equality of two study groups

LACTATION PERSISTENCY

Lactation performance is a function of two interrelated factors: peak yield and lactation persistency. Maximum lactation performance is associated with a high initial rate of milk secretion and a high degree of persistency, defined as the change in milk yield as lactation advances (Park and Jacobson, 1993). The number of secretory cells is one of the basic elements that limits milk yield. For high milk yields throughout lactation cycles, an animal must possess more mammary epithelial cells, more synthetic activity per cell, and greater longevity of the cells. Although most proliferation of secretory cells occurs before the end of pregnancy, mammary tissues continue to grow until peak lactation. During early lactation, most proliferation of mammary cells is in alveolar epithelial cells (Joshi *et al.*, 1986). As shown in Table 27.8, the cell proliferation rate in rat mammary tissues from the compensatory-growth group was 2.7-fold greater compared with those from the control.

Table 27.8 LABELING INDEX OF RAT MAMMARY CELLS EXHIBITING CELL PROLIFERATION AND APOPTOSIS DURING LACTATION (%)

		Control		Stair-step	
Item	*n*	*Mean*	*SE*	*Mean*	*SE*
Cell proliferation					
Early lactation	5	2.90	0.03	7.81*	0.06
Apoptosis					
Late lactation	5	4.59	0.34	3.97	0.24

Source: Kim *et al.* (1998)
*Mean values are significantly different from that of the control group (P<0.05)

In addition to cell proliferation, persistency of lactation may also be affected by cell death (apoptosis). Apoptosis is a mode of physiological cell death that occurs naturally in rodent mammary tissue during involution (Walker *et al.*, 1989). As mammary alveolar secretary cells are lost, and synthetic activity per cell declines, milk yield gradually decreases. Although, what triggers the onset of cell death after the peak of lactation is not known, change in endocrine secretion is a contributing factor (Walker *et al.*, 1989). In recent studies mammary tissues from the compensatory-nutrition group have been found to have 0.15 less apoptotic cells than those from the control group (Table 27.8). The inhibition of apoptosis increases the longevity of alveolar secretory cells in the mammary gland (Li *et al.*, 1996) and may partially explain the overall enhancement of lactation persistency found in compensatory-nutrition animals (Kim *et al.*, 1998; Moon and Park, 1999). It is further hypothesised that this inhibition of apoptosis is a physiological consequence of greatly increased endocrine and metabolic activity.

Working model for heifer rearing

It has been repeatedly said that high feeding intensity (i.e. unregulated excessively high plane of nutrition), imposed during the prepubertal phase in particular, casues a severe reduction in milk yield potential (Little and Kay, 1979; Sejrsen *et al.*, 1982). However, other studies have shown either a positive (Park *et al.*, 1987, 1989, 1998; Choi *et al.*, 1997; Ford and Park, 2001) or no (Gardner *et al.*, 1988; Van Amburgh, *et al.*, 1998) relationship between prepubertal accelerated growth and lactation performance. These discrepancies may be due to differences in growth model (e.g. regulated vs uncontrolled growth rate) or type of nutrition regimen (e.g energy intake vs total feed intake), as well as age and hormonal state (e.g. prepuberty, puberty or gestation) during which the nutrition regimen in question was examined. We, as well as others (Barash *et al.*, 1994; Choi *et al.*, 1997; Mantysaari *et al.*, 1999; Peri *et al.*, 1993; Yambayamba and Price, 1997), have shown that heifers raised on a well-controlled nutrition regimen (i.e. energy realimentation following a period of energy restriction) during certain hormone-sensitive growth stage(s) can significantly affect mammary development and lactation potential.

While our multi-step nutrition regimen has been proven effective for heifer development and life-long performance, there have been demands by livestock (dairy and beef) producers and animal scientists for a simplified compensatory growth nutrition programme. Accordingly, we have begun to investigate one-step models focusing on the last two trimesters of gestation. We believe that the gestational period is the most critical stage of mammary development because the majority of mammary growth occurs during this time and, furthermore, compensatory growth during the last trimester of gestation may improve overall metabolic status of prepartum heifers (i.e. health during transition period).

In summary, key considerations for implementing a successful stair-step regimen for rearing replacement heifers are as follows:

(1)   The model should parallel an allometric and hormone-dependent developmental stagel i.e. a straight-forward system would be a one-step gestational model inclusive of the final 6 to 7 months of gestation.
(2)   Resources that are uniquely available to a particular geographical area should be fully utilised; i.e. feeding good quality roughages during the restricted feeding phase and a high energy concentrate during the refeeding period (e.g. straw and oil seeds in the Midwestern region of the USA).

Conclusions

Successful dairy and beef operations begin with sound feeding and management of replacement heifers to produce the best possible cows. Because of the actions of compensatory growth imposed during peripuberty and gestation, a stair-step nutrition regimen significantly improves not only general heifer development, but also the growth and differentiation of the mammary gland and the ensuing milk-yield potential. Moreover, this regimen can be adapted to operations and management practices of average to large sized farms.

Findings to date provide conclusive evidence that a time-dependent and nutritionally-induced compensatory growth favourably alters the physiological development and differentiation of the mammary gland as well as lactation potential. Further studies are required to determine the mechanisms responsible for the effect of nutritionally-directed compensatory growth upon enhanced galactopoiesis and persistency of lactation in relation to the control of the cell cycle and apoptosis of mammary epithelial cells.

Acknowledgments

I am thankful to Drs. Y. Choi, M. Baik, S. Kim, Y. Moon, R. Maddock and J. Ford for their direct scientific contribution to these studies. I am grateful to Ms. W. Keller for her assistance on most aspects of these studies including laboratory analysis, data collection, and manuscript preparation. Special thanks is given to Ms. J. Berg for secretarial assistance.

Financial support from U.S. Department of Agriculture-National Research Initiative, North Dakota Agricultural Products Utilization Commission, Hoffmann LaRoche Pharmaceutical Company, and American Institute for Cancer Research is gratefully acknowledged.

References

Barash, H., Bar-Meir, Y. and Bruckental, I. (1994). *Livestock Production Science,* **39**, 263-268

Bassett, J. M. (1974). *Australian Journal of Biological Science,* **27**, 167-174

Bauman, D. E., Eisemann, J. H. and Currie, W. B. (1982). *Federation Proceedings,* **41**, 2538-2544

Blum, J. W., Schnyder, W., Kunz, P. L., Blom, A. K., Bickel, H. and Schürch, A. (1985). *Journal of Nutrition.* **115**, 417-424

Choi, Y. J., Han, I. K., Woo, J. H., Lee, H. J., Jang, K., Myung, K. H. and Kim, Y. S. (1997). *Journal of Dairy Science,* **80**, 519-524

Crenshaw, J. D., Park, C. S., Swantek, P. M., Keller, W. L. and Zimprich, R. C. (1989). *Journal of Animal Science,* **67** (suppl 2),107

Ford, J. A. (1997). *Role of stair-step compensatory nutrition in heifer growth and mammary development.* M. S. Thesis, North Dakota State University, Fargo, ND

Ford, J. A., Keller, W. L. and Park, C. S. (1996). *FASEB Journal,* **10(3)**, A769

Ford, J. A. and Park, C. S. (2001) *Journal of Dairy Science*, **84**, 1669-1678

Forsyth, I. A. (1996). *Journal of Dairy Science,* **79**, 1085-1096

Gardner, R. W., Smith, L. W. and Park, R. L. (1988). *Journal of Dairy Science,* **71**, 996-999

Gregory, B. T., Cummins, J. T., Francis, H., Sudburry, A. W., McCloud, P. I. and Clarke, I. J. (1991). *Endocrinology, 128*, 1151-1158

Guyette, W. A., Matusik, R. J. and Rosen, J. M. (1979). *Cell, 17*, 1013-1023

Harrison, R. D., Reynolds, J. P. and Little, W. (1983). *Journal of Dairy Research, 50*, 405-412

Houseknecht, K. L., Boggs, D. L., Campion, D. R., Sartin, J.L., Kiser, T. E., Rampacek, G. B. and Amos, H. E. (1988). *Journal of Animal Science, 66*, 2916-2923

Jacobson, D. (1961). In *Milk*, pp. 127-160. Ed. Kon, S. K. and Cowie, A. T., Academic Press, New York, USA

Joshi, K., Ellis, J. T. B., Hughes, C. M., Monaghan, P. and Neville, A. M. (1986). *Laboratory Investigation, 54*, 52-61

Kim, S. H., Moon, Y.S., Keller, W. L. and Park, C. S. (1998). *British Journal of Nutrition, 79*, 177-183

Knight, C. H. and Peaker, M. (1982). *Journal of Reproduction and Fertility, 65*, 521-536

Knight, C. H. and Wilde, C. J. (1993). *Livestock Production Science, 35*, 3-19

Li, M., Hu, J., Heermeier, K., Hennighausen, L. and Furth, P. A. (1996). *Cell Growth and Differentiation, 7*, 13-20

Little, W. and Kay, R. M. (1979). *Animal Production, 29*, 131-142

Maddock, R. J., Park, C.S., Danielson, R. B., Kim, S. H., and Keller, W. L. (1996). *FASEB Journal, 10(3)*, 769

Mantysaari, P., Ingvartsen, K. L. and Toivonen, V. (1999). *Livestock Production, 62*, 29-41

Moon, Y. S. and Park, C. S. (1999) *Journal of Nutrition, 129*, 1156-1160

National Research Council. (1989). *Nutrient Requirements of Dairy Cattle*. National Academy Press, Washington, DC, USA

Newsholme, E. A. (1980). *The New England Journal of Medicine, 302*, 400-405

Park, C. S., Baik, M. G., Keller, W. L., Berg, I. E. and Erickson, G. M. (1989). *Growth, Development and Aging, 53*, 159-166

Park, C. S., Baik, M. G., Keller, W. L. and Slanger, W. D. (1994). *Journal of Animal Science, 72*, 2319-2324

Park, C. S., Choi, Y. J., Keller, W. L. and Harrold, R. L. (1988). *FASEB Journal, 2*, 2619-2624

Park, C. S., Danielson, R. B., Kreft, B. S., Kim, S.H., Moon, Y.S. and Keller, W. L. (1998). *Journal of Dairy Science, 81*, 243-249

Park, C. S., Erickson, G. M., Choi, Y. J. and Marx, G. D. (1987). *Journal of Animal Science, 64*, 1751 -1758

Park, C. S. and Jacobson, N. L. (1993). In *Dukes' Physiology of Domestic Animals* pp 711-727. Ed. Swenson, M.J., Reece, W.O. Cornell University Press, Ithaca, NY, USA

Peel, C. J., Bauman, D. E., Gorewit, R. C. and Sniffen, C. J. (1981). *Journal of Nutrition*, 111, 1662-1671

Peri, I., Gertler, A., Bruckental, I. and Barash, H. (1993). *Journal of Dairy Science,* **76**, 742-751

Sejrsen, K., Huber, J. T., Tucker, H. A. and Akers, R. M. (1982). *Journal of Dairy Science,* **65**, 793-800

Shetty, P. S. (1990). *Nutrition Research Review,* **3**, 49-74

Swanson, E. W. and Poffenbarger, J. I. (1979). *Journal of Dairy Science,* **62**, 702-714

Topper, Y. J. and Freeman, C. S. (1980). *Physiological Reviews,* **60**, 1049-1106

Van Amburgh, M. E., Galton, D. M., Bauman, D. E., Everett, R. W., Fox, D. G., Chase, L. E. and Erb, H. N. (1998) *Journal of Dairy Science,* **81**, 527-538

Walker, N. I., Bennett, R. E. and Kerr, J. F. R. (1989). *American Journal of Anatomy,* **185**, 19-32

Weindruch, R. and Walford, R. L. (1988). In *The Retardation of Aging and Disease by Dietary Restriction.* Charles Thomas, Springfield, IL USA

Wilson, P. N. and Osbourn, D. F. (1960). *Biological Reviews of the Cambridge Philosophical Society,* **35**, 324-363

Yambayamba, E. S. K. and Price, M. A. (1997) *Livestock Production Science,* **51**, 237-244

This paper was first published in 1998

INDEX